Immune Dysfunction and Immunotherapy in Heart Disease

Immune Dysfunction and Immunotherapy in Heart Disease

EDITED BY

Ronald Ross Watson

Department of Nutritional Sciences, The University of Arizona; *and*
Sarver Heart Center, College of Medicine, The University of Arizona; *and*
Division of Health Promotion Sciences, Mel and Enid Zuckerman Arizona College
of Public Health, The University of Arizona
Tucson, AZ
USA

Douglas F. Larson

Sarver Heart Center
College of Medicine
The University of Arizona
Tucson, AZ
USA

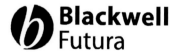

© 2007 by Blackwell Publishing
Blackwell Futura is an imprint of Blackwell Publishing

Blackwell Publishing, Inc., 350 Main Street, Malden, Massachusetts 02148-5020, USA
Blackwell Publishing Ltd, 9600 Garsington Road, Oxford OX4 2DQ, UK
Blackwell Science Asia Pty Ltd., 550 Swanston Street, Carlton, Victoria 3053, Australia

First published 2007

1   2007

ISBN: 978-1-4051-5568-7

Library of Congress Cataloging-in-Publication Data

Immune dysfunction and immunotherapy in heart disease / edited by Ronald
Ross Watson, Douglas F. Larson.
        p. ; cm.
    Includes bibliographical references and index.
    ISBN 978-1-4051-5568-7 (alk. paper)
    1. Heart–Diseases–Immunological aspects.   2. Heart–Diseases–Immunotherapy.
3. Immunologic diseases–Complications.   I. Watson, Ronald R. (Ronald Ross)   II. Larson,
Douglas F.
    [DNLM: 1. Heart Diseases–immunology.   2. Heart Diseases–therapy.   3. Immune System
Diseases–complications.   4. Immune System Diseases–therapy.   5. Immunotherapy–
methods. WG 210 I33 2007]

    RC682.I38 2007
    616.1′207–dc22

                                                                                    2007005644

A catalogue record for this title is available from the British Library

Commissioning Editor: Gina Almond
Development Editor: Fiona Pattison
Editorial Assistant: Victoria Pittman

Set in 9.5/12 Minion and Frutiger by Aptara Inc., New Delhi, India
Printed and bound in Singapore by COS Printers Pte Ltd

For further information on Blackwell Publishing, visit our website:
www.blackwellcardiology.com

Contents

Contributors

Mohsen Araghi-Niknam, MA, PhD
Sr. Clinical Trial Leader
Cardiac Rhythm Disease Management
Minneapolis, MN
USA

Claire Arnaud, PharmD, PhD
Laboratory HP2
University of Grenoble
INSERM ERI 0017
Grenoble
France

Christian Assad-Kottner, MD
The Methodist DeBakey Heart Center
The Methodist Hospital
Houston, TX
USA

Pål Aukrust, MD,PhD
Research Institute for Internal Medicine
University of Oslo; and
Section of Clinical Immunology and Infectious
Rikshospitalet, University of Oslo
Oslo
Norway

Giuseppe Barbaro, MD
Cardiology Unit
Department of Medical Pathophysiology
University "La Sapienza"
Rome
Italy

John Anthony Bauer, PhD
Director, Center for Cardiovascular Medicine
Columbus Childrens Research Institute; and
Sections of Neonatology and Cardiology
Columbus Children's Hospital
Columbus, OH
USA

Zofia T. Bilińska, MD, PhD
Associate Professor of Cardiology
Consultant, 1st Department of Coronary Artery Disease
Institute of Cardiology
Alpejsja 42
Warsaw
Poland

Simin Bolourchi-Vaghefi, PhD, CNS, LNutr.
Emeritus Professor of Nutrition
University of North Florida College of Health
Jacksonville, FL
USA

A. E. Bolton, PhD, DSc
Chief Scientific Officer
Vasogen Ireland Ltd.
Santry
Dublin 9
Ireland

Charles E. Canter, MD
Professor of Pediatrics
Washington University of School of Medicine; and
Medical Director, Heart Transplant Program
St. Louis Children's Hospital
St. Louis, MO
USA

W. L. Chan, PhD, DSc
Biochemical Pharmacology
William Harvey Research Institute
John Vane Science Centre
Queen Mary University of London
Charterhouse Square
London
UK

David Chen, MD
The Methodist DeBakey Heart Center
The Methodist Hospital
Houston, TX
USA

Yinhong Chen, PhD
Scientist
Geron Corporation
Menlo Park, CA
USA

Jonathan Choy, PhD
Boyer Center for Molecular Medicine
Yale University
New Haven
Connecticut
USA

Jack Copeland, MD
Department of Surgery
University of Arizona
USA

Francisco J. Cordova, MD
The Methodist DeBakey Heart Center
The Methodist Hospital
Houston, TX
USA

Jan Kristian Damås, MD,PhD
Research Institute for Internal Medicine
Rikshospitalet
University of Oslo
Oslo
Norway

Betsy B. Dokken, PhD, NP
Departments of Medicine and Surgery
University of Arizona
Tucson, AZ
USA

Jos Domen, PhD
Department of Surgery
University of Arizona
Tucson, AZ
USA

Urs Eriksson, MD
Departments of Internal Medicine
University Hospital
Petersgraben 4
Ch-4031 Basle
Switzerland

Timothy F. Feltes, MD
Center for Cardiovascular Medicine
Columbus Childrens Research Institute; *and*
Chief Section of Pediatric Cardiology
Columbus Children's Hospital
Columbus, OH
USA

Julia R. Gage, PhD
Kendle International, Inc.
Thousand Oaks, CA
USA

Amy Galena, MSH, RD
Clinical Dietitian
Mayo Clinic
Jacksonville
USA

Kimbery Gandy, MD, PhD
Assistant Professor
Department of Surgery
University of Arizona
Tucson, AZ
USA

Mohammad Abraham Kazemizadeh Gol
School of Medicine
University of Minnesota
Minneapolis, MN
USA

Joseph D. Gold, PhD
Director of Stem Cell Biology and Research Operations
Geron Corporation
Menlo Park, CA
USA

Christina Grothusen, MD
Department of Cardiology and Angiology
Medical School of Hannover
Carl-Neuberg Str. 1
30625 Hannover
Germany

Lars Gullestad, MD, PhD
Senior Consultant
Department of Cardiology
University of Oslo
Oslo
Norway

Timothy M. Hoffman, MD
Center for Cardiovascular Medicine
Columbus Childrens Research Institute; *and*
Medical Director, Pediatric Heart Transplant/Heart Failure Program
Columbus Children's Hospital
Columbus, OH
USA

Palle Holmstrup, DDS, PhD, Dr.Odont., Odont.Dr. (h.c.)
Professor and Chairman
Department of Periodontology
School of Dentistry
Faculty of Health Sciences
University of Copenhagen
Denmark

Katherine Horak, PhD
Sarver Heart Center
The University of Arizona
Tucson, AZ
USA

Mandar S. Joshi, PhD
Center for Cardiovascular Medicine
Columbus Childrens Research Institute
Columbus, OH
USA

Ismail Laher, PhD
Department of Pharmacology and Therapeutics
Faculty of Medicine
University of British Columbia
Vancouver
BC, Canada

Douglas F. Larson
Sarver Heart Center
College of Medicine
The University of Arizona
Tucson, AZ
USA

Carl V. Leier, MD
The James W. Overstreet Professor of Medicine and Pharmacology
Division of Cardiovascular Medicine
College of Medicine and Public Health
The Ohio State University
Columbus, OH
USA

Wendy A. Luce, MD
Center for Cardiovascular Medicine
Columbus Childrens Research Institute; *and*
Section of Neonatology
Columbus Children's Hospital
Columbus, OH
USA

François Mach, MD, PhD
Division of Cardiology
Foundation for Medical Research
Faculty of Medicine
Geneva University Hospital
Switzerland

A. Mandel, MD, PhD, DSc
Director of Fundamental & Medical Research
Vasogen Inc.
Mississauga
Ontario
Canada

Paul F. McDonagh, PhD
Professor of Surgery, Physiology and Nutrition
Allan C. Hudson and Helen Lovaas Endowed Chair
of Vascular Biology and Coagulation
The Sarver Heart Center
University of Arizona
Tuscon, AZ
USA

Bruce M. McManus, MD, PhD, FRSC
Director, The James Hogg iCAPTURE Centre
Scientific Director, The Heart Centre
Providence Health Care – University of British Columbia
Vancouver, BC
Canada

Farzad Moien-Afshari, MD, PhD
Department of Pharmacology and Therapeutics
Faculty of Medicine
University of British Columbia
Vancouver
BC, Canada

James P. Morgan, MD, PhD
Chief, Division of Cardiovascular Medicine
Department of Medicine
Caritas St. Elizabeth's Medical Center and Caritas
Carney Hospital *and*
Director, Cardiovascular Center Caritas Christi
Healthcare System
Boston, MA
USA

Samira Najmaii, MT (ASCP), MS
Sarver Heart Center
The University of Arizona
Tucson, AZ
USA

Sota Omoigui, MD
Division of Inflammation and Pain Medicine
LA Pain Clinic
Hawthorne, CA
USA

Carlos Orrego, MD
The Methodist DeBakey Heart Center
The Methodist Hospital
Houston, TX
USA

Oana Madalina Petrescu, MD
Fellow—Cardiovascular Medicine
Department of Medicine
Caritas St. Elizabeth's Medical Center
Boston
USA

Catherine A. Priest, PhD
Associate Director of Transplantation Sciences
Geron Corporation
Menlo Park, CA
USA

Witold Rużyłło, MD, FESC
Professor of Cardiology
Head, 1st Department of Coronary Artery Disease and
Cardiac Catheterization
Laboratory
Institute of Cardiology
Alpejsja 42
04-628 Warsaw
Poland

Bernhard Schieffer, MD
Associate Professor of Medicine
Department of Cardiology and Angiology
Medical School of Hannover
Carl-Neuberg Strasse 1
30625 Hannover
Germany

Guillermo Torre-Amione, MD, PhD, FACC
The Methodist DeBakey Heart Center
The Methodist Hospital
Houston, TX
USA

Donna. L. Vredevoe, PhD
University of California, Los Angeles
School of Nursing
Los Angeles, CA
USA

Ronald Ross Watson, PhD
Department of Nutritional Sciences, The University of
Arizona; *and*
Sarver Heart Center, College of Medicine, The University of
Arizona; *and*
Division of Health Promotion Sciences, Mel and Enid
Zuckerman Arizona College of Public Health,
The University of Arizona
Tucson, AZ
USA

Bo Yang, MD, PhD
Department of Surgery
University of Arizona
Tuscon, AZ
USA

Arne Yndestad, PhD
Research Institute for Internal Medicine
University of Oslo
N-0027 Oslo
Norway

Qianli Yu, MD, PhD
Sarver Heart Center
The University of Arizona
Tucson, AZ
USA

Jin Zhang, PhD
Scientist
Iams Technical Center, The Proctor and Gamble Company
Lewisburg, OH
USA

Sherma Zibadi, MD
Department of Nutritional Sciences
The University of Arizona
Tucson, AZ
USA

Preface

The pathophysiology of cardiovascular disease and current therapeutics designed for disease treatment are primarily based on autonomic nervous system and endocrine pathways. Yet, there are numerous recent reports describing that the immune system may be a fundamental basis of cardiovascular disease processes which is supported by the evidence that immunomodulatory therapeutics have demonstrated therapeutic efficacy. This text systematically describes cardiovascular disease conditions where the immune system appears to play a pivotal role and provides evidence that selective modulation of the immune system can alter the disease processes. This text provides the first compiled evidence that there exists the possibility that the immune system may be a third pathway that directly affects cardiovascular structure and function beyond that of the neuro-endocrine pathways.

The overall goal of this book is to relate various immune disorders caused by toxicants, autoimmune conditions, aging, HIV, and metabolic disorders with cardiovascular pathology and present the current state-of-the art immune based therapeutics to reverse the pathology. Therefore researchers reviewed the following areas:

I. Immune dysfunction and its role in the enzymatic changes leading to cardiac remodeling
II. Immune modulation by transplantation drugs and their cardiotoxic side effects
III. Prevention of cytokine dysregulation in cardiac therapy
IV. Immunosuppression promoting cardiac damage by opportunistic pathogens
V. Immunoregulatory treatments and their role in heart health

About the Editors

Ronald R. Watson, PhD, has edited 65 books, including four on the effects of various dietary nutrients in heart disease. He initiated and directed the Specialized Alcohol Research Center at the University of Arizona College of Medicine for six years. The main theme of this National Institute of Alcohol Abuse and Alcoholism (NIAAA) Center grant was to understand the role of ethanol-induced immunosuppression with increased oxidation and nutrient loss on disease and disease resistance in animals. For 8 years he directed with Douglas F. Larson several NIH grants studying the effects of retroviral-induced immune dysfunction on cardiac structure and function in a model of AIDS.

Dr. Watson is a member of several national and international societies concerned with nutrition, immunology, and cancer research. He has directed a program studying ways to slow aging using nutritional supplements, funded by the Wallace Genetics Foundation for 30 years. Currently, he is the co-principal investigator on an NIH grant studying the role of immune dysfunction to exacerbate heart disease. He has recently completed studies using completary and alternative medicines in clinical trials. Dr. Watson and Dr. Larson are co principal investigators on an NIH grant from the National Center on Complementary and Alternative Medicine to study cytokine dysregulation in cardiac remodeling.

Dr. Watson attended the University of Idaho, but graduated from Brigham Young University in Provo, UT, with a degree in chemistry in 1966. He completed his PhD degree in 1971 in biochemistry at Michigan State University. His postdoctoral education was completed at the Harvard School of Public Health in Nutrition and Microbiology, including a two-year postdoctoral research experience in immunology. He was Assistant Professor of Immunology and did research at the University of Mississippi Medical Center in Jackson from 1973 to 1974. He was an Assistant Professor of Microbiology and Immunology at the Indiana University Medical School from 1974 to 1978 and an Associate Professor at Purdue University in the Department of Food and Nutrition from 1978 to 1982. In 1982, he joined the faculty at the University of Arizona in the Department of Family and Community Medicine. He is also a professor in the University of Arizonas College of Public Health. He has published 450 research papers and review chapters.

Dr Larson has had a research focus in the area of immune dysfunction and cardiac function for a number of years. He has performed research related to immunosuppressive therapies for 20 years in the laboratory and in the clinic. As a member of the heart and lung transplantation team at the University of Arizona, he has seen the relationship of immunosuppression between the development of diastolic dysfunction and hypertension. As a senior research scientist in a large pharmaceutical company in Basel, Switzerland, he was charged with the development of a newer generation of immunosuppressants for use in transplantation and autoimmunity. The key experiment that led to Dr Larson's research motivation to define the relationship between the immune system and cardiac remodeling was the observation that the infarcted site in the SCID mouse heart does not remodel. Subsequently, Dr Larson has applied selective immunomodulatory agents to demonstrate that the T-lymphocyte provides a significant control in the cardiac extracellular matrix remodeling. Furthermore, he has shown that cardiovascular pathological conditions can be adaptively transferred with purified T-lymphocytes—further emphasizing the role of the immune system in cardiac diseases. More specifically, since the current therapeutic armamentarium for systolic heart failure is considered palliative and there are no approved FDA therapeutics for diastolic heart failure, Dr Larson's primary investigational goal has been to develop immunomodulatory therapeutics for the treatment of heart failure.

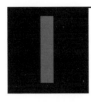

PART I

Immune dysfunction leading to heart disease: induction by physiological changes

CHAPTER 1

Immunosuppression by ultraviolet light-B radiation: a mediator of cardiac remodeling

Sherma Zibadi, Douglas F. Larson & Ronald Ross Watson

Introduction

Heart failure (HF) represents a major public health problem, affecting approximately 5 million patients in the United States and more than 550,000 new cases each year [1]. Heart failure has an extremely complex multidimensional pathophysiology involving structural and functional cardiac disorders and increased neurohormonal activity, primarily mediated through the sympathetic nervous system and the renin–angiotensin–aldosterone axis. Despite the diversity of HF etiologies, a crucial process in the progression of most forms of HF is left ventricular remodeling. Increasing evidence suggests the immune response-mediated regulation of cardiac extracellular matrix (ECM) remodeling.

Ultraviolet (UV) radiation presents one of the most important environmental factors that influence human health. Besides its well-known advantages, UV radiation also has well-documented adverse health effects, including premature skin aging, skin cancer, cataracts, and exacerbation of infectious diseases. Conclusive evidence has demonstrated that exposure to UV-B light induces photoimmunosuppression, which mediates several of these hazardous health effects. Estimation of over 1 million new cases of nonmelanoma skin cancer, and about 50,000 cases of in situ melanoma in the United States in 2006, according to the American Cancer Society [2], suggests the number of people who likely have UV-B exposure with likely enhancement of carcinogenesis with immunosuppression. However, do the UV-induced immunosuppressive changes in the skin become significant enough to have systemic effects that could affect heart structure?

Role of T_H1/T_H2 imbalance in development of cardiac ECM remodeling

Cardiac remodeling, a determinant of the clinical progression of HF, is defined as alternation of genome expression resulting in molecular, cellular, and interstitial changes and manifested clinically as changes in size, shape, and function of the heart [3]. Changes in the myocardial ECM, including the activation of proteolytic enzymes, matrix metalloproteinases (MMPs), and alteration in the myocardial collagen organization, contribute to the remodeling process [4]. Not only neurohormonal and autonomic nervous systems have been described as effector pathways in myocardial ECM reorganization, but also $CD4^+$ T lymphocyte has been shown to play a fundamental regulatory role in cardiac ECM composition through modulation of collagen synthesis and degradation.

$CD4^+$ T helper (T_H) cell subsets can be classified by the pattern of the cytokines they express upon activation. T_H1 cells produce mainly interleukin (IL)-2, -12, -15, and -18, interferon (IFN)-γ, and transforming growth factor (TGF)-β and promote cell-mediated immunity, whereas T_H2 cells secrete IL-4, -5, -6, -10, -13, -17, associated with humoral immune responses [5]. The T_H phenotypes have been shown to differentially alter cardiac

ECM composition. Selective induction of T_H1 lymphocytes in young mice increased left ventricular stiffness, through decreased pro-MMPs expression, MMPs activity, and increased total and cross-linked collagen synthesis. However, T_H2 induction resulted in dilated cardiomyopathy associated with decreased left ventricular stiffness, increased MMPs expression and activity, and decreased myocardial total and cross-linked collagen synthesis [6]. An important observation was the finding that the immune background of the mouse affects the cardiac remodeling processes in response to the induction of hypertension. In this study, T_H2 predominant strain was associated with increase in collagen synthesis and deposition, and ventricular stiffness, whereas no significant changes was observed in T_H1 predominant strain [7]. Moreover, the T_H2 murine model of HIV has been shown to be associated with a significant diastolic dysfunction [6]. Interestingly, in a recent clinical study, increased peripheral T_H2 subtype of $CD4^+$ T lymphocytes has been hypothesized as an immunological pathogenesis underlying dilated cardiomyopathy [8].

Ultraviolet light-B-induced immunosuppression

The immunosuppression results mainly form the effect of UV-B light on skin dendritic cells (DC) and T lymphocytes, which is a consequence of the formation of pyrimidine dimers in UV-irradiated epidermal Langerhans cells [9]. It has been shown that solar-simulated UV radiation induces a defective maturation and an anomalous migratory phenotype of DC, accompanied by decreased expression of molecules involved in antigen capture, diminished endocytic capacity, enhanced expression of molecules involved in antigen presentation, and a significant increase in their capability to stimulate T cells [10]. Moreover, it has been indicated that UV-B exposure impairs antigen presentation to T_H1 cells, whereas enhances the antigen presentation to T_H2 cell [11, 12]. Therefore, a shift in the activation of the T cells from a T_H1- to a T_H2-type immune response may mediate, in part, the immunosuppressive effect. This T_H1/T_H2 imbalance was confirmed in another study in which the pro-inflammatory T_H1 cytokines, IFN-γ and IL-12, were depleted from the murine epidermis by UV-B

by 24 hours, whereas expression of the T_H2 cytokine IL-10 was unregulated, peaking at 72 hours [13].

The UV-B effect has been thought to be mediated, in part, by a subset of T regulatory cells. The UV-B-induced $CD3^+$, $CD4^+$, and $CD8^-$ regulatory T cells mediate their suppressive effects by releasing the immune regulatory cytokines IL-4 and IL-10 [14]. Recently, this subtype of regulatory T cells, with the ability to transfer UV-induced immune suppression to the UV-B unexposed recipient mice, have been shown to express CTLA-4, a negative regulatory T cell-associated molecule [15]. Upon in vitro expansion, $CTLA-4^+$ T cells secrete variety of cytokine, including IL-2, IL-10, TGF-β, and IFN-γ, resembling a T regulatory 1-like cytokine pattern [16]. IL-10 monoclonal antibody not only has been shown to neutralize the suppressive activity of $CTLA-4^+$ T cells in vivo [15], but also to reserve both the failure to present to T_H1 cells and the enhanced presentation to T_H2 cells [17]. These findings suggest the involvement of $CTLA-4^+$ T cells in induction of T_H1/T_H2 imbalance.

Supporting the observed immunosuppressive effect of UV in experimental studies, UV exposure suppresses the induction of immunity in human volunteers [18, 19]. Many of the mechanisms involved in UV-induced immune suppression in humans are similar to those described previously in experimental animals. Induction of delayed-type hypersensitivity and contact hypersensitivity are suppressed after a single or short-term exposure to UV radiation [20], indicative of impaired cell-mediated immunity and T_H1/T_H2 imbalance. Moreover, UV-B irradiation of antigen-presenting cells selectively impairs T_H1-like responses, a phenomenon caused by reduced IL-12 production by human monocyte [21]. There is also evidence that UV-B irradiation in healthy volunteers initiates a rapid proinflammatory response followed by a combined T_H1/T_H2 response in which ultimately T_H2 cytokines, IL-4 and IL-10, predominated after 24 hours [22].

Conclusion

These epidemiologic and experimental animal studies lead us to the hypothesis that UV-B through its immunosuppressive effect may initiate or attenuate the adverse cardiac remodeling, which may in turn contribute to the clinical syndrome of HF. In light of the fact that exposure to UV-B radiation occurs daily and may be increasing due to the effects of atmospheric pollution on the ozone layer, it is critically important to investigate the potential role of UV-B radiation on cardiac ECM remodeling.

Acknowledgment

Supported by grants to RRW from Wallace Research Foundation and to DFL by NIH R01 HL079206-01.

References

1 American Heart Association. *Heart Disease and Stroke Statistics—2006 Update*. American Heart Association, Dallas, 2006.

2 Jemal A, Siegel R, Ward E *et al.* Cancer statistics, 2006. CA Cancer J Clin 2006;56:106–30.

3 Cohn JN, Ferrari R, Sharpe N. Cardiac remodeling—concepts and clinical implications: a consensus paper from an international forum on cardiac remodeling. J Am Coll Cardiol 2000;35:569–82.

4 Gunja-Smith Z, Morales AR, Romanelli R, Woessner JF. Remodeling of human myocardial collagen in idiopathic dilated cardiomyopathy—role of metalloproteinases and pyridinoline cross-links. Am J Pathol 1996;148:1639–48.

5 Rogge L. A genomic view of helper T cell subsets. Ann N Y Acad Sci 2002;975:57–67.

6 Yu Q, Watson RR, Marchalonis JJ, Larson DF. A role for T lymphocytes in mediating cardiac diastolic function. Am J Physiol Heart Circ Physiol 2005;289:H643–51.

7 Yu Q, Horak K, Larson DF. Role of T lymphocytes in hypertension-induced cardiac extracellular matrix remodeling. Hypertension 2006;48:98–104.

8 Kuethe F, Braun RK, Foerster M *et al.* Immunopathogenesis of dilated cardiomyopathy. Evidence for the role of TH2-type CD4$^+$T lymphocytes and association with myocardial HLA-DR expression. J Clin Immunol 2006;26:33–9.

9 Vink AA, Moodycliffe AM, Shreedhar V *et al.* The inhibition of antigen-presenting activity of dendritic cells resulting from UV irradiation of murine skin is restored by *in vitro* photorepair of cyclobutane pyrimidine dimers. Proc Natl Acad Sci U S A 1997;94:5255–60.

10 Mittelbrunn M, Tejedor R, de la Fuente H *et al.* Solar-simulated ultraviolet radiation induces abnormal maturation and defective chemotaxis of dendritic cells. J Invest Dermatol 2005;125:334–42.

11 Ullrich SE. Does exposure to UV radiation induce a shift to a Th-2-like immune reaction? Photochem Photobiol 1996;64:254–8.

12 Gorgun G, Miller KB, Foss FM. Immunologic mechanisms of extracorporeal photochemotherapy in chronic graft-versus-host disease. Blood 2002;100:941–7.

13 Shen J, Bao S, Reeve VE. Modulation of IL-10, IL-12, and IFN-γ in the epidermis of hairless mice by UVA (320–400 nm) and UVB (280–320 nm) radiation. J Invest Dermatol 1999;113:1059–64.

14 Rivas JM, Ullrich SE. The role of IL-4, IL-10, and TNF-alpha in the immune suppression induced by ultraviolet radiation. J Leukoc Biol 1994;56:769–75.

15 Schwarz A, Beissert S, Grosse-Heitmeyer K *et al.* Evidence for functional relevance of CTLA-4 in ultraviolet-radiation-induced tolerance. J Immunol 2000;165: 1824–31.

16 Groux H, O'Garra A, Bigler M *et al.* A CD4$^+$ T-cell subset inhibits antigen-specific T-cell responses and prevents colitis. Nature 1997;389:737–42.

17 Ullrich SE. Mechanism involved in the systemic suppression of antigen-presenting cell function by UV irradiation: keratinocyte-derived IL-10 modulates antigen-presenting cell function of splenic adherent cells. J Immunol 1994;152:3410–6.

18 Cooper KD, Oberhelman L, Hamilton TA *et al.* UV exposure reduces immunization rates and promotes tolerance to epicutaneous antigens in humans: relationship to dose, CD1a$^-$ R$^+$ epidermal macrophage induction, and Langerhans cell depletion. Proc Natl Acad Sci U S A 1992;89:8497–501.

19 Tie C, Golomb C, Taylor JR, Streilein JW. Suppressive and enhancing effect of ultraviolet B radiation on expression of contact hypersensitivity in man. J Invest Dermatol 1995;104:18–22.

20 Ullrich SE. Mechanisms underlying UV-induced immune suppression [review]. Mutat Res 2005;571:185–205.

21 Kremer IB, Hilkens CM, Sylva-Steenland RM *et al.* Reduced IL-12 production by monocytes upon ultraviolet-B irradiation selectively limits activation of T helper-1 cells. J Immunol 1996;157:1913–8.

22 Averbeck M, Beilharz S, Bauer M *et al.* In situ profiling and quantification of cytokines released during ultraviolet B-induced inflammation by combining dermal microdialysis and protein microarrays. Exp Dermatol 2006;15: 447–54.

CHAPTER 2

Immune mechanisms in pediatric cardiovascular disease

Wendy A. Luce, Mandar S. Joshi, Timothy M. Hoffman,
Timothy F. Feltes & John Anthony Bauer

Introduction

It is now well established that the cardiovascular system is vulnerable to immune system modulation and injury. Several, or perhaps most, forms of adult cardiovascular disease have an identified immune system component contributing to its pathogenesis spanning both acute (i.e., myocarditis, myocardial infarction) and chronic (coronary artery disease, heart failure) disease states [1, 2]. Key features of immune modulation in cardiovascular disease include immune cell activation, local or regional inflammation and/or cellular injury, and cardiac and/or vascular dysfunction, which may ultimately result in death [3]. The key aspects of these phenomena in specific settings of adult disease are addressed in many other chapters of this text.

Heart disease in infants, children, and adolescents is a large and relatively under-appreciated public health problem. Diseases range from congenital structural defects to genetic abnormalities of the heart muscle or conduction system as well as forms of acquired heart disease. In addition to clinically evident disease in the pediatric population, many recent studies have demonstrated that adult cardiovascular disease often originates in childhood and adolescence [4]. Because children have a long life ahead, the burden and cost of congenital or acquired heart disease in the pediatric patient are substantial for families and society. In this chapter, we provide some perspectives regarding the roles and mechanisms of immune system involvement in pediatric cardiovascular disease. The central questions addressed in this chapter are: Is the immune system an important contributor to pediatric cardiovascular disease? Are there important aspects of immune system involvement that differ in pediatrics versus adults? Are there important opportunities for better understanding and for therapeutic interventions?

Immune system function in pediatric versus adult populations

When one considers immune system involvement in pediatric disease it is important to recognize the age-dependent features of immune function throughout development to adulthood. Recent literature has demonstrated that the developing immune system of the neonate not only differs significantly from that of the adult, but also varies based on gestational age [5]. Prenatal and perinatal events such as challenges to the maternal immune system and mode of delivery can affect immune responses at birth, and these influences may play a significant role in various disease outcomes. The immune system continues to develop throughout infancy and childhood and is influenced by multiple factors including environmental exposures, immunization status, nutrition, and genetic predispositions [6].

Immune system development begins as early as the seventh to eighth week of gestation with the appearance of lymphocyte progenitors in the liver [7]. The thymus begins to develop around this same time frame, and splenic T-cells can be detected by week 14 [8, 9]. Despite the early identification of T-cells, these cells do not become functional until the end of the second trimester [10]. At birth, the

T-cell population is low in comparison to older children and adults, but the functionality of the T-cells is reasonably well developed [11]. The mechanisms involved and the time course of T-cell maturation in neonates and infants are not well defined. Although there is deficient cytokine production by neonatal lymphocytes, this does not appear to be associated with an inability to respond to supplemental cytokines [12].

Separate from changes in numbers of circulating immune cells in the neonate, polymorphonuclear neutrophils (PMNs), macrophages, and eosinophils have reduced surface-binding components and have defective opsonization, phagocytosis, and antigen-processing capabilities, leading to a generally less robust response to pathogen exposure. PMNs function as the primary line of defense in the cellular immune system. There is an alteration in both neutrophil function and survival in neonates versus adults. Neonates display a pattern of infectious diseases that is similar to those seen in older individuals with severe neutropenia [13] and are more likely to develop neutropenia during systemic infection [14]. Functional deficiencies of neutrophils in preterm and stressed/septic neonates include chemotaxis, endothelial adherence, migration, phagocytosis, and bactericidal potency [13]. The NADPH oxidase system, however, may be a first-line mechanism of innate immunity as there is a direct negative correlation between oxidative burst product generation and gestational age [13]. This could, however, have a detrimental effect on preterm infants as exaggerated oxygen-free radical formation may contribute to the development of such neonatal diseases as retinopathy of prematurity and bronchopulmonary dysplasia, as well as cardiovascular disease.

Inflammatory cytokine responses also differ in the neonate compared to the adult. Intrauterine fetal cord blood samples taken between 21 and 32 weeks gestation have demonstrated significant synthesis of IL-6, IL-8, and TNF-α [13]. Term and preterm infants have been shown to have a higher percentage of IL-6 and IL-8 positive cells than do adults, with preterm infants having the highest percentage of IL-8 positive cells [15]. After stimulation with lipopolysaccharide (LPS), this increased percentage of proinflammatory cells in neonates is more pronounced and occurs faster than in adults. TNF-α levels are also higher in newborns [16] and do not appear to vary based on gestational age [17]. In addition, the compensatory anti-inflammatory response system in neonates appears to be immature with both term and preterm infants demonstrating profoundly decreased IL-10 production and a lower amount of TGF-β positive lymphocytes than do adults after LPS stimulation [16]. These differences in innate immunity and cytokine response may predispose neonates to the harmful effects of proinflammatory cytokines and oxidative stress, leading to severe organ dysfunction and sequelae during infection and inflammation [16].

An important consequence of this diminished immune system responsiveness in early life is an increased vulnerability to pathogen exposures. This is a well-recognized clinical problem, illustrated by a neonate's typically poor ability to mount an immune response to *Streptococcus pneumoniae* or *Haemophilus influenza*. In addition to increased susceptibility to pathogens, the ability to detect pathogen exposures via blood markers of immune system activation is also difficult in the very young. The clinical course of sepsis and severe inflammatory response syndrome is different in neonates, children, and adults and traditional markers of inflammation and disease severity used in adults have not been shown to be helpful in younger age groups [18–20]. Thus, it is clear that there is continued development of acquired immunity concomitant with increased antigen exposure throughout Years 1 and 2 of childhood [5, 21]. Following this critical period of "immune system education," other factors dictate the development of "immunocompetence." During late childhood and adolescence, continuous growth processes and hormonal influences also play an important role in immune development. Although it is clear that the neonatal setting is different from that of the adult, changes occurring throughout childhood and adolescence are less well defined. The ability to more precisely define the critical windows for immune system development in the newborn and pediatric patient is essential for anticipating and identifying risk factors and defining effective therapeutic strategies [5]. Therefore, there is a need for greater understanding of these developmental changes in order to adequately understand

and treat immune-related cardiovascular diseases in the neonatal and pediatric patient.

Defining immune system involvement in pediatric cardiovascular disease

Immune system contributions to a cardiovascular disorder can be identified via several indices in adult disease states, and many of the basic principles and key issues regarding pathogenesis are mirrored in pediatric conditions. A contemporary challenge in this research field, and in related clinical practice, is the criteria one may use to demonstrate the involvement of immune pathways in a disease setting [22]. A classical approach to implicate the immune system in cardiac disease has been to observe an increased prevalence of immune cells in parenchymal tissues. For example, in 1986, the Dallas criteria were developed for histological diagnosis of myocarditis from biopsy samples, wherein the grading system was primarily determined by lymphocyte presence among myocytes [23, 24]. Clinical pathology also often determines evidence of "inflammation" via the presence of neutrophils at a lesion site since this illustrates a site of active tissue remodeling. Although this emphasis on leukocyte prevalence has had value, it is now evident that activation of inflammatory pathways in parenchymal cell types (e.g., cardiac myocytes, vascular smooth muscle cells, endothelium) clearly contributes to cell dysfunction and often occurs at sites remote to or unrelated to leukocyte interactions in vivo. This is particularly true in neonatal disease states wherein total leukocyte numbers may be low. We and others have observed a discordance of immune cell infiltration and cardiac myocyte expression of inflammatory markers in settings of retrovirus-related cardiomyopathy suggesting that newer approaches to implicate the immune system and identify key mechanisms are needed [25–27]. Due to the previously mentioned deficiencies in inflammatory cell numbers, signaling, response and migration, solely using the presence of inflammatory cells in cardiac muscle as a diagnostic criteria and measure of disease severity may overlook cases of severe inflammation and mechanisms of myocyte dysfunction and injury. The issue of immune cell recruitment/infiltration versus evidence of parenchymal cell inflammatory response

as criteria to define a disease state may be important for improved diagnosis and therapy. Furthermore, there may be differences in these features in children versus adults. Some specific pediatric conditions known to involve immune system contributions are discussed below.

Pediatric disease states involving immune mechanisms

Kawasaki disease

This is the leading cause of acquired heart disease in children in developing countries and is now recognized as an important risk factor for subsequent ischemic heart disease in adults and sudden death in early adulthood. Kawasaki disease is an acute vasculitis that is typically self-limiting and of unknown etiology and occurs primarily in the first few years of life [28]. This condition was first described in Japan and is most frequently observed among Asian populations [29]. The clinical presentation typically includes fever, conjunctivitis, mucosal erythema and rash, and elevated markers of systemic inflammation (particularly CRP) [30, 31]. Approximately 20% of untreated children develop coronary artery aneurysms or ectasia, which frequently precipitates ischemic heart disease or sudden death [32]. There is strong evidence that the etiology involves an infectious agent, although no specific pathogen has been determined. The fact that Kawasaki disease is rare in both very young infants protected by maternal antibodies and in adults has led to the theory that the agent causes overt clinical features in only a subset of children infected. There are strong links to Asian racial groups but the genetic basis of susceptibility is not known [28].

Striking evidence of immune activation exists in Kawasaki disease, with elevated levels of cytokines in blood and endothelial cell activation. Although this is a condition of widespread vasculitis, coronary arteries are virtually always involved and autopsy specimens demonstrate a localized "response to injury" vascular lesion [33]. Influx of neutrophils within the first 10 days of onset is followed by increased lymphocytes (particularly CD8+) and IgA plasma cells at coronary lesions, leading to damage to the elastic lamina and fibrosis [34, 35]. Remodeling the lesion site can lead to progressive stenosis and a form of advanced atherosclerosis. Cardiovascular manifestations of this acute condition of immune activation can be prominent and cardiac sites other than the coronary vasculature may be involved; patients may also present with poor myocardial function and/or electrophysiological abnormalities. The risk of aneurysm is highest in patients with long-standing fever and other risk factors including high leukocyte counts ($>12,000/mm^3$) and low platelet counts ($<350,000/mm^3$). Because of the limitations of identifying patients most at risk, recently published guidelines recommend intravenous gamma globulin (IVGG) treatment to all Kawasaki disease cases [28]. If administered early in the disease course, IVGG is valuable in reducing the prevalence of coronary artery abnormalities. The mechanism of this therapy is unclear but seems to provide a nonspecific anti-inflammatory effect. Modulations of cytokine production, binding of bacterial superantigens, suppression of antibody production, and influences on T-cell suppressor activity have all been postulated. A challenge with this therapeutic approach in the United States and other countries is the high cost of the IVGG therapy, especially when administered in high doses. Therefore, further refinement of mechanism-based approaches or better strategies for identifying the approximately 20% of patients who are most vulnerable are warranted.

Myocarditis

This is an inflammatory disease of the myocardium that is diagnosed by established histological, immunological, and immunochemical criteria, and is associated with cardiac dysfunction. The clinical manifestations of myocarditis are varied and some patients present a fully developed disease course with acute heart failure and severe arrhythmias, but most present with minimal symptoms or are entirely asymptomatic [36]. Initial presentation may be with acute or chronic heart failure, suspected acute myocardial infarction, or symptomatic or fatal arrhythmias. A history of flu-like syndrome may be present in up to 90% of patients with myocarditis, accompanied by fever and musculoskeletal pain. Laboratory tests may show leucocytosis, elevated erythrocyte sedimentation rate, eosinophilia, or an elevation in the cardiac fraction of creatine kinase [37, 38]. The electrocardiogram may reveal a variety of conduction disturbances (e.g., ventricular arrhythmias, atrioventricular block), evidence

of myocardial ischemia, acute myocardial infarction, or pericarditis. The relations between these clinical and laboratory findings and the positive biopsy results for the presence of myocarditis are obscure [38]. Therefore, the endomyocardial biopsy remains a "gold standard" for the diagnosis of myocarditis. However, because of its limited sensitivity and specificity, a negative biopsy does not rule out myocarditis [36]. PCR testing has been accomplished on endomyocardial biopsies and tracheal aspirates simultaneously. Both samples amplified the same viral genome, therefore suggesting that tracheal aspirate PCR testing is a comparable test to endomyocardial biopsy for the determination of a viral etiology [39].

Previous data from necropsy studies suggest that undiagnosed or asymptomatic myocarditis is a cause of death with the prevalence of up to 1% [40]. Infectious agents are thought to play a central role in acute myocarditis as evident by various viral, serological, and molecular biological methods. In spite of growing evidence from animal models, clinical data are limited. Many modern techniques such as RNA isolation and PCR have been utilized for defining the role of a pathogen but the results have been highly variable. On the other hand, noninfectious myocarditis, which often affects patients with latent or symptomatic autoimmune disease, denotes cardiac inflammation with no evidence of myocardial infection and carries a very poor prognosis [41].

The true incidence of myocarditis is unknown but in the largest myocarditis trial (Myocarditis Treatment Trial), 9.6% of 2333 patients with recent onset of heart failure met pathological criteria for myocarditis [42]. The difficulties in detecting infectious agents and evidence of ongoing infection in patients with clinical myocarditis have led to the speculation that there might also be an autoimmune component in the disease pathology and progression. Animal models support the involvement of autoimmune interactions in development and progression of myocarditis [43, 44] and there is some recent evidence to suggest that an autoimmune response constitutes an important role in myocarditis in humans [45].

Release of viral particles can lead to activation of macrophages and release of IFN-γ by natural killer (NK) cells. Uncontrolled activation of the NK cells may lead to myocyte injury and contribute to cardiac dysfunction. The proinflammatory cytokines are essential for "clearing" of the viral particles but more importantly may also play a central role in the development of chronic disease. These agents may contribute to the progression of acute to chronic myocarditis eventually leading to dilated cardiomyopathy (DCM). It is important to note that the setting of myocarditis is a temporal sequence of disease progression. This includes viral infection in myocardium, infiltration of immune cells, activation of inflammatory pathways in infiltrates and/or parenchymal cells, tissue remodeling, and eventual resolution. Defining the time course of various inflammatory and immune mechanisms, and identifying key mechanistic targets and therapeutic windows is critical for improving outcomes.

Despite evidence of an inflammatory response in acute myocarditis, the use of immunosuppressive agents does not clearly change the outcome in this disease. In children, administration of intravenous immunoglobulin may improve outcome and is therefore commonly used [46]. Such a response has not been demonstrated in adults. Other immunosuppressive agents such as steroids have not been shown to be beneficial. In general, the reversibility of impaired ventricular function observed in myocarditis tends to be greater in the younger patient but the mechanism for this observation is unknown.

Dilated cardiomyopathy

Cardiomyopathies in children are rare overall, with roughly 1 per 100,000, but rates are much higher (8- to 12-fold) in infants. Nearly, 40% of children with symptomatic cardiomyopathy receive a transplant or die within 2 years, and survival has only slightly improved over the last decade [47]. DCM, characterized by cardiac dilatation and impaired contraction of the left ventricle or both ventricles [48], represents the majority of the cases of cardiomyopathy (versus restrictive, hypertrophic, and mixed forms) and is most commonly linked to immune system and/or inflammatory processes.

An important precursor to DCM is often an acute episode of myocarditis, and this is most commonly related to viral presence in myocardial tissue [49]. A recent report by the pediatric cardiomyopathy registry showed that 51% of the DCM cases with known etiology were shown to involve a viral pathogen. Viral infections have frequently been implicated in idiopathic dilated cardiomyopathy (IDCM), and several studies have found increased levels of antibodies to viruses (e.g., Coxsackie B) in many cases of IDCM [50]. Studies using very sensitive PCR have also reported variable results for detection of enteroviral RNA. A recent study examining myocardial biopsy viral PCR genome testing noted that virus was noted in 20% of patients with DCM, and only adenovirus and enterovirus were detected with adenovirus being the most common pathogen [51]. The true frequency of viral myocarditis as an initiator of later DCM might be much higher, owing to the issues of endocardial biopsy sampling infrequency and detection limits for some viral suspects. The histological evidence of myocarditis can also regress quickly, making detection of the active phase difficult. Whether detection of virus or viral RNA in patients with DCM is proof of viral etiology or rather should be considered a possible nonspecific observation also remains to be clarified. For these and other reasons, only one-third of all DCM cases in pediatrics have a known cause, whereas the remaining two-thirds have unknown etiology and are therefore considered "idiopathic" DCM.

Several studies have suggested that autoimmune mechanisms play an important role in the development of pediatric DCM. A number of autoantibodies against various cellular and subcellular components have been reported to be present in patients. However, these types of autoantibodies have been reported to be present in both patients with myocarditis and in asymptomatic individuals [38]. Whether there is a causative role for these autoantibodies and its significance remain to be elucidated. The recent observations that immunoadsorption and immunosuppression may cause a reduction in these circulating autoantibodies and result in a clinical improvement strongly support the etiological importance of such autoantibodies and the relevance of adaptive immunity mechanisms in some cases of DCM progression [52–54]. Familial analysis has shown that idiopathic DCM may have a genetic or inherited basis. Reduced cardiac function and cardiomegaly have been described in 20% of first-degree relatives of IDCM patients. A similar high prevalence of cardiac dysfunction in first-degree relatives of IDCM patients has been reported by other investigators. Furthermore, it has been reported that mutations in genes that encode for such proteins as dystrophin, endothelin, and desmin appear to be genetic risk factors for the disease. In IDCM, a linkage between disease frequency and genes of the major histocompatibility complex (MHC) has also been proposed. The most frequently described linkage between IDCM and MHC genes has been in class II alleles. Four out of five independent studies identified a positive association of IDCM with HLA-DR4. An association between HLA-DR4 and anti-cardiac autoantibodies has also been demonstrated. These studies strongly implicate genetically controlled immunological factors in the pathogenesis of IDCM. Molecular resemblance between the microbial antigen and self-structures may induce the immune system to activate autoreactive T-cells and build up a cytotoxic immune response [55]. Chagas disease is an example of molecular mimicry wherein autoantibodies from Chagasic patients recognize the carboxyl terminal part of the ribosomal P0 protein of *Trypanosoma cruzi* and the second extracellular loop of the human beta-1-adrenergic receptor. These autoantibodies bind to the beta-adrenergic receptors and modulate their activity [38, 56].

The autoimmune process in pediatric IDCM could be triggered by diverse causes of cardiac injury, such as an initial viral infection, trauma, and ischemia. Likewise, there may be a specific predisposing genetic background and development of humoral and/or cell-mediated organ-specific autoimmunity, which could lead to IDCM in the presence of a precipitating factor such as a viral or toxic insult. Abnormality in a regulatory mechanism of the immune system, such as deficient natural killer cell activity, has been observed in approximately 50% of IDCM patients, demonstrating an ongoing antiviral defense mechanism. In a case study, Gerli *et al.* reported an abnormal T-cell population in peripheral blood from IDCM patients, in which there was an increase in the number of helper-induced cells and a decrease in the number of suppressor/cytotoxic T cells [57]. The abnormal expression of HLA class II antigens may lead to an autoimmune stage that is correlated to the prevalence of circulating autoantibodies, such as antibodies to beta-adrenergic receptor.

The studies described above demonstrate the important role for immune system activation in pediatric dilated cardiomyopathies. Although a minority of cases has a known etiology, initiating episodes of myocarditis or autoimmune mechanisms are most often suspected. Thus, adaptive as well as innate immunity pathways likely contribute to DCM progression. Strategies to develop therapy to modulate these mechanisms and improve outcomes in this patient group are clearly warranted.

Postpericardiotomy syndrome

Postpericardiotomy syndrome (PPS) is a cluster of symptoms and physical signs observed in as high as 15% of pediatric patients within the first week or two following open heart surgery. PPS is marked clinically by the presence of low-grade fever, irritability, chest pain, and loss of appetite associated with pleural and pericardial effusions. These effusions commonly require intervention. An inflammatory response marked by leukocytosis and elevated erythrocyte sedimentation rate is evident. PPS responds to treatment with anti-inflammatory agents, such as acetyl salicylic acid and nonsteroidal anti-inflammatory agents, but its occurrence is not prevented by these agents and may actually be exaggerated by a short-treatment course of steroids (24 hours) following open heart surgery [58].

Allograft rejection

Availability of pulmonary and aortic allografts (homografts) has greatly aided in the surgical repair of congenital heart disease. Because these grafts are biopreserved and are a variety of sizes, they may be stored and used as needed. These grafts often last an extensive period of time requiring replacement only after the child outgrows the size of the graft. But implantation has been associated with an immunologic response [59] and may be responsible for graft failure often within months of initial implantation. High plasma reactive antibody titers can be observed following allograft placement which may not only jeopardize graft viability but may also impact the future option for cardiac transplantation [60]. Use of decellularized or tissue engineered grafts may in the long run be superior to cyropreserved allografts in minimizing the inflammatory response [61, 62].

Inflammation in chronic heart failure

Regardless of the etiology of heart failure, several mechanisms are involved in the progression of myocardial dysfunction and failure. Myocardial remodeling is associated with an increase in myocardial mass, hypertrophy, induction of fetal gene expression, and changes in function and structure. Injury to the myocardium triggers a cascade of events that involve neuroendocrine activation, release of growth factors, cytokines, integrins, and adhesion molecules causing remodeling events and progression of disease. Persistent immune activation has been demonstrated in patients with chronic heart failure [63]. Irrespective of the initiating factors, increased serum levels of inflammatory cytokines have been described (e.g., TNF-α, IL-1-β, and IL-6), and enhanced expression of various inflammatory mediators within the myocardium has been observed during heart failure [64,65]. Thus, regardless of etiology, the failing myocardium is characterized by a state of chronic inflammation, as evident by infiltration of mononuclear cells and/or activation of inflammatory cytokine gene expression in myocardium. Of note is that this chronic state of inflammation ultimately leads to increased cellular "oxidative stress," wherein specific reactive oxygen and nitrogen intermediates cause cellular injury via protein oxidation and DNA damage. We and others have shown that these reactive species are important contributors to cardiac and vascular dysfunction and can occur in numerous settings of nonischemic heart disease [66–71]. Thus, the presence of an inflammatory reaction in the myocardium may be considered a cause as well as a consequence of myocardial dysfunction and failure.

Sepsis

Sepsis is characterized by systemic inflammation, cardiovascular dysfunction, inability of oxygen delivery to meet oxygen demand, altered substrate metabolism, and ultimately multiorgan failure and death. The mortality rate from sepsis doubles in patients who develop cardiovascular dysfunction and septic shock [72]. Cardiac dysfunction and cardiovascular collapse result from increased myocyte production of TNF-α, nitric oxide, and peroxynitrite, which leads to further DNA damage and ATP depletion resulting in secondary energy failure [73]. In addition, serum from patients with septic shock directly causes decreased maximum extent and peak velocity of contraction, activates transcription factors for proinflammatory cytokines, and induces apoptosis in cultured myocytes [74]. As discussed previously, immune function and inflammatory responses to pathogens differ in neonates and children from adults; their cardiovascular response to sepsis is also different and less well understood.

In adults, septic shock is characterized by a hyperdynamic phase with decreased left ventricular ejection fraction (LVEF), decreased systemic vascular resistance (SVR), and an increased cardiac index [75]. Underlying coronary artery disease, cardiomyopathy, and congestive heart failure may contribute to the systolic and diastolic ventricular dysfunction described in the setting of adult sepsis. Myocardial dysfunction in childhood septic shock, however, reaches its maximum within hours and is the main cause of mortality [76]. In comparison to adults, children more often present in a non-hyperdynamic state with decreased cardiac output (CO) and increased SVR [77]. This low CO is associated with an increase in mortality [78]. Since children are more able to maximize SVR and maintain a normal blood pressure despite decreased CO, hypotension is a late and ominous sign of septic shock.

Due to a limited number of research studies in the very young, the hemodynamic response of premature infants and neonates is not well understood, and the presenting hemodynamic abnormalities are more variable than in older children and adults [77]. Infants and young children have a limited ability to increase stroke volume or myocardial contractility as they have relatively decreased ventricular muscle mass and are already functioning at the top of the Frank–Starling curve; therefore, increases in CO are highly dependent on heart rate. LPS-induced production of TNF-α has been associated with increased apoptosis and cell death in adult cultured cardiomyocytes [81], and this ventricular myocyte apoptosis has been linked to cardiovascular dysfunction in adult whole animal experiments [79, 80]. Neonatal cardiomyocytes, however, do not exhibit an increase in apoptosis despite an increase in TNF-α production after LPS exposure, suggesting another mechanism for sepsis-associated cardiovascular dysfunction in neonates [82]. Complicating the cardiovascular response to sepsis in the neonate are additional morbidities including reopening of a patent ductus arteriosus and the development of persistent pulmonary hypertension of the newborn (PPHN) due to the cytokine elaboration, acidosis, and hypoxia in the setting of sepsis [78].

Therapeutic issues and opportunities

The pediatric disease states described previously highlight some key features of this population relative to adults and provide important opportunities for research and therapeutics. The classical large coronary artery obstruction, myocardial infarction, and ischemia infarct-related heart failure, which is the most common form of adult cardiovascular sequelae, is exceedingly uncommon in children. Rather, most forms of heart disease in children are considered nonischemic and implicate other processes, particularly infectious and/or inflammatory etiologies. Given the strong evidence that immune system competence and phenotypes are variability is different in children relative to adults (and most different in neonates and infants), it is likely that there are discrete differences in pediatric cardiovascular disease, even when the disease state appears generally similar. Overall, much of the therapeutic approaches used in children have been derived from trials conducted in adults, and this is true of cardiovascular medicine as well. Some recent studies have suggested that the use of nonspecific anti-inflammatory strategies such as IVGG may have value in at least some of the conditions described above, but large-scale randomized trials in children are generally lacking. Further research to define the mechanisms and immuno-inflammatory oxidative pathways involved in these disease states is clearly warranted and will help to define new therapeutic strategies for an underserved population.

References

1 Lange LG, Schreiner GF. Immune mechanisms of cardiac disease. N Engl J Med April 21, 1994;330(16):1129–35.

2 Taqueti VR, Mitchell RN, Lichtman AH. Protecting the pump: controlling myocardial inflammatory responses. Annu Rev Physiol 2006;68:67–95.

3 Barry WH. Mechanisms of immune-mediated myocyte injury. Circulation May 1994;89(5):2421–32.

4 Groner JA, Joshi M, Bauer JA. Pediatric precursors of adult cardiovascular disease: noninvasive assessment of early vascular changes in children and adolescents. Pediatrics October 2006;118(4):1683–91.

5 West LJ. Defining critical windows in the development of the human immune system. Hum Exp Toxicol September–October 2002;21(9–10):499–505.

6 Holt PG, Jones CA. The development of the immune system during pregnancy and early life. Allergy August 2000;55(8):688–97.

7 Haynes BF, Denning SM, Singer KH, Kurtzberg J. Ontogeny of T-cell precursors: a model for the initial stages of human T-cell development. Immunol Today March 1989;10(3):87–91.

8 Hannet I, Erkeller-Yuksel F, Lydyard P, Deneys V, DeBruyere M. Developmental and maturational changes in human blood lymphocyte subpopulations. Immunol Today June 1992;13(6):215–8.

9 Hulstaert F, Hannet I, Deneys V et al. Age-related changes in human blood lymphocyte subpopulations. II: Varying kinetics of percentage and absolute count measurements. Clin Immunol Immunopathol February 1994;70(2):152–8.

10 Royo C, Touraine JL, de Bouteiller O. Ontogeny of T lymphocyte differentiation in the human fetus: acquisition of phenotype and functions. Thymus 1987;10(1–2):57–73.

11 Hayward AR. The human fetus and newborn: development of the immune response. Birth Defects Orig Artic Ser 1983;19(3):289–94.

12 Demeure CE, Wu CY, Shu U et al. In vitro maturation of human neonatal CD4 T lymphocytes. II. Cytokines present at priming modulate the development of lymphokine production. J Immunol May 15, 1994;152(10):4775–82.

13 Strunk T, Temming P, Gembruch U, Reiss I, Bucsky P, Schultz C. Differential maturation of the innate immune response in human fetuses. Pediatr Res August 2004;56(2):219–26.

14 Molloy EJ, O'Neill AJ, Grantham JJ et al. Granulocyte colony-stimulating factor and granulocyte-macrophage colony-stimulating factor have differential effects on neonatal and adult neutrophil survival and function. Pediatr Res June 2005;57(6):806–12.

15 Schultz C, Rott C, Temming P, Schlenke P, Moller JC, Bucsky P. Enhanced interleukin-6 and interleukin-8 synthesis in term and preterm infants. Pediatr Res March 2002;51(3):317–22.

16 Schultz C, Temming P, Bucsky P, Gopel W, Strunk T, Hartel C. Immature anti-inflammatory response in neonates. Clin Exp Immunol January 2004;135(1):130–6.

17 Dembinski J, Behrendt D, Martini R, Heep A, Bartmann P. Modulation of pro- and anti-inflammatory cytokine

production in very preterm infants. Cytokine February 21, 2003;21(4):200–6.

18 Carr R. Neutrophil production and function in newborn infants. Br J Haematol July 2000;110(1):18–28.

19 Gessler P, Luders R, Konig S, Haas N, Lasch P, Kachel W. Neonatal neutropenia in low birthweight premature infants. Am J Perinatol January 1995;12(1): 34–8.

20 Gladstone IM, Ehrenkranz RA, Edberg SC, Baltimore RS. A ten-year review of neonatal sepsis and comparison with the previous fifty-year experience. Pediatr Infect Dis J November 1990;9(11):819–25.

21 Wilson CB. Immunologic basis for increased susceptibility of the neonate to infection. J Pediatr January 1986;108(1):1–12.

22 Baughman KL. Diagnosis of myocarditis: death of Dallas criteria. Circulation January 31, 2006;113(4):593–5.

23 Aretz HT. Myocarditis: the Dallas criteria. Hum Pathol June 1987;18(6):619–24.

24 Aretz HT, Billingham ME, Edwards WD et al. Myocarditis. A histopathologic definition and classification. Am J Cardiovasc Pathol January 1987;1(1):3–14.

25 Chaves AA, Baliga RS, Mihm MJ et al. Bacterial lipopolysaccharide enhances cardiac dysfunction but not retroviral replication in murine AIDS: roles of macrophage infiltration and toll-like receptor 4 expression. Am J Pathol March 2006;168(3):727–35.

26 Chaves AA, Mihm MJ, Basuray A, Baliga R, Ayers LW, Bauer JA. HIV/AIDS-related cardiovascular disease. Cardiovasc Toxicol 2004;4(3):229–42.

27 Chaves AA, Mihm MJ, Schanbacher BL et al. Cardiomyopathy in a murine model of AIDS: evidence of reactive nitrogen species and corroboration in human HIV/AIDS cardiac tissues. Cardiovasc Res October 15, 2003;60(1):108–18.

28 Newburger JW, Takahashi M, Gerber MA et al. Diagnosis, treatment, and long-term management of Kawasaki disease: a statement for health professionals from the Committee on Rheumatic Fever, Endocarditis and Kawasaki Disease, Council on Cardiovascular Disease in the Young, American Heart Association. Circulation October 26, 2004;110(17):2747–71.

29 Kawasaki T. Acute febrile mucocutaneous syndrome with lymphoid involvement with specific desquamation of the fingers and toes in children. Arerugi March 1967;16(3):178–222.

30 Anderson MS, Burns J, Treadwell TA, Pietra BA, Glode MP. Erythrocyte sedimentation rate and C-reactive protein discrepancy and high prevalence of coronary artery abnormalities in Kawasaki disease. Pediatr Infect Dis J July 2001;20(7):698–702.

31 Burns JC, Kushner HI, Bastian JF et al. Kawasaki disease: a brief history. Pediatrics August 2000;106(2):E27.

32 Kato H, Sugimura T, Akagi T et al. Long-term consequences of Kawasaki disease. A 10- to 21-year follow-up study of 594 patients. Circulation September 15, 1996;94(6):1379–85.

33 Naoe S, Takahashi K, Masuda H, Tanaka N. Kawasaki disease. With particular emphasis on arterial lesions. Acta Pathol Jpn November 1991;41(11):785–97.

34 Brown TJ, Crawford SE, Cornwall ML, Garcia F, Shulman ST, Rowley AH. CD8 T lymphocytes and macrophages infiltrate coronary artery aneurysms in acute Kawasaki disease. J Infect Dis October 1, 2001;184(7):940–3.

35 Rowley AH, Shulman ST, Mask CA et al. IgA plasma cell infiltration of proximal respiratory tract, pancreas, kidney, and coronary artery in acute Kawasaki disease. J Infect Dis October 2000;182(4):1183–91.

36 Burian J, Buser P, Eriksson U. Myocarditis: the immunologist's view on pathogenesis and treatment. Swiss Med Wkly June 25, 2005;135(25–26):359–64.

37 Feldman AM, McNamara D. Myocarditis. N Engl J Med November 9, 2000;343(19):1388–98.

38 Hjalmarson A, Fu M, Mobini R. Who are the enemies? Inflammation and autoimmune mechanisms. Eur Heart J Suppl 2002;4(suppl G):G27–32.

39 Akhtar N, Ni J, Stromberg D, Rosenthal GL, Bowles NE, Towbin JA. Tracheal aspirate as a substrate for polymerase chain reaction detection of viral genome in childhood pneumonia and myocarditis. Circulation April 20, 1999;99(15):2011–8.

40 Pauschinger M, Doerner A, Kuehl U et al. Enteroviral RNA replication in the myocardium of patients with left ventricular dysfunction and clinically suspected myocarditis. Circulation February 23, 1999;99(7): 889–95.

41 Cooper LT, Jr, Berry GJ, Shabetai R, for Multicenter Giant Cell Myocarditis Study Group Investigators. Idiopathic giant-cell myocarditis—natural history and treatment. N Engl J Med June 26, 1997;336(26):1860–6.

42 Mason JW, O'Connell JB, Herskowitz A et al., for The Myocarditis Treatment Trial Investigators. A clinical trial of immunosuppressive therapy for myocarditis. N Engl J Med August 3, 1995;333(5):269–75.

43 Neumann DA, Lane JR, Allen GS, Herskowitz A, Rose NR. Viral myocarditis leading to cardiomyopathy: do cytokines contribute to pathogenesis? Clin Immunol Immunopathol August 1993;68(2):181–90.

44 Rose NR, Hill SL. The pathogenesis of postinfectious myocarditis. Clin Immunol Immunopathol September 1996;80(3, pt 2):S92–9.

45 Frustaci A, Chimenti C, Calabrese F, Pieroni M, Thiene G, Maseri A. Immunosuppressive therapy for active lymphocytic myocarditis: virological and immunologic profile of responders versus nonresponders. Circulation February 18, 2003;107(6):857–63.

46 Drucker NA, Colan SD, Lewis AB *et al.* Gamma-globulin treatment of acute myocarditis in the pediatric population. Circulation January 1994;89(1):252–7.

47 Cox GF, Sleeper LA, Lowe AM *et al.* Factors associated with establishing a causal diagnosis for children with cardiomyopathy. Pediatrics October 2006;118(4):1519–31.

48 Richardson P, McKenna W, Bristow M *et al.* Report of the 1995 World Health Organization/International Society and Federation of Cardiology Task Force on the definition and classification of cardiomyopathies. Circulation March 1, 1996;93(5):841–2.

49 Kawai C. From myocarditis to cardiomyopathy: mechanisms of inflammation and cell death: learning from the past for the future. Circulation March 2, 1999;99(8):1091–100.

50 Muir P, Nicholson F, Tilzey AJ, Signy M, English TA, Banatvala JE. Chronic relapsing pericarditis and dilated cardiomyopathy: serological evidence of persistent enterovirus infection. Lancet April 15, 1989;1(8642):804–7.

51 Bowles NE, Ni J, Kearney DL *et al.* Detection of viruses in myocardial tissues by polymerase chain reaction. Evidence of adenovirus as a common cause of myocarditis in children and adults. J Am Coll Cardiol August 6, 2003;42(3):466–72.

52 Felix SB, Staudt A, Dorffel WV *et al.* Hemodynamic effects of immunoadsorption and subsequent immunoglobulin substitution in dilated cardiomyopathy: three-month results from a randomized study. J Am Coll Cardiol May 2000;35(6):1590–8.

53 Gullestad L, Aass H, Fjeld JG *et al.* Immunomodulating therapy with intravenous immunoglobulin in patients with chronic heart failure. Circulation January 16, 2001;103(2):220–5.

54 Muller J, Wallukat G, Dandel M *et al.* Immunoglobulin adsorption in patients with idiopathic dilated cardiomyopathy. Circulation February 1, 2000;101(4):385–91.

55 Albert LJ, Inman RD. Molecular mimicry and autoimmunity. N Engl J Med December 30, 1999;341(27):2068–74.

56 Ferrari I, Levin MJ, Wallukat G *et al.* Molecular mimicry between the immunodominant ribosomal protein P0 of Trypanosoma cruzi and a functional epitope on the human beta 1-adrenergic receptor. J Exp Med July 1, 1995;182(1):59–65.

57 Gerli R, Rambotti P, Spinozzi F *et al.* Immunologic studies of peripheral blood from patients with idiopathic dilated cardiomyopathy. Am Heart J August 1986;112(2):350–5.

58 Mott AR, Fraser CD, Jr, Kusnoor AV *et al.* The effect of short-term prophylactic methylprednisolone on the incidence and severity of postpericardiotomy syndrome in children undergoing cardiac surgery with cardiopulmonary bypass. J Am Coll Cardiol May 2001;37(6):1700–6.

59 Baskett RJ, Nanton MA, Warren AE, Ross DB. Human leukocyte antigen-DR and ABO mismatch are associated with accelerated homograft valve failure in children: implications for therapeutic interventions. J Thorac Cardiovasc Surg July 2003;126(1):232–9.

60 Shaddy RE, Hunter DD, Osborn KA *et al.* Prospective analysis of HLA immunogenicity of cryopreserved valved allografts used in pediatric heart surgery. Circulation September 1, 1996;94(5):1063–7.

61 Bechtel JF, Muller-Steinhardt M, Schmidtke C, Brunswik A, Stierle U, Sievers HH. Evaluation of the decellularized pulmonary valve homograft (SynerGraft). J Heart Valve Dis November 2003;12(6):734–9; discussion 9–40.

62 Cebotari S, Lichtenberg A, Tudorache I *et al.* Clinical application of tissue engineered human heart valves using autologous progenitor cells. Circulation July 4, 2006;114(1, suppl):I132–7.

63 Sasayama S, Matsumori A, Kihara Y. New insights into the pathophysiological role for cytokines in heart failure. Cardiovasc Res June 1999;42(3):557–64.

64 Aukrust P, Ueland T, Lien E *et al.* Cytokine network in congestive heart failure secondary to ischemic or idiopathic dilated cardiomyopathy. Am J Cardiol February 1, 1999;83(3):376–82.

65 Levine B, Kalman J, Mayer L, Fillit HM, Packer M. Elevated circulating levels of tumor necrosis factor in severe chronic heart failure. N Engl J Med July 26, 1990;323(4):236–41.

66 Mihm MJ, Bauer JA. Peroxynitrite-induced inhibition and nitration of cardiac myofibrillar creatine kinase. Biochimie October 2002;84(10):1013–9.

67 **67** Mihm MJ, Coyle CM, Schanbacher BL, Weinstein DM, Bauer JA. Peroxynitrite induced nitration and inactivation of myofibrillar creatine kinase in experimental heart failure. Cardiovasc Res March 2001;49(4):798–807.

68 Mihm MJ, Jing L, Bauer JA. Nitrotyrosine causes selective vascular endothelial dysfunction and DNA damage. J Cardiovasc Pharmacol August 2000;36(2):182–7.

69 Mihm MJ, Schanbacher BL, Wallace BL, Wallace LJ, Uretsky NJ, Bauer JA. Free 3-nitrotyrosine causes striatal neurodegeneration in vivo. J Neurosci June 1, 2001;21(11):RC149.

70 Mihm MJ, Wattanapitayakul SK, Piao SF, Hoyt DG, Bauer JA. Effects of angiotensin II on vascular endothelial cells: formation of receptor-mediated reactive nitrogen species. Biochem Pharmacol April 1, 2003;65(7):1189–97.

71 Mihm MJ, Yu F, Reiser PJ, Bauer JA. Effects of peroxynitrite on isolated cardiac trabeculae: selective impact on myofibrillar energetic controllers. Biochimie June 2003;85(6):587–96.

72 Vincent JL, Sakr Y, Sprung CL *et al.* Sepsis in European intensive care units: results of the SOAP study. Crit Care Med February 2006;34(2):344–53.

73 Carcillo JA. Pediatric septic shock and multiple organ failure. Crit Care Clin July 2003;19(3):413–40, viii.

74 Kumar A, Kumar A, Michael P *et al.* Human serum from patients with septic shock activates transcription factors STAT1, IRF1, and NF-kappaB and induces apoptosis in human cardiac myocytes. J Biol Chem December 30, 2005;280(52):42619–26.

75 Maeder M, Fehr T, Rickli H, Ammann P. Sepsis-associated myocardial dysfunction: diagnostic and prognostic impact of cardiac troponins and natriuretic peptides. Chest May 2006;129(5):1349–66.

76 von Rosenstiel N, von Rosenstiel I, Adam D. Management of sepsis and septic shock in infants and children. Paediatr Drugs 2001;3(1):9–27.

77 McKiernan CA, Lieberman SA. Circulatory shock in children: an overview. Pediatr Rev December 2005;26(12):451–60.

78 Carcillo JA, Fields AI. Clinical practice parameters for hemodynamic support of pediatric and neonatal patients in septic shock. Crit Care Med June 2002;30(6):1365–78.

79 Lancel S, Joulin O, Favory R *et al.* Ventricular myocyte caspases are directly responsible for endotoxin-induced cardiac dysfunction. Circulation May 24, 2005;111(20):2596–604.

80 Lancel S, Petillot P, Favory R *et al.* Expression of apoptosis regulatory factors during myocardial dysfunction in endotoxemic rats. Crit Care Med March 2005;33(3):492–6.

81 Comstock KL, Krown KA, Page MT *et al.* LPS-induced TNF-alpha release from and apoptosis in rat cardiomyocytes: obligatory role for CD14 in mediating the LPS response. J Mol Cell Cardiol December 1998;30(12):2761–75.

82 Hickson-Bick DL, Jones C, Buja LM. The response of neonatal rat ventricular myocytes to lipopolysaccharide-induced stress. Shock May 2006;25(5):546–52.

CHAPTER 3

Heart failure–role of autoimmunity

Urs Eriksson

Introduction

In developed countries, ischemic heart disease represents the most common cause of heart failure. In young patients and children, however, most cases of heart failure result from dilated cardiomyopathy or myocarditis [1]. Furthermore, clinical and epidemiological data suggest that many cases of dilated cardiomyopathy also evolve from myocarditis [1–3]. Myocarditis, defined by the Dallas criteria as "the presence of an inflammatory infiltrate in the myocardium with necrosis and/or degeneration of adjacent myocytes" remains an etiologic dilemma and a diagnostic and therapeutic problem [4, 5]. First, disease course and severity are both highly variable. In fact, epidemiologic data suggest that myocarditis can be entirely asymptomatic and its true prevalence is most likely underestimated [6]. But even asymptomatic cardiac inflammation puts patients at risk for sudden death or may slowly progress to heart failure, reflecting chronic myocarditis [7]. Subacute myocarditis, on the other hand, reflects a symptomatic and persistent process that results in progressive heart failure [8]. Moreover, chronic myocarditis sometimes evolves to dilated cardiomyopathy, a disease often requiring cardiac transplantation. Fulminant myocarditis denotes immediate life-threatening heart failure due to extensive tissue damage and inflammation. Interestingly, affected patients surviving the acute phase of fulminant myocarditis usually recover after clearance of the inciting infection [9].

Second, myocarditis appears as a heterogenous disease triggered by many different agents, which can cause the same pathologic picture [1]. We believe that etiologic uncertainties mainly account for many controversies regarding our current views on disease pathogenesis, diagnostic and thera-peutic approaches in patients with myocarditis and dilated cardiomyopathy resulting from cardiac inflammation.

A growing body of evidence supports the view that autoimmune responses play an important pathogenic role in many forms of human myocarditis and, consequently, dilated cardiomyopathy [10–17]. In this chapter, we will provide a common mechanistic concept of autoimmune heart failure, which can explain major aspects of the etiologic, histologic, and clinical diversity observed in patients with myocarditis and dilated cardiomyopathy resulting from it. In addition, we will summarize recent progresses in the diagnostic and therapeutic approach to patients with myocarditis or dilated cardiomyopathy following cardiac inflammation.

Etiology

Worldwide, infection with the parasitic protozoan *Trypanosoma cruzi* (Chagas disease), which is endemic in Southern America, is the leading cause of myocarditis [18]. In Europe and North America, enteroviruses, such as coxsackievirus B3 (CVB3) and to a lesser extent adenovirus, have been suggested as the most important microorganisms inducing inflammatory heart disease [1, 19–21]. Other common cardiotropic microorganisms include cytomegalovirus [22], parvovirus [23], hepatitis C-virus [24], human immunodeficiency virus [25], and Epstein-Barr virus [26]. In addition, recent findings suggest that bacteria such as *Chlamydia pneumoniae* and *Borrelia burgdorferi* might play a yet underestimated role in the development of heart failure following myocarditis [21]. Noninfectious myocarditis denotes cardiac inflammation with no evidence of infection, for example, in the context of autoimmune diseases, drug-induced hypersensitivity, neoplasia and/or other systemic disorders [1]. Giant-cell myocarditis, on the other hand, is a rare, idiopathic, and histologically distinct disease entity with a very poor prognosis, which often affects patients with latent or symptomatic autoimmune diseases [27]. So far, there is no evidence for an inciting infectious agent triggering giant cell myocarditis.

Evidence for autoimmunity in heart failure

How is the myocardium affected by viral infections? First, virus infection directly contributes to cardiac tissue destruction by cleaving the cytoskeletal protein dystrophin, leading to a disruption of the dystrophin–glycoprotein complex [28]. This mechanism is hypothesized to be crucial for enteroviral replication in the heart and development of virus-associated chronic cardiomyopathy. In the presence of extensive tissue damage, it is conceivable that the heart is functionally impaired and heart failure develops. This is the case during fulminant myocarditis and might explain why patients with fulminant myocarditis surviving acute disease and probably clearing the virus do not develop progressive heart failure [9]. Evidence from murine models that in both mouse strains, susceptible and resistant to chronic myocarditis, viral genome and transcript are present indicates that the persistence of virus alone may not be the single determining factor in development of chronic cardiomyopathy and that the viral damage itself may not be as important as the viral-associated immune response [29]. Indeed it appears that progression to overt heart failure reflects an ongoing process due to the development of heart-specific autoimmunity, virus persistence, or both. In this context, clinical observations and insights from animal models indeed provide evidence that autoimmunity plays a relevant pathogenetic role in most cases of human myocarditis and in many patients with dilated cardiomyopathy [15–17].

Autoimmune features include familiar aggregation, abnormal expression of HLA-class II on cardiac endothelial cells, a weak but significant association with HLA-DR4 and the detection of organ- and disease-specific autoantibodies of the Ig G class by indirect immunofluorescence (IFL) in approximately 30% of patients with myocarditis and dilated cardiomyopathy [12, 14, 30, 31]. Two of the autoantigens recognized by the antibodies found by IFL could be identified as alpha- and beta-myosin heavy chain isoforms [31]. The low frequency of cardiac-specific autoantibodies in patients with heart failure not due to myocarditis or dilated cardiomyopathy, the decrease of autoantibody titers during disease progression in dilated cardiomyopathy and the deterioration of cardiac function in myosin antibody-positive patients indicate that these antibodies are not merely an epiphenomenon but represent specific markers of immune pathogenesis [32].

Animal models further support the idea that autoimmune mechanisms, triggered by viral infections contribute to the pathogenesis of myocarditis and dilated cardiomyopathy. In fact, myocarditis can be induced in specific mouse strains and rats by infection with enteroviruses [29], but the associated autoimmune response can be duplicated sufficiently by immunization of the same mouse strains with a well-characterized antigen, cardiac myosin, together with a strong adjuvant (experimental autoimmune myocarditis) [33–35]. Comparable to human myocarditis, experimental autoimmune myocarditis progresses to heart failure [36]. In rats and mice, the development of myocarditis is associated with polyclonal cardiac autoantibody responses and heart-specific, autoaggressive CD4$^+$ T-cell responses [34, 37–40]. The evidence available indicates a key role for alpha-myosin as a target antigen in development of myocarditis and dilated cardiomyopathy as the same susceptible mouse strains develop autoimmune myocarditis in the absence of virus infection after either injection of activated dendritic cells loaded with alpha-myosin peptide or after immunization with alpha-myosin peptide and a strong nonspecific adjuvant [41]. The finding that in the susceptible mouse strain BALB/c virus or myosin-peptide-induced myocarditis is T-cell-mediated [41–43], whereas in other strains, such as DBA/2 mice, it is an antibody-mediated disease [44, 45] may also apply to humans which means that the heart-specific antibodies may be directly pathogenic in some, but not all patients with myocarditis and dilated cardiomyopathy [31, 32].

In conclusion, clinical observations, coupled with insights from animal models, have led to the widely held proposition that chronic myocarditis and many cases of dilated cardiomyopathy are the consequences of an autoimmune response that represents a common pathogenetic pathway of various infectious and noninfectious injuries.

A unifying theory explaining autoimmune heart disease

Genetic susceptibility, environmental triggers, and infectious agents have all been implicated in the development of potential autoimmune responses. So far, we do not know how exactly various viral or bacterial infections are linked to the generation of heart-specific T cells mediating autoimmune inflammation. One hypothesis postulates that specific structures of certain pathogens mimic defined cardiac self-antigens (= molecular mimicry) [46, 47]. Thus, depending on the individual structure of the antigen-presenting MHC class II molecule, T-cell responses against such microorganisms include the expansion of self-reactive T cells with the potential to attack the myocardium. In men, post-streptococcal rheumatic fever represents a well-known cause of pan-carditis including myocarditis due to molecular mimicry between streptococcal proteins and alpha-myosin of the heart [47]. Experimentally, immunization of Lewis rats with the streptococcal M protein results in valvulitis and myocarditis [48]. In addition, M protein-specific T cells isolated from diseased animals proliferate in vitro in response to cardiac alpha-myosin and could adoptively transfer autoimmune myocarditis into healthy rats [49]. Furthermore, structural proteins from several bacterial strains including *Chlamydia* spp., and viral proteins from hepatitis C viruses show a striking homology to pathogenic myosin-derived self-antigens known to mediate experimental autoimmune myocarditis in mice. Accordingly, immunizing mice with chlamydia-derived peptides induces myocarditis [50].

However, the most common cause of myocarditis in humans is viral infection [1, 15, 16]. In the context of viral infections, antigenic mimicry would im-

plicate similarities between the MHC-viral peptide and the MHC-self-protein complex presented to the T-cell receptor. Indeed, alpha-myosin and the VP1 coxsackievirus B4 protein are sharing a common epitope [51]. This epitope, however, does not belong to the most pathogenic myosin peptide sequences triggering myocarditis in mice [27, 28, 35]. Obviously, cross-reactivity between pathogen-derived and self-derived antigens presented on antigen-presenting cell is not a "conditio sine qua non" for the development of heart-specific autoimmunity.

In order to prime efficient T-cell responses, dendritic cells need to be in an activated maturation status expressing high levels of MHC class I and II molecules as well as costimulatory molecules. In the presence of an inciting microbial infection, dendritic cell activation is largely mediated by Toll-like receptors (TLRs). TLRs represent a family of evolutionarily conserved transmembrane receptors [52]. Importantly, different TLRs exhibit different specificities for microbial patterns such as lipopolysaccharide (LPS) or double-stranded RNA, as well as for some endogenous products such as heat-shock proteins and other stimulatory signals released by dying cells [53–56]. Because antigen-presenting dendritic cells process not only foreign antigens but also damaged self-tissue, we would expect that activation of self-antigen-loaded dendritic cells beyond a certain threshold would overcome counter-regulatory mechanisms of peripheral tolerance and result in the expansion of autoreactive, self-aggressive T cells (Figure 3.1). This has been termed the "adjuvant effect" of infection in the pathogenesis of autoimmunity [17, 46]. Accordingly, we have been able to show that alpha-myosin-peptide-loaded dendritic cells activated through TLR ligands such as LPS or CpG can induce autoimmune myocarditis and heart failure in susceptible mice [41]. Furthermore, mice lacking the common adaptor molecule MyD88 for different TLRs are protected from autoimmune myocarditis [57]. The idea that non-antigen-specific activation of self-antigen-loaded dendritic cells is sufficient to induce autoreactive T cells does not exclude antigenic mimicry in putting the organism at risk for autoimmunity; it is conceivable that an immune system that was exposed to symptomatic or subclinical infections with any microorganisms containing

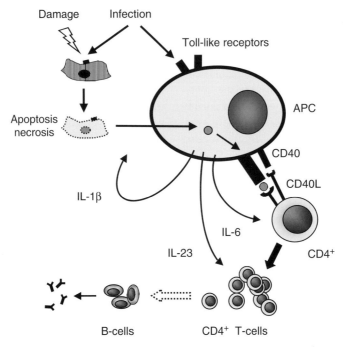

Figure 3.1 *Pathogenesis of heart-specific autoimmunity.* Infections result in tissue damage and release of self-antigens. Antigen-presenting cells (APC) enter the myocardium and take up self-antigens. APC become activated through Toll-like receptors. The combined effect of tissue damage and infection finally activates self-peptide-loaded APC and triggers the generation of heart-specific CD4$^+$ T cells in genetically predisposed subjects. Key cytokines promoting the generation and expansion of self-reactive, pathogenic CD4 T-cells include IL-6 and IL-23.

self-antigen-like structures is more susceptible to boost an autoreactive T-cell response after a second hit that releases self-antigen on the background of a nonspecific inflammatory response. The model of dendritic cell-induced heart failure offers a useful tool to dissect the role of antigen-presenting cells and effector cells while studying mechanisms of autoimmune-mediated cardiomyopathy. Furthermore, the concept nicely fits well-known, mainly experience-based, clinical observations. First, it might explain why some patients are prone to heart-specific autoimmunity after noninfectious tissue damage, i.e., after cardiac surgery or myocardial infarction [58–60]. Here, we expect that tissue damage result in release of self-antigen and uptake by dendritic cells. If self-antigen-loaded dendritic cells become activated via TLR by endogenous heat-shock proteins this might be sufficient for the initiation of an autoimmune response depending in a genetically susceptible individual [41]. Second, infections often worsen the condition of patients with dilated cardiomyopathy, i.e., result in sustained impairment of cardiac contractility. Here, we expect that the activation of self-antigen-loaded dendritic cells boost autoreactive T-cells aggravating cardiac inflammation.

Diagnostic approach to patients with autoimmune heart failure

There are no easily available diagnostic tests, which may be used to diagnose myocarditis. Because of limited sensitivity or specificity, the value of autoantibody measurements is rather hypothetical. Autoantibodies are present in the serum of up to 60% of patients with myocarditis and 20% of samples from patients with dilated cardiomyopathy [31, 61–65], whereas serum from individuals with no history of heart disease usually is negative or reacts only in low titer. Most cardiac autoantibodies of patients with myocarditis or cardiomyopathy express specificity against myosin and were identified in sera by immunofluorescence on frozen heart tissues [65]. Both, the specificity and the sensitivity of the test are highly variable. In fact, patients recovering from many viral infections have antibodies to myosin. Generally, however, these antibodies are not specific for cardiac myosin, appear transiently, and are often of the IgM class. In contrast, patients with myocarditis characteristically develop heart-specific autoantibodies that are usually of the IgG class [65]. Despite low sensitivity and indeterminate specificity, however, anti-myosin antibody measurements might be helpful to assess prognosis and the extent of cardiac damage [64]. Of note, Caforio *et al.* found that cardiac antibodies detected by immunofluorescence in symptom-free relatives of patients with dilated cardiomyopathy were associated with echocardiographic changes suggestive of early disease [66, 67]. Therefore, autoantibodies might be useful as predictive markers of disease susceptibility in healthy subjects at risk of myocarditis or dilated cardiomyopathy, such as first-degree relatives of patients [67]. Antibodies with specificity to cardiac antigens other than myosin include autoantibodies to the beta-1 adrenoceptor found in patients with dilated cardiomyopathy [68], which are strongly associated with specific HLA haplotypes, HLA DR4 and HLA DR1 [69]. Other autoantibodies show specificity to mitochondrial antigens, such as the adenine nucleotide (*ADPI* ATP) translocator (ANT) [70] or the branched chain alphaketoacid dehydrogenase (BCKD) [71]. However, these antigens are not unique for the heart, they may well be more accessible in heart tissue than in other sites. Taken together, autoantibodies lack sensitivity and specificity as diagnostic markers for myocarditis and their measurements make no sense except in the context of clinical studies.

Recent progresses in the development of new cardiovascular magnetic resonance imaging techniques allow the visualization of small myocardial injuries and tissue inflammation [72, 73]. Cardiac magnetic resonance studies might therefore become a useful tool to discriminate between inflammatory and noninflammatory cardiac lesions in the future. At the moment, however, the sensitivity and specificity of cardiac magnetic resonance imaging for the diagnosis of acute and chronic myocarditis are not validated yet.

Despite its low sensitivity, mainly due to sampling errors, endomyocardial biopsy still represents the diagnostic gold standard [1, 4], as a definite diagnosis of myocarditis requires the detection of inflammatory infiltrates and myocyte damage according to the Dallas criteria [4, 5]. However, the role of endomyocardial biopsies in patients with clinically suspected acute myocarditis, myocarditis in the past, and dilated cardiomyopathy is discussed controversially. In fact, it is still a matter of debate whether information obtained from endomyocardial biopsies is relevant for further clinical decisions. Nevertheless, immunohistochemistry and molecular techniques can increase the sensitivity to detect and quantify activated heart infiltrating cells. Yet, there are no universally accepted diagnostic criteria based on immunostaining for activation markers on inflammatory cells. Furthermore, the increasing sensitivity of molecular techniques, such as polymerase chain reaction, gene sequencing, and real time PCR, allows the detection of viral genomes not only in small endomyocardial biopsies from patients with myocarditis but also in some with dilated cardiomyopathy with otherwise no evidence for inflammatory infiltrates [19, 20]. The latter finding reflects both, the low sensitivity of the histological analysis to detect subtle inflammatory infiltrates in endomyocardial biopsies and the fact that viral genomes can persist in the absence of ongoing inflammation. In future, the additional use of new cell isolation techniques like the laser capture microdissection (LCM) that offers the selection of antibody-targeted T lymphocytes and cardiomyocytes from a section of complex, heterogeneous cardiac tissue [74] may ameliorate the read-out of endomyocardial biopsies combining the sensitivity of PCR analysis with the option for cell localization of the infectious agent.

In conclusion, the diagnosis of myocarditis or inflammatory cardiomyopathy largely remains a diagnosis of exclusion. Furthermore, there are no validated tests available to assess the extent of the contribution of autoimmune mechanisms to cardiac inflammation in an individual patient. Autoantibody measurements are of some help but lack sensitivity and specificity. Endomyocardial biopsy including staining for immune activation markers and search for viral genome can be of help to identify patients, which take advantage of immunosuppression or immunomodulation.

Management of patients with autoimmune heart failure

Over the last years, myocarditis therapy has been restricted to supportive options facing the clinical syndromes of heart failure or arrhythmias [75], including basic medications with angiotensin-converting enzyme (ACE) inhibitors or angiotensin-receptor blocking agents, diuretics, nitrates, and beta-blockers. Patients with persistently impaired cardiac ejection fraction and/or life-threatening arrhythmias take survival advantage from ventricular assist devices and implantable cardiac defibrillators (ICD). In severe and rapidly progressive cases, however, heart transplantation still represents the only therapeutic option.

Of note, several commonly used cardiovascular drugs also exhibit immunomodulatory properties. Data on rats and mice with autoimmune myocarditis suggest anti-inflammatory and disease ameliorating potency for the beta-blocking agent carvedilol [76], the antiarrhythmic drug amiodarone [77], and for the ACE inhibitor captopril but not for other ACE inhibitors [78, 79]. Furthermore, a prospective clinical study on patients with idiopathic dilated cardiomyopathy has shown significant improvement in NYHA classification and left ventricular function after a 14-week treatment with the HMG-CoA-reductase-inhibitor simvastatin [80]. The effect of improved cardiac function might be due to changes in inflammatory cytokine patterns as decreased plasma concentrations for TNF-alpha and interleukin-6 have been found.

The idea that autoimmune mechanisms play an important role in the pathogenesis of myocarditis or postviral cardiomyopathy has suggested a potential beneficial effect of immunosuppression in affected patients. Accordingly, a number of clinical studies addressed the effects of various, mostly nonspecific, methods of immunosuppression in patients with myocarditis or dilated cardiomyopathy. In general, the outcome of these studies has been disappointing [81, 82]. In the largest trial so far, Mason *et al.* [82] found no significant effects of a combined immunosuppressive regimen on primary endpoints such as left ventricular function

or survival in patients with myocarditis diagnosed on the basis of the Dallas criteria. A more critical analysis, however, showed that groups of patients did in fact improve after immunosuppression, whereas others actually deteriorated. In contrast, several just recently published studies showed beneficial effects of immunosuppressive treatment for certain subgroups of patients with myocarditis. A large retrospective multicenter study suggested that an immunosuppressive treatment regimen combining cyclosporine and/or azathioprine with corticosteroids improved outcome such as time to death or transplantation for patients with histologically proven giant-cell myocarditis [27]. In a prospective single center study immunosuppression together with a gluten-free diet improved left ventricular function and clinical status of patients with celiac disease-associated myocarditis [83]. A large randomized, prospective 2-center study on patients with dilated cardiomyopathy carried out by Wojnicz *et al.* [84] used up-regulation of HLA in heart biopsies to identify a subgroup of patients with probably autoimmune-mediated heart failure [84]. Immunosuppressive treatment of the subgroup of patients with HLA up-regulation indeed resulted in an improvement of the left ventricular function as well as NYHA scores after 24 month of treatment. Importantly, functional improvement always became evident within the first months of immunosuppressive treatment in most responders. Frustaci *et al.* [26] showed that combined treatment of active myocarditis with prednisone and azathioprine for 6 months is most likely to improve cardiac function when there are circulating cardiac autoantibodies and no viral genome in the myocardium. Within 1 year, 21 of 41 patients with active myocarditis showed prompt improvement in left ventricular ejection fraction and evidence of healed myocarditis on follow-up biopsy. Of the 20 nonresponders, 12 remained the same, 3 required transplantation, and 5 died. Polymerase chain reaction studies of frozen heart tissue showed evidence of entero-, adeno-, parvo B19 virus genome in 17 of the 20 nonresponders. These results strongly suggest that the presence of circulating cardiac autoantibodies, as evaluated by indirect immunofluorescence, and the absence of viral genome is helpful for the identification of patients, which might benefit from immunosuppression. Of note, the same study revealed a good response to immunosuppressive therapy for patients with hepatitis C virus-related myocarditis. Despite these encouraging data, however, there is still no evidence so far that immunosuppression has a significant beneficial effect on primary endpoints, such as heart transplantation or death.

Recent studies have suggested that immunoadsorption designed to remove circulating autoantibody produces clinical benefit [85]. In these experiments, patients with idiopathic dilated cardiomyopathy were treated by extracorporeal adsorption of immunoglobulin with anti-IgG columns. In a preliminary study, antibody titers in patients who benefited from the treatment remained low for long periods of time. In contrast, patients whose cardiac function deteriorated had rising antibody titers [85, 86]. Immunoadsorbent columns coated with protein A rather than anti-IgG failed to remove IgG3 subclass antibody and had little therapeutic value, suggesting that autoantibodies in this subclass are pathogenic [87]. Although these investigations show that depletion of immunoglobulin improves cardiac function, it cannot be with certainty stated which antibody has been removed by the treatment. Therefore, further studies examining the therapeutical value of antibody-specific plasmapheresis and affinity absorption are clearly needed.

Based on findings from animal models of viral or autoimmune myocarditis, it was tempting to speculate that strategies either specifically targeting proinflammatory cytokines or specifically enhancing the anti-viral immune response might affect the outcome of patients with myocarditis or postinflammatory dilated cardiomyopathy [88]. In this context, a prospective single center phase II study recently found that Interferon-beta treatment of patients with dilated cardiomyopathy and myocardial enteroviral or adenoviral persistence resulted in elimination of viral genomes in all patients and improvement of cardiac function in more than 60% of the study population, mainly if suffering from a moderately decreased left ventricular function, after 24 weeks of treatment [89, 90]. Patients with advanced heart failure show increased serum levels of the proinflammatory cytokine TNF-alpha. TNF-alpha is crucial for the development of autoimmune myocarditis in animal models [91]. Given the clinical availability of potent TNF-alpha

antagonists it has been expected that these drugs might offer a promising therapeutical option for patients with myocarditis or dilated cardiomyopathy. Unfortunately, two large-scale, randomized clinical trials evaluating the TNF-alpha-antagonists etanercept and infliximab for the treatment of dilated cardiomyopathy had to be stopped early because of excessive mortality in the treatment arms [92]. Therefore, the effect of TNF-alpha antagonists has never been assessed in patients with biopsy-proven myocarditis. Nevertheless, TNF-alpha antagonists cannot be recommended for the treatment of patients with myocarditis and are clearly contraindicated for patients with dilated cardiomyopathy. However, these negative findings do not exclude the possibility that strategies blocking other proinflammatory cytokines, such as interleukin 1β, IL-17, or IL-23 [95–97] might become of interest in the future. In fact, experimental data on the mouse model of autoimmune myocarditis recently suggested that heart-specific autoimmunity is mediated by a distinct population of autoreactive T-cells characterized by IL-17 production [97]. Another recent study reported beneficial effects of Peroxisome proliferator-activated receptor-gamma (PPAR-gamma) activator treatment in rats with experimental autoimmune myocarditis. The cardioprotective effect was associated with NF-kappa B blockade and thereby inhibition of inflammatory cytokine expressions [98].

Taken together, recent clinical and experimental data suggest that immunosuppression might become a reasonable option for defined subgroups of patients with myocarditis or dilated cardiomyopathy. These subgroups enclose the patients in which autoimmune mechanisms are supposed to play an important role in disease progression. Because the selection of potential treatment responders requires invasive diagnostic approaches, elaborated immunological and microbiological analysis and thorough clinical evaluation, we recommend a multidisciplinary workup [99]. Whenever possible, patients should be enrolled in ongoing treatment trials.

Conclusion

The precise etiology of human myocarditis remains obscure, but circumstantial evidence indicates that infections act as an initiating cause in many cases.

Clinical studies and experimental models suggest that autoimmune mechanisms play an important role in the development of chronic myocarditis and dilated cardiomyopathy in genetically susceptible individuals [100]. In fact, autoimmunity represents a final common pathogenetic pathway of multiple infections and even noninfectious etiologies. Understanding the detailed mechanisms of heart-specific autoimmunity will be critical for the development of refined, novel, and innovative treatment strategies in the future.

References

1 Feldman AM, McNamara D. Myocarditis. N Engl J Med 2000;343:1388–98.

2 Kawai C. From myocarditis to cardiomyopathy: mechanisms of inflammation and cell death: learning from the past for the future. Circulation 1999;99:1091–100.

3 Figulla HR. Transformation of myocarditis and inflammatory cardiomyopathy to idiopathic dilated cardiomyopathy: facts and fiction. Med Microbiol Immunol 2003;42:219–25.

4 Aretz HT. Myocarditis: the Dallas criteria. Hum Pathol 1987;18:619–24.

5 Aretz HT, Billingham ME, Edwards WD et al. Myocarditis, a histopathologic definition and classification. Am J Cardiovasc Pathol 1987;1:3–14.

6 Drory Y, Turetz Y, Hiss Y et al. Sudden unexpected death in persons less than 40 years of age. Am J Cardiol 1991;68:1388–92.

7 Wesslen L, Pahlson C, Lindquist O et al. An increase in sudden unexpected cardiac deaths among young Swedish orienteers during 1979–1992. Eur Heart J 1996; 17:902–10.

8 Strauer BE, Kandolf R, Mall G et al. Myocarditis-cardiomyopathy. Consensus Report of the German Association for Internal Medicine, presented at the 100th annual meeting, Wiesbaden, April 13, 1994. Acta Cardiol 1996;51:347–71.

9 McCarthy RE, 3rd, Boehmer JP, Hruban RH et al. Long-term outcome of fulminant myocarditis as compared with acute (nonfulminant) myocarditis. N Engl J Med 2000;342:690–5.

10 Liu P, Martino T, Opavsky MA, Penninger J. Viral myocarditis: balance between viral infection and immune response. Can J Cardiol 1996;12:935–43.

11 Fairweather D, Kaya Z, Shellam GR, Lawson CM, Rose NR. From infection to autoimmunity. J Autoimmun 2001;16:175–86.

12 Caforio AL, Stewart JT, Bonifacio E et al. Inappropriate major histocompatibility expression on cardiac tissue in dilated cardiomyopathy. Relevance for autoimmunity? J Autoimmun 1990;3:187–200.

13 Caforio AL. Role of autoimmunity in dilated cardiomyopathy. Br Heart J 1994;72(suppl):S30–4.

14 Neumann DA, Burek CL, Baughman KL, Rose NR, Herskowitz A. Circulating heart-reactive antibodies in patients with myocarditis or cardiomyopathy. J Am Coll Cardiol 1990;16:839–46.

15 Liu P, Mason J. Advances in the understanding of myocarditis. Circulation 2001;104:1076–82.

16 Eriksson U, Penninger JM. Autoimmune heart failure: new understandings of pathogenesis. Int J Biochem Cell Biol 2005;37:27–32.

17 Rose NR. The significance of autoimmunity in myocarditis. Ernst Schering Res Found Workshop 2006;55: 141–54.

18 Schofield CJ, Dias JC. The Southern Cone Initiative against Chagas disease. Adv Parasitol 1999;42:1–27.

19 Pauschinger M, Doerner A, Kuehl U et al. Enteroviral RNA replication in the myocardium of patients with left ventricular dysfunction and clinically suspected myocarditis. Circulation 1999;99:889–95.

20 Jin O, Sole MJ, Butany JW et al. Detection of enterovirus RNA in myocardial biopsies from patients with myocarditis and cardiomyopathy using gene amplification by polymerase chain reaction. Circulation 1990;82:8–16.

21 Koelsch S, Pankuweit S, Hufnagel G, Maisch B, for the ESETCID Investigators. The European Study of Epidemiology and Treatment of cardiac inflammatory diseases (ESETCID)—epidemiological results after 6 years. Annual Meeting of the AHA, New Orleans, November 2004.

22 Cohen JI, Corey GR. Cytomegalovirus infection in the normal host. Medicine (Baltimore) 1985;64:100–14.

23 Pankuweit S, Moll R, Baandrup U, Portig I, Hufnagel G, Maisch B. Prevalence of the parvovirus B 19 genome in endomyocardial biopsy specimens. Hum Pathol 2003;34:497–503.

24 Matsumori A, Yutani C, Ikeda Y, Kawai S, Sasayama S. Hepatitis C virus from the hearts of patients with myocarditis and cardiomyopathy. Lab Invest 2000;80:1137–42.

25 Lipshultz SE, Easley KA, Orav EJ et al. Left ventricular structure and function in children infected with human immunodeficiency virus: the prospective P2C2 HIV Multicenter study. Circulation 1998;97:1246–56.

26 Frustaci A, Chimenti C, Calabrese F, Pieroni M, Thiene G, Maseri A. Immunosuppressive therapy for active lymphocytic myocarditis: virological and immunologic profile of responders versus nonresponders. Circulation 2003;107:857–63.

27 Cooper LT, Jr, Berry GJ, Shabetai R, for Multicenter Giant Cell Myocarditis Study Group Investigators. Idiopathic

giant-cell myocarditis-natural history and treatment. N Engl J Med 1997;336:1860–6.

28 Badorff C, Lee GH, Lamphear BJ *et al*. Enteroviral protease 2A cleaves dystrophin: evidence of cytoskeletal disruption in an acquired cardiomyopathy. Nat Med 1999;5:320–6.

29 Lodge PA, Herzum M, Olszewski J, Huber SA. Coxsackievirus B-3 myocarditis. Acute and chronic forms of the disease caused by different immunopathogenic mechanisms. Am J Pathol 1987;128:455–63.

30 Caforio AL, Bonifacio E, Stewart JT *et al*. Novel organ-specific circulating cardiac autoantibodies in dilated cardiomyopathy. J Am Coll Cardiol 1990;15:1527–34.

31 Caforio AL, Mahon NJ, Tona F, McKenna WJ. Circulating cardiac autoantibodies in dilated cardiomyopathy and myocarditis: pathogenic and clinical significance. Eur J Heart Fail 2002;4:411–7.

32 Lauer B, Schannwell M, Kuhl U, Strauer BE, Schultheiss HP. Antimyosin autoantibodies are associated with deterioration of systolic and diastolic left ventricular function in patients with chronic myocarditis. J Am Coll Cardiol 2000;35:11–8.

33 Neu N, Rose NR, Beisel KW, Herskowitz A, Gurri-Glass G, Craig SW. Cardiac myosin induces myocarditis in genetically predisposed mice. J Immunol 1987;139:3630–6.

34 Kishimoto C, Hiraoka Y, Takamatsu N, Takada H, Kamiya H, Ochiai, H. An in vivo model of autoimmune post-coxsackievirus B3 myocarditis in severe combined immunodeficiency mouse. Cardiovasc Res 2003;60:397–403.

35 Pummerer CL, Luze K, Grassl G *et al*. Identification of cardiac myosin peptides capable of inducing autoimmune myocarditis in BALB/c mice. J Clin Invest 1996; 97:2057–62.

36 Afanasyeva M, Georgakopoulos D, Belardi DF *et al*. Quantitative analysis of myocardial inflammation by flow cytometry in murine autoimmune myocarditis: correlation with cardiac function. Am J Pathol 2004; 164:807–15.

37 Smith SC, Allen PM. Myosin-induced acute myocarditis is a T-cell mediated disease. J Immunol 1991;147:2141–7.

38 Smith SC, Allen PM. The role of T cells in myosin-induced autoimmune myocarditis. Clin Immunol Immunopathol 1993;68:100–6.

39 Kodama M, Matsumoto Y, Fujiwara M, Masani F, Izumi T, Shibata A. A novel experimental model of giant cell myocarditis induced in rats by immunization with cardiac myosin fraction. Clin Immunol Immunopathol 1990;57:250–62.

40 Inomata T, Hanawa H, Miyanishi T *et al*. Localisation of porcine cardiac myosin epitopes that induce experimental autoimmune myocarditis. Circ Res 1995;76:726–33.

41 Eriksson U, Ricci R, Hunziker L *et al*. Dendritic cell-induced autoimmune heart failure requires cooperation between adaptive and innate immunity. Nat Med 2003;9:1484–90.

42 Eriksson U, Kurrer MO, Schmitz N *et al*. IL-6 deficient mice resist development of autoimmune myocarditis associated with impaired up-regulation of Complement C3. Circulation 2003;107:320–5.

43 Malkiel S, Factor S, Diamond B. Autoimmune myocarditis does not require B cells for antigen presentation. J Immunol 1999;163:5265–8.

44 Liao L, Sindhwani R, Rojkind M, Factor S, Leinwand L, Diamond B. Antibody-mediated autoimmune myocarditis depends on genetically determined target organ sensitivity. J Exp Med 1995;181:1123–31.

45 Kuan AP, Zucker L, Liao L, Factor SM, Diamond B. Immunoglobulin isotype determines pathogenicity in antibody-mediated myocarditis in naive mice. Circ Res 2000;86:281–5.

46 Rose NR. Infections, mimics, and autoimmune disease. J Clin Invest 2001;107:943–4.

47 Cunningham MW. T cell mimicry in inflammatory heart disease. Mol Immunol 2004;40:1121–7.

48 Fae KC, da Silva DD, Oshiro SE *et al*. Mimicry in recognition of cardiac myosin peptides by heart-intralesional T cell clones from rheumatic heart disease. J Immunol 2006;176:5662–70.

49 Ellis NM, Li Y, Hildebrand W, Fischetti VA, Cunningham MW. T cell mimicry and epitope specificity of cross-reactive T cell clones from rheumatic heart disease. J Immunol 2005;175:5448–56.

50 Bachmaier K, Neu N, de la Maza LM, Pal S, Hessel A, Penninger JM. Chlamydia infections and heart disease linked through antigenic mimicry. Science 1999;283:1335–9.

51 Beisel KW, Srinivasappa J, Prabhakar BS. Identification of a putative shared epitope between Coxsackie virus B4 and α cardiac myosin heavy chain. Clin Exp Immunol 1991;86:49–55.

52 Akira S, Hemmi H. Recognition of pathogen-associated molecular patterns by TLR family. Immun Lett 2003; 85:85–95.

53 Tsan MF, Gao B. Endogenous ligands of toll-like receptors. J Leukoc Biol 2004;76:514–9.

54 Millar DG, Garza KM, Odermatt B *et al*. Hsp70 promotes antigen-presenting cell function and converts T-cell tolerance to autoimmunity in vivo. Nat Med 2003;9:1469–76.

55 Schett G, Metzler B, Kleindienst R *et al*. Myocardial injury leads to a release of heat shock protein (hsp) 60 and a suppression of the anti-hsp65 immune response. Cardiovasc Res 1999;42:685–95.

56 Foti M, Granucci F, Ricciardi-Castagnoli P. A central role for tissue-resident dendritic cells in innate responses. Trends Immunol 2004;25:650–4.

57 Marty RR, Dirnhofer S, Mauermann N et al. MyD88 signaling controls autoimmune myocarditis induction. Circulation 2006;113:258–65.

58 Maisel A, Cesario D, Baird S, Rehman J, Haghighi P, Carter S. Experimental autoimmune myocarditis produced by adoptive transfer of splenocytes after myocardial infarction. Circ Res 1998;82:458–63.

59 Moraru M, Roth A, Keren G, George J. Cellular autoimmunity to cardiac myosin in patients with a recent myocardial infarction. Int J Cardiol 2006;107:61–6.

60 Dybdahl B, Slordahl SA, Waage A, Kierulf P, Espevik T, Sundan A. Myocardial ischaemia and the inflammatory response: release of heat shock protein 70 after myocardial infarction. Heart 2005;9:299–304.

61 Caforio AL, McKenna WJ. Recognition and optimum management of myocarditis. Drugs 1996;52:515–25.

62 Caforio AL, Bonifacio E, Stewart JT et al. Novel organ-specific circulating cardiac autoantibodies in dilated cardiomyopathy. J Am Coll Cardiol 1990;15:1527–34.

63 Konstanoulakis MM, Kroumbouzou H, Tsiamis E, Trikas A, Toutouzas P. Clinical significance of antibodies against tropomyosin, actin, and myosin in patients with dilated cardiomyopathy. J Clin Lab Immunol 1993;40:61–7.

64 Mobini R, Maschke K, Waagstein F. New insights into the pathogenesis of dilated cardiomyopathy: possible underlying autoimmune mechanisms and therapy. Autoimmun Rev 2004;3:277–84.

65 Lauer B, Padberg K, Schultheiss HP, Strauer BE. Autoantibodies against human ventricular myosin in sera of patients with acute and chronic myocarditis. J Am Coll Cardiol 1994;23:146–53.

66 Caforio ALP, Keeling PJ, Zachara E et al. Evidence from family studies for autoimmunity in dilated cardiomyopathy. Lancet 1994;344:773–7.

67 Mahon NG, Madden BP, Caforio ALP et al. Immuno-histologic evidence of myocardial disease in apparently healthy relatives of patients with dilated cardiomyopathy. J Am Coll Cardiol 2002;39:455–62.

68 Limas CJ, Goldenberg IF, Limas C. Influence of anti-beta receptor antibodies on cardiac adenylate cyclase in patients with idiopathic dilated cardiomyopathy. Am Heart J 1990;119:1322–8.

69 Limas CJ, Limas C. Beta-adrenoreceptor antibodies and genetics in dilated cardiomyopathy, an overview and review. Eur Heart J 1999;12:175–7.

70 Schulze K, Becker BF, Schauer R, Schultheiss P. Antibodies to ADP-ATP carrier—an autoantigen in myocarditis and dilated cardiomyopathy-impair cardiac function. Circulation 1990;81:959–69.

71 Ansari AA, Neckelmann N, Villinger F et al. Epitope mapping of the branched chain alpha-ketoacid dehydrogenase dihydrolipoyl transacylase (BCKD-E2) protein that reacts with sera from patients with idiopathic dilated cardiomyopathy. J Immunol 1994;153:4754–65.

72 Mahrholdt H, Goedecke C, Wagner A et al. Cardiovascular magnetic resonance assessment of human myocarditis: a comparison to histology and molecular pathology. Circulation 2004;109:1250–8.

73 De Cobelli F, Pieroni M, Esposito A et al. Delayed gadolinium-enhanced cardiac magnetic resonance in patients with chronic myocarditis presenting with heart failure or recurrent arrhythmias. J Am Coll Cardiol 2006;47:1649–54.

74 Chimenti C, Russo A, Pieroni M et al. Intramyocyte detection of Epstein-Barr virus genome by laser capture microdissection in patients with inflammatory cardiomyopathy. Circulation 2004;110:3534–9.

75 Louis A, Cleland JG, Crabbe S et al. Clinical Trials Update: CAPRICORN, COPERNICUS, MIRACLE, STAF, RITZ-2, RECOVER and RENAISSANCE and cachexia and cholesterol in heart failure. Highlights of the Scientific Sessions of the American College of Cardiology, 2001. Eur J Hear Fail 2001;3:381–7.

76 Yuan Z, Shioji K, Kihara Y, Takenaka H, Onozawa Y, Kishimoto C. Cardioprotective effects of carvedilol on acute autoimmmune myocarditis: antiinflammatory effects associated with antioxidant property. Am J Physiol Heart Circ Physiol 2004;286:H83–90.

77 Matsui S, Zong ZP, Han JF, Katsuda S, Yamaguchi N, Fu ML. Amiodarone minimizes experimental autoimmune myocarditis in rats. Eur J Pharmacol 2003;469:165–73.

78 Godsel LM, Leon JS, Wang K, Fornek JL, Molteni A, Engman DM. Captopril prevents experimental autoimmune myocarditis. J Immunol 2003;171:346–52.

79 Godsel LM, Leon JS, Engman DM. Angiotensin converting enzyme inhibitors and angiotensin II: receptor antagonists in experimental myocarditis. Curr Pharm Des 2003;9:723–35.

80 Node K, Fujita M, Kitakaze M, Hori M, Liao JK. Short-term statin therapy improves cardiac function and symptoms in patients with idiopathic dilated cardiomyopathy. Circulation 2003;108:839–43.

81 Parrillo JE, Cunnion RE, Epstein SE et al. A prospective, randomized, controlled trial of prednisone for dilated cardiomyopathy. N Engl J Med 1989;321:1061–8.

82 Mason JW, O'Connell JB, Herskowitz A et al., for The Myocarditis Treatment Trial Investigators. A clinical trial of immunosuppressive therapy for myocarditis. N Engl J Med 1995;333:269–75.

83 Frustaci A, Cuoco L, Chimenti C et al. Celiac disease associated with autoimmune myocarditis. Circulation 2002;105:2611–8.

84 Wojnicz R, Nowalany-Kozielska E, Wojciechowska C et al. Randomized, placebo-controlled study for immunosuppressive treatment of inflammatory dilated cardiomyopathy: two-year follow-up results. Circulation 2001;104:39–45.

85 Dorffel WV, Wallukat G, Dorffel Y, Felix SB, Baumann G. Immunoadsorption in idiopathic dilated cardiomyopathy, a three year follow-up. Int J Cardiol 2004;97:529–34.

86 Felix SB, Staudt A, Friedrich GB. Improvement of cardiac function after immunoadsorption in patients with dilated cardiomyopathy. Autoimmunity 2001;34:211–5.

87 Staudt A, Böhm M, Knebel F et al. Potential role of autoantibodies belonging to the immunoglobulin G3 subclass in cardiac dysfunction among patients with dilated cardiomyopathy. Circulation 2002;106:2448–53.

88 Kurrer MO, Kopf M, Penninger JM, Eriksson U. Cytokines that regulate autoimmune myocarditis. Swiss Med Wkly 2002;132:408–13.

89 Kühl U, Pauschinger M, Schwimmbeck PL et al. Interferon-beta treatment eliminates cardiotropic viruses and improves left ventricular function in patients with myocardial persistence of viral genomes and left ventricular dysfunction. Circulation 2003;107:2793–8.

90 Lenzo JC, Mansfield JP, Sivamoorthy S, Cull VS, James CM. Cytokine expression in murine cytomegalovirus-induced myocarditis: modulation with interferon-alpha therapy. Cell Immunol 2003;223:77–86.

91 Bachmaier K, Pummerer C, Kozieradzki I et al. Low-molecular-weigh tumor necrosis factor receptor p55 controls induction of autoimmune heart disease. Circulation 1997;95:655–61.

92 Kwon HJ, Cote TR, Cuffe MS, Kramer JM, Braun MM. Case reports of heart failure after therapy with a tumor necrosis factor antagonist. Ann Intern Med 2003;138:807–11.

93 Muller-Ehmsen J, Schwinger RH. TNF and congestive heart failure: therapeutic possibilities. Expert Opin Ther Targets 2004;8:203–9.

94 Anker SD, Coats AJ. How to RECOVER FROM RENAISSANCE? The significance of the results of RECOVER, RENAISSANCE, RENEWAL and ATTACH. Int J Cardiol 2002;86:123–30.

95 Eriksson U, Kurrer MO, Sonderegger I et al. Activation of dendritic cells through the interleukin 1 receptor 1 is critical for the induction of autoimmune myocarditis. J Exp Med 2003;197:323–31.

96 Afanasyeva M, Georgakopoulos D, Rose NR. Autoimmune myocarditis: cellular mediators of cardiac dysfunction. Autoimmun Rev 2004;3:476–86.

97 Rangachari M, Mauermann N, Marty RR et al. T-bet is a negative regulator of autoimmune heart disease. J Exp Med 2006;203:2009–19.

98 Yuan Z, Liu Y, Zhang J et al. Cardioprotective effects of PPAR-gamma activators in autoimmune myocarditis: anti-inflammatory actions associated with NF-kappa B blockade. Heart 2005;91:1203–8.

99 Burian J, Buser P, Eriksson U. Myocarditis: the immunologist's view on pathogenesis and treatment. Swiss Med Wkly 2005;135:359–64.

100 Marty RR, Eriksson U. Dendritic cell-induced autoimmune heart failure. Int J Cardiol 2006;112:34–39.

CHAPTER 4

Immune basis of hypertension in humans

Katherine Horak & Douglas F. Larson

Introduction

Primary hypertension affects 50% of the individuals older than 60 years; however, the etiology is understood for only 10% of these cases. The incidence of primary hypertension increases with age, with 50% of individuals at the age of 60 and 60–70% of individuals over the age of 70 suffering from high blood pressure [1]. Currently the factors contributing to hypertension are considered to be alterations in renal function, including perturbations in the renin–angiotensin system and sodium balance, increased sympathetic tone, and vascular dysfunction. However, there is compelling evidence that altered immune function is involved in the pathogenesis of most forms of hypertension. Therefore, we contend that there is a direct involvement of the adaptive immune system (T lymphocytes) in the evolution of primary hypertension. This review will support the association between adaptive immune system and the development of hypertension in humans.

Primary hypertension related to cytokines

Essential hypertension or primary hypertension, as it has recently been termed, has historically been defined as an increase in blood pressure with no known etiology, although it is often accompanied by immune activation. Moreover, aging is associated with a dysregulation of the immune response [2]. Since aging is a major risk factor for the development of hypertension, it follows, therefore, that if immune system plays a role in the etiology of hypertension, aging may increase the incidence of hypertension.

Barbieri *et al.* investigated the correlation between pro-inflammatory cytokines and essential hypertension in 537 human subjects with a mean age of 74 years [3]. In this study, systolic blood pressure was associated with age and plasma IL-6 concentration. Diastolic blood pressure was found to be associated with plasma IL-6 and IL-1 receptor antagonist (IL-1ra) concentrations and negatively associated with IL-1β [3]. This study supports that immune activation is positively correlated with the incidence of essential hypertension. Another study assessed the concentrations of IL-1β, IL-6, TNF-α, and IL-1ra in patients with essential hypertension. IL-1ra was significantly greater in patients with essential hypertension compared with normotensive controls. These studies do not provide direct evidence that these pro-inflammatory cytokines induce the essential hypertension or are merely a product of the strain on vessels due to the increased blood pressure.

Hypertension associated with immunoglobulins

In addition to alterations in inflammatory cytokines, individuals with essential hypertension have increased activity of T lymphocytes reactive against human arterial antigen [4]. Also, essential hypertension is associated with increased serum levels of IgG and IgM. No changes were reported in the levels of IgA or the number of circulating T lymphocytes in patients with essential hypertension when compared to normotensive controls [4]. Suryaprabha *et al.* also reported a significant increase of IgG in essential hypertension patients compared to controls. In this study there was no gender difference in IgG concentration with essential hypertension [5].

In light of the above-mentioned studies, the involvement of the humoral immune system in the pathogenesis of essential hypertension has yet to be fully understood. The reported increase in serum antibody concentrations could be secondary to damage of the vascular endothelium caused by an increase in blood pressure. However, increased activity of T lymphocytes reactive against arterial antigen suggests that T lymphocytes may be involved in the pathophysiology of essential hypertension and the associated vascular damage.

Immunosuppression and hypertension

Hypertension is a major complication of organ transplantation, affecting 63% of pediatric heart transplant recipients and 90% of cardiac transplant recipients overall [6, 7]. Posttransplant hypertension is often attributed to the use of immunosuppressive therapeutics. Moreover, hypertension has been reported to occur in 70–90% of renal transplant recipients and 33% of liver transplant recipients treated with either cyclosporine (CsA) or tacrolimus (FK506) [8, 9]. CsA and, more recently, tacrolimus have become primary immunosuppressants for organ transplant recipients. CsA and tacrolimus have similar mechanisms of action converging at the inhibition of the phosphotase calcineurin, and thereby both drugs inhibit T-lymphocyte activation and IL-2 gene expression [10]. The drugs differ in their effect on the TH2 cytokine expression [11]. CsA was shown to decrease IL-6 while increasing IL-4. Moreover, tacrolimus inhibits IL-10 production to a greater extent than CsA [12]. Also, CsA has been shown to induce dysfunction of the vascular endothelium [13] and pronounced hypertension; however, tacrolimus-induced hypertension has been shown to be less severe than that resulting from CsA [14]. Although immunosuppression-induced hypertension is almost ubiquitous in transplant recipients, its etiology still remains unclear.

Recent evidence has suggested that CsA-induced hypertension and endothelial dysfunction is a result of decreased levels of nitric oxide (NO) [15]. The administration of L-arginine, the amino acid substrate used in the synthesis of NO, was shown to decrease blood pressure in CsA-induced hypertensive rats and primates [16]. L-arginine also attenuated the increase in blood pressure in pediatric cardiac transplant recipients [17]. Additionally, CsA induced a decrease in acetylcholine-mediated relaxation in resistance vessels of rats [18]. Impaired NO production and decreased vasorelaxation—both of which induce hypertension—are possible mechanisms of CsA-induced endothelial dysfunction.

Immunosuppression and induction of autoimmunity

Related to its immunosuppressive properties, CsA increases the number of autoreactive T lymphocytes by interfering with their deletion [19, 20]. Administration of CsA to newborn mice caused organ-specific autoimmune diseases, while thymectomy immediately following CsA administration increased the prevalence of autoimmune diseases. From these findings, it was concluded that CsA induces autoimmune conditions by interfering with the thymus/T-lymphocyte-dependent control of autoreactive T lymphocytes [21]. The autoreactive T lymphocytes may affect the vascular endothelium, causing the reported vascular dysfunction and increase in blood pressure. Furthermore, cytokines released from immune cells are also involved in the regulation of blood pressure and fibrosis. TGF-β is a known potent fibrogenic mediator and has been reported to induce fibrosis in the kidney, liver, and lung [22]. CsA, but not tacrolimus, has been shown to induce TGF-β [23]. The difference in the induction of TGF-β may account for the variation in the severity of the hypertension induced by CsA and tacrolimus. Therefore, an alternative mechanism of CsA- and tacrolimus-induced hypertension resides in the effect of altered lymphocyte cytokine production, such as TGF-β, on the adventitial fibroblasts. This concept suggests that vascular dysfunction may occur due to an increased collagen deposition in the vasculature, which not only impairs NO function and diffusion but also alters vascular mechanics.

Moreover, CsA administration has been shown to decrease the number of T regulatory cells [24]. T regulatory cells are responsible for the suppression of T-lymphocyte function, preferentially autoreactive T lymphocytes. In addition to CD4, T regulatory cells express CD25 (IL-2 receptor, α chain) on their cell surface. Therefore, it is logical that because CsA affects IL-2 gene expression, it also has an effect on the production of T regulatory cells. Our laboratory is investigating the role of specifically CD4$^+$ lymphocytes on cardiac and vascular remodeling. These studies will help elucidate the possible role of T regulatory cells in hypertension.

Preeclampsia, hypertension, and the immune response

Preeclampsia is a common complication during pregnancy, affecting up to 5% of pregnant women [25]. This condition is defined by elevated blood pressure and excess protein in the urine after 20 weeks of pregnancy. There is no known specific treatment, although traditional measures such as antihypertensive drugs, magnesium, steroids, and early delivery improve outcomes. This lack of definite treatment is a result of the unknown etiology of the condition. Endothelial cell dysfunction is often present in preeclampsia and therefore is considered a contributing factor in the pathology [26]. Since medical interventions aimed at the treatment of preeclampsia and the underlying endothelial cell dysfunction have not been completely successful, it is likely that preeclampsia is multifactorial in origin. Since the report by Wegman *et al.* that TH2 cytokines are essential for successful pregnancy [27], it has been hypothesized that alterations in the maternal immune balance contribute to the development of preeclampsia.

It has been shown that during normal pregnancy the production of TH2 cytokines is increased with a concomitant decrease in TH1 cytokines [28]. In other studies the numbers of both INF-γ- and IL-4-producing cells have been shown to increase [29]. Saito *et al.* address this contradiction by using flow cytometry to quantify INF-γ (TH1)- and IL-4 (TH2)-producing cells in blood from women with normal pregnancies and those with preeclampsia. In this study, normal pregnant women had a decrease in the number of TH1 cells in the third trimester and an increase in the number of TH2 cell in the first trimester. In the peripheral blood from women with preeclampsia, TH1 cells were increased and TH2 cells decreased throughout the pregnancy,

giving rise to a larger TH1/TH2 ratio than that in women with normal pregnancies [30].

Other immune responses and cytokines in addition to IFN-γ and IL-4 have been investigated as possible mediators of preeclampsia. Systemic activation of the innate immune system occurs in both normal pregnancy and pregnancies with preeclampsia, perhaps as a compensatory mechanism for the other immune changes [31]. However, the degree of activation is exaggerated in preeclampsia, producing an inflammatory response [32]. The cytokine IL-10 has both immunosuppressive and anti-inflammatory effects. IL-10 inhibits proliferation and cytokine synthesis of TH1 lymphocytes [33], which, under the current paradigm, is beneficial to the maintenance of pregnancy [34]. To elucidate the correlation between preeclampsia, IL-10, and other cytokines, Jonsson *et al.* analyzed blood samples from women with preeclampsia and those with normal pregnancy. They reported a decreased secretion of TH2 cytokines, IL-5, and IL-10 from cells in the blood of women with preeclampsia when compared with normal controls [25]. The reduction in IL-10 levels is indicative of decreased immunosuppression and correlated with previous reports of increased inflammation derived from TH1 cells. The reported decrease of IL-5 is supportive of the decreased number of basophils in women with preeclampsia as IL-5 regulates basophil differentiation [35]. The TH1/TH2 balance reported in this study is in agreement with previous reports of TH1 predominance in preeclampsia [36]; however, the characterization of IL-5, IL-10, and other cytokines increases the validity of the proposed involvement of the immune system in preeclampsia.

Numerous factors have been reported to be involved in the pathogenesis of preeclampsia, although many reports now support the participation of immune cells in the perturbation of normal pregnancy seen in preeclampsia. As mentioned earlier, preeclampsia is often accompanied by endothelial cell dysfunction. Inflammatory cytokines—those secreted from TH1 cells—react with the vascular endothelium, causing the endothelial dysfunction. TH1 cell numbers increase in preeclampsia and therefore these cells represent possible mediators of reported endothelial cell dysfunction. A decrease in TH2 cytokines is also associated with preeclampsia.

This is a deviation from normal pregnancy when the mother's lymphocytes are predominantly TH2 subset.

Conclusion

The current understanding of the mechanisms involved in the development of hypertension is partially a result of studies on human cases of hypertension. Primary hypertension, immunosuppressive-induced hypertension, and preeclampsia are all associated with underlying changes in immune function (Table 4.1). Transplant recipients with CsA-induced hypertension have increased numbers of autoreactive T lymphocytes and pro-fibrotic cytokine secretion. It is possible that these lymphocytes interact with the vascular endothelium, causing injury and increased blood pressure. Individuals with essential hypertension have highly activated immune systems as supported by elevated concentrations of pro-inflammatory cytokines and high serum levels of antibodies. In addition, individuals with essential hypertension have increased levels of T lymphocytes reactive to arterial antigens, again possibly causing injury to the vasculature. Another type of hypertension, preeclampsia, is correlated with deviations from the immune profile of normal pregnant women. As in essential hypertension, women with preeclampsia exhibit an increased inflammatory response. They also have a shift from TH2 predominance, found in normal pregnancy, to TH1. Preeclampsia is associated with a decrease in the immunosuppressive cytokine IL-10. Since IL-10 is capable of decreasing the activity of lymphocytes

and specifically the TH1 subset, the decrease in IL-10 levels associated with preeclampsia further augments the inflammation and TH1 predominance reported in preeclampsia. All three of these examples of human hypertension are associated with either self-reactive T lymphocytes or inflammation, although neither of these are being addressed in current therapeutic regimes.

New therapeutics are being designed to modify the immune system in an array of autoimmune diseases. In future, these techniques may demonstrate efficacy in the treatment of many forms of hypertension. The use of hematopoietic stem cells in the treatment of lupus is in clinical trials by the National Institute of Allergy and Infectious Diseases. The working hypothesis is that since hematopoietic stem cells can develop into immune cells, they will normalize the immune system of people suffering from lupus, slowing or stopping the progression of the disease. Immune treatment of multiple sclerosis using interferon β-1β (INFβ-1 β) is also being investigated. The injection of INF β-1β was reported to decrease the development of multiple sclerosis by 50% in patients who had previously presented with early signs of multiple sclerosis [37]. Also, treatment of people suffering from Crohn's disease and ulcerative colitis with soluble TNF-α receptors (etanercept) has been shown to induce remission [38]. Therefore, the treatment of these chronic diseases with immunomodulatory agents makes the treatment of hypertension in this manner a viable option. As in other diseases, the immune component of hypertension is not fully understood, but the development of immunomodulatory

Table 4.1 Immune involvement in human hypertension.

	Pathology	Alterations in immune function	Reference number
Primary hypertension	50% adults $\geq$60 yr; endothelial damage	Increase IL-6, IL-1ra, decrease TNF-α levels	[3, 4]
		Autoreactive T lymphocytes	[5]
		Increase immunoglobulin levels	[5, 6]
Immunosuppression-induced hypertension	90% cardiac recipients; endothelial damage	Autoreactive T lymphocytes	[20–22]
		Increase TGF-β	[23, 24]
		Decreased T regulatory cells	[25]
Preeclampsia	5% pregnant women; endothelial cell damage	Increase TH1	[31, 37]
		Decrease TH2	[31, 36]
		Induction of inflammation	[26, 32, 33]

treatments may enable the physicians to modify the underlying causes of hypertension, not simply alleviate the symptoms.

Research in our laboratory and others will help elucidate the role of the immune system in hypertension and accompanying alterations in cardiovascular extracellular matrix. T-lymphocyte-derived cytokines are known to increase collagen synthesis, inducing fibrosis. The increase in blood pressure in essential hypertension may be a result of fibrotic processes, resulting in a less compliant vasculature. There appears to be an unsubstantiated relationship between age-associated hypertension and age-mediated immune dysfunction. Therefore, further definition of this connection in models of immunosuppression may reveal causal relationship. Modulation of specific immune components, such as T lymphocytes, will help determine the mechanisms through which they influence cardiovascular disease. An understanding of the interactions of the immune and cardiovascular systems will hopefully introduce new possible targets for the pharmaceutical treatment of hypertension and cardiovascular disease.

References

1 Staessen JA, Wang J, Bianchi G, Birkenhager WH. Essential hypertension. Lancet May 10, 2003;361(9369): 1629–41.

2 Bruunsgaard H, Pedersen M, Pedersen BK. Aging and proinflammatory cytokines. Curr Opin Hematol May 2001;8(3):131–6.

3 Barbieri M, Ferrucci L, Corsi AM *et al.* Is chronic inflammation a determinant of blood pressure in the elderly? Am J Hypertens July 2003;16(7):537–43.

4 Gudbrandsson T, Hansson L, Herlitz H, Lindholm L, Nilsson LA. Immunological changes in patients with previous malignant essential hypertension. Lancet February 21, 1981;1(8217):406–8.

5 Suryaprabha P, Padma T, Rao UB. Increased serum IgG levels in essential hypertension. Immunol Lett 1984; 8(3):143–5.

6 Lim DS, Gomez CA, Goldberg CS, Crowley DC, Rocchini AP, Charpie JR. Systemic arterial pressure and brachial arterial flow-mediated dilatation in young cardiac transplant recipients. Am J Cardiol November 1, 2002;90(9): 1035–7.

7 Ventura HO, Mehra MR, Stapleton DD, Smart FW. Cyclosporine-induced hypertension in cardiac transplantation. Med Clin North Am November 1997;81(6):1347–57.

8 Midtvedt K, Hartmann A. Hypertension after kidney transplantation: are treatment guidelines emerging? Nephrol Dial Transplant July 2002;17(7):1166–9.

9 Gonzalez-Pinto IM, Rimola A, Margarit C *et al.* Five-year follow-up of a trial comparing Tacrolimus and cyclosporine microemulsion in liver transplantation. Transplant Proc May 2005;37(4):1713–5.

10 Wiederrecht G, Lam E, Hung S, Martin M, Sigal N. The mechanism of action of FK-506 and cyclosporin A. Ann N Y Acad Sci November 30, 1993;696:9–19.

11 Plosker GL, Foster RH. Tacrolimus: a further update of its pharmacology and therapeutic use in the management of organ transplantation. Drugs February 2000;59(2):323–89.

12 Fujimura T, Yang XF, Soriano R, Ogawa T, Kobayashi M, Jiang H. Cellular surface molecular and cytokine gene expression in rat heart allografts under optimal doses of cyclosporine and FK 506. Transplant Proc June 1998;30(4): 1023–6.

13 Zoja C, Furci L, Ghilardi F, Zilio P, Benigni A, Remuzzi G. Cyclosporin-induced endothelial cell injury. Lab Invest October 1986;55(4):455–62.

14 Henry ML. Cyclosporine and tacrolimus (FK506): a comparison of efficacy and safety profiles. Clin Transplant June 1999;13(3):209–20.

15 Akita K, Dusting GJ, Hickey H. Suppression of nitric oxide production by cyclosporin A and FK506A in rat vascular smooth muscle cells. Clin Exp Pharmacol Physiol March 1994;21(3):231–3.

16 Bartholomeusz B, Hardy KJ, Nelson AS, Phillips PA. Modulation of nitric oxide improves cyclosporin A-induced hypertension in rats and primates. J Hum Hypertens December 1998;12(12):839–44.

17 Lim DS, Mooradian SJ, Goldberg CS *et al.* Effect of oral L-arginine on oxidant stress, endothelial dysfunction, and systemic arterial pressure in young cardiac transplant recipients. Am J Cardiol September 15, 2004;94(6): 828–31.

18 Roullet JB, Xue H, McCarron DA, Holcomb S, Bennett WM. Vascular mechanisms of cyclosporin-induced hypertension in the rat. J Clin Invest May 1994;93(5):2244–50.

19 Jenkins MK, Schwartz RH, Pardoll DM. Effects of cyclosporine A on T cell development and clonal deletion. Science September 23 1988;241(4873):1655–8.

20 Gao EK, Lo D, Cheney R, Kanagawa O, Sprent J. Abnormal differentiation of thymocytes in mice treated with cyclosporin A. Nature November 10, 1988;336(6195):176–9.

21 Sakaguchi N, Sakaguchi S. Causes and mechanism of autoimmune disease: cyclosporin A as a probe for

the investigation. J Invest Dermatol June 1992;98(6 Suppl):70S–6S.

22 Terrell TG, Working PK, Chow CP, Green JD. Pathology of recombinant human transforming growth factor-beta 1 in rats and rabbits. Int Rev Exp Pathol 1993;34 Pt B:43–67.

23 Mohamed MA, Robertson H, Booth TA, Balupuri S, Kirby JA, Talbot D. TGF-beta expression in renal transplant biopsies: a comparative study between cyclosporin-A and tacrolimus. Transplantation March 15, 2000;69(5): 1002–5.

24 Mantel PY, Ouaked N, Ruckert B *et al.* Molecular mechanisms underlying FOXP3 induction in human T cells. J Immunol March 15, 2006;176(6):3593–602.

25 Jonsson Y, Matthiesen L, Berg G, Ernerudh J, Nieminen K, Ekerfelt C. Indications of an altered immune balance in preeclampsia: a decrease in in vitro secretion of IL-5 and IL-10 from blood mononuclear cells and in blood basophil counts compared with normal pregnancy. J Reprod Immunol June 2005;66(1):69–84.

26 Roberts JM, Redman CW. Pre-eclampsia: more than pregnancy-induced hypertension. Lancet June 5, 1993; 341(8858):1447–51.

27 Wegmann TG, Lin H, Guilbert L, Mosmann TR. Bidirectional cytokine interactions in the maternal-fetal relationship: is successful pregnancy a TH2 phenomenon? Immunol Today July 1993;14(7):353–6.

28 Marzi M, Vigano A, Trabattoni D *et al.* Characterization of type 1 and type 2 cytokine production profile in physiologic and pathologic human pregnancy. Clin Exp Immunol October 1996;106(1):127–33.

29 Matthiesen L, Ekerfelt C, Berg G, Ernerudh J. Increased numbers of circulating interferon-gamma- and interleukin-4-secreting cells during normal pregnancy. Am J Reprod Immunol June 1998;39(6):362–7.

30 Saito S, Sakai M, Sasaki Y, Tanebe K, Tsuda H, Michimata T. Quantitative analysis of peripheral blood Th0, Th1, Th2 and the Th1:Th2 cell ratio during normal human pregnancy and preeclampsia. Clin Exp Immunol September 1999;117(3):550–5.

31 Sacks G, Sargent I, Redman C. An innate view of human pregnancy. Immunol Today March 1999;20(3):114–8.

32 Redman CW, Sacks GP, Sargent IL. Preeclampsia: an excessive maternal inflammatory response to pregnancy. Am J Obstet Gynecol February 1999;180(2 Pt 1):499–506.

33 Mills KH. Regulatory T cells: friend or foe in immunity to infection? Nat Rev Immunol November 2004;4(11): 841–55.

34 Hanna N, Hanna I, Hleb M *et al.* Gestational age-dependent expression of IL-10 and its receptor in human placental tissues and isolated cytotrophoblasts. J Immunol June 1, 2000;164(11):5721–8.

35 Borish LC, Steinke JW. 2: Cytokines and chemokines. J Allergy Clin Immunol February 2003;111(2 Suppl):S460–S475.

36 Wilczynski JR, Tchorzewski H, Glowacka E *et al.* Cytokine secretion by decidual lymphocytes in transient hypertension of pregnancy and pre-eclampsia. Mediators Inflamm April 2002;11(2):105–11.

37 PRISMS (Prevention of Relapses and Disability by Interferon beta-1a Subcutaneously in Multiple Sclerosis) Study Group. Randomised double-blind placebo-controlled study of interferon beta-1a in relapsing/remitting multiple sclerosis. Lancet November 7, 1998;352(9139):1498–504.

38 Schreiber S. Experimental immunomodulatory therapy of inflammatory bowel disease. Neth J Med December 1998;53(6):S24–31.

CHAPTER 5

Immune dysregulation: potential mediator of metabolic syndrome-induced cardiac remodeling

Sherma Zibadi, Douglas F. Larson & Ronald Ross Watson

Introduction

Metabolic syndrome (MetS) has emerged as a public health problem worldwide, with increasing prevalence rate in recent years. MetS is a cluster of several metabolic disorders related to a state of insulin resistance, which together lead to a significantly increased cardiovascular morbidity and mortality. The mechanisms underlying the increased cardiovascular risk may in part be due to the development of more pronounced left ventricular (LV) remodeling and cardiac dysfunction. Although the contribution of neurohormonal overactivity has been studied broadly, the role of adaptive immune system in the pathophysiology of myocardial remodeling and dysfunction associated with MetS has not been elucidated yet.

Definition and prevalence of MetS

The concept of the MetS (also known as syndrome X or insulin resistance syndrome) has been in existence since 1988. At least five organizations have recommended the clinical criteria for the diagnosis of MetS [1]. Although these criteria are similar in many aspects, there are some differences concerning the predominant etiology of MetS, definition of obesity, and cutpoint values of diagnostic criteria. According to the operational definition outlined by the National Cholesterol Education Program (NCEP) Adult Treatment Panel (ATP) III, MetS is defined

by the co-occurrence of any three of the five criteria (Table 5.1) [2].

The prevalence of MetS varies depending on the definition used and population studied. However, MetS is very common in adults in many parts of the world, typically being found from one in six to one in three adults (sometimes more), rising with age and being higher in men than women [3]. A recent population-based study in the United States, using NCEP-ATP III criteria, had found the age-adjusted prevalence of MetS to be 23.7%. The prevalence was shown to increase with age. However, no significant difference was observed between genders. Applying the age-specific prevalence rates to the US census counts from 2000 results in an estimate of approximately 47 million persons with MetS in the United States [4].

Pathophysiology of MetS

Insulin resistance is the central pathophysiologic feature of MetS, and once the hyperglycemia develops, it couples with the genetic predisposition and produces the other manifestation of the syndrome. Significant evidence supports a key role for insulin resistance in the development of the dyslipidemia associated with MetS. It has been shown that insulin resistance state is associated with increased adipose tissue lipolysis and hepatic de novo lipogenesis. Subsequent overproduction of very low density lipoproteins (VLDL) by hepatocytes results

Table 5.1 NCEP-ATP III clinical criteria for the diagnosis of the MetS [2].

Criteria	Defining level
Abdominal obesity (waist circumference)	>102 cm (40 in.) in men; >88 cm (35 in.) in women
TG	≥150 mg/dL (1.7 mM/L); or treated hypertriglyceridemia
HDL-C	<40 mg/dL (1.0 mM/L) in men; <50 mg/dL (1.3 mM/L) in women
BP	Systolic BP ≥130 mmHg or diastolic BP ≥85 mmHg; or documented use of antihypertensive medication
FPG	≥110 mg/dL (6.1 mM/L); or diagnosed type-2 diabetes

MetS, metabolic syndrome; TG, triglycerides; HDL-C, high-density lipoprotein cholesterol; BP, blood pressure; FPG, fasting plasma glucose.

in hypertriglyceridemia, which in turn leads to increased activity of plasma cholesteryl ester transfer protein (CETP). CETP mediates heteroexchange of cholesteryl ester from high-density lipoprotein (HDL) for triglyceride (TG) from apo B-100-containing lipoproteins such as VLDL, chylomicron (CM), and low-density lipoprotein (LDL). Subsequently, hepatic lipase (HL), also elevated in insulin-resistance state, hydrolyzes the TG-enriched HDL, shedding apo A-I and releasing HDL remnant particles, which can be degraded by liver and kidney. Further increase in catabolism rate of apo A-I and decrease in lipoprotein lipase (LPL) activity, which impair pre-β HDL formation and HDL particles maturation, result in reduced plasma HDL concentration. In a similar fashion, CETP-mediated exchange of LDL cholesteryl ester and VLDL or CM TG generates cholesteryl ester-depleted, TG-enriched LDL particles. Lipolysis of these LDL particles by LPL or HL generates small, dense LDL particles that bind to hepatic LDL receptor with low affinity and are cleared slowly, therefore increasing the level of small, dense LDL particle concentration [5, 6] (Figure 5.1).

Although a number of potential mechanisms have been proposed to explain the association between hypertension and insulin resistance, it is unclear whether insulin resistance or compensatory

hyperinsulinemia induce hypertension. Abnormalities in endothelium-dependent vasodilation have been suggested to provide a link between hypertension and insulin resistance. Impaired nitric oxide (NO)-mediated vasodilation, documented in patients and animal models of insulin resistance, may be induced by hypercholesterolemia and hyperglycemia, which are metabolic consequences of insulin resistance. One putative mechanism could be the hyperglycemia-induced overproduction of superoxide radicals by mitochondria, which results in degradation of bioactive NO into the deleterious compound peroxynitrite, favoring vasoconstriction [7]. High glucose concentration has also been shown to inhibit expression of endothelial NO synthase, the enzyme that catalyzes the conversion of arginine to NO [8]. Furthermore, LDL promotes the uncoupling of the endothelial nitric oxide synthase, a condition in which the endothelial nitric oxide synthase produces superoxide anions instead of generating NO [9]. In addition, patients with MetS hypertriglyceridemia and hyperinsulinemia have been shown to stimulate endothelin-1 release, an endothelium-derived vasoconstrictive peptide [10]. Overactivity of sympathetic nervous system may also play a role in the association between insulin resistance and elevated blood pressure [11]. Insulin-induced antinatriuresis may also contribute by increasing the sodium and water reabsorption by renal proximal tubules, and hence, promoting a volume-dependent hypertension [12].

Left ventricular remodeling and myocardial dysfunction

Individual components of MetS, including abdominal obesity, insulin resistance, hypertension, and dyslipidemia are known to increase cardiovascular morbidity and mortality. However, evidence continues to emerge in support of the additional cardiovascular risk in patients with MetS, exceeding that expected from its individual components [13]. This increased cardiovascular risk may be due to the development of more pronounced LV structural and geometric remodeling and subsequent impairment of myocardial function [14]. It is well known that arterial hypertension leads to structural remodeling of the myocardium, interstitial

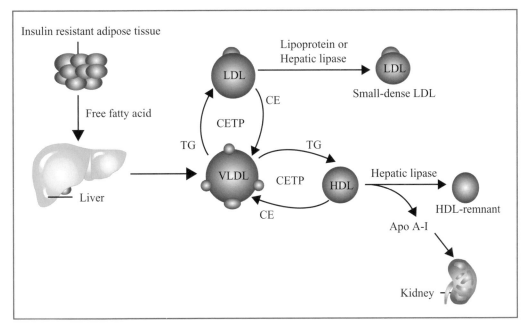

Figure 5.1 Role of insulin resistance in pathogenesis of dyslipidemia associated with MetS. Increased free fatty acid release from insulin resistant adipocytes results in increased hepatic assembly and secretion of VLDL. Subsequent hypertriglyceridemia increases the heteroexchange of CE from HDL and LDL for TG from VLDL by CETP. Enhanced activity of hepatic lipase in insulin resistance state results in dissociation of apo A-I from TG-enriched HDL, which is then filtered by kidneys, and hence decreases HDL level. TG-enriched LDL can undergo lipolysis and forms small, dense LDL. HDL, high-density lipoprotein; LDL, low-density lipoprotein; VLDL, very low density lipoprotein; CETP, cholesteryl ester transfer protein; CE, cholesteryl ester; TG, triglyceride.

fibrosis, and hypertrophy, resulting in diastolic dysfunction [15]. Furthermore, several studies have pointed out the role of insulin resistance, obesity, and atherosclerosis in the development of LV remodeling, as well as diastolic dysfunction [16–19].

Several clinical trials have investigated the effects of the MetS on LV geometry and function. In a cross-sectional study, investigating never-treated Italian hypertensive subjects, higher prevalence of LV concentric remodeling and hypertrophy with no significant LV systolic and diastolic dysfunction was detected in subjects with the MetS [20]. Several recent studies are in support of the association between MetS and diastolic dysfunction. The MetS has been shown to be associated with more pronounced alteration of LV geometry, preserved systolic function, and impaired diastolic function in nondiabetic subjects with MetS [14]. The result of a small-scale study also indicated that the MetS is associated with significant decrease in E/A ratio, an index of diastolic function, in men with well-controlled, un-complicated, type-2 diabetes [21]. Furthermore, evidence of coexistence of systolic and diastolic dysfunction has also been obtained. A cross-sectional study within the Strong Heart Study cohort, a study of cardiovascular disease in American Indians, was in agreement with previous studies in the higher prevalence of LV hypertrophy in the group with MetS. However, an impairment of systolic function and abnormal early diastolic LV relaxation were also observed in participants with MetS [22]. Likewise, a recent study has shown a significant reduction of both systolic and diastolic function even in the absence of LV hypertrophy [23].

T$_H$1/T$_H$2 imbalance: a potential mediator of LV remodeling in MetS

Essential role of maladaptive neurohormonal activation, in particular the renin–angiotensin–aldosterone and sympathetic nervous systems, and pathogenic molecular and cellular changes that accompany insulin resistance and coronary atherosclerosis have been studied extensively in cardiac remodeling. However, recently attention has turned to the $CD4^+$ T helper (T_H) lymphocytes and their potential role in LV extracellular matrix (ECM) remodeling, which contribute to the myocardial stiffness and diastolic and systolic dysfunction. The T_H phenotypes have been shown to affect cardiac ECM structure differently. Predominance of T_H1 immunity in mice leads to profibrotic activity, increased ventricular stiffness, and diastolic dysfunction, whereas T_H2 immune condition results in dilated cardiomyopathy coincided with decreased ventricular collagen content and stiffness and impaired both diastolic and systolic function [24]. Therefore, imbalance of the pro- versus anti-inflammatory and T_H1 versus T_H2 cytokine may play an important role in the development of maladaptive myocardial ECM remodeling.

Recent evidence indicates the association of some components of MetS with T_H1 dominant phenotype. A substantial body of evidence suggests an important role for T_H1-mediated immune responses in pathogenesis of atherosclerotic lesions [25]. Alterations of serum cytokine balance with predominance of T_H1 immunity have also been observed both in preeclampsia and animal model of hypertension [26, 27]. Although a large number of studies have been carried out on innate immunity, only limited number have been devoted to the adaptive immune system in MetS. There is now a consistent body of cross-sectional studies showing that a variety of inflammatory markers, including C-reactive protein and cytokines such as interleukin-6 (IL-6) and tumor necrosis factor-α cluster with MetS traits. Recent evidence also indicates that IL-18, a T_H1 proinflammatory cytokine, is associated with features of the MetS [28]. Whereas circulating levels of the T_H2 anti-inflammatory cytokine IL-10 have been shown to decrease in the MetS [29]. These results suggest a shift in the T_H1/T_H2 balance toward a T_H1-type immune response in MetS. The association of MetS and its component with T_H1-related responses suggests a potential role for T_H1 cells in the pathogenesis of diastolic dysfunction associated with MetS.

Conclusion

Although the interpretation of these studies is limited by relatively small number of evidence-based reports clearly defining the immune phenotype in MetS and by the complex and multifactorial nature of pathogenesis of myocardial remodeling, these studies led us to propose a hypothesis of potential role of T_H1 immunity in promoting the adverse cardiac ECM remodeling and diastolic dysfunction seen in MetS. Further investigation may reveal the contributory role of T_H1 predominant profile in the progression of LV remodeling and modulation of T_H lymphocyte as a potential novel therapeutic target.

Acknowledgment

This work was supported by grants to RRW from Wallace Research Foundation and to DFL by NIH R01 HL079206-01.

References

1 Tsouli SG, Liberopoulos EN, Mikhailidis DP, Athyros VG, Elisaf MS. Elevated serum uric acid levels in metabolic syndrome: an active component or an innocent bystander? Metabolism 2006;55:1293–301.

2 Executive summary of the Third Report of the National Cholestrol Education Program (NCEP) Expert Panel on Detection, Evaluation, and Treatment of High Blood Cholesterol in Adults (Adult Treatment Panel III). JAMA 2001;285:2486–97.

3 Cameron AJ, Shaw JE, Zimmet PZ. The metabolic syndrome: prevalence in worldwide populations. Endocrinol Metab Clin North Am 2004;33:351–75.

4 Ford ES, Giles WH, Dietz WH. Prevalence of the metabolic syndrome among US adults. Findings from the Third National Health and Nutrition Examination Survey. JAMA 2002;287:356–9.

5 Ginsberg HN, Zhang YL, Hernandez-Ono A. Regulation of plasma triglycerides in insulin resistance and diabetes. Arch Med Res 2005;36:232–40.

6 Lewis GF. Determinants of plasma HDL concentrations and reverse cholesterol transport. Curr Opin Cardiol 2006;21:345–52.

7 Nishikawa T, Edelstein D, Du XL et al. Normalizing mitochondrial superoxide production blocks three pathways of hyperglycemic damage. Nature 2000;404:787–90.

8 Du XL, Edelstein D, Dimmeler S, Ju Q, Sui C, Brownlee M. Hyperglycemia inhibits endothelial nitric oxide synthase

activity by posttranslational modification at the Akt site. J Clin Invest 2001;108:1341–8.

9 Stepp DW, Ou J, Ackerman AW, Welak S, Klick D, Pritchard KA, Jr. Native LDL and minimally oxidized LDL differentially regulate superoxide anion in vascular endothelium in situ. Am J Physiol Heart Circ Physiol 2002;283:H750–9.

10 Piatti PM, Monti LD, Conti M et al. Hypertriglyceridemia and hyperinsulinemia are potent inducers of endothelin-1 release in humans. Diabetes 1996;45:316–21.

11 Reaven GM, Lithell H, Landsberg L. Hypertension and associated metabolic abnormalities: the role of insulin resistance and the sympathoadrenal system. N Engl J Med 1996;334:374–81.

12 Muscelli E, Natali A, Bianchi S et al. Effect of insulin on renal sodium and uric acid handling in essential hypertension. Am J Hypertens 1996;9:746–52.

13 Reilly MP, Rader DJ. The metabolic syndrome. More than the sum of its parts? Circulation 2003;108:1546–51.

14 Grandi AM, Maresca AM, Giudici E et al. Metabolic syndrome and morphofunctional characteristics of the left ventricle in clinically hypertensive nondiabetic subjects. Am J Hypertens 2006;19:199–205.

15 Izzo JL, Jr, Gradman AH. Mechanisms and management of hypertensive heart disease: from left ventricular hypertrophy to heart failure. Med Clin North Am 2004;88:1257–71.

16 Lee KW, Lip GY. Insulin resistance and vascular remodelling, in relation to left ventricular mass, geometry and function: an answer to LIFE? J Hum Hypertens 2003;17:299–304.

17 Di Bello V, Santini F, Di Cori A et al. Obesity cardiomyopathy: is it a reality? An ultrasonic tissue characterization study. J Am Soc Echocardiogr 2006;19:1063–71.

18 Roman MJ, Pickering TJ, Schwartz JE, Pini R, Devereux RB. Association of carotid atherosclerosis and left ventricular hypertrophy. J Am Coll Cardiol 1995;25:83–90.

19 Rydberg E, Willenheimer R, Erhardt L. The prevalence of impaired left ventricular diastolic filling is related to the extent of coronary atherosclerosis in patients with stable coronary artery disease. Coron Artery Dis 2002;13:1–7.

20 Cuspidi C, Meani S, Fusi V et al. Metabolic syndrome and target organ damage in untreated essential hypertensives. J Hypertens 2004;22:1991–8.

21 Diamant M, Lamb HJ, Smit JW, de Roos A, Heine RJ. Diabetic cardiomyopathy in uncomplicated type 2 diabetes is associated with the metabolic syndrome and systemic inflammation. Diabetologia 2005;48:1669–70.

22 Chinali M, Devereux RB, Howard BV et al. Comparison of cardiac structure and function in American Indians with and without the metabolic syndrome (The Strong Heart Study). Am Heart J 2004;93:40–4.

23 Wong CY, O'Moore-Sullivan T, Fang ZY et al. Myocardial and vascular dysfunction and exercise capacity in the metabolic syndrome. Am J Cardiol 2005;96:1686–91.

24 Yu Q, Watson RR, Marchalonis JJ, Larson DF. A role for T lymphocytes in mediating cardiac diastolic function. Am J Physiol Heart Circ Physiol 2005;289:H643–51.

25 Hansson GK, Libby P, Schonbeck U, Yan ZQ. Innate and adaptive immunity in the pathogenesis of atherosclerosis. Circ Res 2002;91:281–91.

26 Dong MY, Shi XL, He J, Wang ZP, Xie X, Wang HZ. Imbalance of serum T helper 1- and 2-type cytokines in preeclampsia and gestational hypertension. Zhejiang Da Xue Xue Bao Yi Xue Ban 2005;34:488–91.

27 Pascual DW, Pascual VH, Bost KL, McGhee JR, Oparil S. Nitric oxide mediates immune dysfunction in the spontaneously hypertensive rat. Hypertension 1993;21:185–94.

28 Hung J, McQuillan BM, Chapman CM, Thompson PL, Beilby JP. Elevated interleukin-18 levels are associated with the metabolic syndrome independent of obesity and insulin resistance. Arterioscler Thromb Vasc Biol 2005;25:1268–73.

29 Esposito K, Pontillo A, Giugliano F et al. Association of low interleukin-10 levels with the metabolic syndrome in obese women. J Clin Endocrinol Metab 2003;88:1055–8.

CHAPTER 6

T helper 2 cell cytokines in remodeling of aortic wall

W. L. Chan

Introduction

Atherosclerosis is an important chronic inflammatory disease of the vascular system, characterized by intense immunological activity [1]. Atherosclerosis involves the formation of lesions, chiefly in large elastic and muscular arteries that are characterized by inflammation, lipid accumulation, cell death, and fibrosis. Being a slow dynamic progressive disease, the earliest lesion, the fatty streak, which is common in infants and young children [2], consists only of monocyte-derived macrophages, which are lipid-laden, and T lymphocytes [3]. The influx of these cells is preceded by the extracellular deposition of amorphous and membranous lipids in people with hypercholesterolemia [2, 3] and over time these lesions, known as atherosclerotic plaques, mature and gain new characteristics leading to clinical complications with advancing age. These can arise from plaques expanding into the lumen to limit blood flow with stenoses and leading ultimately to plaque rupture, which exposes the pro-thrombotic material in the plaque to the blood and causes sudden thrombotic occlusion of the artery at the site of disruption. In the heart, atherosclerosis can lead to heart attack and failure, whereas atherosclerosis in the arteries of the brain can cause ischemic stroke and transient ischemic attacks. Atherosclerosis in other arterial branches can result in hypertension, abdominal aortic aneurysms (AAA), renal impairment, and critical limb impairment. However, only 50% of patients with cardiovascular disease have hypercholesterolemia [4]. Thus, atherosclerosis is clearly an inflammatory disease that does not result simply from the accumulation of lipids but from an interplay of multiple factors including cytokines, chemokines, growth factors, free radicals caused by cigarette smoking, hypertension, diabetes mellitus, genetic alterations, and infectious microorganisms that can cause endothelial injury and dysfunction [1].

Atherosclerosis initiates because of endothelial dysfunction with the accumulation of immune cells and lipid droplets in the intima, which is the innermost layer of the arterial wall, leading to asymmetrical focal thickening. The early plaque contains mainly macrophages and T cells from the blood, as well as endothelial cells (ECs), smooth muscle cells, extracellular matrix, lipids, and acellular lipid-rich debris [5]. Lipid-laden macrophages, known as foam cells, outnumber other cells in early nascent plaques. Prevalent in young individuals, these fatty streaks never cause symptoms of atherosclerosis and can disappear with time or progress slowly into mature atherosclerotic plaques, indicating that this is a complex disease with no simple answer to what arm of the adaptive immune response promotes or retards atherogenesis. Current evidences point to a yin and yang effect of the adaptive immune response at various times and places in the evolution of this complex and lengthy disease.

The mature human plaque or atheroma has a more complex immune cell structure than the fatty streak. Apart from T cells and macrophages, dendritic cells (DCs) [6], mast cells [7], and a few B cells [8] are also present in plaques. In addition, we have recently demonstrated the presence of natural killer (NK) T and NK cells in atherosclerotic AAA [9]. In the center of the plaque, foam cells and extracellular lipid droplets form a core region that is surrounded by a cap of smooth muscle cells and extracellular matrix rich in collagen [8]. There is an abundance of T cells and macrophages in the shoulder region of the plaque, which is where it grows, and in the interface between the cap and the core [8]. As the plaque progresses in complexity with time, the fibrous cap, which is of varying thickness, prevents the lipid core rich in cholesterol and cellular debris containing pro-thrombotic material from contact with the blood.

Initiation of inflammation and atherogenesis

Modified low-density lipoprotein (LDL)—a major cause of injury and dysfunction to the endothelium and underlying vascular smooth muscle cells (VSMCs)—can activate ECs to express leukocyte adhesion molecules, in particular vascular cell adhesion molecule 1 (VCAM-1) [10], and produce growth factors, cytokines, and chemoattractants [11, 12], leading to monocyte adhesion and extravasation. Further increased adherence of leukocytes and platelets to the endothelium will lead to an influx of macrophages and lymphocytes into the arterial wall [8, 13], migration and proliferation of VSMCs, accumulation of extracellular matrix, and expansion of the arterial intima [14]. Thus, removal of modified LDL by ingestion is an important part of the initial protective role of macrophages. However, once ingested, these lipids can activate the resultant lipid-laden foam cells to produce pro-inflammatory cytokines, including IL-1, tumor necrosis factor-α (TNF-α) and macrophage colony stimulating factor (MCSF) which can increase the binding of LDL to ECs and VSMCs [15, 16]. If the inflammatory response cannot neutralize or remove the offending agents, it can continue indefinitely. Up to a point the lumen remains unaltered as the arterial wall compensates by gradual dilation [17]. Continual activation of the inflammatory macrophages and lymphocytes results in the release of hydrolytic enzymes, cytokines, chemokines, and growth factors that lead eventually to focal necrosis [1]. The balance of migration and proliferation of VSMCs over death by apoptosis has an important impact on the final size and stability of the plaque. While all aspects of VSMC behavior are under coordinated control by growth factors, inflammatory mediators, cell–matrix, and cell–cell interactions, evidence suggests that matrix-degrading metallo-

proteinases (MMPs) regulate migration, proliferation, and survival of VSMCs by cleaving both matrix and nonmatrix substrates such as cadherin [18]. For VSMCs to migrate, several signal transduction pathways are activated to reorganize the cytoskeleton and to form reversible contacts with existing and newly expressed cell surface and extracellular matrix components, while integrin-mediated pathways as well as growth-factor-induced signaling pathways are essential in stimulating VSMC proliferation [19]. A broad range of MMPs are coordinately induced by pro-inflammatory cytokines such as IL-1 and TNF-α [20] which can act synergistically with growth factors. However, the activity of MMPs is limited physiologically by binding to endogenous tissue inhibitors of MMPs (TIMPs) [21] which are either constitutive or upregulated by fibrogenic cytokines. A range of MMPs and TIMPs are elevated in human atherosclerotic plaques especially at the macrophage-rich shoulder regions and also in aneurysms. Thus, cycles of accumulation of mononuclear cells, migration and proliferation of smooth muscle cells, and formation of fibrous tissue lead to further enlargement and restructuring of the lesion to eventually become covered by a fibrous cap that overlies a core of lipid and necrotic tissue [1]. The advanced lesion may then intrude into the lumen, when the artery can no longer compensate by dilation, and alter the flow of blood. This could lead to thrombosis when the plaque ruptures [22] as a result of VSMC apoptosis [23], and we have recently shown that NKT cells derived from plaques can induce VSMC apoptosis via Fas/FasL interaction and Caspase I/ICE activity induced by CD40 ligation [9].

Importance of mouse models to elucidate the immunology of atherosclerosis

It is not practical to directly analyze the early phases of human atherosclerosis. Therefore, animal models of the disease are used to systematically investigate the mechanisms that initiate atherosclerosis. This is possible as there is substantial overlap between disease development in these animal models and the human disease. The availability of two strains of genetically modified mice susceptible to atherosclerosis has been very useful in this respect. Apolipoprotein E-(apoE, a key component in cholesterol metabolism) deficient mice develop spontaneous atherosclerotic disease that is exacerbated by an atherogenic high-fat diet, and this can progress to myocardial infarction and stroke. Low-density-lipoprotein receptor (LDLR)-deficient mice develop atherosclerotic plaques on a cholesterol diet [24–27]. The lesions in these animals share many features of human atherosclerosis and have been particularly useful in facilitating attempts to study the role of pro-inflammatory T-cell subsets and their secreted mediators in atheroma formation.

Role of T lymphocytes in atherosclerosis

There is compelling evidence that T lymphocytes are a fundamental component of the histopathology of early and late lesions of atherosclerosis and antibody responses to modified lipids in atheroma are characteristic of the disease. Both $CD4^+$ and $CD8^+$ T cells are present in the lesions at all stages of atherosclerosis [1], with the majority being $\alpha\beta$ T cells and a small proportion of $\gamma\delta$ T cells. Analyses of human lesions indicate that many of the plaque T cells express activation markers like HLA-DR, IL-2R, CD45RO, CD38, VLA-1 [28], and the costimulatory molecules CD27, CD28, B7-1, and CD40 [29, 30]. In addition, there is evidence that plaque T cells are actively dividing [31] and the T-cell cytokines, such as IL-2 and IFN-γ, are expressed within human plaques [32]. Heat shock protein (HSP)-60 and oxidized LDL-specific $CD4^+$ T-cell clones have been isolated from human carotid lesions [33, 34]. The HSP60-specific T cells isolated from human plaques from patients with positive serology and PCR for *Chlamydia pneumoniae* DNA also recognized *C. pneumoniae* HSP60, suggesting that the autoreactive T cells arose from molecular mimicry, since the presence of *Chlamydia* in blood vessels and increased antibody levels to these pathogens have been associated with atherosclerosis [35]. T cells are also the principal activators of macrophages, one of the key players in the pathogenesis of atherosclerosis, as well as ECs and VSMCs mainly via the cytokines they produce. We have recently demonstrated using human-plaque-derived T cells and VSMCs that $CD4^+$ T cells can en-

hance VSMC proliferation on cell–cell contact [9]. Although T lymphocytes have been implicated in atherosclerosis, the type and distribution of T-cell subset response, how and when they influence the disease process, is still not clear since this is a slow and dynamic progressive disease that is also influenced by the presence of Th2 and regulatory T (Treg) cells that produce the anti-inflammatory cytokines IL-4, IL-13, IL-10, and TGF-β. Thus the balance of Th1 to Th2/Treg response in the plaque would determine the state and progress of the disease.

Role of pro-inflammatory cytokines in atherosclerosis

The chronic inflammatory and fibroproliferative responses within lesions that are central to atherogenesis are affected by cytokines/chemokines, multipotent mediators of inflammation and immunity [36]. Cytokines participate as autocrine or paracrine mediators in atherogenesis, as cells in lesions can both produce and respond by activation and growth to these mediators [37]. IFN-γ is a potent activator of macrophages, causing them to produce more nitric oxide, pro-inflammatory cytokines like TNF and IL-1, and pro-thrombotic and vasoactive mediators. It is a promoter of type 1 helper T-cell (Th1) responses and its early colocalization with T cells to atherosclerotic lesions suggests that IFN-γ contributes to atherogenesis [32]. IFN-γ induces and modulates chemokine production in a variety of cell types, including ECs and mononuclear phagocytes, to produce monocyte chemotactic protein-1 (MCP-1), known to direct monocyte migration into the intima [38, 39]. In addition, IFN-γ has recently been shown to act directly on VSMCs to potentiate growth-factor-induced mitogenesis [40]. The importance of IFN-γ driving the disease is shown in the mouse model of atheroma formation, where serological neutralization or genetic absence of IFN-γ or its receptor or the Th1-cell-inducing transcription factor T-bet markedly reduces the plaque size [41–43]. IL-12 produced by macrophages in the plaque can indirectly affect plaque development by promoting naive T (Th0) cells differentiation to Th1 cells that produce IFN-γ, IL-2, TNF, and lymphotoxin. IFN-γ production in Th1 cells is induced by IL-18 (formerly called IFN-γ-inducing factor), a macrophage-produced cytokine with pleiotropic activities that play an important role primarily in promoting proliferation and IFN-γ production by Th1, CD8+, and NK cells in mice and humans [44, 45].

Although T cells are the major source of IFN-γ, it is also produced by macrophagic cells responding to the synergistic effect of IL-12 and IL-18 [46]. As receptors of IL-18 are stably expressed by Th1 cells, IL-18R-expressing T cells are abundant in the lesions [9, 47]. Thus, through its effect on IFN-γ induction, IL-18 aggravates atherosclerosis. Therefore, atherosclerosis is reduced when a plasmid encoding a soluble, recombinant IL-18-binding protein (IL-18BP) that neutralizes IL-18 is administrated for 9 weeks to apoE-deficient mice fed normal chow diet [48]. In addition, treatment of apoE-deficient mice on normal chow diet with recombinant IL-18 led to an increased size of atherosclerotic lesions [49] and IL-18 and apoE double-deficient (IL-18$^{-/-}$ apoE$^{-/-}$) mice fed normal chow diet showed reduced atherosclerosis compared with apoE-deficient mice [50].

A Th1 cytokine like IFN-γ or TNF-α also directly accelerates the disease through its action on macrophages and VSMCs. TNF-α triggers vascular inflammation by inducing the production of reactive oxygen and nitrogen species and prothrombotic tissue factors by ECs, and it modulates the fibrinolytic capacity of VSMCs with the induction of proteolytic enzymes [51–53]. TNF-α also has profound effect on lipid metabolism by suppression of lipoprotein lipase, leading to accumulation of triglyceride-rich lipoprotein in the blood, which has been associated with heart disease [54].

Anti-inflammatory cytokines

Atherogenesis involves the complex interactions between the inflammatory cells and vascular cells (EC and VSMC), and the response of the vascular cells during the inflammatory process is critical. The multiple cytokines and growth factors present at sites of inflammation can each influence the nature of the inflammatory response. So the vascular cells integrate these signals to regulate their immunoinflammatory responses through the expression of adhesion molecules, cytokines, chemokines, growth factors, and MMPs. Much re-

cent work shows that vascular inflammation can be limited by anti-inflammatory counter-regulatory mechanisms involving anti-inflammatory external signals and intracellular mediators to maintain the integrity and homeostasis of the vascular wall. Here we focus on the local cellular immunity that predominantly promotes atherosclerosis through cell–cell surface interaction and cytokines (such as IFN-γ and TNF), and only the counter balancing external factors that function to dampen the disease activity will be discussed. As anti-inflammatory Th2 and Treg cytokines, IL-10 and TGF-β, provide particularly important atheroprotective signals, while the effect of IL-13 and the prototypic Th2-cytokine IL-4 is inconclusive.

IL-10

IL-10 is a pleiotropic cytokine that inhibits Th1 cell cytokine production, antigen presentation, and T-cell proliferation. It is also produced by B cells and macrophages and has potent anti-inflammatory properties on macrophages. IL-10 downregulates TNF-α and IL-1 production by lipopolysaccharide-stimulated monocytes, and this is demonstrated in in vivo studies that showed that TNF-α levels are higher and remained elevated longer in IL-10-deficient mice injected with lipopolysaccharide than in IL-10-competent mice [55]. IL-10 downregulates the expression of adhesion molecules (ICAM-1 and VCAM-1) induced by IL-1 on EC [56] and inhibits TNF-induced fibroblast growth factor-2 (FGF-2) [57]. The IL-10 receptor (IL-10R) is composed of two distinct subunits. The IL-10R α chain (IL-10R1) plays a dominant role in mediating high-affinity ligand binding and signal transduction [58]. IL-10 functions to block NF-kB activity through the suppression of IkB kinase activity, by preventing IkB-α degradation, and the suppression of NF-kB DNA-binding activity [59]. In vivo, IL-10 exerts its anti-inflammatory effects on the vascular system through inhibition of EC–leukocyte interactions [60–62] and also the pro-inflammatory cytokine and chemokine production by macrophages and lymphocytes [63–65]. The atheroprotective role of IL-10 starts at the initial stage of atherogenesis as illustrated by the reports using IL-10-deficient C57BL/6 mice that do not develop lesions similar to human clinical disease. When these IL-10-deficient mice were fed a fatty diet, they developed an increased quantity of fatty streaks compared with IL-10-competent C57BL/6 mice or IL-10-transgenic C57BL/6 mice, which do not develop fatty streaks [65, 66]. When IL-10 and apoE double deficient mice were used, the mice developed increased atherosclerosis compared with apoE-deficient mice [67], showing an atheroprotective role for IL-10.

TGF-β

TGF-β is a pluripotent cytokine with many effects on a diverse range of cell types and is produced by Treg cells, ECs, and VSMCs [68–70]. It mediates pleiotropic functions both inside and outside the immune system. Recent reports on the role of TGF-β show that it participates in suppression of effector T-cell (both Th1 and Th2) function and modulates T-cell differentiation by inhibiting differentiation of Th1 and Th2 but promotes Treg differentiation [70]. In addition, TGF-β has an important role in repair responses that lead to matrix deposition and tissue remodeling. TGF-β promotes collagen production, which could increase plaque stability. It was first reported to have a deactivating effect on macrophages by suppressing inducible nitric oxide synthase protein expression [71]. TGF-β also has potent anti-inflammatory effects on vascular cells. It downregulates cytokine-induced expression of VCAM-1 and E-selectin in ECs [72, 73] and also VCAM-1 in VSMCs [74]. MCP-1 produced by ECs stimulated with TNF-α or IL-1 is significantly decreased in the presence of TGF-β as it downmodulates the expression of TNF-α receptors [75]. Furthermore, by inhibiting IL-8 production by TNF-activated ECs, it inhibits IL-8-dependent migration of neutrophils through activated EC monolayer [76]. TGF-β is able to restore endothelial-dependent vasodilation impaired by TNF-α [77]. TGF-β produced by vascular cells may act as a paracrine anti-inflammatory factor by inhibiting the production of pro-inflammatory cytokines by emigrated macrophages as demonstrated with glomerular mesangial cells [78]. Studies with animal models show that TGF-β can inhibit atherosclerosis at least as well as IL-10. Administration of TGF-β-specific blocking antibodies or decoy receptors for TGF-β increases

atherosclerotic plaque formation in LDLR-deficient mice [79, 80]. TGF-β can also exert its atherosclerotic effects by modulating T-cell activation. This is shown when mice carrying dominant negative TGFRβ receptors expressed under the control of the CD4 promoter were crossbred with apoE-deficient mice. It led to a fivefold increase in plaque size with increased inflammation and fewer interstitial collagen fibers in the crossbred mice [81]. In another study, when bone marrow from mice that expressed a dominant-negative form of the type II TGF-β receptor, which is expressed under the control of the CD2 promoter, was transplanted to irradiated LDLR-deficient mice, their plaques showed signs of substantial inflammation with a poorly developed collagenous matrix [82]. As Treg produce TGF-β, activation of Treg could be atheroprotective, and this was confirmed recently by showing that the transfer of natural CD4$^+$ CD25$^+$ Treg cells reduces atherosclerosis, whereas depletion of CD25$^+$ cells increases disease in apoE-deficient mice [83].

Th2 anti-inflammatory cytokines IL-4 and IL-13

Th2 cytokines IL-4 and IL-13 are considered anti-inflammatory because they suppress the production of inflammatory cytokines by macrophages and monocytes. IL-4 and IL-13 mediate anti-inflammatory response via the induction of 15-lipoxygenase that catalyzes the hydroperoxidation of arachidonic acid to lipoxin A4, which can suppress leukocyte activation, adherance, and chemotaxis [84]. IL-4 can inhibit VSMC proliferation [85]. IL-4 and IL-13 can protect porcine ECs from killing by complement or apoptosis induced by TNF-α [86]. However, IL-4 and IL-13 have been reported to selectively induce VCAM-1 expression on ECs and VSMCs [87, 88]. Furthermore, IL-13 markedly enhances IL-8 and MCP-1 release by cytokine-stimulated human VSMCs [89], and in vivo studies show that IL-4 and IL-13 are capable of promoting angiogenesis [90]. Thus, IL-4 displays a complex range of biological activities. Therefore, it is no wonder that data from animal models on the role of IL-4 in atherogenesis are inconclusive. Some studies have shown that IL-4 is atheroprotective, whereas others found reduced disease in the absence of IL-4 [91, 92]. Further study is required to define the role of Th2 cell, which is complicated by IL-4, the prototype Th2 cytokine, being also produced by NK T cells and NK cells. These cells are present in abundance in advanced atherosclerotic AAA [9].

In conclusion, the Th2-cytokine IL-10 and TGF-β produced by Treg are anti-inflammatory cytokines that may be considered for use in remodeling aortic wall. It is noteworthy that chronic production of high levels in the systemic circulation or long-term usage may lead to complications arising from susceptibility to microbial infection. An alternate possible approach is to block the proinflammatory cytokines with, for example, anti-TNF or anti-IFN-γ monoclonal antibodies, soluble receptors or binding proteins, and receptor antagonist. This is evident with IL-1, one of the most potent pro-inflammatory cytokines acting on both ECs and VSMCs [1]. Although IL-1 has a naturally secreted receptor antagonist (IL-1Ra) and the intracellular form is expressed in ECs and VSMCs [93, 94], in vivo studies show that IL-1Ra is vascular protective, as treatment of apoE-deficient mice with recombinant IL-Ra reduces atherosclerosis [95].

References

1 Ross R. Atherosclerosis—an inflammatory disease [see comments]. N Engl J Med 1999;340:115–26.

2 Napoli C, D'Armiento FP, Mancini FP et al. Fatty streak formation occurs in human fetal aortas and is greatly enhanced by maternal hypercholesterolemia. Intimal accumulation of low density lipoprotein and its oxidation precede monocyte recruitment into early atherosclerotic lesions. J Clin Invest 1997;100:2680–90.

3 Stary HC, Chandler AB, Glagov S et al. A definition of initial, fatty streak, and intermediate lesions of atherosclerosis. A report from the Committee on Vascular Lesions of the Council on Arteriosclerosis, American Heart Association. Circulation 1994;89:2462–78.

4 Braunwald E. Shattuck lecture. Cardiovascular medicine at the turn of the millennium: triumphs, concerns, and opportunities [see comments]. N Engl J Med 1997;337: 1360–9.

5 Ross R. The pathogenesis of atherosclerosis: a perspective for the 1990s. Nature 1993;362:801–9.

6 Bobryshev YV, Lord RS. S-100 positive cells in human arterial intima and in atherosclerotic lesions. Cardiovasc Res 1995;29:689–96.

7 Kovanen PT, Kaartinen M, Paavonen T. Infiltrates of activated mast cells at the site of coronary atheromatous erosion or rupture in myocardial infarction. Circulation 1995;92:1084–8.

8 Jonasson L, Holm J, Skalli O, Bondjers G, Hansson GK. Regional accumulations of T cells, macrophages, and smooth muscle cells in the human atherosclerotic plaque. Arteriosclerosis 1986;6:131–8.

9 Chan WL, Pejnovic N, Hamilton H et al. Atherosclerotic abdominal aortic aneurysm and the interaction between autologous human plaque-derived vascular smooth muscle cells, type 1 NKT, and helper T cells. Circ Res 2005; 96: 675–83.

10 Cybulsky MI, Gimbrone MA, Jr. Endothelial expression of a mononuclear leukocyte adhesion molecule during atherogenesis. Science 1991;251:788–91.

11 Rajavashisth TB, Andalibi A, Territo MC et al. Induction of endothelial cell expression of granulocyte and macrophage colony-stimulating factors by modified low-density lipoproteins. Nature 1990;344:254–7.

12 Leonard EJ, Yoshimura T. Human monocyte chemoattractant protein-1 (MCP-1). Immunol Today 1990;11: 97–101.

13 Gerrity RG, Goss JA, Soby L. Control of monocyte recruitment by chemotactic factor(s) in lesion-prone areas of swine aorta. Arteriosclerosis 1985;5:55–66.

14 Munro JM, Cotran RS. The pathogenesis of atherosclerosis: atherogenesis and inflammation. Lab Invest 1988; 58:249–61.

15 Stopeck AT, Nicholson AC, Mancini FP, Hajjar DP. Cytokine regulation of low density lipoprotein receptor gene transcription in HepG2 cells. J Biol Chem 1993;268: 17489–94.

16 Hajjar DP, Haberland ME. Lipoprotein trafficking in vascular cells. Molecular Trojan horses and cellular saboteurs. J Biol Chem 1997;272:22975–8.

17 Glagov S, Weisenberg E, Zarins CK, Stankunavicius R, Kolettis GJ. Compensatory enlargement of human atherosclerotic coronary arteries. N Engl J Med 1987; 316:1371–5.

18 Newby AC. Matrix metalloproteinases regulate migration, proliferation, and death of vascular smooth muscle cells by degrading matrix and non-matrix substrates. Cardiovasc Res 2006;69:614–24.

19 Morla AO, Mogford JE. Control of smooth muscle cell proliferation and phenotype by integrin signaling through focal adhesion kinase. Biochem Biophys Res Commun 2000;272:298–302.

20 Galis ZS, Muszynski M, Sukhova GK et al. Cytokine-stimulated human vascular smooth muscle cells synthesize a complement of enzymes required for extracellular matrix digestion. Circ Res 1994;75:181–9.

21 Sternlicht MD, Werb Z. How matrix metalloproteinases regulate cell behavior. Annu Rev Cell Dev Biol 2001; 17:463–516.

22 Davies MJ, Thomas A. Thrombosis and acute coronary-artery lesions in sudden cardiac ischemic death. N Engl J Med 1984;310:1137–40.

23 Bennett MR. Apoptosis of vascular smooth muscle cells in vascular remodelling and atherosclerotic plaque rupture. Cardiovasc Res 1999;41:361–8.

24 Zhang SH, Reddick RL, Piedrahita JA, Maeda N. Spontaneous hypercholesterolemia and arterial lesions in mice lacking apolipoprotein E. Science 1992;258:468–71.

25 Plump AS, Smith JD, Hayek T et al. Severe hypercholesterolemia and atherosclerosis in apolipoprotein E-deficient mice created by homologous recombination in ES cells. Cell 1992;71:343–53.

26 Ishibashi S, Brown MS, Goldstein JL, Gerard RD, Hammer RE, Herz J. Hypercholesterolemia in low density lipoprotein receptor knockout mice and its reversal by adenovirus-mediated gene delivery [see comments]. J Clin Invest 1993;92:883–93.

27 Ishibashi S, Herz J, Maeda N, Goldstein JL, Brown MS. The two-receptor model of lipoprotein clearance: tests of the hypothesis in "knockout" mice lacking the low density lipoprotein receptor, apolipoprotein E, or both proteins. Proc Natl Acad Sci U S A 1994;91:4431–5.

28 Stemme S, Holm J, Hansson GK. T lymphocytes in human atherosclerotic plaques are memory cells expressing CD45RO and the integrin VLA-1. Arterioscler Thromb 1992;12:206–11.

29 de Boer OJ, Hirsch F, van der Wal AC, van der Loos CM, Das PK, Becker AE. Costimulatory molecules in human atherosclerotic plaques: an indication of antigen specific T lymphocyte activation. Atherosclerosis 1997;133:227–34.

30 Mach F, Schonbeck U, Libby P. CD40 signaling in vascular cells: a key role in atherosclerosis? Atherosclerosis 1998;137(suppl):S89–95.

31 Rekhter MD, Gordon D. Active proliferation of different cell types, including lymphocytes, in human atherosclerotic plaques. Am J Pathol 1995;147:668–77.

32 Hansson GK, Holm J, Jonasson L. Detection of activated T lymphocytes in the human atherosclerotic plaque. Am J Pathol 1989;135:169–75.

33 de Boer OJ, van der Wal AC, Houtkamp MA, Ossewaarde JM, Teeling P, Becker AE. Unstable atherosclerotic plaques contain T-cells that respond to Chlamydia pneumoniae. Cardiovasc Res 2000;48:402–8.

34 Stemme S, Faber B, Holm J, Wiklund O, Witztum JL, Hansson GK. T lymphocytes from human atherosclerotic plaques recognize oxidized low density lipoprotein. Proc Natl Acad Sci U S A 1995;92:3893–7.

35 Benagiano M, D'Elios MM, Amedei A et al. Human 60-kDa heat shock protein is a target autoantigen of T cells derived from atherosclerotic plaques. J Immunol 2005;174:6509–17.

36 Terkeltaub R, Boisvert WA, Curtiss LK. Chemokines and atherosclerosis. Curr Opin Lipidol 1998;9:397–405.

37 Libby P, Sukhova G, Lee RT, Galis ZS. Cytokines regulate vascular functions related to stability of the atherosclerotic plaque. J Cardiovasc Pharmacol 1995;25:S9–12.

38 Weiss JM, Cuff CA, Berman JW. TGF-beta downmodulates cytokine-induced monocyte chemoattractant protein (MCP)-1 expression in human endothelial cells. A putative role for TGF-beta in the modulation of TNF receptor expression. Endothelium 1999;6:291–302.

39 Penton-Rol G, Polentarutti N, Luini W et al. Selective inhibition of expression of the chemokine receptor CCR2 in human monocytes by IFN-gamma. J Immunol 1998;160:3869–73.

40 Tellides G, Tereb DA, Kirkiles-Smith NC et al. Interferon-gamma elicits arteriosclerosis in the absence of leukocytes. Nature 2000;403:207–11.

41 Buono C, Come CE, Stavrakis G, Maguire GF, Connelly PW, Lichtman AH. Influence of interferon-gamma on the extent and phenotype of diet-induced atherosclerosis in the LDLR-deficient mouse. Arterioscler Thromb Vasc Biol 2003;23:454–60.

42 Gupta S, Pablo AM, Jiang X, Wang N, Tall AR, Schindler C. IFN-gamma potentiates atherosclerosis in ApoE knockout mice. J Clin Invest 1997;99:2752–61.

43 Buono C, Binder CJ, Stavrakis G, Witztum JL, Glimcher LH, Lichtman AH. T-bet deficiency reduces atherosclerosis and alters plaque antigen-specific immune responses. Proc Natl Acad Sci U S A 2005;102:1596–601.

44 Okamura H, Nagata K, Komatsu T et al. A novel costimulatory factor for gamma interferon induction found in the livers of mice causes endotoxic shock. Infect Immun 1995;63:3966–72.

45 Barbulescu K, Becker C, Schlaak JF, Schmitt E, Meyer zum Buschenfelde KH, Neurath MF. IL-12 and IL-18 differentially regulate the transcriptional activity of the human IFN-gamma promoter in primary CD4$^+$ T lymphocytes. J Immunol 1998;160:3642–7.

46 Munder M, Mallo M, Eichmann K, Modolell M. Murine macrophages secrete interferon gamma upon combined stimulation with interleukin (IL)-12 and IL-18: a novel pathway of autocrine macrophage activation. J Exp Med 1998;187:2103–8.

47 Chan WL, Pejnovic N, Lee CA, Al-Ali NA. Human IL-18 receptor and ST2L are stable and selective markers for the respective type 1 and type 2 circulating lymphocytes. J Immunol 2001;167:1238–44.

48 Mallat Z, Silvestre JS, Le Ricousse-Roussanne S et al. Interleukin-18/interleukin-18 binding protein signaling modulates ischemia-induced neovascularization in mice hindlimb. Circ Res 2002;91:441–8.

49 Whitman SC, Ravisankar P, Daugherty A. Interleukin-18 enhances atherosclerosis in apolipoprotein E(−/−)

mice through release of interferon-gamma. Circ Res 2002;90:E34–8.

50 Elhage R, Jawien J, Rudling M *et al.* Reduced atherosclerosis in interleukin-18 deficient apolipoprotein E-knockout mice. Cardiovasc Res 2003;59:234–40.

51 van Hinsbergh VW, van den Berg EA, Fiers W, Dooijewaard G. Tumor necrosis factor induces the production of urokinase-type plasminogen activator by human endothelial cells. Blood 1990;75:1991–8.

52 Lee E, Vaughan DE, Parikh SH *et al.* Regulation of matrix metalloproteinases and plasminogen activator inhibitor-1 synthesis by plasminogen in cultured human vascular smooth muscle cells. Circ Res 1996;78:44–9.

53 Saren P, Welgus HG, Kovanen PT. TNF-alpha and IL-1beta selectively induce expression of 92-kDa gelatinase by human macrophages. J Immunol 1996;157:4159–65.

54 Jovinge S, Hamsten A, Tornvall P *et al.* Evidence for a role of tumor necrosis factor alpha in disturbances of triglyceride and glucose metabolism predisposing to coronary heart disease. Metabolism 1998;47:113–8.

55 Berg DJ, Kuhn R, Rajewsky K *et al.* Interleukin-10 is a central regulator of the response to LPS in murine models of endotoxic shock and the Shwartzman reaction but not endotoxin tolerance. J Clin Invest 1995;96:2339–47.

56 Krakauer T. IL-10 inhibits the adhesion of leukocytic cells to IL-1-activated human endothelial cells. Immunol Lett 1995;45:61–5.

57 Selzman CH, Meldrum DR, Cain BS *et al.* Interleukin-10 inhibits postinjury tumor necrosis factor-mediated human vascular smooth muscle proliferation. J Surg Res 1998;80:352–6.

58 Liu Y, Wei SH, Ho AS, de Waal Malefyt R, Moore KW. Expression cloning and characterization of a human IL-10 receptor. J Immunol 1994;152:1821–9.

59 Schottelius AJ, Mayo MW, Sartor RB, Baldwin AS, Jr. Interleukin-10 signaling blocks inhibitor of kappaB kinase activity and nuclear factor kappaB DNA binding. J Biol Chem 1999;274:31868–74.

60 Downing LJ, Strieter RM, Kadell AM *et al.* IL-10 regulates thrombus-induced vein wall inflammation and thrombosis. J Immunol 1998;161:1471–6.

61 Morise Z, Eppihimer M, Granger DN, Anderson DC, Grisham MB. Effects of lipopolysaccharide on endothelial cell adhesion molecule expression in interleukin-10 deficient mice. Inflammation 1999;23:99–110.

62 Henke PK, DeBrunye LA, Strieter RM *et al.* Viral IL-10 gene transfer decreases inflammation and cell adhesion molecule expression in a rat model of venous thrombosis. J Immunol 2000;164:2131–41.

63 Pugin J, Ulevitch RJ, Tobias PS. A critical role for monocytes and CD14 in endotoxin-induced endothelial cell activation. J Exp Med 1993;178:2193–200.

64 Mallat Z, Heymes C, Ohan J, Faggin E, Leseche G, Tedgui A. Expression of interleukin-10 in advanced human atherosclerotic plaques: relation to inducible nitric oxide synthase expression and cell death. Arterioscler Thromb Vasc Biol 1999;19:611–6.

65 Mallat Z, Besnard S, Duriez M *et al.* Protective role of interleukin-10 in atherosclerosis. Circ Res 1999;85:e17–24.

66 Pinderski Oslund LJ, Hedrick CC, Olvera T *et al.* Interleukin-10 blocks atherosclerotic events in vitro and in vivo. Arterioscler Thromb Vasc Biol 1999;19:2847–53.

67 Caligiuri G, Rudling M, Ollivier V *et al.* Interleukin-10 deficiency increases atherosclerosis, thrombosis, and low-density lipoproteins in apolipoprotein E knockout mice. Mol Med 2003;9:10–7.

68 Axel DI, Riessen R, Athanasiadis A, Runge H, Koveker G, Karsch KR. Growth factor expression of human arterial smooth muscle cells and endothelial cells in a transfilter coculture system. J Mol Cell Cardiol 1997;29:2967–78.

69 Kirschenlohr HL, Metcalfe JC, Weissberg PL, Grainger DJ. Adult human aortic smooth muscle cells in culture produce active TGF-beta. Am J Physiol 1993;265:C571–6.

70 Schmidt-Weber CB, Blaser K. Regulation and role of transforming growth factor-beta in immune tolerance induction and inflammation. Curr Opin Immunol 2004;16:709–16.

71 Vodovotz Y, Bogdan C, Paik J, Xie QW, Nathan C. Mechanisms of suppression of macrophage nitric oxide release by transforming growth factor beta. J Exp Med 1993;178:605–13.

72 DiChiara MR, Kiely JM, Gimbrone MA, Jr, Lee ME, Perrella MA, Topper JN. Inhibition of E-selectin gene expression by transforming growth factor beta in endothelial cells involves coactivator integration of Smad and nuclear factor kappaB-mediated signals. J Exp Med 2000;192:695–704.

73 Park SK, Yang WS, Lee SK *et al.* TGF-beta(1) down-regulates inflammatory cytokine-induced VCAM-1 expression in cultured human glomerular endothelial cells. Nephrol Dial Transplant 2000;15:596–604.

74 Gamble JR, Bradley S, Noack L, Vadas MA. TGF-beta and endothelial cells inhibit VCAM-1 expression on human vascular smooth muscle cells. Arterioscler Thromb Vasc Biol 1995;15:949–55.

75 Honda HM, Leitinger N, Frankel M *et al.* Induction of monocyte binding to endothelial cells by MM-LDL: role of lipoxygenase metabolites. Arterioscler Thromb Vasc Biol 1999;19:680–6.

76 Smith WB, Noack L, Khew-Goodall Y, Isenmann S, Vadas MA, Gamble JR. Transforming growth factor-beta 1 inhibits the production of IL-8 and the transmigration of

neutrophils through activated endothelium. J Immunol 1996;157:360–8.

77 Lefer AM, Tsao P, Aoki N, Palladino MA, Jr. Mediation of cardioprotection by transforming growth factor-beta. Science 1990;249:61–4.

78 Kitamura M, Suto T, Yokoo T, Shimizu F, Fine LG. Transforming growth factor-beta 1 is the predominant paracrine inhibitor of macrophage cytokine synthesis produced by glomerular mesangial cells. J Immunol 1996;156:2964–71.

79 Mallat Z, Gojova A, Marchiol-Fournigault C et al. Inhibition of transforming growth factor-beta signaling accelerates atherosclerosis and induces an unstable plaque phenotype in mice. Circ Res 2001;89:930–4.

80 Lutgens E, Gijbels M, Smook M et al. Transforming growth factor-beta mediates balance between inflammation and fibrosis during plaque progression. Arterioscler Thromb Vasc Biol 2002;22:975–82.

81 Robertson AK, Rudling M, Zhou X, Gorelik L, Flavell RA, Hansson GK. Disruption of TGF-beta signaling in T cells accelerates atherosclerosis. J Clin Invest 2003;112:1342–50.

82 Gojova A, Brun V, Esposito B et al. Specific abrogation of transforming growth factor-beta signaling in T cells alters atherosclerotic lesion size and composition in mice. Blood 2003;102:4052–8.

83 Ait-Oufella H, Salomon BL, Potteaux S et al. Natural regulatory T cells control the development of atherosclerosis in mice. Nat Med 2006;12:178–80.

84 Nassar GM, Morrow JD, Roberts LJ, II, Lakkis FG, Badr KF. Induction of 15-lipoxygenase by interleukin-13 in human blood monocytes. J Biol Chem 1994;269:27631–4.

85 Vadiveloo PK, Stanton HR, Cochran FW, Hamilton JA. Interleukin-4 inhibits human smooth muscle cell proliferation. Artery 1994;21:161–81.

86 Grehan JF, Levay-Young BK, Fogelson JL, Francois-Bongarcon V, Benson BA, Dalmasso AP. IL-4 and IL-13 induce protection of porcine endothelial cells from killing by human complement and from apoptosis through activation of a phosphatidylinositide 3-kinase/Akt pathway. J Immunol 2005;175:1903–10.

87 Barks JL, McQuillan JJ, Iademarco MF. TNF-alpha and IL-4 synergistically increase vascular cell adhesion molecule-1 expression in cultured vascular smooth muscle cells. J Immunol 1997;159:4532–8.

88 Bochner BS, Klunk DA, Sterbinsky SA, Coffman RL, Schleimer RP. IL-13 selectively induces vascular cell adhesion molecule-1 expression in human endothelial cells. J Immunol 1995;154:799–803.

89 Jordan NJ, Watson ML, Williams RJ, Roach AG, Yoshimura T, Westwick J. Chemokine production by human vascular smooth muscle cells: modulation by IL-13. Br J Pharmacol 1997;122:749–57.

90 Fukushi J, Ono M, Morikawa W, Iwamoto Y, Kuwano M. The activity of soluble VCAM-1 in angiogenesis stimulated by IL-4 and IL-13. J Immunol 2000;165:2818–23.

91 Davenport P, Tipping PG. The role of interleukin-4 and interleukin-12 in the progression of atherosclerosis in apolipoprotein E-deficient mice. Am J Pathol 2003;163:1117–25.

92 King VL, Szilvassy SJ, Daugherty A. Interleukin-4 deficiency decreases atherosclerotic lesion formation in a site-specific manner in female LDL receptor−/− mice. Arterioscler Thromb Vasc Biol 2002;22:456–61.

93 Beasley D, McGuiggin ME, Dinarello CA. Human vascular smooth muscle cells produce an intracellular form of interleukin-1 receptor antagonist. Am J Physiol 1995;269:C961–8.

94 Dewberry R, Holden H, Crossman D, Francis S. Interleukin-1 receptor antagonist expression in human endothelial cells and atherosclerosis. Arterioscler Thromb Vasc Biol 2000;20:2394–400.

95 Elhage R, Maret A, Pieraggi MT, Thiers JC, Arnal JF, Bayard F. Differential effects of interleukin-1 receptor antagonist and tumor necrosis factor binding protein on fatty-streak formation in apolipoprotein E-deficient mice. Circulation 1998;97:242–4.

7 CHAPTER 7

Effects of TNF-α on cardiac function

Bo Yang & Douglas F. Larson

Introduction

The pro-inflammatory cytokine, tumor necrosis factor (TNF, TNF-α, cachectin), has been found elevated in many heart-disease conditions and is implicated in the pathogenesis of numerous cardiovascular diseases, including heart failure [1]. The direct administration of TNF-α to rodent and human myocardial tissues has consistently shown negative inotropic effects [2–5]. Recently, a cytokine (TNF-α) hypothesis related to heart failure was proposed [6]. Evidence has shown that TNF-α causes its effects through two independent pathways: (1) an immediate sphingosine, nitric oxide (NO)-independent pathway [7] and (2) a delayed NO-dependent pathway [8]. In this chapter, we will discuss how TNF-α acutely affects cardiac function and possible mechanisms, supporting our claims by our original data.

TNF-α and TNF-α receptors

There are two isoforms of TNF-α: a 26-kDa transmembrane pro-TNF and a 17-kDa secreted mature TNF [9]. Newly synthesized pro-TNF is inserted into the plasma membrane and thereafter proteolytically cleaved by a TNF-α-converting enzyme that releases the mature TNF-α. The major resources of TNF-α are immune cells, such as monocytes and macrophages; however, other cells, such as cardiomyocytes [10], smooth muscle cells, and vascular endothelial cells, can also produce TNF-α. The production of TNF-α can be regulated by cytokines and endogenous mediators. TNF-α itself, IL-Iβ, IFN-γ, GM-CSF, IL-2, TGF-β, and platelet-activating factor can upregulate the levels of TNF-α. Conversely, prostaglandins, corticosteroids, IL-4,

IL-6, and TGF-β downregulate the production of TNF-α [11].

There are two distinct TNF-α receptors on multiple cell surfaces: a 55-kDa (TNF-Rl) and a 75-kDa (TNF-R2) protein. The TNF-Rl receptor transduces most of the activity of TNF-α, including cytotoxicity, antiviral activity [12], initiating transcription of pro-inflammatory cytokines [13], and activation of sphingosinase [7]. The TNF-R2 receptor affects T-cell proliferation and dermal necrosis. The cytoplasmic domains of the two receptors are structurally different, suggesting distinctive, evolutionary signal-transduction pathways [6]. Both receptors have been localized in the human myocardium [10]. In addition, there is another TNF-α receptor, the soluble TNF-α receptor, that comes from the ectodomain cleavage of TNF-Rl and TNF-R2. These soluble TNF-α receptors maintain the ability to bind TNF-α, therefore neutralizing the biologic activity of TNF-α. However, since the binding is reversible and the complexes of TNF with soluble receptors are less readily cleared than is free TNF, soluble TNF receptors can also prolong TNF-α retention in the body [14, 15].

TNF-α and cardiac contractile function

Clinical evidence has shown that cytokines are important mediators of cardiac disease and heart failure, and TNF-α is now known to be the most pleiotropic of all cytokines [1, 6]. TNF-α is a pro-inflammatory cytokine that has been implicated in the pathogenesis of cardiovascular diseases, including acute myocardial infarction, unstable angina pectoris, ischemia and reperfusion injury, atherosclerosis, inflammatory myocarditis, cardiac allograft rejection, sepsis-associated cardiac dysfunction, dilated cardiomyopathy, and chronic heart failure [6, 9, 16, 17]. In the murine model of myocarditis, TNF-α was induced rapidly in the myocardium and continued to express during the chronic stage when the heart assumed the typical pattern of dilated cardiomyopathy in the absence of inflammatory processes [17]. Patients with severe chronic heart failure always had elevated levels of TNF-α, independent of disease etiology [6]. The TNF-α transgenic mice showed dilated left ventricles, decreased stoke volumes, cardiac output, and ejection fractions, and died within 4 months after birth [18, 19]. The results indicated that overproduction of TNF-α by myocytes was sufficient to cause severe heart disease and depression of cardiac-contractile function.

The effects of TNF-α have also been investigated with the administration of TNF-α directly to animal models. Eichenholz et al. gave different intravenous doses of human recombinant TNF-α (30, 60, and 120 μg/kg) to three groups of conscious dogs for more than 1 hour [20]. All the groups receiving TNF-α had decreased left ventricle ejection fraction at 2 hours. The depression of LV contractility and the time required for cardiac performance to return to normal were dose dependent. Murray et al. found that after infusing recombinant TNF-α, 40 μg/kg into conscious dogs for 1 hour, the left-ventricle, systolic performance declined from 19 to 35% of baseline value, including decreased dP/dt max and stroke work [21]. Bozkurt et al. placed osmotic infusion pumps into the peritoneal cavity of rats [2]. The continuous infusion of TNF-α led to a time-dependent depression of LV contractility and progressive dilation. However, the removal of infusion and treatment of a soluble TNF-α antagonist partially restored the cardiac function. These reports suggest that administration of TNF-α in both acute and chronic models depresses cardiac function and leads to dilated cardiomyopathy.

To further define the effect of TNF-α on cardiac function, we injected an acute bolus of murine TNF-α 10 μg/kg into mice via the extrajugular vein and simultaneously acquired pressure–volume loops. Table 7.1 shows that within 10 minutes of

Table 7.1 Hemodynamics of TNF-α treated C57BL/6 mice.

Parameter	Unit	Baseline	10 min	20 min	30 min
Ped	mmHg	3.99 ± 0.37	3.74 ± 0.39	3.67 ± 0.42	3.60 ± 0.47
SV	μL	9.91 ± 0.79	8.62 ± 0.85**	7.29 ± 0.90**	6.23 ± 0.62***
EF	%	63.3 ± 3.26	57.4 ± 4.4*	55.4 ± 4.7*	48.3 ± 5.1**
CO	μL	5763 ± 532	4846 ± 553**	4091 ± 569**	3347 ± 383***
SW	mmHg*μL	800 ± 68	582 ± 81***	438 ± 75***	338 ± 54***
Ea	mmHg*μL	8.97 ± 0.81	7.95 ± 0.56	8.73 ± 0.75	8.46 ± 0.90
			Contractility		
dP/dt_{max}	mmHg/s	9904 ± 888	7245 ± 727**	6279 ± 731**	5032 ± 605***
Ees	mmHg/μL	30.2 ± 3.2	19.4 ± 2.71	13.8 ± 1.80*	11.9 ± 1.41**
PRSW	mmHg	101 ± 7.1	74.2 ± 3.76***	63.1 ± 7.49**	46.7 ± 4.99**
dP/dt_{max} −Ved	mmHg/s/μL	776 ± 119	475 ± 71**	394 ± 77**	231 ± 42**
			Relaxation		
dP/dt_{min}	mmHg/s	−6751 ± 519	−5286 ± 542***	−4285 ± 441***	−3771 ± 425***
τ_{Weiss}	ms	5.85 ± 0.30	6.30 ± 0.37**	6.82 ± 0.46**	8.00 ± 0.57***
β	mmHg/μL	0.27 ± 0.01	0.29 ± 0.04	0.33 ± 0.03	0.26 ± 0.05

* $p < 0.05$, ** $p < 0.01$, *** $p < 0.001$ vs baseline.
Ped, end-diastolic pressure; SV, stroke volume; EF, ejection fraction; CO, cardiac output; SW, stroke work; Ees, elastance of end systole; PRSW, preload recruitable stroke work; Ved, end-diastolic volume; τ_{Weiss}, time constant of isovolumic relaxation; β, stiffness of left ventricle.

injection in this in vivo model, there was a significant decrease in most hemodynamic parameters, including (a) the load-dependent parameters: stroke volume, ejection fraction, cardiac output, stroke work, dP/dt max and (b) the load-independent parameters: Ees (elastance of end systole—the slope of end systolic pressure volume relationship), PRSW (preload recruitable stroke work), and the slope of dP/dt max versus end-diastolic volume. These data demonstrate that acute administration of TNF-α affects both contractile and diastolic functions without decreasing vascular tone (Ea: elastance of artery). Figure 7.1a compares the pressure–volume loops at 0 and 20 minutes after TNF-α administration. Most striking was the time-dependent decrease in PRSW, which is the stroke work plotted against the end-diastolic volume (Figure 7.1b).

In support of our findings, the cardiosuppressive effects of TNF-α also have been found on contractility heart tissue and cultured myocytes in vitro. The perfusion of TNF-α (20 ng/mL) under a constant flow (10 mL/min) in the isolated rat heart decreased left ventricular developed pressure [22]. Cain *et al.* used human myocardial trabeculae to test the effects of TNF-α [3]. The developed force of the myocardial trabeculae decreased with concentrations of 125 and 250 pg/mL of TNF-α. Alloatti *et al.* found that TNF-α (1–10 ng/mL) reduced the contractility and the action-potential duration of guinea pig papillary muscle in a concentration-dependent manner [23]. Exposure of myocytes to TNF-α or TNF-α plus IL-1β produced a concentration-dependent increase of intracellular cGMP and parallel decrease of cardiac myocytes shortening [2, 4, 5, 24]. In spontaneously beating cardiomyocytes, TNF-α blocked α- and β-adrenoceptor-stimulated increase in contractility and intracellular cAMP accumulation; in addition, it impaired the impact of high extracellular calcium on contractile performance [25].

In summary, the accumulated evidence supports the concept that TNF-α inhibits cardiac function in a dose-dependent manner and inhibits catecholamine-receptor stimulation through a cGMP–PKG (protein kinase G) pathway. The TNF-α pathway appears to be additive, with endocrine mediators such as norepinephrine, angiotensin II, and endothelin that ultimately lead to cardiac dysfunction and progressive heart failure [6].

(a)

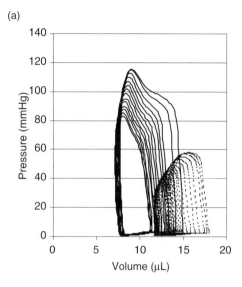

(b)

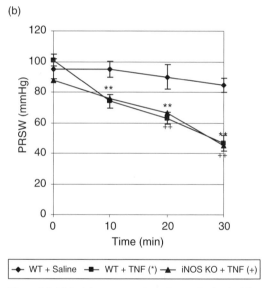

— WT + Saline — WT + TNF (*) — iNOS KO + TNF (+)

Figure 7.1 (a) Serial pressure–volume loops obtained with Millar conductance catheter by compressing inferior vena cava in a C56-black, wild-type mouse. Solid line: baseline; dotted line: 20 minutes after TNF-α intravenous administration. (b) Change of PRSW (preload recruitable stroke work, a load-independent parameter to describe left-ventricle contractility) in three different groups. No significant change of PRSW in WT mice treated with saline. WT, wild type; KO, knockout; **, $p < 0.01$ compared to baseline in WT + TNF-α treatment group; ++, $p < 0.01$ compared to baseline in iNOS KO + TNF-α treatment group.

Mechanisms of TNF-α induced contractile dysfunction

The depression of myocardial contractility induced by TNF-α has a biphasic (immediate and delayed) nature. The immediate depressive effects of TNF-α have been found within minutes in isolated perfused rat hearts (<25 min) [22], isolated hamster papillary muscles, intact left ventricle (10–30 min) [26], cultured myocytes (5–30 min) [7, 24], and mouse hearts in vivo (10 min), as shown in Table 7.1. This immediate effect was correlated with the increased intracellular concentration of sphingosine, which could be abolished by N-oleoylethanolamine, the inhibitor of ceramidase, that catalyzes the reaction to produce sphingosine [7, 22]. Moreover, inducible nitric oxide synthase (iNOS or NOS II) inhibitors could not block the immediate response, further confirming that the immediate response is NO-independent [7]. We also observed that acute cardiosuppressive effects of TNF-α on iNOS-knockout mice were similar to that on the wild-type mice (Figure 7.1b). As a further support, the administration of exogenous sphingosine mimiced the cardiodepressive effects of TNF-α on myocardial contractility [27]. Taken togethers, all those data support the sphingosine pathway (NO-independent pathway) mediates the immediate cardiodepressive effects of TNF-α on myocardial contractility. In contrast, the delayed phase appeared to require hours of TNF-α exposure [1]. Prolonged exposure to TNF-α was found to induce iNOS expression in myocytes [5]. However, iNOS inhibitors were able to effectively block this delayed effect of TNF-α [8, 24]. In summary, acute TNF-α exposure induces a sphingosine-dependent cardiodepression and chronic TNF-α exposure initiates a NO-dependent pathway which leads to cardiac depression and dilation.

Sphingosine pathway (NO-independent pathway)

TNF-α and sphingosine

After TNF-α binding with TNF-α receptor 1 (TNFRI) on the cell surface, myocytes rapidly produce sphingosine which mediates the suppressive effects of TNF-α on cardiac contractility [28, 29]. Wiegmann et al. transfected murine 70Z/3 pre-B cells with a cDNA coding for the human TNFRI, which stably expressed the TNFRI. When these cells were treated with TNF-α, the concentration of diacylglycerol (DAG) and ceramide increased within 2 minutes [29]. By triggering TNFRI, TNF-α activates phosphotidylcholine-specific phospholipase and results in the production of DAG [30–32]. DAG subsequently activates acidic sphingomyelinases, which degrade sphingomyelin to ceramide and phosphocholine [33, 34]. TNF-α can also induce activation of phospholipase Az and results in the release of arachidonic acid (AA) within 5–10 minutes [29, 35]. AA can then directly activate cytosolic sphingomyelinase (neutral sphingomyelinase) which can also produce ceramide [35]. The acute change in ceramide concentration occurs within seconds to minutes by TNF-α stimulation [36]. The accumulated ceramide can activate ceramidase to produce high levels of sphingosine. Sugishita et al. found that sphingosine content was increased to 70% with a concomitant decrease in contractility in hearts perfused with TNF-α (500 U/mL) solution for 5 minutes [27]. The exogenous sphingosine (5 μmol/L) can also mimic the negative inotropic effects of TNF-α within 5 minutes [12]. The ceramidase inhibitor, N-oleoylethanolamine, can completely abrogate the negative inotropic effects of TNF-α in isolated, contracting cardiac myocytes or isolated rat hearts [7, 22]. Taken together, the present findings indicate that sphingosine mediates the immediate negative inotropic effects of TNF-α.

Sphingosine and intracellular Ca^{2+} homeostasis

Sphingosine decreases calcium transients by inhibiting the L-type, calcium-channel current (I_{Ca}) and blocking the ryanodine receptor, which mediates calcium-induced calcium release (CICR) from sarcoplasmic reticulum (SR) [37–40]. The calcium transient represents the transition from the resting state to contraction. It occurs when a small amount of calcium enters the cytosol via voltage-gated, L-type calcium channels, which results in a much greater release of calcium from the ryanodine receptor, calcium-release channel on the SR. These two calcium channels communicate wherever calcium entry through one influences the other [41]. McDonough et al. found that in cardiac myocytes, sphingosine can directly inhibit the I_{Ca}, reducing the entry of trigger Ca^{2+} [38]. The reduction of I_{Ca}

was associated with a reduced rate and magnitude of the Ca^{2+} transient.

Sphingosine can also act on the ryanodine receptor to modulate myocyte-beating behaviors independent of the protein kinase C.

First, sphingosine can significantly block the CICR from isolated cardiac and skeletal SR membranes containing the ryanodine receptor, but cannot modulate the calcium efflux in SR vesicles devoid of the ryanodine receptor [39, 40]. Second, sphingosine had no effects on the SR calcium pump itself [37, 40]. Third, sphingosine significantly reduced [³H]-ryanodine binding to the high-affinity site of the ryanodine receptor in a dose-dependent manner, increasing the K_d for binding by several fold and decreasing B_{max} by half [37, 39]. The binding of [³H]-ryanodine to the high-affinity site on the ryanodine receptor correlates with the abilities of various physiological and pharmacological agents to open the calcium-release channel, including the ability of calcium itself to facilitate channel opening. Conversely, an inhibition of [³H]-ryanodine binding produced by a ligand is likely associated with closure of the calcium-release channel. Therefore, sphingosine can close the calcium-release channel by inhibiting calcium binding with ryanodine receptors to block CICR [37]. Both the inhibition of L-type channels and the blocking of ryanodine receptors cannot be induced by sphingomyelin and its other derivatives such as cerimade and sphinganine, which indicates the specific effects of sphingosine on CICR [37, 39, 40].

The effects of sphingosine on calcium transients are also biphasic. Submicromolar sphingosine can significantly decrease calcium transients, reduce myocyte-beat frequency, and inhibit the spread of activation from sarcomere to sarcomere in myocytes. High concentrations of sphingosine (30–50 μM) were able to induce calcium release by themselves [39, 40]. An explanation is that sphingosine at low concentration could act directly on the channel (negative modulation), but at higher levels it may produce the opposite effects via protein kinase C or CaM kinase [40]. Physiologically, cytoplasmic sphingosine levels are about 0.5 μM because of the degradation of sphingomyelin from the terminal cisternae (TC) membrane, not from the SR membrane [37, 38]. Since sphingosine is pro-

duced by the T-tubule membrane where the L-type calcium channel (DHPR) is located, the level of endogenous sphingosine seen by DHPR could be substantially higher than that seen by the ryanodine receptor. Furthermore, L-type channels may be more sensitive to sphingosine than ryanodine receptors. Therefore, it is possible that physiological levels of sphingosine in the cytosol may be too low to block the ryanodine receptor directly, yet high enough in the surface membrane to substantially affect I_{Ca} [38]. Taken together, sphingosine produced by the sphingomyelin signal-transduction pathway could be physiologically relevant regulators of cardiac-calcium transients and therefore cardiac contractility [38].

If sphingosine serves as a second message for TNF-α to depress myocardial contractility, TNF-α should be able to decrease myocardial calcium transients. It has already been confirmed by several laboratories that TNF-α decreases calcium transients within 5 minutes [26, 27, 42]. Furthermore, in myocytes after 5-minute exposure, TNF-α caused a significant and rapid inhibition of the L-type calcium channel and a progressive decrease in the amplitude of the calcium transients to 43% of control amplitude. Importantly, the time course of TNF-α action on peak calcium transients was similar to that exhibited by TNF-α on the I_{Ca}. In summary, physiologically, sphingosine may serve as a second message to modulate calcium transients by inhibiting L-type calcium channels and ryanodine receptors. In addition, by triggering TNFRI, TNF-α can rapidly activate sphingomyelinase through DAG and AA to produce more sphingosine. Sphingosine mediates the immediate phase (NO-independent) of TNF-α negative inotropic effects in minutes by decreasing calcium transients.

TNF-α also causes cardiac dysfunction through iNOS–NO pathways as a delayed effect. It is well known that the expression of iNOS is transcriptionally regulated by TNF-α [43]. The cloning of a 1.7-kb fragment flanking the transcriptional start site of the murine gene reveals several putative, transcription-factor binding sequences including 10 IFN-γ response elements, 3 γ-activated sites, 2 consensus sequences for nuclear factor-κB (NF-κB) binding and 4 for NF-IL6, 2 TNF-α response elements 2 activating protein-1 binding motifs, 3

IFN-α stimulated response elements, and a basal transcription recognition site (TATA box). Many of these elements are also present in human iNOS promoters [31, 44]. Of all these promoters, the NF-κB site is essential for LPS-induced iNOS transcription, and TNF-α promotes NF-κB expression. Extensive evidence shows that all nucleated cells in the cardiovascular system can express iNOS, including endothelial cells, endocardial cells, fibroblasts, smooth muscle cells, and cardiac myocytes [32]. Once expressed, the cytokine-inducible iNOS produces high levels of NO, which is independent in intracellular calcium and acts for a prolonged time [43, 45]. Therefore, the regulation of iNOS expression is the key step to modulate its activity and effects since posttranscriptional and posttranslational regulation have minor effects on iNOS activity. High doses (μM) of NO, such as NO produced by iNOS, are deleterious to the heart through negative inotropic effects [46–48]. The molecular mechanism of high levels of NO in the heart can be summarized as cGMP-dependent and cGMP-independent pathways, which was reviewed in detail by Yang *et al.* [49].

Clinical trials of targeting TNF-α in heart failure patients

One of the first successful trials of treating heart failure patients by using pentoxifylline to target TNF-α was done by Sliwa *et al.* [50]. Pentoxifylline was found to inhibit the production of TNF-α in both in vivo and in vitro studies [51]. In Sliwa's study, 28 patients with idiopathic, dilated cardiomyopathy were assigned pentoxifylline, 400 mg three times daily or a matching placebo. After 6 months of treatment, the TNF-α plasma concentrations were significantly lower in the pentoxifylline-treated group than in the placebo group (2.1 versus 6.5 pg/mL, $p = 0.001$). The proportion of patients in NYHA functional class I or II was higher in the pentoxifylline group than in the placebo group (14/14 versus 10/14, $p = 0.01$), and ejection fraction was higher in the pentoxifylline group than in the placebo group (mean 38.7% versus 26.8%, $p = 0.04$). After that Sliwa continued adding pentoxifylline to the standard heart failure treatment in patients with peripartum cardiomyopathy [52], de-

compensated congestive heart failure secondary to idiopathic dilated cardiomyopathy [51], and ischemic cardiomyopathy [50]. All these clinical trials showed decreased plasma TNF-α levels, increased left-ventricular ejection fractions, and improved clinical outcomes.

Besides pentoxifylline trials, a soluble TNF antagonist (etanercept) was used clinically to neutralize TNF-α in patients with heart failure. (This antagonist consists of the extracellular domains of the sTNFR2 fused in duplicate to the Fc portion of the IgG molecule.) Deswal *et al.* studied 18 patients with NYHA, class-III heart failure by adding a single dose of etanercept to the standard treatment of heart failure they were receiving, including digitalis, diuretics, and ACE inhibitors [53]. Fourteen days after the treatment, there was a significant decrease in TNF bioactivity and a significant improvement of ejection fraction, 6-minute walking distance, and quality of life.

Based on the positive results of those small studies, two larger randomized clinical trials in which patients with moderate to severe heart failure were treated repeatedly with etanercept over longer periods of time were launched in the United States (Randomized Etanercept North American Strategy to Study Antagonism of Cytokines [RENAISSANCE]) and in Europe and Australia (Research into Etanercept Cytokine Antagonism in Ventricular Dysfunction [RECOVER]). However, both studies failed to show efficacy [54].

It is unclear why etanercept did not show any efficacy in these two large trials. As mentioned above, TNF-α is a strong stimulant of iNOS expression in the myocardium, which produces a high concentration of NO. Besides inhibiting ventricular contractility, high concentrations of NO can also cause cell death by forming peroxynitrite, ONOO⁻ [49]. With chronic exposure to TNF-α, myocardial cell death could be significant. Although TNF-α could be neutralized by etanercept, it could not reverse myocyte death. TNF-α stimulates the myocardial matrix metalloproteinase (MMP) activity and can lead to degradation of the extracellular matrix in the myocardium [55]. In idiopathic, dilated cardiomyopathy patients, circulating TNF-α, MMP-1, MMP-3, and MMP-9 were all increased. There was a strong association between the circulating level of MMPs and TNF-α [56]. For the same reason, the degradation of the extracellular matrix cannot be easily reversed by neutralization of TNF-α with etanercept. TNF-α also stimulates endothelial nitric oxide synthase (eNOS) expression. eNOS produces a low concentration of NO, which is beneficial to the heart [49]. Eliminating TNF-α with etanercept may decrease eNOS expression, canceling the beneficial effects of low doses of NO made by eNOS. Though anti-TNF-α therapy was not efficacious in the RENAISSANCE and RECOVER studies, it demonstrated decreased rates of myocardial infarction and mortality due to cardiovascular diseases in rheumatoid arthritis patients [57, 58].

In summary, TNF-α can acutely or directly cause cardiac dysfunction through sphingosine pathways. TNF-α can cause chronic damage to the heart by stimulating iNOS and MMP expression. Disappointingly, eliminating TNF-α with a soluble TNF-α receptor did not show beneficial effects on heart failure patients. More studies need to be done on modulating cytokines (TNF-α) in heart failure patients.

References

1 Meldrum DR. Tumor necrosis factor in the heart. Am J Physiol 1998;274(3 Pt 2):R577–95.

2 Bozkurt B, Kribbs SB, Clubb FJ *et al.* Pathophysiologically relevant concentrations of tumor necrosis factor-alpha promote progressive left ventricular dysfunction and remodeling in rats. Circulation 1998;97(14):1382–91.

3 Cain BS, Meldrum DR, Dinarello CA *et al.* Tumor necrosis factor-alpha and interleukin-1beta synergistically depress human myocardial function. Crit Care Med 1999;27(7):1309–18.

4 Kumar A, Thota V, Dee L, Olson J, Uretz E, Parrillo JE. Tumor necrosis factor alpha and interleukin 1beta are responsible for in vitro myocardial cell depression induced by human septic shock serum. J Exp Med 1996;183(3):949–58.

5 Kumar A, Brar R, Wang P *et al.* Role of nitric oxide and cGMP in human septic serum-induced depression of cardiac myocyte contractility. Am J Physiol 1999;276(1 Pt 2):R265–76.

6 Francis GS. TNF-alpha and heart failure: the difference between proof of principle and hypothesis testing. Circulation 1999;99(25):3213–14.

7 Oral H, Dorn GW, Mann DL. Sphingosine mediates the immediate negative inotropic effects of tumor necrosis factor-alpha in the adult mammalian cardiac myocyte. J Biol Chem 1997;272(8):4836–42.

8 Panas D, Khadour FH, Szabo C, Schulz R. Proinflammatory cytokines depress cardiac efficiency by a nitric oxide-dependent mechanism. Am J Physiol 1998;275(3 Pt 2):H1016–23.

9 Ferrari R. The role of TNF in cardiovascular disease. Pharmacol Res 1999;40(2):97–105.

10 Torre-Amione G, MacLellan W, Kapadia S *et al.* Tumor necrosis factor-alpha is persistently expressed in cardiac allografts in the absence of histological or clinical evidence of rejection. Transplant Proc 1998;30(3):875–7.

11 Neta R, Sayers TJ, Oppenheim JJ. Relationship of TNF to interleukins. Immunol Ser 1992;56:499–566.

12 Tartaglia LA, Ayres TM, Wong GH, Goeddel DV. A novel domain within the 55 kd TNF receptor signals cell death. Cell 1993;74(5):845–53.

13 Ashkenazi A, Dixit VM. Death receptors: signaling and modulation. Science 1998;281(5381):1305–8.

14 Aderka D, Engelmann H, Maor Y, Brakebusch C, Wallach D. Stabilization of the bioactivity of tumor necrosis factor by its soluble receptors. J Exp Med 1992;175(2):323–9.

15 Engelmann H, Aderka D, Rubinstein M, Rotman D, Wallach D. A tumor necrosis factor-binding protein purified to homogeneity from human urine protects cells from tumor necrosis factor toxicity. J Biol Chem 1989;264(20):11974–80.

16 Cain BS, Meldrum DR, Joo KS *et al.* Human SERCA2a levels correlate inversely with age in senescent human myocardium. J Am Coll Cardiol 1998;32(2):458–67.

17 Sasayama S, Matsumori A, Kihara Y. New insights into the pathophysiological role for cytokines in heart failure. Cardiovasc Res 1999;42(3):557–64.

18 Bryant D, Becker L, Richardson J *et al.* Cardiac failure in transgenic mice with myocardial expression of tumor necrosis factor-alpha. Circulation 1998;97(14):1375–81.

19 Franco F, Thomas GD, Giroir B *et al.* Magnetic resonance imaging and invasive evaluation of development of heart failure in transgenic mice with myocardial expression of tumor necrosis factor-alpha. Circulation 1999;99(3):448–54.

20 Eichenholz PW, Eichacker PQ, Hoffman WD *et al.* Tumor necrosis factor challenges in canines: patterns of cardiovascular dysfunction. Am J Physiol 1992;263(3 Pt 2):H668–75.

21 Murray DR, Freeman GL. Tumor necrosis factor-alpha induces a biphasic effect on myocardial contractility in conscious dogs. Circ Res 1996;78(1):154–160.

22 Edmunds NJ, Lal H, Woodward B. Effects of tumour necrosis factor-alpha on left ventricular function in the rat isolated perfused heart: possible mechanisms for a decline in cardiac function. Br J Pharmacol 1999;126(1):189–96.

23 Alloatti G, Penna C, De Martino A, Montrucchio G, Camussi G. Role of nitric oxide and platelet-activating factor in cardiac alterations induced by tumor necrosis factor-alpha in the guinea-pig papillary muscle. Cardiovasc Res 1999;41(3):611–9.

24 Goldhaber JI, Kim KH, Natterson PD, Lawrence T, Yang P, Weiss JN. Effects of TNF-alpha on [Ca2+]i and contractility in isolated adult rabbit ventricular myocytes. Am J Physiol 1996;271(4 Pt 2):H1449–55.

25 Kumar A, Kosuri R, Kandula P, Dimou C, Allen J, Parrillo JE. Effects of epinephrine and amrinone on contractility and cyclic adenosine monophosphate generation of tumor necrosis factor alpha-exposed cardiac myocytes. Crit Care Med 1999;27(2):286–92.

26 Yokoyama T, Vaca L, Rossen RD, Durante W, Hazarika P, Mann DL. Cellular basis for the negative inotropic effects of tumor necrosis factor-alpha in the adult mammalian heart. J Clin Invest 1993;92(5):2303–12.

27 Sugishita K, Kinugawa K, Shimizu T et al. Cellular basis for the acute inhibitory effects of IL-6 and TNF-alpha on excitation-contraction coupling. J Mol Cell Cardiol 1999;31(8):1457–67.

28 Kim MY, Linardic C, Obeid L, Hannun Y. Identification of sphingomyelin turnover as an effector mechanism for the action of tumor necrosis factor alpha and gamma-interferon. Specific role in cell differentiation. J Biol Chem 1991;266(1):484–9.

29 Wiegmann K, Schutze S, Kampen E, Himmler A, Machleidt T, Kronke M. Human 55-kDa receptor for tumor necrosis factor coupled to signal transduction cascades. J Biol Chem 1992;267(25):17997–8001.

30 Xie QW, Whisnant R, Nathan C. Promoter of the mouse gene encoding calcium-independent nitric oxide synthase confers inducibility by interferon gamma and bacterial lipopolysaccharide. J Exp Med 1993;177(6):1779–84.

31 Nunokawa Y, Ishida N, Tanaka S. Promoter analysis of human inducible nitric oxide synthase gene associated with cardiovascular homeostasis. Biochem Biophys Res Commun 1994;200(2):802–7.

32 Stoclet JC, Muller B, Gyorgy K, Andriantsiothaina R, Kleschyov AL. The inducible nitric oxide synthase in vascular and cardiac tissue. Eur J Pharmacol 1999; 375(1–3):139–55.

33 Kolesnick RN. Sphingomyelin and derivatives as cellular signals. Prog Lipid Res 1991;30(1):1–38.

34 Schutze S, Machleidt T, Kronke M. The role of diacylglycerol and ceramide in tumor necrosis factor and interleukin-1 signal transduction. J Leukoc Biol 1994; 56(5):533–41.

35 Jayadev S, Linardic CM, Hannun YA. Identification of arachidonic acid as a mediator of sphingomyelin hydrolysis in response to tumor necrosis factor alpha. J Biol Chem 1994;269(8):5757–63.

36 Hannun YA. Functions of ceramide in coordinating cellular responses to stress. Science 1996;274(5294):1855–9.

37 Dettbarn CA, Betto R, Salviati G, Palade P, Jenkins GM, Sabbadini RA. Modulation of cardiac sarcoplasmic reticulum ryanodine receptor by sphingosine. J Mol Cell Cardiol 1994;26(2):229–42.

38 McDonough PM, Yasui K, Betto R et al. Control of cardiac Ca^{2+} levels. Inhibitory actions of sphingosine on Ca^{2+} transients and L-type Ca^{2+} channel conductance. Circ Res 1994;75(6):981–9.

39 Sabbadini RA, Betto R, Teresi A, Fachechi-Cassano G, Salviati G. The effects of sphingosine on sarcoplasmic reticulum membrane calcium release. J Biol Chem 1992;267(22):15475–84.

40 Webster RJ, Sabbadini RA, Dettbarn CA, Paolini PJ. Sphingosine effects on the contractile behavior of skinned cardiac myocytes. J Mol Cell Cardiol 1994;26(10):1273–90.

41 Meldrum DR, Cleveland JC, Jr, Cain BS, Meng X, Harken AH. Increased myocardial tumor necrosis factor-alpha in a crystalloid-perfused model of cardiac ischemia-reperfusion injury. Ann Thorac Surg 1998;65(2):439–43.

42 Krown KA, Yasui K, Brooker MJ et al. TNF alpha receptor expression in rat cardiac myocytes: TNF alpha inhibition of L-type Ca2+ current and Ca2+ transients. FEBS Lett 1995;376(1–2):24–30.

43 Sanders DB, Larson DF, Jablonowski C, Olsen L. Differential expression of inducible nitric oxide synthase in septic shock. J Extracorporeal Tech 1999;31:118–24.

44 Lowenstein CJ, Alley EW, Raval P et al. Macrophage nitric oxide synthase gene: two upstream regions mediate induction by interferon gamma and lipopolysaccharide. Proc Natl Acad Sci U S A 1993;90(20):9730–4.

45 Xie QW, Kashiwabara Y, Nathan C. Role of transcription factor NF-kappa B/Rel in induction of nitric oxide synthase. J Biol Chem 1994;269(7):4705–8.

46 Drexler H, Kastner S, Strobel A, Studer R, Brodde OE, Hasenfuss G. Expression, activity and functional significance of inducible nitric oxide synthase in the failing human heart. J Am Coll Cardiol 1998;32(4):955–63.

47 Paulus WJ, Bronzwaer JG. Myocardial contractile effects of nitric oxide. Heart Fail Rev 2002;7(4):371–83.

48 Drexler H. Nitric oxide synthases in the failing human heart: a doubled-edged sword? Circulation 1999;99(23): 2972–5.

49 Yang B, Larson DF, Watson RR. Inducible nitric oxide synthase (iNOS) and heart failure. In: Watson RR, Preedy VR, eds. Nutrition and heart disease. CRC Press, New York, 2004:333–50.

50 Sliwa K, Woodiwiss A, Kone VN et al. Therapy of ischemic cardiomyopathy with the immunomodulating agent pentoxifylline: results of a randomized study. Circulation 2004;109(6):750–5.

51 Sliwa K, Woodiwiss A, Candy G *et al.* Effects of pentox-ifylline on cytokine profiles and left ventricular perfor-mance in patients with decompensated congestive heart failure secondary to idiopathic dilated cardiomyopathy. Am J Cardiol 2002;90(10):1118–22.

52 Sliwa K, Skudicky D, Candy G, Bergemann A, Hopley M, Sareli P. The addition of pentoxifylline to conventional therapy improves outcome in patients with peripartum cardiomyopathy. Eur J Heart Fail 2002;4(3):305–9.

53 Deswal A, Bozkurt B, Seta Y *et al.* Safety and efficacy of a soluble P75 tumor necrosis factor receptor (Enbrel, etanercept) in patients with advanced heart failure. Cir-culation 1999;99(25):3224–6.

54 Mann DL, McMurray JJ, Packer M *et al.* Targeted anti-cytokine therapy in patients with chronic heart failure: results of the Randomized Etanercept Worldwide Evalu-ation (RENEWAL). Circulation 2004;109(13):1594–602.

55 Siwik DA, Chang DL, Colucci WS. Interleukin-1beta and tumor necrosis factor-alpha decrease collagen syn-thesis and increase matrix metalloproteinase activity in cardiac fibroblasts in vitro. Circ Res 2000;86(12): 1259–65.

56 Ohtsuka T, Hamada M, Saeki H *et al.* Serum levels of matrix metalloproteinases and tumor necrosis factor-alpha in patients with idiopathic dilated cardiomyopa-thy and effect of carvedilol on these levels. Am J Cardiol 2003;91(8):1024–7, A8.

57 Dixon WG, Watson K, Lunt M, Hyrich KL, Silman AJ, Symmons DP. Rates of serious infection, including site-specific and bacterial intracellular infection, in rheuma-toid arthritis patients receiving anti-tumor necrosis factor therapy: results from the British Society for Rheumatol-ogy Biologics Register. Arthritis Rheum 2006;54(8):2368–76.

58 Marzo-Ortega H, McGonagle D, Haugeberg G, Green MJ, Stewart SP, Emery P. Bone mineral density improvement in spondyloarthropathy after treatment with etanercept. Ann Rheum Dis 2003;62(10):1020–1.

CHAPTER 8

Immunosuppression in promotion of cardiac allograft vasculopathy

Farzad Moien-Afshari, Jonathan Choy,
Bruce M. McManus & Ismail Laher

Introduction

Heart transplantation is one of the few effective means of treating end-stage heart disease and as of June 2003, more than 63,000 heart transplantations had been performed worldwide [1]. The main clinical conditions requiring heart transplantation are (i) dilated cardiomyopathy (56%), (ii) coronary artery disease (32%), (iii) retransplantation (5%), and (iv) other reasons (7%) [2]. Due largely to improved clinical management, the survival rates for cardiac transplant patients have increased significantly as compared with statistics two decades ago. However, patient survival is only 50% within 10 years of transplantation and of great concern is that most cardiac allografts will fail within 20 years. This is especially critical in pediatric heart transplantation. The main reason for graft failure is allograft vascular disease; malignancy and infections are also responsible for some late deaths in recipients [3]. Cardiac allograft vasculopathy (CAV) is a rapidly progressive and unique form of atherosclerosis, which is clinically apparent in up to 60% of transplant recipients within the first 5 years following surgery [4]. By the end of the first-year post-transplantation, intimal thickening occurs in 75% of cardiac transplant arteries as assessed by intravascular coronary ultrasound techniques [5]. CAV is a limiting factor in the long-term success of cardiac transplantation, since it is the main cause of death in long-term survivors [6]. Importantly, myocardial ischemia and related infarction occurring secondary to CAV in such patients is usually silent due to the lack of cardiac innervation. Therefore, instead of chest pain, more serious events such as congestive heart failure, ventricular arrhythmias, and sudden death are commonly the first clinical manifestations [7]. Even if CAV is diagnosed early, routine cardiologic methods of treatment such as balloon angioplasty or coronary bypass grafting will be less effective in cardiac transplant recipients than in the nontransplant patients since these patients suffer from both proximal and distal arteriopathy [8, 9].

Insufficient immunosuppression is recognized as contributing to allograft vascular disease. However, greater immunosuppression is limited by several factors including increased risk of malignancy and infection, and cytotoxicity to target organs [3]. Early CAV manifests as a dysfunction of arterial endothelial and smooth muscle cells (SMCs), and as such, changes in arterial function including endothelium-dependent relaxation and myogenic tone are apparent and can be monitored to assess the early progression of CAV [10–12]. Myogenic tone is an inherent ability of the vascular smooth muscle of small arteries and arterioles to constrict in response to an increase in transmural pressure, and is a critical determinant of coronary autoregulation of blood flow. Recent studies demonstrate that in allograft rat coronary septal arteries, myogenic tone is profoundly inhibited compared with site- and size-matched isograft arteries, resulting in greatly increased arterial diameters at all pressures [11, 12]. Vasodilatation of resistance arteries will increase coronary flow, which can lead to deterioration of coronary circulatory homeostasis and cause interstitial edema. The resulting edema decreases cardiac muscle compliance and contractile ability sufficiently enough to cause ventricular failure [13].

This chapter summarizes the key concepts related to CAV and is followed by a discussion of changes that occur in cardiac transplant resistance arteries, the clinical outcome, and the effects of immunosuppression.

Cardiac allograft vasculopathy

Although CAV resembles atherosclerosis, there are several differences between this phenomenon and the native form of atherosclerosis (Table 8.1). In CAV, the lesions are diffuse and generally concentric, and involve all portions of coronary vessels. These lesions ultimately affect the entire length of the artery. Calcification is typically uncommon in these lesions until very late, damage to the internal elastic lamina is comparatively mild, a low-grade vasculitis (under the influence of immunosuppression) is at times observed, and the disease develops quickly. This contrasts with traditional forms of atherosclerosis where lesions are focal, eccentric, and geometrically complex, and are prominent in the proximal portion of major epicardial coronary arteries. Calcium deposits are typically present in these lesions when mature, the internal elastic lamina is often severely disrupted, and it takes years for lesions to develop in absence of major single gene defects [14]. Although CAV lesions are diffuse, occasionally focal atherosclerotic plaques with traditional characteristics can also be present and may represent an underlying superimposed native atherosclerotic process, native heart vascular disease [18], or late-stage degeneration.

Frank atherosclerotic changes of CAV are initiated early after transplantation. During the early stages, CAV involves intimal infiltration and proliferation of T lymphocytes and macrophages, migration and proliferation of SMCs, and the circumferential insudation and accumulation of lipids in the intima. Cellular hyperproliferation, along with lipid insudation [19] and matrix alterations, results in intimal thickening, which ultimately causes decreased lumen size and distal vessel occlusion. The distal occlusions do not reflect more severe disease biologically, but rather the comparative geometric consequences of a given amount of intimal thickening on the relatively smaller original lumen of distal vessels and their branch points. While intimal thickening may be prominent, the media of these vessels rarely shows proliferative changes and indeed the media in these arteries becomes thinner and with much more matrix than present in normal arteries [20]. The unique type of vascular lesion characteristic of CAV is not limited to cardiac transplant vasculature and may occur almost with similar characteristics in renal allograft arteries and in arteries of other solid organ allografts [21–23].

Table 8.1 A comparison between histopathological findings in CAV and CAD.

Histopathology	CAV	CAD
Development period	Months	Years
Vascular localization	Diffuse	Focal and proximal
Lipid*	Prominent, early and late	Prominent, generally later
Prominent accumulated lipid[†]	Apolipoproteins a, B, and E	Apolipoprotein B and E
Intimal proliferation	Concentric	Eccentric
Calcium deposit	In late stages	Frequent
Vasculitis	Occasionally	Generally absent
Internal elastic lamina	Mildly disrupted	Disrupted and frequently reduplicated
Main inflammatory cell involved/mechanism of death[††]	Macrophages, CD4[+] and CD8[+] T cells/Fas and granule-mediated apoptosis	Macrophages and CD4[+] T cells/apoptosis
Prominent proteoglycan[†]	Biglycan, versican	Decorin

CAD, coronary artery disease; CAV, coronary allograft vasculopathy [14].
*Reference [15].
[†]Reference [16].
[††]Reference [17].

The detailed pathogenesis of CAV is incomplete, but both immunologic and nonimmunologic mechanisms are major contributors. The evidence suggesting a primary immunologic basis for CAV is as follows: First, proliferative vascular disease is limited to allograft arteries and does not involve the host's vessels. Second, the nature of allograft vascular involvement is usually diffuse. Third, in animal models, CAV develops severely and is accelerated with greater allograft histocompatibility mismatch. Fourth, under matching conditions of nonimmunologic risk factors and duration of ischemia–reperfusion, CAV occurs only in allografts whereas isograft arteries are spared [7, 20]. The nonimmunologic risk factors that may contribute to the development of CAV include peritransplantation ischemia [24], age, sex, obesity, hypertension, dyslipidemia, smoking, diabetes, and donor characteristics [25].

The host's T-lymphocyte interactions with endothelial- and antigen-presenting cells displaying alloantigens start and sustain the inflammatory response against the graft tissue [26]. Host T cells are triggered by two signals: (a) foreign MHC plus peptide and (b) costimulatory signals. The antigen presenting cells, which present the foreign antigen in the context of MHC-peptide molecules, can be either of donor origin (direct antigen presentation) or of recipient origin (indirect antigen presentation) [4]. The principal costimulatory signals from the antigen-presenting cells are CD80 and CD86, which interact with a receptor on the T cell called CD28 [27]. Other costimulatory molecules have been described and also contribute to transplant rejection [28]. The appropriate signals from the antigen-presenting cell, together with foreign antigen (MHC plus peptide), activate T cells (Figure 8.1). Upon activation CD4+ lymphocytes produce IL-2, and either IFNγ or IL-4 and -5. IL-2 and IFNγ further activate CD4+ lymphocytes and also assist in CD8+ differentiation (direct cytotoxicity) [30]. IL-4 and -5 activate B cells (humoral immunity), and other cytokines increase vascular permeability and regional accumulation of mononuclear cells (Figure 8.1).

Endothelial cell dysfunction and damage is an initial event in the development of CAV. Thus, an early initiating event of CAV may be subclinical graft coronary endothelial injury. Functional studies show that endothelial cell response to acetylcholine (ACh) is compromised and therefore loss of ACh dilation is a useful early marker of CAV [31–33]. Studies in animal models of CAV have demonstrated early loss of endothelial integrity, which is inhibited by cyclosporine A (CsA) [34]. Also, histological studies of human CAV specimens reveal a significant level of endothelial cell apoptosis early during the development of CAV, which appears to subside with time [15]. Such endothelial injury has also been documented in kidney transplants [35]. An intact endothelium is required for the normal regulation of vascular wall function, which includes the inhibition of leukocyte adhesion, thrombus formation, vascular SMC proliferation, and regulation of vasomotor function [36]. Thus, endothelial damage/loss could alter any or all of these functions and lead to lymphocyte and macrophage adhesion to the vascular wall and induction of inflammation, thrombosis, smooth muscle proliferation, and vasoconstriction [37].

The host immune response is a key contributor to endothelial damage following transplantation. In response to infected or foreign cells/tissues, cytotoxic T cells of the host immune system can induce cell death of target cells through the Fas/FasL and/or granzyme/perforin pathways [38]. Histological studies of human CAV specimens indicate that endothelial cells undergoing apoptosis also express Fas (the death ligand for FasL), suggesting that this pathway is involved in inducing endothelial cell apoptosis [15]. Furthermore, perforin-expressing T cells have been observed immediately adjacent to damaged and/or dysfunctional endothelium in human CAV [39].

Animal models of CAV have further illustrated that both the Fas/FasL and granzyme/perforin pathways play an important role in the development of this disease. In mouse models of allograft vasculopathy, there is reduced intimal hyperplasia when vessels are transplanted into mice deficient in functional FasL or when FasL is inhibited by overexpression of soluble Fas within the vasculature [40, 41]. In the latter report, the inhibition of apoptosis within the vessel wall was suggested to be the mechanism by which blockade of FasL inhibited allograft vasculopathy. In addition to the FasL cytotoxic pathway, the granzyme/perforin pathway may also contribute to the pathogenesis

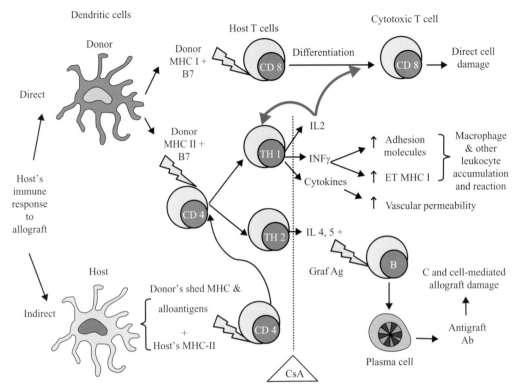

Figure 8.1 Schematic representation of the direct and indirect pathways of the events that lead to the destruction of allograft tissue and the possible modulation by cyclosporine A (CsA). Donor class I and class II MHC antigens along with B7 molecules on the surface of donor's dendritic cells are recognized by host CD8+ cytotoxic T cells and CD4+ helper T cells, respectively. In response to MHC class II antigens, CD4+ cells proliferate and differentiate to TH1 and TH2 cells. TH1 releases IL-2, thereby causing further proliferation of CD4+ cells and signaling the differentiation of CD8+ cytotoxic cells. TH1 cells also secrete interferon-γ (INF-γ) and other cytokines, which potentiate the expression of MHC molecules on graft ETCs and increase vascular permeability, respectively. TH1 cells are also responsible for the induction of a local delayed hypersensitivity reaction. Activation of TH2-type CD4+ cells generates IL-4 and IL-5, which promote B-cell differentiation. Eventually, the following mechanisms act in concert to destroy allograft tissue: (1) lysis of cells bearing MHC class I by CD8+ cytotoxic T cells; (2) antigraft antibodies produced by plasma cells; and (3) nonspecific damage induced by macrophages and other leukocytes, which accumulate as a result of the delayed hypersensitivity reaction. CsA blocks the production of cytokines by T cells. Ag, antigen; Ab, antibody; C, complement. (With permission from Reference [29].)

of CAV. In a minor histocompatibility mismatch model of cardiac transplantation, there is an early loss of endothelial integrity and significant apoptosis within the endothelial layer of allograft arteries [42]. Transplantation of hearts into mice that are deficient in perforin ameliorates the loss of endothelial integrity in allograft, reduces the number of apoptotic cells in the endothelial layer of allograft arteries, and significantly reduces intimal thickening [42]. Similar results were also observed in mice deficient in granzyme B [43].

Together, these studies demonstrate that the FasL and granzyme/perforin pathways are important inducers of endothelial injury in cardiac transplantation, and that these pathways and associated events contribute to the pathogenesis of CAV.

In addition to immune-mediated endothelial damage, a "smoldering" immune response within the vasculature may be important in the pathogenesis of CAV through the production of cytokines, which have the ability to influence vascular cell proliferation and activation [44]. Interferon-γ is a particularly important cytokine in this process as is evident by the amelioration of CAV in hearts transplanted into mice deficient in IFNγ in a MHC class II mismatch model of cardiac transplant rejection [45]. Tellides *et al.* [46] have also shown, using a humanized mouse model of vascular disease, that IFNγ is sufficient for the induction of intimal hyperplasia and that the mechanism involves an indirect stimulation of SMC proliferation. Other cytokines, such as TNF, also contribute to the pathogenesis of CAV [47]. As such, the accumulation of T cells within the vasculature of allograft arteries may induce intimal hyperplasia through the secretion of cytokines.

In addition to the above-mentioned cell-mediated processes involved in the pathogenesis of CAV, antibody-mediated processes may also play a role by inducing endothelial damage and/or activation [48]. Circulating antibodies to several host antigens have been detected in patients with CAV [49, 50]. Also, CAV is reduced in hearts transplanted into hosts lacking a functional complement cascade [51]. The mechanisms through which antibodies induce CAV remain an area of active study but are likely to involve endothelial lysis and/or activation.

Nonimmunologic factors are also involved in endothelial cell damage during the course of allograft rejection. Ischemia and reperfusion injury may be an important nonimmunologic injury during the initial transplantation process, which results in the activation of the endothelium of small vessels to produce oxygen-free radicals, which in turn activates host leukocytes passing through the vessel [52]. Activated leukocytes release mediators that cause acute inflammation, leading to endothelial dysfunction [53].

At both early and late stages posttransplantation, the host's immune response is the major source of endothelial dysfunction.

Cyclosporine A

CsA is a potent immunosuppressive agent that revolutionized clinical transplantation in the early 1980s. It has since received widespread clinical use and represents the prototypical immunosuppressive agent. Its molecular structure consists of a cyclic polypeptide having 11 amino acids, and it is derived as a metabolite of the fungus *Beauveria nivea* [31]. The relative advantage of CsA over cytotoxic immunosuppressants is its selectivity (although not absolutely—e.g., CsA can also affect the mitochondrial permeability pore, an important regulator of cell function in a number of cell types) for interaction with the immune system, particularly T lymphocytes, thereby not destroying other rapidly proliferating cells.

CsA is able to suppress immune responses by inhibiting the signal transduction pathway responsible for the activation of B- and T lymphocytes. The mechanism whereby CsA produces immunosuppression includes the following steps [54] and is illustrated in Figure 8.2:

1 Following entry into the T-cell cytoplasm, CsA binds to the binding protein "cyclophilin," a protein from the immunophilin family [62].

2 This causes the formation of an intra-cytoplasmic CsA/cyclophilin complex.

3 The cytoplasmic CsA/cyclophilin complex acts as a composite surface able to inhibit the phosphatase activity of calcineurin [63, 64]. Calcineurin is a calmodulin-dependent serine/threonine phosphatase and is a key participant in T-cell activation.

4 Calcineurin inhibition prevents the dephosphorylation of nuclear factor of activated T cells (NFAT), leading to full blockade of the translocation of NFAT from the cytoplasm to the nucleus. NFAT is a multisubunit protein consisting of a cytosolic fraction (NF-Atc) and a nuclear subunit (NF-Atn). NFAT expression occurs mainly in cells of the immune system where it has a key role in the regulation of a large number of inducible genes during the immune response such as activation of the IL-2 gene [65].

5 Blockade of activation of the genes regulated by the NFAT/transcription factor activator protein-1 in lymphocytes, such as those required for B lymphocytes recruitment (e.g., CD40 ligand) as well as those necessary for T-helper and T-cytotoxic lymphocyte proliferation, for example, IL-2.

There is also evidence that CsA participates in the expansion of the T-suppressor (T-regulatory cell) population [66]. Finally, CsA disrupts lymphokine-dependent T-cell-macrophage interactions [67].

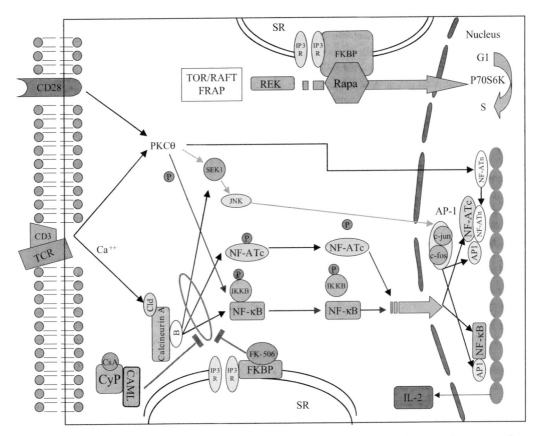

Figure 8.2 The inhibitory effect of CsA and FK506 is mediated through the blockade of several calcineurin-mediated transcription pathways that act on the IL-2 gene. TCR/CD3 stimulation, together with Ca^{2+} binding to calmodulin, activates calcineurin, which dephosphorylates cytoplasmic NFAT (cNFAT). Upon dephosphorylation, cNFAT migrates to the nucleus and forms a dimer after binding to activated nNFAT. This complex activates IL-2 gene transcription. Nuclear NFAT becomes activated directly by PKCθ, and its activation is not dependent on calcineurin. CsA and FK506 bind to their associated cytoplasmic immunophilins (cyclophilin and FKBP, respectively). These complexes make a composite surface that will block calcineurin dephosphorylation and thereby decrease IL-2 production. TCR signals alone can activate calcineurin; however, a secondary signal from CD28 is necessary to activate PKCθ. PKCθ is able to activate IKKB (dark-blue arrows) and SEK1/JNK (green arrows) and these two pathways will activate NF-κB and c-Jun/cFos (AP-1), respectively. Finally, the transcription factors bind to their binding site on the IL-2 gene and will increase its product, IL-2. Potential drugs (to be invented) that could block PKCθ function selectively could induce T-cell suppression and thereby protect allograft tissue NF-κB normally bound to IKKB in the cytoplasm of noninduced cells. Phosphorylation of IKKB by PKC in the presence of Ca^{2+} and calcineurin, followed by proteolysis, will allow NF-κB to enter the nucleus and stimulate transcription. Inhibition of calcineurin function via CsA will prevent NF-κB to enter the nucleus. As can also be seen in the figure, FKBP is linked to IP3 receptor and modifies its function. Similar to FK506, rapamycin also binds to FKBP but possesses a different mechanism of immunosuppression. Rapamycin-FKBP complex binds to rapamycin effector kinases, RAFT/TOR and FRAP [55–57], which are kinases on the pathway whereby cytokines trigger the cell cycle. This makes an even larger complex that is not able to enter the nucleus where it normally activates other kinases, such as p70S6K [58, 59]. Activation of p70S6K is involved in cell-cycle progression [60, 61]. Therefore, in the presence of rapamycin, T cells cannot become activated in response to cytokines (e.g., IL-2). AP-1, activating protein-1; CN, calcineurin; CsA, cyclosporine A; IKKB, Ikappa B kinase beta; IL-2, interleukin 2; IP3, inositol triphosphate; JNK, c-Jun N-terminal kinase; NFAT, nuclear factor of activated T cells; NF-κB, nuclear factor kappa B; OCT-1, octamer binding protein-1; PKC, protein kinase C; PKCθ, protein kinase Cθ; SEK1, SPAK kinase; TCR, T-cell receptor. (With permission from Reference [29].).

Endothelium-dependent and endothelium-independent relaxation in septal coronary arteries of transplanted hearts: a progressive dysfunction without treatment

CsA treatment and endothelial function

We recently demonstrated that the endothelium-mediated vasodilatory response to ACh was significantly lower at day 21 posttransplantation and not at earlier time points (e.g., day 4 posttransplantation) in untreated allograft rat-isolated coronary arteries [11] (Figure 8.3). This observation is in agreement with other studies demonstrating endothelial cell malfunction in allograft arteries as manifested by a blunted vasodilator response to ACh [68, 69]. However, coronary arteries from CsA-treated allograft recipient rats maintained their ability to dilate to ACh to a similar extent as in arteries from an

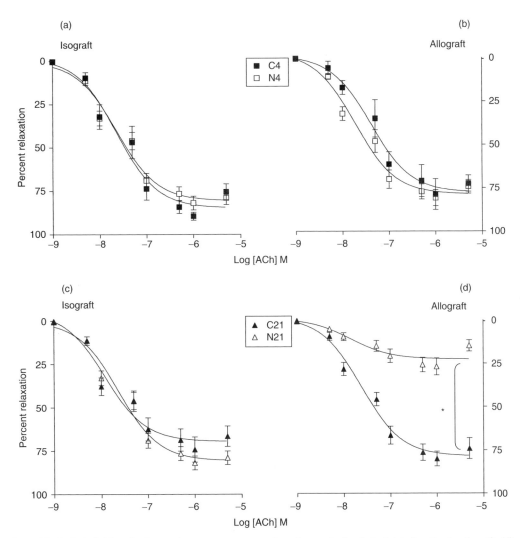

Figure 8.3 Endothelial function is septal coronary arteries of grafted hearts. Endothelial dysfunction does not exist on day 4 posttransplantation in both isograft and allograft hearts (a, b). On day 21 posttransplantation, although endothelial function is intact in isografts (c), there is a marked endothelial dysfunction in allografts (d) (*$p < 0.01$). CsA treatment (5 mg/kg) prevents endothelial function in allografts up to day 21 posttransplantation. (With permission from Reference [11].)

isograft recipient rat (Figure 8.3). The vasodilatation due to ACh occurs through enzymatic activation of endothelial nitric oxide synthase (eNOS) [70]. Endothelial-dependent vasodilation occurs through the release of NO that diffuses to the underlying SMCs to increase intracellular cyclic guanosine monophosphate (cGMP) content and causing the opening of potassium channels and the inhibition of other intracellular mechanisms that regulate smooth muscle tone. There is an additional NO-independent dilatory mechanism for ACh in resistance arteries, which occurs through the release of endothelium-derived hyperpolarizing factor (EDHF), the nature of which remains elusive [71]. There are at least two likely reasons for the weaker ACh-induced vasodilatation in allograft arteries: there may be a defect in endothelial cell activity (synthesis or release of NO) and/or a reduced SMC responsiveness to NO. An additional possibility is that ACh induces vasoconstriction by direct stimulation of muscarinic receptors on vascular SMCs [72, 73]. In allograft tissue, ACh is able to directly stimulate the subendothelial SMC layer and cause constriction. Electron micrographs and silver staining methods indicate some degree of endothelial cell denudation at day 20 posttransplantation [74, 75]. This will promote ACh-induced vasoconstriction in allograft arteries, which would counterbalance its NO-mediated dilatory effects.

CsA treatment and smooth muscle sensitivity to NO

Recent studies conducted by Moien-Afshari et al. [11] in a rat model of cardiac transplantation confirm that allograft arteries at day 21 and not day 4 posttransplantation have an attenuated response to cumulative additions of various concentrations of sodium nitroprusside (SNP) (Figure 8.4). However, this defective response was completely relieved by CsA treatment so that no differences in vasodilation were observed between coronary arteries of CsA-treated allograft and -untreated isograft recipients (Figure 8.4). The vasodilatory responses to SNP occur by a direct mechanism that is endothelium-independent; SNP acts to release NO directly within arterial SMC after its metabolism [76]. Since both ACh and SNP use common

NO-mediated mechanisms to cause vasodilatation, the weak relaxatory response to both compounds in allograft heart arteries strongly suggests a defect in the cGMP-mediated component of smooth muscle relaxation. However, Moien-Afshari et al. were unable to ascertain whether there could be specific defect in endothelial cell production of NO in allograft arteries based on the observation that the magnitude of endothelium-based vasorelaxation (ACh-induced) was not significantly reduced compared to endothelium-independent (SNP-induced) dilation in these vessels. Koh et al. [77] studied the function of human allograft arteries undergoing cell-mediated rejection in a humanized mouse model of allograft vasculopathy. In these experiments using human cells and tissues, there is early endothelial dysfunction characterized by a reduction in endothelial-mediated relaxation. This endothelial dysfunction is a result of an IFNγ-mediated decrease in eNOS expression by the graft endothelium. Furthermore, there is a desensitization of the vascular smooth muscle to NO-mediated vasodilation in these arteries, which is caused by increased expression and activity of inducible nitric oxide synthase (iNOS) within these grafts. Taken together, these investigations highlight the importance and extent of functional abnormalities in allograft arteries.

Smooth muscle cell function in septal coronary arteries of transplanted hearts: a progressive dysfunction without treatment

As discussed earlier, Moien-Afshari et al. [11] studied coronary artery function from rat allografts at day 21 and not at day 4 post-cardiac transplantation; in terms of vasoconstriction, they reported that KCl depolarization-induced reduction in luminal diameter of coronary resistance arteries was significantly lower in arteries from allograft recipients. Since these experiments were performed after iNOS blockade, the results led them to conclude that the weaker response to KCl was unlikely to be due to the increased expression of iNOS and its associated unregulated production of NO in the arterial walls. Thus, it is clear that CsA treatment also preserved depolarization-induced contractions in allograft arteries (Figure 8.5).

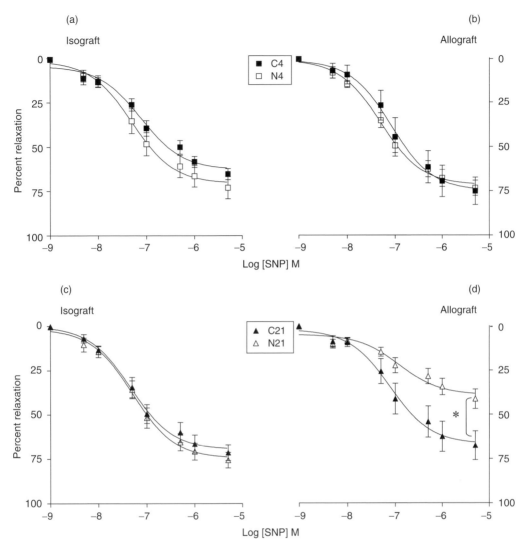

Figure 8.4 Endothelium-independent relaxation is septal coronary arteries of grafted hearts.
Endothelium-independent relaxation is intact on day 4 posttransplantation in both isograft and allograft hearts (a, b). On day 21 posttransplantation, although endothelium-independent relaxation is intact in isografts (c), there is a marked decline in smooth muscle vasodilatory response to NO release from NO donor SNP in allografts (d) (*$p < 0.01$). CsA treatment (5 mg/kg) preserves smooth muscle relaxation to NO in allografts up to day 21 posttransplantation. (With permission from Reference [11].)

Myogenic tone in transplant arteries

Studies in a rat model of heterotopic cardiac transplantation clearly demonstrate that the extent of myogenic tone in allograft coronary septal resistance arteries is significantly inhibited in comparison with site- and size-matched isograft arteries [11, 12] (Figures 8.6, 8.7A, and 8.8). One consequence of

this inhibition of myogenic tone is that it will result in greatly increased arterial diameters at all pressure steps. As discussed earlier, the regulation of constitutive and inducible NO bioavailability is an important component in the modulation of arterial diameters during the process of CAV. Endothelial NOS is constitutively expressed in cells of the intimal layer with nearly all (>90%) being membrane-associated [78] and localizes predominantly to subdomains of

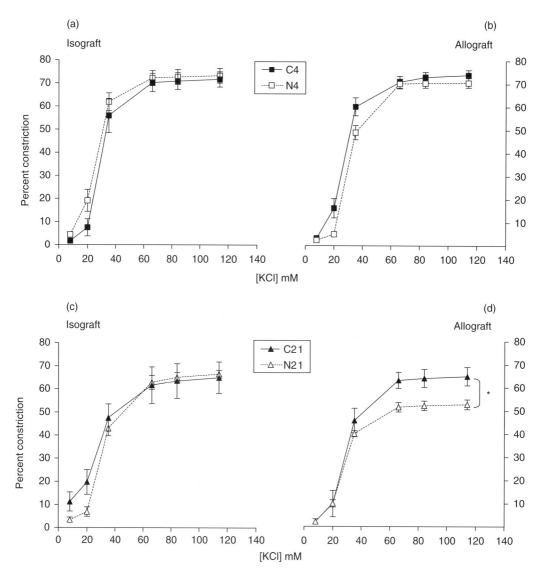

Figure 8.5 Arteriolar smooth muscle function is septal coronary arteries of grafted hearts. Smooth muscle dysfunction does not exist on day 4 posttransplantation in both isograft and allograft hearts (a, b). On day 21 posttransplantation, although smooth muscle function is intact in isografts (c), there is a marked smooth muscle dysfunction in allografts (d) (*$p < 0.01$). CsA treatment (5 mg/kg) prevents smooth muscle function in allografts up to day 21 posttransplantation. (With permission from Reference [11].)

the plasma membrane termed caveolae [79], small plasmalemmal invaginations characterized by the transmembrane protein caveolin [80].

There are three mechanisms of dysregulation of myogenic tone that are manifest in this model of allograft rejection. During the early stages of transplant vascular disease, there is an inhibition of vascular tone that occurs via an enhanced basal release of constitutive nitric oxide synthase (eNOS)-based NO due to increased endothelial Ca^{2+} availability (Figure 8.9). This is apparent in arteries from allografts at day 4 posttransplantation which have less myogenic tone than matched isograft arteries. Selective iNOS inhibition with aminoguanidine did not increase tone in either group, and no iNOS protein was identified using immunohistochemical

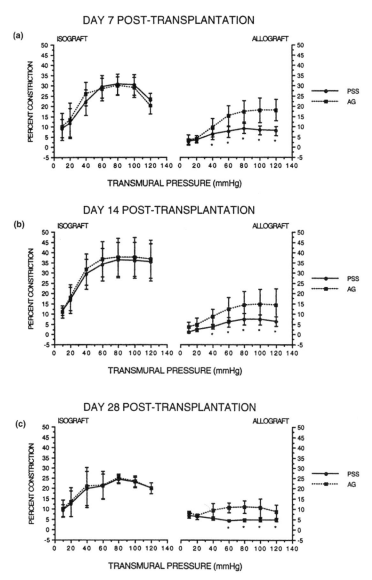

Figure 8.6 Days 7–28 posttransplantation. Myogenic tone in isograft and allograft vessels before and after iNOS inhibition for days 7 (a), 14 (b), and 28 (c). $*p < 0.05$. (With permission from Reference [12].)

detection. However, the differences in coronary artery tone were abolished after nonselective NOS inhibition with L-NAME, indicating significantly greater basal release of eNOS-based NO from the allograft endothelium. Immune-based alterations in BH4 or L-arginine requirements were not causally implicated on the basis of a lack of vasoactive responses by these cofactors, thus reducing the possibility that eNOS activity is rate-limiting. However, using fluorescent recordings of intracellular-free Ca levels in coronary endothelial cells, we demonstrated that resting intracellular Ca^{2+} concentrations ($[Ca^{2+}]_i$) were elevated in isolated allograft endothelial cells; since eNOS is very highly regulated by $[Ca^{2+}]_i$, this provides a mechanistic basis for the enhanced basal release of eNOS-based NO early (day 4 posttransplantation) in the process of alloimmune injury. However, the causal role of this early but transient increase in endothelial $[Ca^{2+}]_i$ remains unclear although reductions

(a)

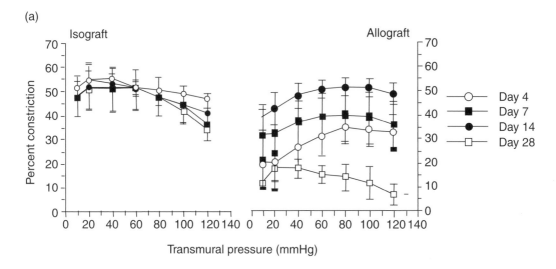

(b)

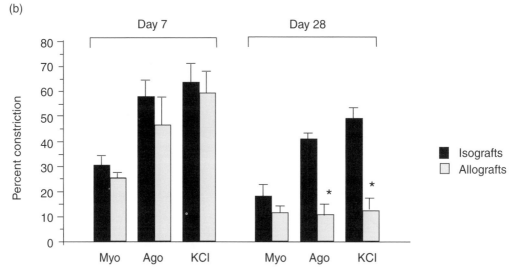

Figure 8.7 Smooth muscle contractile defect in mature allografts. (a) Myogenic tone in isograft and allograft vessels after L-NAME showing graded deterioration in allografts. (b) Constrictions of pressurized allograft and isograft vessels by myogenic, agonist-induced, and depolarization-induced mechanisms reveal a time-dependent, parallel deterioration of constriction by all three mechanisms. Myo indicates myogenic; Ago, agonist; and KCl, depolarization. Statistical comparison by Student's t test, $*p < 0.05$. (With permission from Reference [12].)

in extrusion through the plasmalemmal Ca-ATPase may represent an underlying mechanism [12].

The decline in myogenic tone, which occurs in septal coronary arteries of allograft hearts, has a progressive pattern involving changes in $[Ca^{2+}]_i$, cofactors, and substrate availability. An important rate-limiting step is eNOS activity, which is mainly regulated by $[Ca^{2+}]_i$ under physiological conditions. In disease states, in addition to $[Ca^{2+}]_i$, cofac-

tors and substrate availability can also contribute to eNOS regulation. Intracellular levels of Ca^{2+} in endothelial cells are mainly regulated by the basal leak, remediated activation [81], and mechanical factors such as shear stress and intraluminal flow. Shear stress, presumably operating via the shear stress response element, upregulates both eNOS activity and eNOS expression [82, 83]. While basal Ca^{2+} influx occurs largely through a passive Ca^{2+} "leak" [84],

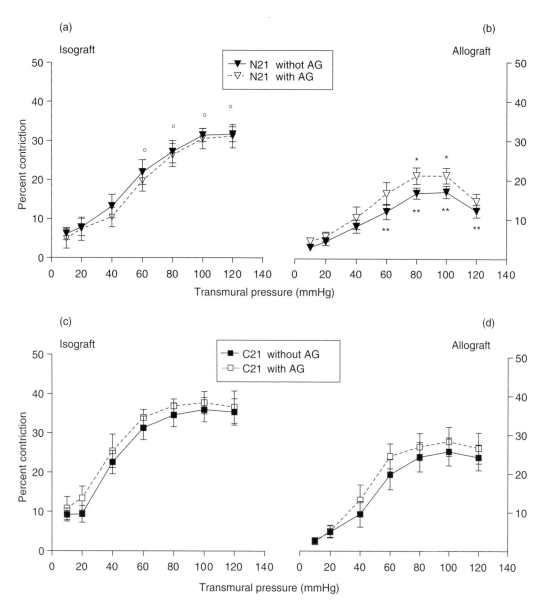

Figure 8.8 Myogenic tone in coronary arteries of CsA-treated or CsA-untreated recipients of allograft or isograft hearts in the presence or absence of aminoguanidine. In the absence of AG, there is a significant decline in myogenic tone in untreated allograft arteries (b) compared to isograft vessels (a) ($p < 0.05$, $n = 8 - 9$ repeated measurement ANOVA). Treating allograft vessels with AG (b) have improved the tone (*$p < 0.05$ repeated measurement ANOVA), indicating iNOS-based NO-mediated tone suppression in these arteries. CsA treatment in graft recipient had no effect on isograft arteries (c) but improved the myogenic tone reduction in allografts arteries (d) in comparison with their untreated counterparts (b) (**$p < 0.05$, $n = 6$ repeated measure ANOVA), so that the response is not different from the isograft tissue. In both CsA-treated isograft and allograft arteries, incubation with AG potentiates the tone but not significantly. C, CsA treated; N, no treatment; 21, day 21 posttransplantation; AG, aminoguanidine. (With permission from Reference [11].)

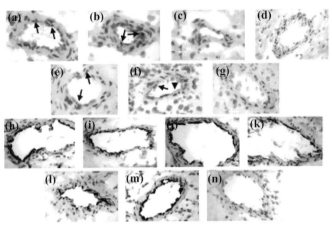

Figure 8.9 iNOS and eNOS expression in allograft and isograft coronary arteries. (a, b) Day 2 isograft and allograft arteries; in most cases, immunostaining appears in close proximity to nuclei (arrows), consistent with iNOS positivity in adherent or infiltrating macrophages. (c, d) Day 4 isograft and allograft vessels. (e, f) Day 14 vessels, showing minimal iNOS expression in isograft intima (e, arrow) but impressive expression of iNOS antigen in allograft intima (f); these day 14 examples are representative of matched grafts for days 7–28. (g) Day 14 allograft negative control. eNOS positivity is evident in allograft and isograft arteries at all time points. (h, i) Day 2 isograft and allograft. (j, k) Day 4 isograft and allograft. (l, m) Day 14 isograft and allograft. (n) eNOS-negative control. (With permission from Reference [12].)

additional influx also occurs through second messenger-operated channels [85] and possibly stores depletion pathways, so-called capacitative Ca^{2+} entry [81]. These mechanisms are counteracted by SR Ca^{2+} release and refilling and plasmalemmal Ca^{2+} extrusion to determine $[Ca^{2+}]_i$ [86, 87]. In the Mn^{2+} quenching experiments of Skarsgard et al. [12], the rate of Ca^{2+} influx was similar in the isograft and allograft endothelium. However, in the allograft endothelium, inhibition of SR refilling with cyclopiazonic acid (an inhibitor of sarcoplasmic/endoplasmic reticulum Ca^{2+}-ATPase) caused a greater increase in $[Ca^{2+}]_i$. The sustained elevation of $[Ca^{2+}]_i$ after tetraethylammonium incubation (which minimizes the Ca^{2+} "leak" via depolarization) was suggestive of a defect in Ca^{2+} extrusion involving plasmalemmal Na^+/Ca^{2+} exchange or Ca^{2+}-ATPase pumping. The hypothetical model, then, will be of an early defect in Ca^{2+} extrusion in allograft endothelial cells, with a resultant increase in basal $[Ca^{2+}]_i$ and SR filling; enhanced basal $[Ca^{2+}]_i$ increases eNOS activity and NO release from the endothelium. Appropriately, the physical location of this early defect in allograft physiology, the endothelial plasma membrane, is also the interface between donor tissue and the host immune cells. The second mechanism of tone reduction is iNOS-based. When iNOS is expressed, tone inhibition occurs through Ca^{2+}-independent release of iNOS-based NO (Figures 8.6 and 8.8). The role of iNOS-based pathophysiology in CAV is untested under clinical conditions although it provides a plausible explanation of coronary hemodynamics in the rodent model. Mouse and rat cells express iNOS with relative ease while iNOS expression is difficult to induce in most human cells in culture, where the levels of induction are not nearly as high as those in mouse or rat cells. Thus, it is likely that iNOS expression in humans and mice/rats is different and the relevance of iNOS findings in mice/rats may not reflect the human situation.

There is some evidence that iNOS may be constitutively expressed in some cells as part of their normal physiology [88]. This includes macrophages, endothelial cells, vascular SMCs, cardiac myocytes, epithelial cells (lung, kidney, and intestine), and neuronal cells (for review, see Kroncke et al.) [89]. iNOS was originally believed to exist only in a cytosol-soluble form; however, this notion was based almost entirely on studies conducted in transformed cell lines. In primary mouse macrophages, almost 50% of iNOS activity is membrane-associated but not lysosome- or peroxisome-associated [90]. iNOS is induced in many mouse/rat cell types in response to inflammatory cytokines or noxious physical stimuli [91, 92], although whether human cells similarly induce iNOS expression is not clear [93–95]. Since iNOS activity is Ca^{2+}-independent, the expression level of iNOS protein is the most important regulator of iNOS activity [96]. Cellular iNOS expression is dependent on NF-κB activation and IFNγ response factors [97] and has been identified in numerous inflammatory diseases including transplantation, atherosclerosis, and ischemia/reperfusion. From day 7 posttransplantation, inhibition of myogenic tone in rat allograft arteries parallels the expression of iNOS protein. In these vessels, selective inhibition of iNOS with aminoguanidine (a relatively specific blocker of iNOS) potentiated tone. Thus, iNOS-based NO is vasoactive and manifests as an important mechanism of tone inhibition. A similar theme has been addressed in other models using lipopolysaccharide (LPS) induction of iNOS. Following a report that LPS activates an L-arginine-dependent pathway in vascular tissue [98], Rees et al. [99] showed that the attendant vasodilation, hyporesponsiveness to vasoconstrictors, and elevation in cyclic GMP were due to induction of a Ca^{2+}-independent NOS and could be reversed by L-arginine analogues. Similarly, in the isolated rabbit heart (with constant flow), LPS treatment attenuated agonist-induced increases in coronary perfusion pressure for treated hearts, consistent with a relative excess of NO production [100]. As shown by Skarsgard et al. [12], selective inhibitors of iNOS ameliorate the vascular changes due to iNOS induction. In an LPS-treated rat model, 100 μmol/L aminoguanidine completely reverses vascular hyporesponsiveness [101, 102] and NOS hyperactivity [102] to control levels, while having no effect on control tissues or on stimulated NO release with ACh.

Expression of iNOS occurs in human and experimental cardiac transplantation. Yang et al. [92] demonstrated iNOS mRNA and iNOS protein in ventricular homogenates of acutely rejecting cardiac allografts but not in matched isografts. Immunostains showed iNOS localized to infiltrating macrophages, endothelial cells, and cardiac myocytes. Using a rodent model of chronic rejection, Russell et al. [103] showed early and persistent iNOS

positivity in adherent and infiltrating macrophages; mature grafts (>75 days posttransplantation) manifest striking iNOS positivity in intimal and medial SMCs. In human grafts, iNOS positivity is similarly localized to macrophages, cardiac myocytes, and vascular SMCs [104, 105]. iNOS expression is not limited to cardiac transplantation and also occurs in lung, liver, kidney, small bowel, and bone marrow transplantation [106–110]. In each of these examples, iNOS expression is accompanied by evidence of enhanced NO synthesis. Immunosuppression by CsA can prevent iNOS induction in coronary arteries of the rat cardiac allograft [11].

Another important mechanism that compounds changes seen with NO-dependent vasodilation mechanisms is the time-dependent, concordant loss of pressure-, agonist-, and depolarization-induced tone in coronary artery allograft vessels. These changes strongly implicate progressive loss of intrinsic regulatory mechanisms of vascular smooth muscle contraction (Figures 8.5, 8.6, and 8.7). It is likely that this defect involves either common events in the signal transduction pathway or a loss in the number of viable, contractile SMCs. The potential alterations in the signal transduction pathway are likely to reside in events that regulate the distal common pathway such as Ca^{2+} influx, calmodulin, myosin light chain kinase, contractile filaments, and phosphatases, supporting a role for inflammatory and possibly allogeneic alteration in contractile filaments. Hansson et al. [111] described inhibition of α-actin protein and mRNA expression in cultured SMCs exposed to INF-γ. Of equal importance is the possibility that impaired vasoconstriction in mature allograft vessels may be due to a decrease in the number of viable contractile SMCs. An apparent loss of medial cells has been observed in human coronary arteries, strongly suggesting that apoptosis may play a key role in CAV. Szabolcs et al. [112] used DNA laddering, terminal deoxynucleotidyl transferase mediated biotinylated UTP nick end-labeling (TUNEL), and in situ nick-translation to identify apoptotic cells in Lewis to Wistar–Furth allografts. Apoptotic nuclei were identified in cardiac myocytes, endothelial cells, and infiltrating monocytes; iNOS protein was also identified in the same cell types. Importantly, the temporal pattern of apoptosis paralleled that of iNOS expression, NOS activity, and nitrotyrosine staining, suggesting that apoptosis may be triggered by iNOS and peroxynitrite. Indeed, exogenous NO can induce apoptosis in macrophages, vascular SMCs, cardiac myocytes, and endothelium [113, 114]. NO-induced apoptosis occurring with coexpression of Fas (vascular SMC) and P53 (macrophages) provides a signaling pathway whereby iNOS-based NO can alter cell viability [115, 116]. With this in mind, it is possible that the effect of iNOS expression on allograft arteries is twofold and time-dependent: an early phase due to vasodilation by NO itself and a delayed phase due to smooth muscle apoptosis by NO and (or) NO adducts. There is an emerging theme that susceptibility to NO-mediated apoptosis hinges on the expression of iNOS within the target cell itself. For example, while mesangial, epithelial, and endothelial cells undergo apoptosis in response to exogenous NO, these cells are resistant to endogenous NO when iNOS is induced [113]. Similarly, heterogeneous expression of iNOS by INF-γ and LPS in cultured mesangial cells is associated with apoptosis only in cells not expressing iNOS. In contrast, iNOS expression in macrophages does not confer apoptotic self-protection [117]. This suggests that in some cells, expression of iNOS may be accompanied by corecruitment of protective pathways. If so, the intense iNOS staining in vascular smooth muscle identified by Russell *et al.* [103] in late rejection may have vastly different consequences compared with perivascular cells expressing iNOS, which occurs predominantly during the early stages.

Effect of CsA treatment on allograft coronary artery myogenic tone

Loss of tone in cardiac allograft arteries has, at least in part, an immune basis, since it can be prevented by immunosuppression with CsA [11]. Our recent study demonstrates that when allograft recipients are treated with CsA (5 mg/kg), myogenic tone in graft arteries at day 21 posttransplantation is preserved and is similar to tone in isograft vessels [11] (Figure 8.8). Moreover, incubation with aminoguanidine did not significantly increase the magnitude of myogenic tone in these arteries. Therefore, treating cardiac transplant recipients with CsA prevents iNOS induction. Thus, fewer apoptotic vascular SMCs are expected to exist

in this tissue, as confirmed by the lower number of TUNEL-positive cells and higher magnitude of medial thickness in CsA-treated allograft arteries [11]. One plausible hypothetical explanation for these observations is that mediators released by immune cells during the course of allograft rejection will increase iNOS in vascular SMCs. The host's immune system also damages SMCs in allograft tissue directly by lysing myocytes or altering their function. Similarly, the host's immune cells infiltrating allograft interstitial space can produce cytokines that hamper SMC contractility. CsA inhibits the production of interleukin-2 and other lymphokines by T-helper lymphocytes, which act as inducers of iNOS or damage the graft myocytes by activating the rest of the host antigraft immune cascade. The role of CsA in CAV is reviewed elsewhere [29].

Clinical significance of changes in myogenic tone has been hypothesized based in the recorded reduction in coronary artery myogenic tone in transplant vessels. The experimental observations of Skarsgard *et al.* [12] provide a mechanistic basis for several clinical observations. In the absence of fixed distal disease, a pattern of enhanced arterial diameter due to myogenic tone inhibition would predict a hemodynamic profile of supranormal coronary flow and reduced flow reserve. In nonrejecting human cardiac grafts, resting coronary flow is indeed elevated, with a proportional decrease in flow reserve [118, 119]. These findings have been attributed to increased cardiac work in recipients with systolic hypertension and tachycardia, and when corrected for this, coronary flow is appropriate. However, during biopsy-proven acute rejection, corrected coronary flow is significantly elevated (and coronary resistance depressed) when compared with flow after successful recovery on immunosuppression [120], indicating that vasodilatation accompanies uncontrolled graft rejection. Interestingly, corrected coronary flow remains significantly elevated after a single episode of rejection as compared with patients without prior rejection episodes, consistent with a persistent defect in resistance vessel tone due to the rejection event. Since iNOS expression in cardiac allografts is inhibited by immunosuppression [121], it is possible that the residual elevation in resting corrected coronary flow in transplant patients after rejection is due to an iNOS-independent event such as enhanced endothelial $[Ca^{2+}]_i$ and NO or a smooth muscle contractile defect as we have shown. If so, these alterations in resistance vessel function may be irreversible (Figure 8.9).

Elevated coronary flow in the face of an unrestrained immune assault may, at first consideration, appear to be an appropriate and beneficial response. However, normal coronary myogenic behavior is necessary not only to regulate myocardial blood flow but also to provide graded vascular resistance. Appropriate vascular resistance protects the microvasculature from central arterial pressures and so preserves the important balance of hydrostatic and oncotic forces at the capillary and venular level [122]. A massively dilated coronary circulation, predicted by our results, would transmit abnormally high perfusion pressures to nutritive vessels, distorting the balance of intravascular oncotic and hydrostatic pressure and favoring a net movement of fluid into the myocardial interstitium. In support of this hypothetical pathogenesis, Skarsgard et al. [12] measured a greater wet to dry ratio in allograft hearts, reflecting greater myocardial-free water content. Since endothelial permeability to serum proteins is enhanced in allograft rejection (also an iNOS-dependent event) [123], these two mechanisms could act synergistically to cause significant myocardial edema, thereby compromising ventricular compliance and performance. This general theme may also be operative after myocardial infarction or reperfusion (both of which are followed by iNOS expression) [124, 125]. In the rabbit heart with regional infarction, poor contractility and elevated left ventricular filling pressures were improved by selective iNOS inhibition [126]. The detrimental effect of iNOS expression on ventricular performance in human grafts has been confirmed [105]. In support of our hypothesis that altered allograft coronary physiology (in part due to iNOS-based NO) would favor myocardial edema, ventricular stiffness, and poor performance. Lewis et al. [105] reported that expression of iNOS correlates with cGMP levels and systolic and diastolic left ventricular contractile dysfunction. Importantly, iNOS expression did not associate with the rejection grade as determined by the criteria set by the International Society for Heart and Lung Transplantation. These key observations, coupled with the results of Skarsgard et al. [12], indicate that current techniques of rejection assessment

(International Society for Heart and Lung Transplantation classification) ignore coexistent physiologic mechanisms of allograft dysfunction.

Conclusions

Cardiac transplantation is currently the best method of therapy for end-stage heart failure; however, long-term survival of graft recipients is limited by CAV. Early CAV manifests as some important functional changes in the arteries of the transplanted heart. One example of these functional changes is the profound inhibition of myogenic tone. Myogenic tone provides an underlying constriction allowing the fine-tuning of basal tone by other mechanisms, which leads to appropriate matching of tissue demand with tissue perfusion. Myogenic tone inhibition in cardiac allograft arteries is caused in part by excess vasoactive NO and in part by a defect in vascular SMC contractility. Excess NO can be derived from eNOS and iNOS isoforms. These changes predict a hemodynamic pattern within the rejecting heart that would favor myocardial edema, ventricular stiffness, and poor myocardial performance. Deterioration of myogenic tone in the resistance arteries of the transplant is extremely important, since it provides a pathway of allograft injury that is not accounted for by the current methods of identifying allograft rejection. CsA immunosuppressive therapy has a significant effect on the alleviation of myogenic- and depolarization-induced tone in coronary allograft arteries by preventing iNOS induction, smooth muscle dysfunction, or apoptosis. Importantly, immunosuppressive therapy largely restores endothelial function in the coronary circulation of coronary arteries in a rejection model of cardiac transplantation, where the immune barrier has been breached.

However, immunosuppressive therapy does not alleviate the prevalence of CAV, especially at late stages of the disease—this is the case even with the optimization of immunosuppressive regimens (mostly involving CsA) that effectively prevent graft loss due to acute rejection. Thus, the pathological determinants that drive CAV in humans may involve processes that are not inhibited by CsA. For instance, only 5–10% of T cells in laboratory mice are memory T cells while up to 50–60% of human T cells are of the memory phenotype. As such, many rodent models are not able to accurately assess the role of memory T cells in graft rejection, although these types of T cells are likely very important in graft rejection in humans. Importantly, memory T-cell functions are much more refractory to inhibition by CsA than are naïve T cells [127]. In addition to differences between naïve and memory T cells, CD8$^+$ T cells are less sensitive to inhibition by CsA than are CD4$^+$ T cells [128]. Finally, CAV in humans may be caused by a "smoldering" immune response that is not rigorous enough to cause acute rejection. While CsA may affect the immune processes, this distinct response observed in the arterial wall may also represent the unique ability of vascular cells to effect T-cell functions [44].

The persistent prevalence of CAV may also represent suboptimal immunosuppression by CsA, most likely due to the inability to provide higher doses of the drug due to side effects. In nonhuman primates, high doses of CsA were able to prevent both acute rejection and CAV, while suboptimal dosing led to a delay in acute rejection and arterial inflammation [129]. Also, in a rat model of CAV, Lai *et al.* [34] have observed early endothelial damage that is inhibited by CsA. Treatment of rats with CsA in a model of heterotopic cardiac transplantation also reduces apoptosis within the vascular wall and this protective property of CsA is associated with a preservation of vascular function [11].

Although more modern immunosuppressive regimens, such as CTLA4-Ig, are currently undergoing clinical trials in the hopes of more effectively and specifically inhibiting transplant rejection, immunosuppression with tacrolimus and/or everolimus may be beneficial in treating CAV [130]. In a randomized, double-blind clinical trial, Eisen *et al.* [131] showed that immunosuppression with everolimus significantly reduced both acute rejection episodes and CAV 12 months after transplantation. Also, immunosuppression with rapamycin can prevent allograft vasculopathy in a nonhuman primate model of aortic transplantation and can also inhibit this disorder in a chimeric human–SCID mouse model of vascular transplant rejection [132, 133]. In addition to being able to inhibit allograft vasculopathy, studies in nonhuman primates suggest that rapamycin can partially reverse allograft vasculopathy [134].

Acknowledgments

Work from the authors' laboratories has been supported by the Heart and Stroke Foundation of Canada, the Canadian Institutes of Health Research, and Genome Canada. We also acknowledge the collaboration of many colleagues who have engaged in many aspects of the work described in this chapter.

References

1 Taylor DO, Edwards LB, Mohacsi PJ et al. The registry of the International Society for Heart and Lung Transplantation: twentieth official adult heart transplant report—2003. J Heart Lung Transplant 2003;22(6):616–24.

2 Harringer W, Haverich A. Heart and heart-lung transplantation: standards and improvements. World J Surg 2002;26(2):218–25.

3 Taylor DO. Immunosuppressive therapies after heart transplantation: best, better, and beyond. Curr Opin Cardiol 2000;15(2):108–14.

4 Wahlers T, Mugge A, Oppelt P et al. Coronary vasculopathy following cardiac transplantation and cyclosporine immunosuppression: preventive treatment with angiopeptin, a somatostatin analog. Transplant Proc 1994;26(5):2741–2.

5 Yeung AC, Davis SF, Hauptman PJ et al. Incidence and progression of transplant coronary artery disease over 1 year: results of a multicenter trial with use of intravascular ultrasound. Multicenter Intravascular Ultrasound Transplant Study Group. J Heart Lung Transplant 1995;14(6 Pt 2):S215–20.

6 Hosenpud JD, Bennett LE, Keck BM, Fiol B, Boucek MM, Novick RJ. The Registry of the International Society for Heart and Lung Transplantation: fifteenth official report—1998. J Heart Lung Transplant 1998;17(7):656–68.

7 Weis M, von Scheidt W. Cardiac allograft vasculopathy: a review. Circulation 1997;96(6):2069–77.

8 Halle AA, III, DiSciascio G, Massin EK et al. Coronary angioplasty, atherectomy and bypass surgery in cardiac transplant recipients. J Am Coll Cardiol 1995;26(1):120–8.

9 Musci M, Pasic M, Meyer R et al. Coronary artery bypass grafting after orthotopic heart transplantation. Eur J Cardiothorac Surg 1999;16(2):163–8.

10 Hollenberg SM, Klein LW, Parrillo JE et al. Coronary endothelial dysfunction after heart transplantation predicts allograft vasculopathy and cardiac death. Circulation 2001;104(25):3091–6.

11 Moien-Afshari F, Choy JC, McManus BM, Laher I. Cyclosporine treatment preserves coronary resistance

artery function in rat cardiac allografts. J Heart Lung Transplant 2004;23(2):193–203.

12 Skarsgard PL, Wang X, McDonald P *et al*. Profound inhibition of myogenic tone in rat cardiac allografts is due to eNOS- and iNOS-based nitric oxide and an intrinsic defect in vascular smooth muscle contraction. Circulation 2000;101(11):1303–10.

13 Szabo G, Batkai S, Dengler TJ *et al*. Systolic and diastolic properties and myocardial blood flow in the heterotopically transplanted rat heart during acute cardiac rejection. World J Surg 2001;25(5):545–52.

14 Billingham ME. Histopathology of graft coronary disease. J Heart Lung Transplant 1992;11(3 Pt 2):S38–44.

15 Dong C, Wilson JE, Winters GL, McManus BM. Human transplant coronary artery disease: pathological evidence for Fas-mediated apoptotic cytotoxicity in allograft arteriopathy. Lab Invest 1996;74(5):921–31.

16 Wilson JE, Wood S, McDonald P, Kenyon J, Dong C, McManus BM. Contribution of lipids to the pathogenesis of transplant vascular sclerosis. Transpl Immunol 1997;5(4):247–50.

17 McDonald PC, Kenyon JA, McManus BM. The role of lipids in transplant vascular disease. Lab Invest 1998;78(10):1187–201.

18 Johnson DE, Gao SZ, Schroeder JS, DeCampli WM, Billingham ME. The spectrum of coronary artery pathologic findings in human cardiac allografts. J Heart Transplant 1989;8(5):349–59.

19 McManus BM, Horley KJ, Wilson JE *et al*. Prominence of coronary arterial wall lipids in human heart allografts. Implications for pathogenesis of allograft arteriopathy. Am J Pathol 1995;147(2):293–308.

20 Hamano K, Ito H, Fujimura Y, Tsuboi H, Esato K. Changes in the morphology and components of the coronary arteries during the progression of coronary arteriosclerosis following cardiac transplantation in rats. Cardiovas Surg 1998;6(3):296–301.

21 Busch GJ, Galvanek EG, Reynolds ES, Jr. Human renal allografts. Analysis of lesions in long-term survivors. Hum Pathol 1971;2(2):253–98.

22 Liu G, Butany J, Wanless IR, Cameron R, Greig P, Levy G. The vascular pathology of human hepatic allografts. Hum Pathol 1993;24(2):182–8.

23 Radio S, Wood S, Wilson J, Lin H, Winters G, McManus B. Allograft vascular disease: comparison of heart and other grafted organs. Transplant Proc 1996;28(1):496–9.

24 Tilney NL, Paz D, Ames J, Gasser M, Laskowski I, Hancock WW. Ischemia-reperfusion injury. Transplant Proc 2001;33(1–2):843–4.

25 Ventura HO, Mehra MR, Smart FW, Stapleton DD. Cardiac allograft vasculopathy: current concepts. Am Heart J 1995;129(4):791–9.

26 Libby P, Swanson SJ, Tanaka H, Murray A, Schoen FJ, Pober JS. Immunopathology of coronary arteriosclerosis in transplanted hearts. J Heart Lung Transplant 1992;11(3 Pt 2):S5–6.

27 Linsley PS, Greene JL, Brady W, Bajorath J, Ledbetter JA, Peach R. Human B7-1 (CD80) and B7-2 (CD86) bind with similar avidities but distinct kinetics to CD28 and CTLA-4 receptors. Immunity 1994;1(9):793–801.

28 Clarkson MR, Sayegh MH. T-cell costimulatory pathways in allograft rejection and tolerance. Transplantation 2005;80(5):555–63.

29 Moien-Afshari F, McManus BM, Laher I. Immunosuppression and transplant vascular disease: benefits and adverse effects. Pharmacol Ther 2003;100(2):141–56.

30 Potter BVL. Structure-activity relationships of adenophostin A and related molecules at the 1-D-myo-inositol 1,4,5-trisphosphate receptor. Phosphoinositides 1999:158–79.

31 Borel JF, Feurer C, Gubler HU, Stahelin H. Biological effects of cyclosporin A: a new antilymphocytic agent. Agents Actions 1976;6(4):468–75.

32 Hosenpud JD, Bennett LE, Keck BM, Fiol B, Boucek MM, Novick RJ. The Registry of the International Society for Heart and Lung Transplantation: fifteenth official report—1998. J Heart Lung Transplant 1998;17(7):656–68.

33 Marti V, Romeo I, Aymat R *et al*. Coronary endothelial dysfunction as a predictor of intimal thickening in the long term after heart transplantation. J Thorac Cardiovasc Surg 2001;122(6):1174–80.

34 Lai JC, Tranfield EM, Walker DC *et al*. Ultrastructural evidence of early endothelial damage in coronary arteries of rat cardiac allografts. J Heart Lung Transplant 2003;22(9):993–1004.

35 Ishii Y, Sawada T, Kubota K, Fuchinoue S, Teraoka S, Shimizu A. Injury and progressive loss of peritubular capillaries in the development of chronic allograft nephropathy. Kidney Int 2005;67(1):321–32.

36 Aranda JM, Jr, Hill J. Cardiac transplant vasculopathy. Chest 2000;118(6):1792–800.

37 Treasure CB, Alexander RW. Relevance of vascular biology to the ischemc syndromes of coronary atherisclerosis. Cardiovasc Drugs Ther 1995;9:13–9.

38 Raja SM, Metkar SS, Froelich CJ. Cytotoxic granule-mediated apoptosis: unraveling the complex mechanism. Curr Opin Immunol 2003;15(5):528–32.

39 Fox WM, III, Hameed A, Hutchins GM *et al*. Perforin expression localizing cytotoxic lymphocytes in the intimas of coronary arteries with transplant-related accelerated arteriosclerosis. Hum Pathol 1993;24(5):477–82.

40 Subbotin V, Sun H, Aitouche A *et al*. Marked mitigation of transplant vascular sclerosis in FasLgld (CD95L) mutant recipients. The role of alloantibodies

in the development of chronic rejection. Transplantation 1999;67(10):1295–300.

41 Wang T, Dong C, Stevenson SC et al. Overexpression of soluble fas attenuates transplant arteriosclerosis in rat aortic allografts. Circulation 2002;106(12):1536–42.

42 Choy JC, Kerjner A, Wong BW, McManus BM, Granville DJ. Perforin mediates endothelial cell death and resultant transplant vascular disease in cardiac allografts. Am J Pathol 2004;165(1):127–33.

43 Choy JC, Cruz RP, Kerjner A et al. Granzyme B induces endothelial cell apoptosis and contributes to the development of transplant vascular disease. Am J Transplant 2005;5(3):494–9.

44 Libby P, Pober JS. Chronic rejection. Immunity 2001;14(4):387–97.

45 Nagano H, Mitchell RN, Taylor MK, Hasegawa S, Tilney NL, Libby P. Interferon-gamma deficiency prevents coronary arteriosclerosis but not myocardial rejection in transplanted mouse hearts. J Clin Invest 1997;100(3):550–7.

46 Tellides G, Tereb DA, Kirkiles-Smith NC et al. Interferon-gamma elicits arteriosclerosis in the absence of leukocytes. Nature 2000;403(6766):207–11.

47 Suzuki J, Cole SE, Batirel S et al. Tumor necrosis factor receptor-1 and -2 double deficiency reduces graft arterial disease in murine cardiac allografts. Am J Transplant 2003;3(8):968–76.

48 Moll S, Pascual M. Humoral rejection of organ allografts. Am J Transplant 2005;5(11):2611–8.

49 Lawson C, Holder AL, Stanford RE, Smith J, Rose ML. Anti-intercellular adhesion molecule-1 antibodies in sera of heart transplant recipients: a role in endothelial cell activation. Transplantation 2005;80(2):264–71.

50 Rodriguez ER, Skojec DV, Tan CD et al. Antibody-mediated rejection in human cardiac allografts: evaluation of immunoglobulins and complement activation products C4d and C3d as markers. Am J Transplant 2005;5(11):2778–85.

51 Qian Z, Hu W, Liu J, Sanfilippo F, Hruban RH, Baldwin WM, III. Accelerated graft arteriosclerosis in cardiac transplants: complement activation promotes progression of lesions from medium to large arteries. Transplantation 2001;72(5):900–6.

52 Boros P, Bromberg JS. New cellular and molecular immune pathways in ischemia/reperfusion injury. Am J Transplant 2006;6(4):652–8.

53 Day JD, Rayburn BK, Gaudin PB et al. Cardiac allograft vasculopathy: the central pathogenetic role of ischemia-induced endothelial cell injury. J Heart Lung Transplant 1995;14(6 Pt 2):S142–9.

54 Ho S, Clipstone N, Timmermann L et al. The mechanism of action of cyclosporin A and FK506. Clin Immunol Immunopathol 1996;80(3 Pt 2):S40–5.

55 Sabatini DM, Erdjument-Bromage H, Lui M, Tempst P, Snyder SH. RAFT1: a mammalian protein that binds to FKBP12 in a rapamycin- dependent fashion and is homologous to yeast TORs. Cell 1994;78(1):35–43.

56 Brown EJ, Albers MW, Shin TB et al. A mammalian protein targeted by G1-arresting rapamycin-receptor complex. Nature 1994;369(6483):756–8.

57 Kunz J, Henriquez R, Schneider U, Deuter-Reinhard M, Movva NR, Hall MN. Target of rapamycin in yeast, TOR2, is an essential phosphatidylinositol kinase homolog required for G1 progression. Cell 1993;73(3):585–96.

58 Calvo V, Crews CM, Vik TA, Bierer BE. Interleukin 2 stimulation of p70 S6 kinase activity is inhibited by the immunosuppressant rapamycin. Proc Natl Acad Sci U S A 1992;89(16):7571–5.

59 Chung J, Kuo CJ, Crabtree GR, Blenis J. Rapamycin-FKBP specifically blocks growth-dependent activation of and signaling by the 70 kd S6 protein kinases. Cell 1992;69(7):1227–36.

60 Erikson RL. Structure, expression, and regulation of protein kinases involved in the phosphorylation of ribosomal protein S6. J Biol Chem 1991;266(10):6007–10.

61 Sturgill TW, Wu J. Recent progress in characterization of protein kinase cascades for phosphorylation of ribosomal protein S6. Biochim Biophys Acta 1991;1092(3):350–7.

62 Handschumacher RE, Harding MW, Rice J, Drugge RJ, Speicher DW. Cyclophilin: a specific cytosolic binding protein for cyclosporin A. Science 1984;226(4674):544–7.

63 Liu J, Farmer JD, Jr, Lane WS, Friedman J, Weissman I, Schreiber SL. Calcineurin is a common target of cyclophilin-cyclosporin A and FKBP- FK506 complexes. Cell 1991;66(4):807–15.

64 Friedman J, Weissman I. Two cytoplasmic candidates for immunophilin action are revealed by affinity for a new cyclophilin: one in the presence and one in the absence of CsA. Cell 1991;66(4):799–806.

65 Macian F, Lopez-Rodriguez C, Rao A. Partners in transcription: NFAT and AP-1. Oncogene 2001;20(19):2476–89.

66 Cohen DJ, Loertscher R, Rubin MF, Tilney NL, Carpenter CB, Strom TB. Cyclosporine: a new immunosuppressive agent for organ transplantation. Ann Intern Med 1984;101(5):667–82.

67 Kahan BD. Cyclosporine. N Engl J Med 1989;321(25):1725–38.

68 Andriambeloson E, Pally C, Hengerer B et al. Transplantation-induced endothelial dysfunction as studied in rat aorta allografts. Transplantation 2001;72(12):1881–9.

69 Hollenberg SM, Klein LW, Parrillo JE *et al.* Coronary endothelial dysfunction after heart transplantation predicts allograft vasculopathy and cardiac death. Circulation 2001;104(25):3091–6.

70 Moncada S, Higgs EA. Molecular mechanisms and therapeutic strategies related to nitric oxide. FASEB J 1995;9(13):1319–30.

71 Woodman OL, Wongsawatkul O, Sobey CG. Contribution of nitric oxide, cyclic GMP and K+ channels to acetylcholine-induced dilatation of rat conduit and resistance arteries. Clin Exp Pharmacol Physiol 2000;27(1–2):34–40.

72 Nasa Y, Kume H, Takeo S. Acetylcholine-induced vasoconstrictor response of coronary vessels in rats: a possible contribution of M2 muscarinic receptor activation. Heart Vessels 1997;12(4):179–91.

73 Tsuji T, Cook DA. Mechanism of acetylcholine-induced constriction enhanced by endothelial removal in isolated, perfused canine basilar arteries. J Cardiovasc Pharmacol 1995;25(6):940–6.

74 Andriambeloson E, Pally C, Hengerer B *et al.* Transplantation-induced endothelial dysfunction as studied in rat aorta allografts. Transplantation 2001;72(12):1881–9.

75 Gohra H, McDonald TO, Verrier ED, Aziz S. Endothelial loss and regeneration in a model of transplant arteriosclerosis. Transplantation 1995;60(1):96–102.

76 Bates JN, Baker MT, Guerra R, Jr, Harrison DG. Nitric oxide generation from nitroprusside by vascular tissue. Evidence that reduction of the nitroprusside anion and cyanide loss are required. Biochem Pharmacol 1991;42(suppl):S157–65.

77 Koh KP, Wang Y, Yi T *et al.* T cell-mediated vascular dysfunction of human allografts results from IFN-gamma dysregulation of NO synthase. J Clin Invest 2004;114(6):846–56.

78 Forstermann U, Pollock JS, Schmidt HH, Heller M, Murad F. Calmodulin-dependent endothelium-derived relaxing factor/nitric oxide synthase activity is present in the particulate and cytosolic fractions of bovine aortic endothelial cells. Proc Natl Acad Sci U S A 1991; 88(5):1788–92.

79 Feron O, Belhassen L, Kobzik L, Smith TW, Kelly RA, Michel T. Endothelial nitric oxide synthase targeting to caveolae. Specific interactions with caveolin isoforms in cardiac myocytes and endothelial cells. J Biol Chem 1996;271(37):22810–4.

80 Anderson RG. Caveolae: where incoming and outgoing messengers meet. Proc Natl Acad Sci U S A 1993; 90(23):10909–13.

81 Putney JW, Jr. Capacitative calcium entry revisited. Cell Calcium 1990;11(10):611–24.

82 Lamontagne D, Pohl U, Busse R. Mechanical deformation of vessel wall and shear stress determine the basal release of endothelium-derived relaxing factor in the intact rabbit coronary vascular bed. Circ Res 1992;70(1):123–30.

83 Nishida K, Harrison DG, Navas JP *et al.* Molecular cloning and characterization of the constitutive bovine aortic endothelial cell nitric oxide synthase. J Clin Invest 1992;90(5):2092–6.

84 Demirel E, Laskey RE, Purkerson S, van Breemen C. The passive calcium leak in cultured porcine aortic endothelial cells. Biochem Biophys Res Commun 1993;191(3):1197–203.

85 Luckhoff A, Clapham DE. Inositol 1,3,4,5-tetrakisphosphate activates an endothelial Ca(2+)-permeable channel. Nature 1992;355(6358):356–8.

86 Daniel EE, van Breemen C, Schilling WP, Kwan CY. Regulation of vascular tone: cross-talk between sarcoplasmic reticulum and plasmalemma. Can J Physiol Pharmacol 1995;73(5):551–7.

87 Lee CH, Poburko D, Kuo KH, Seow CY, van Breemen C. Ca(2+) oscillations, gradients, and homeostasis in vascular smooth muscle. Am J Physiol Heart Circ Physiol 2002;282(5):H1571–83.

88 Guo FH, De Raeve HR, Rice TW, Stuehr DJ, Thunnissen FB, Erzurum SC. Continuous nitric oxide synthesis by inducible nitric oxide synthase in normal human airway epithelium in vivo. Proc Natl Acad Sci U S A 1995;92(17):7809–13.

89 Kroncke KD, Fehsel K, Kolb-Bachofen V. Inducible nitric oxide synthase and its product nitric oxide, a small molecule with complex biological activities. Biol Chem Hoppe Seyler 1995;376(6):327–43.

90 Vodovotz Y, Russell D, Xie QW, Bogdan C, Nathan C. Vesicle membrane association of nitric oxide synthase in primary mouse macrophages. J Immunol 1995;154(6):2914–25.

91 Xie QW, Whisnant R, Nathan C. Promoter of the mouse gene encoding calcium-independent nitric oxide synthase confers inducibility by interferon gamma and bacterial lipopolysaccharide. J Exp Med 1993;177(6):1779–84.

92 Yang X, Chowdhury N, Cai B *et al.* Induction of myocardial nitric oxide synthase by cardiac allograft rejection. J Clin Invest 1994;94(2):714–21.

93 Chan GC, Fish JE, Mawji IA, Leung DD, Rachlis AC, Marsden PA. Epigenetic basis for the transcriptional hyporesponsiveness of the human inducible nitric oxide synthase gene in vascular endothelial cells. J Immunol 2005;175(6):3846–61.

94 Chesrown SE, Monnier J, Visner G, Nick HS. Regulation of inducible nitric oxide synthase mRNA levels by LPS, INF-gamma, TGF-beta, and IL-10 in murine

macrophage cell lines and rat peritoneal macrophages. Biochem Biophys Res Commun 1994;200(1):126–34.

95 Schneemann M, Schoedon G, Hofer S, Blau N, Guerrero L, Schaffner A. Nitric oxide synthase is not a constituent of the antimicrobial armature of human mononuclear phagocytes. J Infect Dis 1993;167(6):1358–63.

96 Loscalzo J, Welch G. Nitric oxide and its role in the cardiovascular system. Prog Cardiovasc Dis 1995;38(2):87–104.

97 Xie QW, Kashiwabara Y, Nathan C. Role of transcription factor NF-kappa B/Rel in induction of nitric oxide synthase. J Biol Chem 1994;269(7):4705–8.

98 Fleming I, Gray GA, Julou-Schaeffer G, Parratt JR, Stoclet JC. Incubation with endotoxin activates the L-arginine pathway in vascular tissue. Biochem Biophys Res Commun 1990;171(2):562–8.

99 Rees DD, Palmer RM, Schulz R, Hodson HF, Moncada S. Characterization of three inhibitors of endothelial nitric oxide synthase in vitro and in vivo. Br J Pharmacol 1990;101(3):746–52.

100 Smith RE, Palmer RM, Moncada S. Coronary vasodilatation induced by endotoxin in the rabbit isolated perfused heart is nitric oxide-dependent and inhibited by dexamethasone. Br J Pharmacol 1991;104(1):5–6.

101 Joly GA, Ayres M, Chelly F, Kilbourn RG. Effects of NG-methyl-L-arginine, NG-nitro-L-arginine, and aminoguanidine on constitutive and inducible nitric oxide synthase in rat aorta. Biochem Biophys Res Commun 1994;199(1):147–54.

102 Scott JA, Machoun M, McCormack DG. Inducible nitric oxide synthase and vascular reactivity in rat thoracic aorta: effect of aminoguanidine. J Appl Physiol 1996;80(1):271–7.

103 Russell ME, Wallace AF, Wyner LR, Newell JB, Karnovsky MJ. Upregulation and modulation of inducible nitric oxide synthase in rat cardiac allografts with chronic rejection and transplant arteriosclerosis. Circulation 1995;92(3):457–64.

104 Lafond-Walker A, Chen CL, Augustine S, Wu TC, Hruban RH, Lowenstein CJ. Inducible nitric oxide synthase expression in coronary arteries of transplanted human hearts with accelerated graft arteriosclerosis. Am J Pathol 1997;151(4):919–25.

105 Lewis NP, Tsao PS, Rickenbacher PR et al. Induction of nitric oxide synthase in the human cardiac allograft is associated with contractile dysfunction of the left ventricle. Circulation 1996;93(4):720–9.

106 Cicalese L, Hierholzer C, Subbotin V, Iyengar A, Rao AS, Stanko RT. Protective effect of pyruvate during acute rejection of intestinal allografts: accompanied by upregulation of inducible nitric oxide synthase mRNA. Transplant Proc 1997;29(3):1813–4.

107 Kuo PC, Alfrey EJ, Krieger NR et al. Differential localization of allograft nitric oxide synthesis: comparison of liver and heart transplantation in the rat model. Immunology 1996;87(4):647–53.

108 Langrehr JM, Hoffman RA, Billiar TR, Lee KK, Schraut WH, Simmons RL. Nitric oxide synthesis in the in vivo allograft response: a possible regulatory mechanism. Surgery 1991;110(2):335–42.

109 Salahudeen A, Wang C, McDaniel O, Lagoo-Denadayalan S, Bigler S, Barber H. Antioxidant lazaroid U-74006F improves renal function and reduces the expression of cytokines, inducible nitric oxide synthase, and MHC antigens in a syngeneic renal transplant model. Partial support for the response-to-injury hypothesis. Transplantation 1996;62(11):1628–33.

110 Worrall NK, Boasquevisque CH, Misko TP, Sullivan PM, Ferguson TB, Jr, Patterson GA. Inducible nitric oxide synthase is expressed during experimental acute lung allograft rejection. J Heart Lung Transplant 1997;16(3):334–9.

111 Hansson GK, Hellstrand M, Rymo L, Rubbia L, Gabbiani G. Interferon gamma inhibits both proliferation and expression of differentiation-specific alpha-smooth muscle actin in arterial smooth muscle cells. J Exp Med 1989;170(5):1595–608.

112 Szabolcs M, Michler RE, Yang X et al. Apoptosis of cardiac myocytes during cardiac allograft rejection. Relation to induction of nitric oxide synthase. Circulation 1996;94(7):1665–73.

113 Muhl H, Sandau K, Brune B, Briner VA, Pfeilschifter J. Nitric oxide donors induce apoptosis in glomerular mesangial cells, epithelial cells and endothelial cells. Eur J Pharmacol 1996;317(1):137–49.

114 Pollman MJ, Yamada T, Horiuchi M, Gibbons GH. Vasoactive substances regulate vascular smooth muscle cell apoptosis. Countervailing influences of nitric oxide and angiotensin II. Circ Res 1996;79(4):748–56.

115 Fukuo K, Nakahashi T, Nomura S et al. Possible participation of Fas-mediated apoptosis in the mechanism of atherosclerosis. Gerontology 1997;43(suppl 1):35–42.

116 Messmer UK, Ankarcrona M, Nicotera P, Brune B. p53 expression in nitric oxide-induced apoptosis. FEBS Lett 1994;355(1):23–6.

117 Nitsch DD, Ghilardi N, Muhl H, Nitsch C, Brune B, Pfeilschifter J. Apoptosis and expression of inducible nitric oxide synthase are mutually exclusive in renal mesangial cells. Am J Pathol 1997;150(3):889–900.

118 Kofoed KF, Czernin J, Johnson J et al. Effects of cardiac allograft vasculopathy on myocardial blood flow, vasodilatory capacity, and coronary vasomotion. Circulation 1997;95(3):600–06.

119 Senneff MJ, Hartman J, Sobel BE, Geltman EM, Bergmann SR. Persistence of coronary vasodilator

responsivity after cardiac transplantation. Am J Cardiol 1993;71(4):333–8.

120 Barry WH. Mechanisms of immune-mediated myocyte injury. Circulation 1994;89(5):2421–32.

121 Cai B, Roy DK, Sciacca R, Michler RE, Cannon PJ. Effects of immunosuppressive therapy on expression of inducible nitric oxide synthase (iNOS) during cardiac allograft rejection. Int J Cardiol 1995;50(3):243–51.

122 Chilian WM, Layne SM, Klausner EC, Eastham CL, Marcus ML. Redistribution of coronary microvascular resistance produced by dipyridamole. Am J Physiol 1989;256(2 Pt 2):H383–90.

123 Worrall NK, Boasquevisque CH, Botney MD et al. Inhibition of inducible nitric oxide synthase ameliorates functional and histological changes of acute lung allograft rejection. Transplantation 1997;63(8):1095–101.

124 Dudek RR, Wildhirt S, Conforto A et al. Inducible nitric oxide synthase activity in myocardium after myocardial infarction in rabbit. Biochem Biophys Res Commun 1994;205(3):1671–80.

125 Liu P, Hock CE, Nagele R, Wong PY. Formation of nitric oxide, superoxide, and peroxynitrite in myocardial ischemia-reperfusion injury in rats. Am J Physiol 1997;272(5 Pt 2):H2327–36.

126 Wildhirt SM, Suzuki H, Wolf WP et al. S-methy- lisothiourea inhibits inducible nitric oxide synthase and improves left ventricular performance after acute myocardial infarction. Biochem Biophys Res Commun 1996;227(2):328–33.

127 Schwinzer R, Siefken R. CD45RA+ and CD45RO+ T cells differ in susceptibility to cyclosporin A mediated inhibition of interleukin-2 production. Transpl Immunol 1996;4(1):61–3.

128 Bishop DK, Li W. Cyclosporin A and FK506 mediate differential effects on T cell activation in vivo. J Immunol 1992;148(4):1049–54.

129 Wieczorek G, Bigaud M, Menninger K et al. Acute and chronic vascular rejection in nonhuman primate kidney transplantation. Am J Transplant 2006;6(6):1285–96.

130 Lechler RI, Sykes M, Thomson AW, Turka LA. Organ transplantation—how much of the promise has been realized? Nat Med 2005;11(6):605–13.

131 Eisen HJ, Tuzcu EM, Dorent R et al. Everolimus for the prevention of allograft rejection and vasculopathy in cardiac-transplant recipients. N Engl J Med 2003;349(9):847–58.

132 Dambrin C, Klupp J, Birsan T et al. Sirolimus (rapamycin) monotherapy prevents graft vascular disease in nonhuman primate recipients of orthotopic aortic allografts. Circulation 2003;107(18):2369–74.

133 Yi T, Cuchara L, Wang Y et al. Human allograft arterial injury is ameliorated by sirolimus and cyclosporine and correlates with suppression of interferon-gamma. Transplantation 2006;81(4):559–66.

134 Ikonen TS, Gummert JF, Hayase M et al. Sirolimus (rapamycin) halts and reverses progression of allograft vascular disease in non-human primates. Transplantation 2000;70(6):969–75.

CHAPTER 9

Immunotherapy for left ventricular dysfunction after heart transplantation

Charles E. Canter

Introduction

Left ventricular dysfunction after heart transplantation has multiple etiologies. Graft failure occurring immediately after the surgical procedure, termed primary graft failure, is correlated with multiple characteristics of the donor as well as perioperative factors mainly associated with the severity of illness in the recipient [1, 2]. With follow-up, left ventricular volumes and ejection fractions tend to remain normal even longer than 10 years after transplantation [3]. Thus the development of left ventricular dysfunction or heart failure in a transplant recipient is abnormal and not an inevitable result of transplantation per se. The most frequent cause of ventricular dysfunction and graft loss in the long term is the progressive ischemia from transplant coronary arteriopathy [4, 5]. Immunologic and nonimmunologic factors contribute to the development of transplant coronary arteriopathy including rejection, CMV infection, donor cause of death and ischemic time, and traditional atherosclerotic risk factors [6–8]. A less well-characterized entity, chronic nonspecific graft failure, may also occur late after transplantation, without a definite association with transplant coronary arteriopathy [9]. Myocarditis [9], especially associated with CMV infection, is a rare cause of left ventricular dysfunction after heart transplantation.

This chapter will focus on left ventricular dysfunction associated with acute rejection of the cardiac allograft. Acute rejection remains a major cause of morbidity and mortality after cardiac transplantation [4, 5]. Left ventricular dysfunction may be directly associated with an episode of acute rejection, so-called rejection with hemodynamic compromise. Cumulative episodes of rejection not associated with hemodynamic compromise may also indirectly lead to left ventricular dysfunction due to the relationship of rejection to the development of transplant coronary arteriopathy and secondary ventricular ischemia [7, 10–11]. Therapy for left ventricular dysfunction associated with rejection, therefore, has two components: (1) acute treatment to reverse left ventricular dysfunction when it occurs with an acute episode of rejection and (2) prevention of rejection to avoid episodes of hemodynamic compromise and decrease the risk for transplant coronary arteriopathy.

Epidemiology of rejection with hemodynamic compromise

Rejection with hemodynamic compromise occurs in only approximately 10–15% of all episodes of acute rejection [12, 13]. However, it is a dangerous complication of heart transplantation, which carries a high mortality rate and may occur anytime after transplantation. Figure 9.1 summarizes the survival of patients after an episode of rejection with hemodynamic compromise within the CTRD (Cardiac Transplant Research Database) and PHTS (Pediatric Heart Transplant Study) databases. The CTRD and PHTS are multi-institutional databases housed at the University of Alabama, Birmingham,

(a)

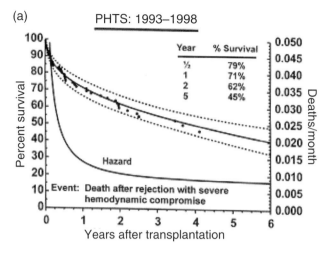

(b)

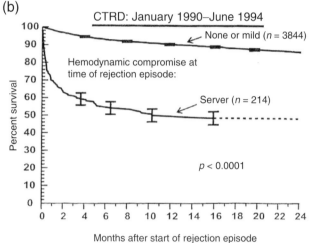

Months after start of rejection episode

Figure 9.1 Actuarial survival curves for pediatric (a) and adult (b) heart transplant recipients after an episode of rejection with severe hemodynamic compromise in the multicenter Pediatric Heart Transplant Study [13] and Cardiac Transplant Research Database [12]. Severe compromise was defined as the need for intravenous inotropic support.

which collect event-driven data including rejection with hemodynamic compromise. The 12-month mortality within both databases is greater than 30% after an episode of rejection with hemodynamic compromise. Cause of death is not just a result of heart failure from left ventricular dysfunction, but may also occur due to infection or other complications from the intense immunosuppression with which it is treated. Most episodes of acute rejection occur within the first 6 months after surgery, but there is an ongoing hazard for rejection in adult and pediatric heart transplant recipients [14,

15]. In adults the proportion of rejection episodes with hemodynamic compromise remains constant over time after transplantation. However, in children, a substantially higher proportion of rejection episodes associated with hemodynamic compromise in rejection occur greater than 1 year after transplant.

Risk factors for development of rejection with hemodynamic compromise are generally similar to those of any episode of acute rejection. In adults, female sex, black race, and a history of diabetes are associated with a greater risk for the development of rejection with hemodynamic compromise [12]. In children, multivariable analysis identifies older age and nonwhite race as risk factors [13]. While cumulative episodes of rejection are associated with a greater risk for recurrent and late (greater than 1 yr after transplant) rejection, they do not confer a greater risk for developing rejection with hemodynamic compromise. Thus, while rejection with hemodynamic compromise carries a high mortality, direct factors that identify a unique risk for its development have not been elucidated.

Acute cellular rejection

Acute T-cell-mediated, or cellular, rejection has primarily been characterized through endomyocardial biopsies evaluated for the presence of lymphocytic infiltration and myocardial necrosis. Multiple mechanisms [16, 17] have been proposed that link the development of left ventricular dysfunction with acute cellular rejection. In vitro studies have found cytotoxic T lymphocytes to be able to injure and lyse myocytes [18, 19]. However, the importance of these studies to in vivo left ventricular dysfunction with acute cellular rejection remains uncertain as left ventricular dysfunction associated with acute cellular rejection is often reversible. However, there is evidence that cytotoxic T lymphocytes may be associated with reversible myocardial dysfunction [20–22]. Inflammatory cytokines produced by infiltrating lymphocytes and macrophages may lead to depression of myocardial function without myocyte destruction through direct negative inotropic effects of increasing nitric oxide production within myocytes [23] and/or by their interplay on catecholamine metabolism to blunt a positive inotropic response to catecholamines [24, 25].

Most acute cellular rejection episodes are associated with normal cardiac hemodynamics and left ventricular ejection fraction [26]. Furthermore, it is unclear what the effects of intensification of immunosuppression have on the prevention of progression of rejection without left ventricular dysfunction or hemodynamic compromise to an episode with these complications. The vast majority of patients with biopsies showing lymphocytic infiltration without myocardial necrosis do not demonstrate clinical or histological deterioration if their immunosuppression is unchanged

[27, 28]. Even patients with biopsies demonstrating lymphocytic infiltration and myocardial necrosis do not necessarily deteriorate without treatment and may demonstrate spontaneous improvement in biopsies in the absence of treatment [29]. The factors or antecedent stimuli that determine if an episode of acute cellular rejection will evolve into an episode associated with left ventricular dysfunction/hemodynamic compromise remain obscure.

Acute humoral rejection

The potential for antibody-mediated rejection to cause graft dysfunction and death is clearly illustrated with hyperacute rejection [30], where the presence of circulating antidonor antibodies in a recipient leads to severe vasculitis and vascular thrombosis with graft destruction within hours after implantation of the allograft. Distinct from this phenomenon, in the late 1980s/early 1990s, a syndrome of left ventricular dysfunction within the first weeks after transplant associated with absent or minimal lymphocytic myocardial infiltration with no myocyte necrosis on endomyocardial biopsy was identified in heart transplant recipients [31, 32]. Associated with this syndrome was the presence of anti-HLA antibodies, usually with donor specificity, in the serum of recipients [11, 33–35]. Histologically, a pattern of endothelial cell swelling, interstitial edema, and acute vasculitis was identified along with detection of IgG, IgM, and IgA, C1q, and/or C3 deposition in capillaries by immunofluorescence [31, 32].

Further studies have demonstrated that the observed endothelial cell "swelling" is infiltration of macrophages demonstrated by positivity of CD68 with immunoperoxidase staining of capillaries [10, 36, 37]. Evidence of deposition of complement activation can be observed by staining, demonstrating C3d and C4d deposition in capillaries [10, 38–40]. The combination of clinical, histologic, and immunopathologic findings as well as the demonstration of circulating antidonor antibodies has defined episodes of what is termed acute antibody-mediated or humoral rejection (Table 9.1) [41].

While the presence of circulating antidonor antibodies and evidence of C4d deposition in capillaries are components of a diagnosis of acute humoral rejection, the combination also defines

Table 9.1 Findings in acute antibody-mediated rejection in cardiac allografts [41].

---

1 Clinical evidence of acute graft dysfunction

2 Histologic evidence of acute capillary injury

Capillary endothelial changes: swelling or denudation with congestion

Macrophages in capillaries

Neutrophils in capillaries (more severe cases)

Interstitial edema and/or hemorrhage (more severe cases)

3 Immunopathologic evidence for antibody-mediated injury (in the absence of OKT3)

Ig (G, M, and/or A) + C3d and/or C4d or C1q (equivalent staining diffusely in capillaries, 2–3+, demonstrated by immunofluorescence

CD68 positivity for macrophages in capillaries (identified using CD31 or CD34) and/or C4d staining of capillaries with 2–3+ intensity by paraffin Immunohistochemistry

Fibrin in vessels (optional; if present, process is reported as more severe)

Serologic evidence of anti-HLA class I and/or class II antibodies or other antidonorantibody (e.g., non-HLA antibody, ABO) at time of biopsy (supports clinical and/or morphologic findings)

---

accommodation, the absence of humoral-mediated injury, and continued function of the graft despite the presence of antidonor antibodies in the circulation [42]. Similarly, deposition of immunoglobulin or complement detected by immunofluorescence may be observed in cardiac allografts from initial ischemic injury [43, 44] or from the presence of antibodies to the murine component of the cytolytic immunosuppressant OKT3 [45]. Thus the pathologic and serologic findings ascribed to acute humoral rejection, in and of themselves, may not define an episode of acute humoral rejection in the absence of ventricular dysfunction [46]. However, deposition of immunoglobulins and activation of complement in the cardiac vascular bed associated with antimurine OKT3 antibodies or graft ischemic injury may be predisposing factors that increase the risk for acute vascular/humoral rejection associated with ventricular dysfunction [44, 45, 47].

In the absence of observable myocardial necrosis and intense lymphocytic infiltration of the myocardium, the mechanism of ventricular dysfunction associated with acute humoral or antibody-mediated rejection has been felt to be sec-

ondary to the consequences of antibody-induced and complement-mediated activation of endothelial cells, secretion of cytokines, and increased endothelial cell adherence of leukocytes [30, 31]. Myocardial dysfunction results from ischemic distress or injury and decreased myocardial compliance due to tissue edema associated with vascular injury. Similar to cellular rejection, cytokine expression by macrophages could lead to direct reversible myocardial dysfunction [16, 17].

While initially described as a phenomena occurring early after transplantation, increasing experience indicates that acute humoral rejection may occur any time after transplantation [10, 12–16]. The prevalence of left ventricular dysfunction associated with these episodes of acute humoral rejection from single-center experiences has been nearly 50% [10]. Within the CTRD and PHTS databases, over 50% of the rejection episodes with hemodynamic compromise are associated with biopsies demonstrating no or low-grade lymphocytic infiltration without myocyte necrosis [12, 13]. Furthermore, studies of patients with rejection with hemodynamic compromise have found histologic evidence of cellular and humoral components, so-called "mixed" rejection [31, 48]. Thus acute humoral rejection after heart transplantation accounts for a substantial, if not a majority, of rejection episodes associated with ventricular dysfunction.

Rescue therapy for an acute episode of rejection with left ventricular dysfunction

Therapy for episodes of acute cellular rejection, sometimes termed rescue therapy [49, 50], has generally involved intensification of immunosuppression. Initial therapy generally entails an acute pulse of high-dose oral or intravenous corticosteroids. However, episodes associated with hemodynamic compromise and/or that are resistant to treatment with corticosteroids are usually treated with intravenous antilymphocytic antibodies [49, 50]. These antibodies may be nonspecific (polyclonal) in their protein target on the lymphocyte or have a specific (monoclonal) target. Polyclonal preparations commonly used are horse antilymphocyte globulin (Atgam) and rabbit antilymphocyte globulin (Thymoglobulin). In renal transplant recipients,

Thymoglobulin has greater efficacy than Atgam for steroid-resistant rejection [51]. While all of these lymphocytic drugs have been shown to be highly effective in the treatment of steroid-resistant rejection, OKT3 has had a reported success rate of 90% or greater even in patients who appeared resistant to antithymocyte globulin [52–56].

While OKT3 is highly successful in treating acute rejection episodes, its use is not without significant adverse effects. Initial administration is associated with a cytokine release phenomenon [57], characterized by lowered systemic vascular resistance and increased capillary permeability, which can easily exacerbate existing heart failure symptoms in heart transplant recipients with rejection with hemodynamic compromise. Prolonged (greater than 1 wk) administration can lead to development of human antimurine antibodies, which in turn can lead to a loss of efficacy and have been associated with the development, as stated earlier, of acute humoral rejection [45, 58]. The profound immunosuppression induced by OKT3 is a risk factor for development of serious infections [59] and/or lymphoproliferative disease [60].

Somewhat paradoxically, use of OKT3 for treatment of rejection has been associated with a greater risk of recurrent episodes of rejection. "Rebound" rejection episodes may occur [61]. In the CTRD [14], use of OKT3 for initial immunosuppression was a significant risk factor for recurrent rejection.

Despite some reports of efficacy [62], rescue therapies initially developed for the treatment of acute cellular rejection proved to be ineffective for the treatment of acute humoral rejection [63, 64]. These therapies were ultimately modified into protocols that have resulted in successful treatment of an episode of acute humoral rejection with resolution of hemodynamic compromise and left ventricular dysfunction. A number of centers (Table 9.2) have reported their results in adult and pediatric heart transplant recipients [32, 63–71]. These protocols, as a group, share three components. First, therapy for acute cellular rejection in the form of high-dose steroids with and without cytolytic antilymphocyte antibody preparations is performed. OKT3, despite experience that suggests its administration can precipitate acute humoral rejection, is used due to its known effectiveness in reversing acute cellular rejection as well as some early evi-

dence that it was effective therapy for acute humoral rejection in kidney transplant recipients [72]. Secondly, cyclophosphamide has been substituted for azothioprine, due to its increased ability over azothioprine to limit B-cell proliferation [73]. In addition, coadministration of cyclophosphamide also has appeared to mitigate the development of human antimurine antibodies to OKT3 [74]. Finally, and likely most importantly, techniques that led to removal of antibody from the circulation, either plasmapheresis or immunoadsorption, were performed. Animal studies [75] and clinical experience [66] have suggested that the key factor leading to reversal of left ventricular dysfunction was antibody removal. Plasmapheresis also had the added benefit of removing cytokines from the circulation, which might contribute to left ventricular dysfunction [76, 77].

Utilization of these protocols has been associated with symptomatic improvement within a few days of initiation of treatment [67, 71, 75]. Improvement of left ventricular dysfunction, however, generally has lagged behind symptomatic improvement. Normalization of left ventricular dysfunction often has not occurred for weeks to months after completion of the acute rescue therapy [63, 68, 71]. Most importantly, while these protocols have led to symptomatic improvement and resolution of left ventricular dysfunction, they have not ameliorated the increased risk of transplant coronary artery disease, graft loss, and/or mortality associated with acute humoral rejection with hemodynamic compromise [10, 65, 68, 69, 71].

More recently, specific antibody preparations with direct effects on B lymphocytes have been utilized as rescue therapy for acute humoral rejection with ventricular dysfunction. Intravenous immune globulin (IVIG) has been utilized for treatment of numerous autoimmune and systemic inflammatory disorders [78]. Its mechanism is complex and may include interference with complement and cytokine activation; activation, differentiation, and effector function of T and B lymphocytes; and provision of anti-idiotypic antibodies [78, 79]. A pilot study [80] utilized IVIG at a total dose of 2 g/kg instead of plasmapheresis along with cyclophosphamide, steroids, and/or anti-T-cell antibodies as rescue therapy in a combined group of 10 heart and kidney transplant recipients with acute humoral

Table 9.2 Experience with rescue therapy for acute humoral rejection.

Study	Number of episodes (patients)	Protocol	Successful treatment	Long-term complications
Olson et al. [65]	13 patients	Plasmapheresis cyclophosphamide steroids OKT3 (6) ALG (2)	12/13 (92%)	5/13 patient died within 2 yr of episode
Miller et al. [32]	5 patients	Plasmapheresis cyclophosphamide steroids	4/5 (80%)	None noted
Olivari et al. [66]	3 patients	Immuoadsorption cyclophosphamide steroids	3/3 (100%)	1/3 died from infection 2 mo after treatment
Berglin et al. [67]	5 patients	Plasmapheresis steroids	5/5 (100%)	None noted
Kobashigawa et al. [63]	7 patients	Plasmapheresis cyclophosphamide steroids OKT3	7/7 (100%)	None noted
Pahl et al. [68]	7 Episodes in 5 patients (pediatric)	Plasmapheresis cyclophosphamide steroids OKT3	7/7 (100%)	3/5 patients developed transplant coronary disease
Grauhan et al. [64]	11 episodes in 6 patients	Plasmapheresis steroids cyclophosphamide OKT3 and/or ATG	11/11 (100%)	None noted Use of cyclophosphamide as maintenance immunosuppression did not prevent recurrences
Uber et al. [69]	20 patients	Plasmapheresis "augmented" immunosuppression	20/20 (100%)	1.7× increased risk for transplant coronary disease 5-yr mortality 50% vs. 80% for patients without humoral rejection
Veiga Barreiro et al. [70]	12 patients	Plasmapheresis steroids	11/12 (92%)	None noted
McOmber et al. [71]	13 episodes in 10 patients (pediatric)	Plasmapheresis cyclophosphamide steroids OKT3	12/13 (92%)	50% survival 24 mo after first episode of acute humoral rejection

rejection. In 3 heart transplant recipients, acute ventricular dysfunction normalized, but, similar to the protocols utilizing plasmapheresis, 2 of the 3 patients died 14 months and 5.5 years after treatment. The efficacy of IVIG to reverse steroid and anti-lymphocyte resistant rejection in renal transplant patients has been confirmed in two recent studies [81, 82].

Rituximab, a murine anti-CD20 B-lymphocyte-specific antibody, has recently been utilized by itself as rescue therapy in a small number of cases [83, 84] of acute humoral rejection in heart transplant recipients. In one case report [85], rituximab successfully reversed a humoral rejection episode

that was resistant to plasmapheresis and anti-T-cell cytolytic therapy. The dose generally used has been 375 mg/m^2 in four doses given weekly, but in one case report [83] a single dose was efficacious. As antibody-producing plasma cells do not express CD20, how rituximab would work to reverse antibody-mediated rejection is unclear. Potential mechanisms include a nonspecific intravenous immunoglobulin effect, depletion of specific anti-donor antibody, or by its ability to eliminate B cells [86]. While these initial results are intriguing, it has yet to be shown that it is efficacious in reducing the long-term risks of transplant coronary arteriopathy and/or graft loss associated with acute humoral rejection. Furthermore, its murine component may have the potential for the development of human antibodies similar to what has been observed with OKT3.

Prevention of rejection in heart transplant candidates with preformed anti-HLA antibodies

The potential for preformed antibodies with donor specificity to precipitate severe graft dysfunction and loss (hyperacute rejection) [30] in the heart transplant recipient has been a dreaded complication. Early [87, 88] experience in heart transplant patients who had positive retrospective crossmatches suggested poorer survival compared to those having a negative crossmatch as well as a greater risk for rejection with hemodynamic compromise. Further experience [89–91] suggested that even with a negative retrospective crossmatch, transplant candidates that exhibited evidence of IgG anti-HLA antibodies to a high percentage of HLA antigens, the panel reactive antibody (PRA) at levels of greater than 10 or 20% had a higher risk of rejection and graft loss compared to candidates with negative or low PRAs. Most of these studies have utilized techniques that required complement-dependent cytotoxicity to detect antibody that are less sensitive than newer techniques utilizing ELISA or flow cytometry [92]. However, even high PRAs and positive T- and B-cell crossmatches detected by flow cytometry have been associated with high rates of rejection [93, 94].

Multiparous females, patients with frequent transfusions, and patients previously transplanted are known to be at high risk for high PRAs, so-called sensitized patients [95]. Patients with previous cardiac surgery that utilized preserved human homograft material for valve or vessel replacement also routinely develop high PRAs [96]. Perhaps most significantly, utilization of ventricular assist devices (VADs) for mechanical support as a bridge to transplantation in adults is associated with the rapid development of high PRAs. The etiology of rapid elevation of PRA has been attributed to blood and platelet transfusion and exposure to blood donor leukocytes [97–99]. These findings led to recommendations to use leukocyte filters for transfusions in VAD patients and/or leukocyte-depleted blood

products. In leukocyte-depleted blood, this activity may not necessarily be due to anti-HLA IgG antibodies, but may be due to antialbumin antibodies, which lead to false-positive results on solid-phase assays [100]. While early single-center studies have noted an increase risk for rejection associated with high PRAs in patients placed on VADs [91], a recent analysis of the International Society for Heart and Lung Transplantation database [101] did not find that the increased frequency of elevated PRAs did not translate into an increased risk for mortality or rejection.

The primary means of prevention of episodes of rejection in heart transplant candidates with pre-existing anti-HLA antibodies is avoidance-utilizing prospective potential donor/recipient crossmatches and proceeding with transplantation only if the crossmatch is negative. The ability of newer techniques that allow identification of antibodies to specific HLA antigens can allow this crossmatch to occur without a donor's serum, the "virtual" crossmatch [102]. However, the likelihood of a negative crossmatch decreases proportionally with higher percentages of PRA positivity, which can make listing for transplantation more of a therapeutic gesture than a true possibility.

A second option is to desensitize high-risk transplant candidates with interventions designed to lower PRA percentages and increase the likelihood of a negative prospective crossmatch with potential donors. Transplant nephrologists have utilized different protocols incorporating IVIG [79, 103] or plasmapheresis [104] prior to transplantation that both effectively lower PRAs and improve transplant rates in sensitized kidney transplant candidates with good graft survival and acceptable rates of rejection. A recent study by Stegall et al. [105] found that a plasmapheresis-based protocol led to more reproducible desensitization and lower rates of humoral rejection compared to an IVIG-based protocol, but neither protocol was effective in completely preventing episodes of humoral rejection. In this study, it appeared that the titer of a specific anti-HLA antibody was critical to the success of any of the therapies. While PRAs give a sense of the broadness of HLA sensitization, it is only with recent techniques that one can determine the magnitude of sensitization for a given HLA antigen. Stegall's study suggests that the depth of sensitization to individual antigens may be the crucial factor that determines success of any desensitizing treatment and/or feasibility of successful transplantation [106].

The importance of relative short graft ischemic times in heart transplantation and the frequent use of nonlocal heart donors have limited the easy attainability of a prospective crossmatch in heart transplantation as opposed to kidney transplantation. This problem has led a number of heart transplant centers to utilize protocols similar to those used as rescue therapy for acute antibody-mediated rejection to perform heart transplantation in highly sensitized patients without a prospective negative crossmatch (Table 9.3) [107–110]. All of these protocols have used plasmapheresis (some in combination with IVIG) for antibody removal and cyclophosphamide to inhibit B-cell proliferation. Early [87] experience found improved survival in patients with positive crossmatches when plasmapheresis was performed in the first week after transplant. Leech *et al.* [110] demonstrated that their

overall group had declines in Class I and II PRA levels with their plasmapheresis and IVIG protocol; however, a substantial minority of the patients did not respond to the treatment with a reduction in PRAs. Also, it has appeared that the rejection frequency from the pediatric experience [108, 109] has been much higher than it has been from the adult experience, though the differences in protocols make any attempt to determine etiology of these differences problematic.

The Columbia University heart transplant group's high frequency of infectious complications with the use of plasmapheresis in presensitized heart transplant candidates [111] led them to abandon the procedure and substitute a protocol [112] of monthly infusions of IVIG at a dose of 2 g/kg coupled with a single pulse of intravenous cyclophosphamide at 0.5–1 g/m^2. Posttransplant, the monthly pulses of intravenous cyclophosphamide were continued for the first 4 months after transplantation. Treatment prior to transplantation reduced, but did

Table 9.3 Experience with performing heart transplantation in highly sensitized candidates without a prospective crossmatch.

Study	Number of patients	Protocol	Survival	Rejection
Pisani *et al.* [107]	16 12 with retrospective + crossmatch	Before transplant: plasmapheresis and IVIG	No difference to control group (PRAs <10%)	No difference to control group
Jacobs *et al.* [108]	8 children 3 with retrospective + crossmatch	Before transplant: plasmapheresis and IVIG After transplant: plasmapheresis anti-T-cell antibodies cyclophosphamide	50% overall mortality compared to 15% or nonsensitized control group $p = 0.043$	2/3 children with + crossmatch died from rejection
Holt *et al.* [109]	17 children 14 with retrospective + crossmatch	Before transplant: plasmapheresis After transplant: plasmapheresis anti-T-cell antibodies cyclophosphamide	91% 12-mo survival 79% 36-mo survival	13/14 patients with + crossmatch had rejection, 5/14 had multiple episodes 50% of rejection episodes associated with hemodynamic compromise
Leech *et al.* [110]	35 patients 17 with retrospective + crossmatch	Before transplant: plasmapheresis and IVIG After transplant: plasmapheresis and IVIG anti-T-cell antibodies cyclophosphamide	No increased mortality compared to nonsensitized transplant recipients	12 patients had rejection episodes, 7/12 humoral rejection

not eliminate, anti-HLA class I and II alloreactivity by 33%. Time to transplantation was reduced due to earlier acquisition of a prospective donor-negative crossmatch. After transplantation, allogeneic T-cell activation, serum anti-HLS alloreactivity, and rejection were reduced with pulsed cyclophosphamide therapy.

Optimizing maintenance immunosuppression to prevent rejection with ventricular dysfunction

The foundation of immunosuppression in heart transplant recipients has been based on "triple" immunosuppression—the combination of a calcineurin inhibitor, a cell proliferation inhibitor, and steroids [49, 50]. Fifteen to 20 years ago, choices were limited to cyclosporine, azathioprine, and steroids. However, in the past decade new immunosuppressants have increased choices. Calcineurin inhibition can be accomplished with tacrolimus as opposed to cyclosporine. While tacrolimus is associated with less hisuitism, gingival hyperplasia, hypertension, and hyperlipidemia than cyclosporine, clinical trials comparing the efficacy of the drugs have been mixed with some studies showing a reduction [113, 114] or no effect [115–117] on prevention of rejection with tacrolimus over cyclosporine. In contrast, mycophenolate mofetil (MMF), a cell proliferation inhibitor that replaces azathioprine, has been shown to have a consistent benefit in reduction of rejection and rejection with hemodynamic compromise in trials comparing it to azathioprine [118, 119]. MMF also appears to be a much more effective inhibitor of antibody production after transplantation [120]. Recent analysis [121] has also demonstrated a reduction in the severity of transplant coronary arteriopathy with MMF. The combination of tacrolimus/MMF has been shown to negate the increased risk of rejection in black heart transplant recipients [122]. When compared to a cyclosporine/MMF regimen, a tacrolimus/MMF regimen reduces overall rejection frequency, but has had no effect on the frequency of rejection with hemodynamic compromise [123].

3-Hydroxy-3-methylglutarylcoenzyme A (HMG-CoA) reductase inhibitors (statins) are a class of drugs whose primary indication is treatment of hy-perlipidemia, not immunosuppression. However, a decade ago, Kobashigawa et al. [124] demonstrated that pravastatin not only reduced cholesterol in heart transplant recipient, but also improved 12-month survival, reduced overall frequency of rejection, and significantly ($p = 0.005$) reduced the frequency of rejection with hemodynamic compromise in a randomized trial. The ability of statins to reduce the development of hemo-dynamically compromising rejection in heart transplant recipients has been confirmed in two other studies [125, 126] using different specific statins. A meta-analysis of the effects of statins on hemodynamically compromising rejection found a nearly fivefold reduction of risk (relative risk = 0.22, 95% confidence intervals 0.08–0.63, $p = 0.004$) [127]. Statin use has also been associated with a retarded development of transplant coronary arteriopathy [124–126]. Statins as a drug class have shown immunomodulating properties, such as a suppression of natural killer cell activity [124, 128]. Other studies [129] have demonstrated statins to directly inhibit major histocompatibility complex (MHC) class II expression with repression of MHC-II-mediated T-cell activation. Statins have also been shown to have anti-inflammatory effect by modulating levels of cytokines interleukin-6 and tumor necrosis factor α [130], as well reducing circulating levels of C-reactive protein in heart transplant recipients [131]. Despite an apparent indirect anti-inflammatory and immunomodulating effects, the demonstrable clinical benefits of statins have made their use a routine component of maintenance immunosuppression therapy [132].

Conclusions

Over the past two decades, steady improvement has occurred in survival after heart transplantation [4, 5]. Newer immunosuppressive drugs and drug protocols have reduced rejection [132]. However, the prevalence of antibody-mediated rejection, which is commonly associated with left ventricular dysfunction, has not declined to the extent observed with cellular rejection [133] and is being observed with increasing frequency in long-term (>5 yr) survivors of heart transplantation [134]. A definitive diagnosis of acute antibody-mediated rejection, especially when it is not associated with ventricular dysfunction, remains elusive. While successful treatment for rejection with ventricular dysfunction can acutely reverse heart failure and the ventricular dysfunction, these treatments often do not reduce the increased risk of earlier mortality associated with rejection with ventricular dysfunction. The overall complexity of the population of heart transplant candidates is increasing. This increase is especially due to an increase in the population of sensitized candidates. Early experience with protocols to inhibit the severe rejection with ventricular dysfunction and permit short-term survival observed in recipients with preformed antibodies is encouraging. However, these protocols reduce, but do not eliminate, rejection and their ability to inhibit early transplant coronary arteriopathy and promote long-term survival remains to be determined.

References

1 Young JB, Hauptman PJ, Naftel DC *et al*. Determinants of early graft failure following cardiac transplantation: a 10-year, multi-institutional, multivariable analysis [abstract]. J Heart Lung Transplant 2001;19:212.

2 Huang J, Trinkaus K, Huddleston CB, Mendeloff EN, Spray TL, Canter CE. Recipient as well as donor characteristics are risk factors for primary graft failure after pediatric cardiac transplantation. J Heart Lung Transplant 2004;23:716–22.

3 Streeter RP, Nichols K, Bergmann SR. Stability of right and left ejection fraction and volumes after heart transplantation. J Heart Lung Transplant 2005;24:815–18.

4 Taylor DO, Edwards LB, Boucek MM, Trulock EP, Keck BM, Hertz MI. Registry of the International Society for Heart and Lung Transplantation: twenty-second official adult heart transplant report. J Heart Lung Transplant 2005;24:945–55.

5 Boucek MM, Edwards LB, Keck BM, Trulock EP, Taylor DO, Hertz MI. Registry of the International Society for Heart and Lung Transplantation: eighth official pediatric report—2005. J Heart Lung Transplant 2005;24:968–82.

6 Costanzo MR, Naftel DC, Pritzker MR *et al*. Heart transplant coronary artery disease detected by coronary angiography: a multiinstitutional study of preoperative donor and recipient risk factors. J Heart Lung Transplant 1998;17:744–53.

7 Mehra MR, Ventura HO, Chambers RB, Ramireddy K, Smart FW, Stapleton DD. The prognostic impact of immunosuppression and cellular rejection on cardiac allo-graft vasculopathy: time for a reappraisal. J Heart Lung Transplant July 1997;16(7):743–51.

8 Johnson MR. Transplant coronary disease: nonimmunologic risk factors. J Heart Lung Transplant 1992;11: S124–32.

9 McNamara D, Di Salvo T, Mathier M, Keck S, Sekigran M, Dec GW. Left ventricular dysfunction after heart transplantation: incidence and role of enhanced immunosuppression. J Heart Lung Transplant 1996;15: 506–15.

10 Michaels PJ, Espejo ML, Kobashigawa J, Alejos JC, Burch C, Takemoto S. Humoral rejection in cardiac transplantation: risk factors, hemodynamic consequences and relationship to transplant coronary artery disease. J Heart Lung Transplant 2003;22:58–69.

11 Taylor DO, Yowell RI, Kfoury AG, Hammond EH, Renlund DG. Allograft coronary artery disease: clinical correlations with circulating anti-HLA antibodies and the immunopathologic pattern of vascular rejection. J Heart Lung Transplant 2000;19:518–21.

12 Mills RM, Naftel DC, Kirklin JK, Van Bakel AB, Jaski BE, Massin EK. Heart transplant rejection with hemodynamic compromise: a multiinstitutional study of the role of endomyocardial cellular infiltrate. J Heart Lung Transplant 1997;16:813–21.

13 Pahl E, Naftel DC, Canter CE, Frazier EA, Kirklin JK, Morrow WR. Death after rejection with severe hemodynamic compromise in pediatric heart transplant recipients: a multi-institutional study. J Heart Lung Transplant 2001;20:279–87.

14 Kubo SH, Naftel DC, Mills RM *et al*. Risk factors for late recurrent rejection after heart transplantation: a multi-institutional, multivariable analysis. J Heart Lung Transplant 1995;14:409–18.

15 Webber SA, Naftel DC, Parker J *et al*. Late rejection episodes more than 1 year after pediatric heart transplantation: risk factors and outcomes. J Heart Lung Transplant 2003;22:869–75.

16 Lange LG, Schreiner GF. Immune mechanisms of cardiac disease. N Eng J Med 1994;330:1129–35.

17 Barry WH. Mechanism of immune-mediated myocyte injury. Circulation 1994;89:2421–32.

18 Bradley J, Bolton E. The T-cell requirements for allograft rejection. Transplant Rev 1992;6:115–29.

19 Strom TB. The cellular and molecular basis of allograft rejection: what do we know? Transplant Proc 1988; 20:143–6.

20 Woodley SL, McMillan M, Shelby J *et al*. Myocyte injury and contraction abnormalities produced by cytoxic T lymphocytes. Circulation 1991;83:1410–8.

21 Young JDE, Hengartner H, Podack ER, Cohn AZ. Purification and characterization of a cytolytic pore-forming protein from granules of cloned lymphocytes

with natural killer activity. Cell 1986;44:849–59.

22 Jones J, Hallett MB, Morgan BP. Reversible cell damage by T-cell perforins. Biochem J 1990;267:303–7.

23 Finkel MS, Oddis CV, Jacob TD, Watkins SC, Hattler BG, Simmons RL. Negative inotropic effects of cytokines on the heart mediated by nitric oxide. Science 1992;257:387–9.

24 Yokoyama T, Vaca L, Rossen RD, Durante W, Hazarika P, Mann D. Cellular basis for the negative inotropic effects of tumor necrosis factor-alpha in the adult mammalian heart. J Clin Invest 1993;92:2303–12.

25 Chung MK, Gulick TS, Rotondo RE, Schreiner GF, Lange LG. Mechanism of cytokine inhibition of β-adrenergic agonist stimulated cyclic AMP generation in cardiac myocytes: impairment of signal transduction. Circ Res 1990;67:753–63.

26 Bolling SF, Putnam JB, Abrams GD, McKay AM, Deeb GM. Hemodynamics versus biopsy findings during cardiac transplant rejection. Ann Thorac Surg 1991;51:52–5.

27 Lloveras J-J, Escourrou G, Delisle MB et al. Evolution of untreated mild rejection in heart transplant recipients. J Heart Lung Transplant 1992;11:751–6.

28 Milano A, Caforio ALP, Livi U et al. Evolution of focal moderate (International Society for Heart and Lung Transplantation Grade 2) rejection of the cardiac allograft. J Heart Lung Transplant 1996;15:456–60.

29 Klingenberg R, Kock A, Schnabel PA et al. Allograft rejection of ISHLT Grade ≥3A occurring late after heart transplantation—a distinct entity? J Heart Lung Transplant 2003;22:1005–13.

30 Platt JL, Fischel RJ, Matas AJ, Reif SA, Bolman RM, Bach FH. Immunopathology of hyperacute xenograft rejection in a swine-to-primate model. Transplantation 1991;52:214–20.

31 Hammond EH, Yowell RL, Nunonda S et al. Vascular (humoral) rejection in heart transplantation: pathologic observations and clinical implications. J Heart Lung Transplant 1989;8:430–43.

32 Miller LW, Wesp A, Jennison SH et al. Vascular rejection in heart transplant recipients. J Heart Lung Transplant 1993;12(suppl):S147–52.

33 Costanzo-Nordin MR, Heroux Al, Radvany R, Koch D. Robinson JA. Role humoral immunity in acute cardiac allograft dysfunction. J Heart Lung Transplant 1993; 12(suppl):S143–6.

34 Cherry R, Nielsen H, Reed E, Reemtsma K, Suciu-Foca N, Marboe CC. Vascular (humoral) rejection in human cardiac allograft biopsies: relation to circulating anti-HLA antibodies. J Heart Lung Transplant 1992;11:24–30.

35 Leprince P, Fretz C, Dorent T et al. Posttransplantation cytoxic immunoglobulin G is associated with a high rate of acute allograft dysfunctions in heart transplant recipients. Am Heart J 1999;138:586–92.

36 Caple JF, McMahon JT, Myles JL, Hook S, Ratliff NB. Acute vascular (humoral) rejection in non-OKT3-treated cardiac transplants. Cardiovasc Pathol 1995; 4:11–8.

37 Lones MA, Czer LS, Trento A, Harasty D, Miller JM, Fishbein MC. Clinico-pathologic features of humoral rejection in cardiac allografts: a study in 81 consecutive patients. J Heart Lung Transplant 1995;14:151–62.

38 Behr TM, Feucht HE, Richter K et al. Detection of humoral rejection in human cardiac allografts by assessing the capillary deposition of complement fragment C4d in endomyocardial antibodies. J Heart Lung Transplant 1999;8:904–12.

39 Rodriguez ER, Skojec DV, Tan CD et al. Antibody-mediated rejection in human cardiac allografts evaluation of immunoglobulin and complement activation products C4d and C3d as markers. Am J Transplant 2005;5:2778–85.

40 Chantranuwat C, Qiao J-H, Kobashigawa J, Hong L, Shintaku P, Fishbein MC. Immunoperoxidase staining for C4d on paraffin-embedded tissues in cardiac allograft endomyocardial biopsies. Appl Immunohistochem Mol Morphol 2004;12:166–71.

41 Reed EF, Demetris AJ, Hammond E et al. Acute antibody-mediated rejection of cardiac transplants. J Heart Lung Transplant 2006;25:153–9.

42 Lin SS, Hanaway MJ, Gonzalez-Stawinski GV et al. The role of anti-Galα1-3Gal antibodies in acute vascular rejection and accommodation of xenografts. Transplantation 2000;70:1667–74.

43 Bonnaud EN, Lewis NP, Masek MA, Billingham ME. Reliability and usefulness of immunofluorescence in heart transplantation. J Heart Lung Transplant 1995;14:163–71.

44 Baldwin WM, III, Samaniego-Picota M, Kasper EK et al. Complement deposition in early cardiac transplant biopsies is associated with ischemic injury and subsequent rejection episodes. Transplantation 1999;68:894–900.

45 Hammond EA, Yowell RL, Greenwood J, Hartung L, Renlund D, Wittwer C. Prevention of adverse clinical outcome by monitoring of cardiac transplant patients for murine monoclonal CD3 antibody (OKT3) sensitization. Transplantation 1993;55:1061–3.

46 Williams JM, Holzknecht ZE, Plummer TB, Lin SS, Brunn GJ, Platt JL. Acute vascular rejection and accommodation: divergent outcomes of the humoral response in organ transplantation. Transplantation 2004;78:1471–8.

47 Saadi S, Takahashi T, Holzknecht RA, Platt JL. Pathways to acute humoral rejection. Am J Pathol 2004;164:1073–80.

48 Book WM, Kelley L, Gravanis MB. Fulminant mixed humoral and cellular rejection in a cardiac transplant recipient: a review of the histologic findings and the literature. J Heart Lung Transplant 2003;22:604–7.

49 Mueller XM. Drug immunosuppression therapy for adult heart transplantation. Part 2: clinical applications and results. Ann Thorac Surg 2004;77:363–71.

50 Lindenfeld J, Miller GG, Shakar SF et al. Drug therapy in the heart transplant recipient. Part I: cardiac rejection and immunosuppressive drugs. Circulation 2004;110:3734–40.

51 Gaber AO, First MR, Tesi RJ et al. Results of the double-blind randomized, multicenter, phase III clinical trail of Thymoglobulin versus ATGAM in the treatment of acute graft rejection episodes after renal transplantation. Transplantation 1998;66:29–37.

52 Deeb GM, Bolling SF, Steimle CN, Dawe JE, McKay AL, Richardson AM. A randomized prospective comparison of MALG with OKT3 for rescue therapy of acute myocardial rejection. Transplantation 1991;51:180–3.

53 Kremer AB, Barnes L, Hirsch RL, Goldstein G. Orthoclone OKT3 monoclonal antibody reversal of hepatic and cardiac allograft rejection unresponsive to conventional immunosuppressive treatments. Transplant Proc 1987;19(suppl 1):54–7.

54 Costanzo-Nordin MR, Silver MA, O'Connell JB et al. Successful reversal of acute cardiac allograft rejection with OKT3 monoclonal antibody. Circulation 1987;76(suppl V):V-71–80.

55 Gilbert EM, Dewitt CC, Eiswirth CC et al. Treatment of refractory rejection with OKT3 monoclonal antibody. Am J Med 1987;82:202–6.

56 Haverty TP, Sanders M, Sheahan M. OKT3 treatment of cardiac allograft rejection. J Heart Lung Transplant 1993;12:591–8.

57 Chatenoud L, Ferran C, Reuter A et al. Systemic reaction to the anti-T-cell monoclonal antibody OKT3 in relation to serum levels of tumor necrosis factor and interferon-gamma [corrected]. N Engl J Med 1989;320:1420–1.

58 Ma H, Hammond EH, Taylor DO et al. The repetitive histologic pattern of vascular cardiac allograft rejection. Increased incidence associated with longer exposure to prophylactic murine monoclonal anti-CD3 antibody (OKT3). Transplantation 1996;62:205–10.

59 Smart FW, Naftel DC, Costanzo MR et al. Risk factors for early, cumulative, and fatal infections after heart transplantation: a multiinstitutional study. J Heart Lung Transplant 1996;15:329–41.

60 Swinnen LJ, Constanzo-Nordin MR, Fisher SG et al. Increased incidence of lymphoproliferative disorder af-ter immunosuppression with the monoclonal antibody OKT3 in cardiac transplant recipients. N Engl J Med 1990;323:1723–8.

61 Wagner FM, Reichenspurner H, Überfuhr P et al. How successful is OKT3 rescue therapy for steroid-resistant acute rejection episodes after heart transplantation? J heart Lung Transplant 1994;13:438–43.

62 Ballester M, Obrador D, Carrió I et al. Reversal of rejection-induced coronary vasculitis detected early after heart transplantation with increased immunosuppression. J Heart Transplant 1989;8:413–7.

63 Kobashigawa JA, Moriguchi JD, Laks H et al. Successful therapy for cardiac transplant recipients with hemodynamic compromising rejection [abstract]. Circulation 1996;94(suppl I):I-479.

64 Grauhan O, Knosalla C, Ewert R et al. Plasmapheresis and cyclophosphamide in the treatment of humoral rejection after heart transplantation. J Heart Lung Transplant 2001;20:316–21.

65 Olsen SL, Wagoner LE, Hammond EH et al. Vascular rejection in heart transplantation: clinical correlation, treatment options, and future considerations. J Heart Lung Transplant 1993;12:S135–42.

66 Olivari MT, May CB, Johnson NA, Ring WS, Stephens MK. Treatment of acute vascular rejection with immunoadsorption. Circulation 1994;90 (part 2):II-70–3.

67 Berglin E, Kjellstrom C, Mantovani V, Stelin G, Svalander C, Wiklund L. Plasmapheresis as a rescue therapy to resolve cardiac rejection with vasculitis and severe heart failure. A report of five cases. Transplant International 1995;8:382–7.

68 Pahl E, Crawford SE, Cohn Ra et al. Reversal of severe late left ventricular failure after pediatric heart transplantation and possible role of plasmapheresis. Am J Cardiol 2000;85:735–9.

69 Uber WI, Padgett SL, VanBakel AB et al. Predictors and outcomes of acute humoral rejection treated with plasmapheresis in heart transplant recipients [abstract]. J Heart Lung Transplant 2002;22:S169.

70 Viego-Barreiro A, Crespo-Leiro M, Domenech-Garcia N et al. Severe cardiac allograft dysfunction without endomyocardial biopsy signs of cellular rejection: incidence and management. Transplant Proc 2004;36:778–9.

71 McOmber D, Ibrahim J, Lublin DM et al. Non-ischemic left ventricular dysfunction after pediatric cardiac transplantation: treatment with plasmapheresis and OKT3. J Heart Lung Transplant 2004;23:552–7.

72 Schroeder TJ, Weiss MA, Smith RD, Stephens GW, First MR. The efficacy of OKT3 in vascular rejection. Transplantation 1991;51:312–5.

73 Zhu L, Cupps TR, Whalen G, Fauci AS. Selective effects of cyclophosphamide therapy on activation, proliferation,

and differentiation of human B cells. J Clin Invest 1987;79:1082–90.

74 Taylor DO, Bristow MR, O'Connell JB et al. A prospective, randomized comparison of cyclophosphamide and azothioprine for early rejection prophylaxis after cardiac transplantation. Decreased sensitization to OKT3. Transplantation 1994;58:645–9.

75 Grauhan O, Müller J, v. Baeyer H et al. Treatment of humoral rejection after heart transplantation. J Heart Lung Transplant 1998;17:1184–94.

76 Nakae H, Asanuma Y, Tajimi K. Cytokine removal by plasma exchange with continuous hemodiafiltration in critically ill patients. Ther Apher 2002;6:419–24.

77 Zachary AA, Lucas DP, Montgomery RA, Warren D, Simpkins C, Leffell MS. Mechanisms of desensitization: the role of plasmapheresis [abstract]. Am J Transplant 2006;World Transplant Congress Supplement:435.

78 Kazatchkine MD, Kaveri SV. Immunomodulation of autoimmune and inflammatory disease with intravenous immune globulin. N Engl J Med 2001;345:747–55.

79 Jordan SC, Vo AA, Peng A, Toyoda M, Tyan D. Intravenous gammaglobulin (IVIG): a novel approach to improve transplant rates and outcomes in highly HLA-sensitized patients. Am J Transplant 2006;6:559–66.

80 Jordan SC, Quartel AW, Czer LSC et al. Posttransplant therapy using high-dose human immunoglobulin (intravenous gammaglobulin) to control acute humoral rejection in renal and cardiac allograft recipients and potential mechanism of action. Transplantation 1998;66:800–5.

81 Casadei DH, del CRM, Opetz G et al. A randomized and prospective study comparing treatment with high-dose intravenous immunoglobulin with monoclonal antibodies for rescue of kidney grafts with steroid-resistant rejection. Transplantation 2001;71:53–8.

82 Luke PP, Scantlebury VP, Jordan ML et al. Reversal of steroid- and anti-lymphocyte antibody-resistant rejection using intravenous immunoglobulin (IVIG) in renal transplant recipients. Transplantation 2001;72:419–22.

83 Baran DA, Lubitz S, Alvi S et al. Refractory humoral cardiac allograft rejection successfully treated with a single dose of rituximab. Transplant Proc 2004;36:3164–6.

84 Garrett HE, Duvall-Seaman D, Helsley B, Groshart K. Treatment of vascular rejection with rituximab in cardiac transplantation. J Heart Lung Transplant 2005;24:1337–42.

85 Aranda JM, Scornik JC, Normann SJ et al. Anti-CD20 monoclonal antibody (rituximab) therapy for acute cardiac humoral rejection: a case report. Transplantation 2002;73:907–10.

86 Pescovitz MD. Rituximab, an anti-CD20 monoclonal antibody: history and mechanism of action. Am J Transplant 2006;6:859–66.

87 Ratkovec RM, Hammond EH, O'Connell JB et al. Outcome of cardiac transplant recipients with a positive donor-specific crossmatch-preliminary results with plasmapheresis. Transplantation 1992;54:651–5.

88 Smith JD, Danskine AJ, Laylor RM, Rose ML, Yacoub MH. The effect of panel reactive antibodies and the donor specific crossmatch on graft survival after heart and heart-lung transplantation. Transplant Immunol 1993;1:60–5.

89 Lavee J, Kormos RL, Duquesnoy RJ et al. Influence of panel-reactive antibody and lymphocytotoxic crossmatch on survival after heart transplantation. J Heart Lung Transplant 1991;10:921–30.

90 Kobashigawa JA, Sabad A, Drinkwater D et al. Pretransplant panel reactive-antibody screens. Are they truly a marker for poor outcome after cardiac transplantation? Circulation 1996;94(suppl II):II-294–7.

91 Itescu S, Tung TC, Burke EM et al. Preformed IgG antibodies against major histocompatibility complex class II antigens are major risk factors for high-grade cellular rejection in recipients of heart transplantation. Circulation 1998;98:786–93.

92 Girnita Al, Webber SA, Zeevi A. Anti-HLA alloantibodies in pediatric solid organ transplantation. Pediatr Transplant 2006;10:146–53.

93 Tambur AR, Bray RA, Takemoto SK et al. Flow cytometric detection of HLA-specific antibodies as a predictor of heart allograft rejection. Transplantation 2000;70:1055–9.

94 Aziz S, Hassantash A, Nelson K et al. The clinical significance of flow cytometry crossmatching in heart transplantation. J Heart Lung Transplant 1998;17:686–92.

95 Mehra MR, Uber PA, Uber WE, Scott RL, Park MH. Allosensitization in heart transplantation: implications and management strategies. Curr Opin Cardiol 2003;18:153–8.

96 Hawkins JA, Breinholt JP, Lambert LM et al. Class I and class II anti-HLA antibodies after implantation of cryopreserved allograft material in pediatric patients. J Thorac Cardiovasc Surg 2000;119:324–30.

97 Massad MG, Cook DJ, Schmitt SK et al. Factors influencing HLA sensitization in implantable LVAD recipients. Ann Thorac Surg 1997;64:1120–5.

98 Moazami N, Itescu S, Williams MR, Argenziano M, Weinberg A, Oz MH. Platelet transfusions are associated with the development of anti-major histocompatibility complex class I antibodies in patients with left ventricular assist support. J Heart Lung Transplant 1998;17:876–80.

99 McKenna DH, Jr, Eastlund T, Segall M, Noreen HJ, Park S. HLA alloimmunization in patients requiring ventricular assist device support. J Heart Lung Transplant 2002;21:1218–24.

100 Newell H, Smith JD, Rogers P *et al.* Sensitization following LVAD implantation using leucodepleted blood is not due to HLA antibodies. Am J Transplant 2006;6:1712–7.

101 Joyce DL, Southard RE, Torre-Amione G, Noon GP, Land GA, Loebe M. Impact of left ventricular assist device (LVAD)-mediated humoral sensitization on post-transplant outcomes. J Heart Lung Transplant 2005;24:2054–9.

102 Zangwill SD, Ellis TM, Zlotocha J *et al.* The virtual crossmatch—a screening tool for sensitized pediatric heart transplant recipients. Pediatr Transplant 2005;10:38–41.

103 Jordan SC, Tyan D, Stablein D *et al.* Evaluation of intravenous immunoglobulin as an agent to lower allosensitization and improve transplantation in highly sensitized adult patients with end-stage renal disease: report of the NIH IG02 Trial. J Am Soc Nephrol 2004;15:3256–62.

104 Montgomery RA, Zachary AA, Racusen LC *et al.* Plasmapheresis and intravenous immune globulin provides effective rescue therapy for refractory humoral rejection and allow kidneys to be successfully transplanted into cross-match-postive recipients. Transplantation 2000;70:887–95.

105 Stegall MD, Gloor J, Winters JL, Moore SB, DeGoey S. A comparison of plasmapheresis versus high-dose IVIG desensitization in renal allograft recipients with high levels of donor specific alloantibody. Am J Transplant 2006;6:346–51.

106 Jordan S. IVIG vs plasmapheresis for desensitization: which is better? Am J Transplant 2006;6:1510–1.

107 Pisani BA, Mullen M, Malinoska K *et al.* Plasmapheresis with intravenous immunoglobulin G is effective in patients with elevated panel reactive antibody prior to cardiac transplantation. J Heart Lung Transplant 1999;18:701–6.

108 Jacobs JA, Quintessenza JA, Boucek RJ *et al.* Pediatric cardiac transplantation in children with high panel reactive antibody. Ann Thorac Surg 2004;78:1703–9.

109 Holt DB, Lublin DM, Phelan DL, Huddleston CB, Saffitz JE, Canter CE. Rejection in presensitized pediatric heart transplant recipients with a positive donor crossmatch utilizing perioperative plasmapheresis and cytolytic therapy [abstract]. J Heart Lung Transplant 2005;24:S113.

110 Leech SH, Lopez-Cepero M, LeFor WM *et al.* Management of the sensitized cardiac recipient: the use of plasmapheresis and intravenous immunoglobulin. Clin Transplant 2006;20:476–84.

111 John R, Lietz K, Burke E *et al.* Intravenous immunoglobulin reduces anti-HLA alloreactivity and shortens waiting time to cardiac transplantation in highly sensitized left ventricular assist device recipients. Circulation 1999;100 (suppl II):II-229–5.

112 Itescu S, Burke E, Lietz K *et al.* Intravenous pulse administration of cyclophosphamide is an effective and safe treatment for sensitized cardiac allograft recipients. Circulation 2002;105:1214–9.

113 Wang CH, KO WJ, Chou NK, Wang SS. Efficacy and safety of tacrolimus versus cyclosporine microemulsion in primary cardiac transplant recipients: 6-month results in Taiwan. Transplant Proc 2004;36:2384–5.

114 Grimm M, Rinaldi M, Yonan NA *et al.* Superior prevention of acute rejection by tacrolimus vs. cyclosporine in heart transplant recipients—a large European trial. Am J Transplant 2006;6:1387–97.

115 Reichart B, Meiser B, Vigano M *et al.* European multicenter tacrolimus (FK506) heart pilot study: one-year results—European Tacrolimus Multicenter Heart Study Group. J Heart Lung Transplant 1998;17:775–81.

116 Taylor DO, Barr ML, Radovancevic B *et al.* A randomized, multicenter comparison of tacrolimus and cyclosporine immunosuppressive regimens in cardiac transplantation: decreased hyperlipidemia and hypertension with tacrolimus. J Heart Lung Transplant 1999;18:336–45.

117 Kobashigawa JA, Patel J, Furukawa H *et al.* Five-year results of a randomized, single-center study of tacrolimus vs microemulsion cyclosporine in heart transplant recipients. J Heart Lung Transplant 2006;25:434–9.

118 Kobashigawa J, Miller L, Renlund D *et al.* A randomized active-controlled trial of mycophenolate mofetil in heart transplant recipients. Transplantation 1998;66:507–15.

119 Kobashigawa J, Meiser BM. Review of major clinical trials with mycophenolate mofetil in cardiac transplantation. Transplantation 2005;80:S235–43.

120 Rose ML, Smith J, Dureau G, Keogh A, Kobashigawa J. Mycophenolate mofetil decreases antibody production after cardiac transplantation. J heart Lung Transplant 2002;21:282–5.

121 Kobashigawa JA, Tobis JM, Mentzer RM *et al.* Mycophenolate mofetil reduces intimal thickness by intravascular ultrasound after heart transplant: reanalysis of the multicenter trial. Am J Transplant 2006;6:993–7.

122 Mehra MR, Uber PA, Scott RL, Park MH. Ethnic disparity in clinical outcome after heart transplantation is abrogated using tacrolimus and mycophenolate mofetil-based immunosuppression. Transplantation 2002;74:1568–73.

123 Kobashigawa JA, Miller LW, Russell SD *et al.* Tacrolimus with mycophenolate mofetil (MMF) or sirolimus vs. cyclosporine with MMF in cardiac transplant patients: 1-year report. Am J Transplant 2006;6:1377–86.

124 Kobashigawa JA, Katznelson S, Laks H *et al.* Effect of pravastatin on outcomes after cardiac transplantation. N Engl J Med 1995;333:621–7.

125 Wenke K, Meiser B, Thiery J *et al.* Simvastatin initiated early after heart transplantation: 8-year prospective experience. Circulation 2003;107:93–7.

126 Stojanovic I, Vrtovec B, Radovancevic B *et al.* Survival, graft atherosclerosis, and rejection incidence in heart transplant recipients treated with statin: 5-year follow-up. J Heart Lung Transplant 2005;24:1235–8.

127 Mehra MR, Raval NY. Metaanalysis of statins and survival in de novo cardiac transplantation. Transplant Proc 2004;36:1539–41.

128 Katznelson S, Wang XM, Chia D *et al.* The inhibitory effects of pravastatin on natural killer cell activity in vivo and on cytotoxic T lymphocyte activity in vitro. J Heat Lung Transplant 1998;17:335–40.

129 Mach F. Statins as immunomodulators. Transpl Immunol 2002;9:197–200.

130 Weis M, Pehlivanli S, Meiser BM, von Scheidt W. Simvastatin treatment is associated with improvement in coronary endothelial function and decreased cytokine activation in patients after heart transplantation. J Am Coll Cardiol 2001;38:814–8.

131 Ventura HO, Mehra MR. C-reactive protein and cardiac allograft vasculopathy: is inflammation the critical link? J Am Coll Cardiol 2003;42:483–5.

132 Kobashigawa JA, Patel JK. Immunosuppression for heart transplantation: where are we now? Nat Clin Pract (Cardiovasc Med) 2006;3:203–12.

133 Fishbein MC, Kobashigawa J. Biopsy-negative cardiac transplant rejection: etiology, diagnosis, and therapy. Curr Opin Cardiol 2004;19:166–9.

134 Haythe J, Dwyer T, Burke E *et al.* The changing pattern of humoral rejection in cardiac transplant recipients [abstract]. J Heart Lung Transplant 2006;25:S109.

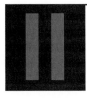

PART II

Immune dysfunction promoting CVD: induction by transplantation drugs

CHAPTER 10

Immunomodulating therapy in chronic heart failure

*Lars Gullestad, Jan Kristian Damås,
Arne Yndestad & Pål Aukrust*

Overview

Evidence from both experimental and clinical trials indicates that inflammatory mediators are of importance in the pathogenesis of chronic heart failure (HF) contributing to cardiac remodeling and peripheral vascular disturbances. Several studies have shown raised levels of inflammatory cytokines such as tumor necrosis factor (TNF)α, interleukin (IL)-1β, and IL-6 in HF patients in plasma, circulating leukocytes, as well as in the failing myocardium itself. Importantly, this rise in inflammatory mediators seems not be accompanied by a corresponding increase in anti-inflammatory cytokines such as IL-10 and transforming growth factor β (TGF-β), resulting in an inflammatory imbalance in the cytokine network. These disturbances are observed in both mild and advanced HF, independently of etiology. Traditional cardiovascular drugs have little influence on the cytokine network in HF patients. Although somewhat disappointing, the negative results of the anti-TNF studies do not necessarily argue against the "cytokine hypothesis." These studies just underscore the challenges in developing treatment modalities that can modulate the cytokine network in HF patients, resulting in beneficial net effects. More broad-based general immunomodulating treatments such as intravenous immunoglobulin (IVIg), thalidomide, and statins have shown promising results in smaller studies, which need to be confirmed in larger studies with hospitalizations and death as endpoints. In addition, further research in this area will have to more precisely identify the most important "actors" in the immunopathogenesis of chronic HF.

Introduction

Heart failure (HF) is a highly complex multistep disorder in which a number of physiological systems participate. Until a few decades ago HF was considered a hemodynamic disorder. In recent years both experimental and clinical studies have clearly demonstrated the involvement of neurohormones in the progression of HF, leading to new treatment modalities such as angiotensin-converting enzyme (ACE) inhibitors and β-blockers. However, despite proper blockade of the neurohumoral system including β-blockers, ACE inhibitors, and aldosterone antagonist, hospital admissions for HF continue to rise and accounts for approximately 5% of medical admissions in Western countries [1]. Moreover, mortality in HF patients is high in these countries, ranging from 5 to 70% per year depending on the severity of the disease [2], suggesting that important pathogenic mechanisms remain active and unmodified by the present treatment modalities. Cytokines and other inflammatory mediators may be such substances.

Rationale for immunomodulating therapy

Increased levels of inflammatory cytokines in HF

Several reports have demonstrated enhanced expression and release of inflammatory cytokines such as tumor necrosis factor (TNF)α, interleukin (IL)-1, IL-6, IL-18, cardiotrophin-1, and Fas ligand (L), as well as several chemokines (e.g., monocyte chemoattractant peptide (MCP)-1, IL-8, and macrophage inflammatory protein (MIP)-1α) in HF patients [3–8]. Plasma levels of inflammatory cytokines and chemokines appear to be elevated in direct relation to deteriorating of functional class (i.e., NYHA classification) and cardiac performance (i.e., left ventricular ejection fraction (LVEF)) [3, 5, 9]. Increased expression of inflammatory cytokines and chemokines in HF patients have also been demonstrated in circulating lymphocytes and monocytes at both the protein and mRNA levels, with particularly enhanced expression in the coronary circulation [10]. Moreover, enhanced expression of inflammatory mediators have also been demonstrated within the failing myocardium (e.g., adhesion molecules, TNFα, IL-6-related cytokines, and chemokines receptors) [11, 12]. Furthermore, these inflammatory mediators may also give important prognostic information in patients with chronic HF. For example, in a substudy to Studies on Left Ventricular Dysfunction (SOLVD), patients with plasma levels of TNFα < 6.5 pg/mL had a better prognosis than those with higher TNFα levels [13]. Furthermore, in a large population of HF patients (1200 patients, the cytokine database from the Vesnarinone trial), circulating levels of inflammatory cytokines (i.e., TNFα and IL-6) and cytokine receptors (i.e., soluble TNF receptors (TNF-Rs)) were found to be independent predictors of mortality in patients with advanced HF [14]. Similarly, we have recently shown that assessment of plasma levels of sTNF-R type I might provide important prognostic information in patients who develop HF during the acute phase following acute myocardial infarction (MI) [15]. Taken together, these clinical data suggest that the raised systemic levels of inflammatory cytokines in HF patients may reflect important pathogenic mechanisms in these patients.

Pathophysiological consequences of immune activation in HF

A series of experimental studies have revealed that the biological effects of cytokines may explain several aspects of the syndrome of chronic HF. The pathogenic role of inflammatory cytokines in congestive heart failure is supported by various transgenic mouse models, and notably, systemic administration of TNFα even in concentrations comparable to those found in circulation of HF patients has been shown to induce a dilated cardiomyopathy-like phenotype in animal models [16], and cardiac-specific overexpression of TNFα has been found to promote a phenotype mimicking several features of clinical HF such as cardiac hypertrophy, ventricular dilation and fibrosis, as well as several biochemical and cellular dysfunctions [17]. Inflammatory cytokines may modulate cardiovascular functions by a variety of mechanisms (Table 10.1). Thus, various cytokines such TNFα and IL-1β have been shown to depress myocardial contractility involving mechanisms such as uncoupling of β-adrenergic signaling, increase in cardiac nitric oxide, or alterations in intracellular calcium homeostasis [18–20]. Moreover, TNFα and members of the IL-6 family may induce structural changes in the failing myocardium such as cardiomyocyte hypertrophy and interstitial fibrosis [21, 22]. TNFα may also promote cardiomyocyte apoptosis [20, 23], as well as activate metalloproteinases (MMPs) and impair the expression of their endogenous tissue inhibitors (TIMPs) [24], possibly contributing to cardiac remodeling.

While several studies have focused on the pathogenic role of TNFα, other inflammatory mediators could also play an important role in the progression of chronic HF. Our research group has been particularly focusing on the potential pathogenic role of chemokines, a family of chemotactic

Table 10.1 Pathophysiological effects of inflammatory.

Left ventricular dysfunction
- Negative inotropic effect
- Hypertrophy
- Fibrosis
- Apoptosis

Endothelial dysfunction
Cachexia
Anemia
Activation of fetal gene program
Promotes tromboembolism
Beta receptor uncoupling from adenylate cyclase
Abnormalities of mitochondrial energetics
Muscular weakness

cytokines causing directed migration of leukocytes into inflamed tissue. These inflammatory mediators could both indirectly (e.g., recruitment and activation of infiltrating leukocytes) and directly (e.g., modulation of apoptosis, fibrosis, and angiogenesis) contribute to myocardial failure [12, 25]. Thus, interstitial monocyte infiltration in the myocardium is associated with cardiac hypertrophy, ventricular dilatation, and depressed contractile function, and is found in transgenic mice with myocardial overexpression of the CC-chemokine MCP-1 [26]. Conversely, MIP-1α knockout mice do not develop cardiac lesions after Coxsackie B virus infection because of attenuated recruitment of activated monocytes into the myocardium [27]. Finally, the observation of high embryonic mortality and organ defects, including cardiac ventricular septum defects in the CXC-chemokine receptor 4 (CXCR4) knockout mice, indicates a crucial and direct dependence of chemokines in the development and function of the myocardium [28].

Besides the classical inflammatory cytokines and chemokines, the numbers of cytokines involved in HF are large and rapidly expanding. IL-18 (a member of the IL-1 family), Activin A, several ligands in the TNF superfamily (e.g., CD40L, TRAIL, LIGHT, and the osteoprotegrin (OPG)/RANKL/RANK axis) are upregulated in HF, potentially contributing to inflammation, apoptosis, and matrix degrading within the failing myocardium.

Immunomodulating therapy

Immunomodulatory effects of traditional cardiovascular therapy

Based on the data outlined above it is conceivable to hypothesize that treatment targeting immune activation and inflammation may have beneficial effects and represent a new therapeutic paradigm for treatment of patients with HF. Based on experimental studies, traditional cardiovascular drugs could potentially attenuate inflammatory responses. Thus, several in vitro studies and studies in animal models have demonstrated a significant cross talk between different neurohormones such as angiotensin II and noradrenalin and inflammatory cytokines. Studies have shown that angiotensin II provokes inflammatory response in different cells and tissue

[29], suggesting an anti-inflammatory potential of cardiovascular drugs such as ACE inhibitors and β-blockers. However, short-time effects during in vitro experiments may not necessarily reflect the effect of long-time exposure to these medications in HF patients in which the immune system is preactivated before start of therapy. In fact, few clinical studies have examined how conventional HF medication influences the immune activation in HF. We have shown that high-dose ACE inhibition with enalapril causes a marked decrease in IL-6 bioactivity, associated with reduction in left ventricular septum thickness [30]. Thus, it is possible that an important "antihypertrophic" mechanism of ACE inhibitors on the myocardium may be a reduction in IL-6 levels and signal transduction. However, except for a favorable effect on IL-6, other immunological parameters were markedly elevated in HF patients and remained unchanged during treatment with an optimal dose of enalapril. In the CONCENSUS trial, enalapril reduced the level of C-reactive protein (CRP), but this decrease was not related to the reduction in mortality [31]. Moreover, although several in vitro studies have shown that β-adrenergic stimulation may modulate cytokine production in myocytes and other cells by increasing intracellular cAMP levels [32–34], the effect of β-blockers on inflammation in HF is mixed and uncertain. Some suppressive effects of β-blockers on plasma levels of both inflammatory and anti-inflammatory cytokines were reported in a nonplacebo controlled study in patients with idiopathic dilated cardiomyopathy (IDCM) [35], while in a substudy of the Metoprolol CR/XL Randomized Intervention Trial in Heart Failure (MERIT) there was no effect of treatment with the β1-selective blocker metoprolol CR/XL on cytokine levels comparing placebo [36]. Nonselective blockade of the β-receptors with carvedilol demonstrated a significant reduction in the transcardial gradient of TNFα, but few patients were included.

In patients with severe HF and ventricular conduction disturbances, cardiac resynchronization therapy (CRT), based on correction of electromechanical dyssynchrony by biventricular pacing, causes an antiremodeling effect, improves symptoms and exercise capacity, reduces the occurrence of ventricular tachyarrhythmias, reduces the

Table 10.2 Immunomodulation in heart failure

Targeted anticytokine therapy
- Soluble TNF receptors (Etanercept)
- Antibodies against TNFα (Infliximab)
- Chemokine modulators
- Interleukin-1 receptor antagonist
- Interleukin-10

Non-specific immunomodulation
- exercise
- antioxidants
- Celacade
- Pentoxyfylline
- Statins
- Immunoadsorption
- Intravenous immunoglobulin
- Thalidomide

Potential immunomodulatory treatment modalities
- TGF-ß superfamily modulators
- Peroxisome proliferator-activated receptor agonists
- Mast cell-stabilizing agent, i.e., tranilast
- Inhibitors of T cell activation (e.g., CTLA4Ig fusion protein)
- Autologous stem cell transplantation

hospitalizations for worsening HF, and improves survival [37]. However, although a prominent reduction in heart size and volume, CRT does not seem to influence inflammatory cytokines [38].

Taken together, although traditional cardiovascular medication may have some immunomodulatory properties, the effects observed in vivo in HF patients are rather modest, suggesting that more potent and specific immunomodulatory treatment modalities should be investigated in this disorder (Table 10.2).

Targeted anticytokine therapy

Given the central role of TNFα in the pathogenesis of HF, therapeutic modulation targeting this cytokine has received particularly much attention. Preliminary reports suggested that TNFα inhibition with recombinant chimeric soluble TNF-R type 2 (etanercept) had beneficial effects on cardiac performance in HF patients [41]. As a result this was followed by the much larger study, designed as two parallel trials (RENAISSANCE and RECOVER), pooled as the Randomized Etanercept Worldwide

Evaluation [RENEWAL] program examining the effect of etanercept on morbidity and mortality in a population of 1500 patients with symptomatic HF and evidence of left ventricular dysfunction (EF < 30%). The trial was stopped early because of futility. There was no evidence of an effect on mortality, hospitalizations, or a clinical composite score [42]. Subanalysis of the trial has suggested an interaction with dosing and outcome, as patients taking the lowest active dose had less hospitalizations/deaths compared with those who received the higher active dose.

A second targeted approach for TNFα was a trial with an anti-TNFα gchimeric monoclonal antibody that binds to human TNF, infliximab. Infliximab has previously been shown to be effective in Crohn's disease and rheumatoid arthritis. The Anti-TNFα Therapy Against CHF (ATTACH) was a placebo controlled phase II trial in 150 patients with symptomatic HF and evidence of left ventricular dysfunction with EF < 35%. Patients were randomized to one of three arms: (1) infusion of infliximab of 5 mg/kg, (2) infusion of infliximab 10 mg/kg, or (3) placebo infusion. The primary endpoint was a clinical composite score that classified the patient as better, worse, or unchanged after intervention. The trial was stopped early because of higher rates of mortality and hospitalization in particular in the active high-dosing group [43].

Why did the anti-TNF therapy fail?

These limitations in anti-TNF therapy may have several explanations (Table 10.3): (1) A recent study in animal models showed that while etanercept decreased plasma cytokine levels, there was no decrease in IL-6 and MCP-1 within the myocardium [44]. (2) The chimeric anti-TNFα antibody (infliximab) directly binds to the transmembrane form

Table 10.3 Why has targeted anti-TNF therapy in HF failed?

Failure to modulate cytokines in the myocardium

Cellular toxicity

From too much to too little of TNFα

Increased molecular stability and half-life of TNFα

Wrong dose of the agent

Failure to modulate other important cytokines

of TNF, resulting in damage of TNF-expressing cells by both antibody-dependent cellular toxicity, complement-dependent cytotoxic effector mechanisms, and by induction of apoptosis [45]. While such mechanisms may be beneficial in inflammatory disorders such as inflammatory bowel disease [45], it may result in deleterious effect in HF leading to damage of TNFα-expressing cardiomyocytes. (3) While etanercept that binds to soluble TNFα can neutralize the effect of this cytokine, the binding of TNFα to this soluble receptor could also potentially result in increased molecular stability and half-life of TNFα [46]. (4) While too much of inflammatory cytokines such as TNFα may be harmful, too little of these mediators may also have adverse effects on the myocardium, reflecting the involvement of these cytokines in both maladaptive and adaptive responses [22, 47]. (5) Compared to previous pilot studies in HF patients (etanercept) and studies in other human disorders (infliximab), the dosage used in the HF studies was rather high and the correct dosage for anti-TNF therapy in HF patients needs to be established before any firm conclusion can be drawn. In particular, recent reports suggest a dose-dependent toxicity during anti-TNF therapy, further underscoring this issue [42]. (6) Finally, and perhaps most importantly, while several studies have focused on the possible pathogenic role of TNFα and targeted therapy against this molecule, further research in this area will have to more precisely identify the most important actors in the immunopathogenesis of chronic HF in order to develop more specific immunomodulating therapy. Thus, although the results of the placebo-controlled anti-TNF trials may seem disappointing, they do not mean the end of the cytokine era even before it has started. For example, although etanercept therapy resulted in increased mortality in patients with septic shock, few, if anyone, question the pathogenic role of inflammation in this disorder.

Nonspecific immunomodulating therapy

Failure of anti-TNF therapy has led to more interest in a more general immunomodulating approach. It is a fact that the rise in inflammatory mediators in HF is not accompanied by a corresponding increase in anti-inflammatory cytokines such as IL-10 and transforming growth factor (TGF)-β resulting in an imbalance in the cytokine network with inflammation net effects. To restore this, inflammatory imbalance could be an important goal for immunomodulating therapy in HF [3].

Exercise

Exercise training has clinically important effects on exercise capacity, quality of life, left ventricular remodeling, and mortality in patients with HF. In recent years it has also been demonstrated that exercise may favorably influence the cytokine network. Endurance training downregulates inflammatory cytokines and decreases local inducible nitric oxide synthase (iNOS) expression as well as intracellular accumulation of NO [48, 49]. However, if the benefit of exercise on left ventricular remodeling and mortality is mediated through, an effect on inflammation remains to be explored.

Antioxidant therapy

Several studies suggest that enhanced lipid oxidation and damage induced by reactive oxygen species play a pathogenic role in HF [50]. Oxidative stress can increase cytokine levels and vice versa, involving nuclear factor (NF)κB-related mechanisms, possibly representing a vicious cycle in HF [50]. Antioxidative therapy could therefore be of potential interest in HF patients, but somewhat disappointing, vitamin E supplementation did not influence cytokine levels, functional indexes, quality of life, or neurohumoral status among 56 patients with advanced HF [51]. However, recent knowledge suggests that combination of several antioxidants particularly focusing on restoring intracellular glutathione redox status could be a therapeutic approach in disorders characterized by enhanced oxidative stress and inflammation such as chronic HF, and future trials will have to investigate other antioxidant treatment regimens.

Celacade

Autologous blood, exposed ex vivo to oxidative stress at an elevated temperature and administrated intramuscularly, induces several biological responses including a decrease in inflammation [52]. Recently a double-blind trial in 75 patients with HF using this approach was published [53]. Compared with no treatment patients using the device (VC7002, Vasogen, Inc.), which exposed blood from patients to oxidative stress, had reduced risk of death and hospitalization and improved a clinical composite score. There was no difference in left ventricular EF or inflammatory markers such as TNFα, IL-6, IL-10, or CRP. The mechanism of benefit of this treatment is at present unclear, but a larger phase III clinical trial (ACCLAIM) has just been stopped. In that study 2414 patients with HF, in NYHA class II–IV and EF < 35%, were randomized to active treatment or placebo. The primary endpoint was death and cardiovascular hospitalization. In a recent press release, the company states that there was no difference in the primary endpoint, but that among a subgroup of 692 patients with NYHA II, active treatment resulted in a 39% reduction in death and cardiovascular hospitalizations. The reason for a discrepant result among different subgroups, and if the benefit of this therapy involves anti-inflammatory effects, remained to be clarified.

Pentoxyfylline

Pentoxyfylline, a xanthine-derived agent known to inhibit the production of TNFα, was the first immunomodulatory agent that showed beneficial effects in HF patients in clinical trials. Sliwa *et al.* have now conducted three trials in chronic HF using pentoxyfylline. The first was a small pilot study among 28 patients with dilated cardiomyopathy [54]. Compared with placebo pentoxyfylline treatment for 6 months resulted in improved functional class and a significant increase in EF associated with a decrease in TNFα [54]. However, the use of ACE inhibitors and β-blockers was not optimal in that trial, and a new prospective, double-blind, randomized, placebo-controlled study in patients with symptomatic IDCM and left ventricular dysfunction with EF < 35% and optimally treated with ACE inhibitors and β-blockers was performed [55]. The study confirmed the result of the first study demonstrating a beneficial effect of pentoxyfylline on symptoms and left ventricular EF [55]. The third study was among 38 patients with ischemic cardiomyopathy who were randomized to pentoxyfylline or corresponding placebo on top of standard cardiovascular treatment for 6 months [56]. Compared with placebo, pentoxyfylline resulted in an improvement in functional class and left ventricular EF. Although these findings were accompanied

by decreased plasma levels of pro-BNP, TNFα, and Fas, this does not necessarily prove any causal relationship. In fact, pentoxyfylline is a nonspecific inhibitor of phosphodiesterases with potential effects on the myocardium unrelated to immunomodulatory properties of this medication.

Statins

Several studies have shown a remarkable improvement in the prognosis of coronary artery disease after treatment with HMG-CoA reductase inhibitors (statins) [57, 58]. Recent data suggest that statins have pleiotropic effects in addition to their cholesterol lowering properties. Several studies have demonstrated immunomodulatory and anti-inflammatory effects as well as antithrombotic effects of these medications [59]. Furthermore, in vitro experiments and studies in animal models have shown that statins may prevent the development of cardiac hypertrophy in a cholesterol-independent manner, involving immunomodulatory as well as antioxidative and MMP-inhibiting effects [60]. In fact, the combination of cholesterol lowering, immunomodulatory, and antioxidative properties suggests that statins should be an interesting therapeutical approach in HF. There is also evidence for a beneficial effect of statins in HF [61]. However, low levels of circulating cholesterol are associated with worse outcome [62], and the loss of the protection that lipoproteins may provide through binding and detoxifying endotoxins entering the circulation via the gut may be potentially harmful in HF patients [63]. There is therefore a need for definitive outcome trials to assess the efficacy and safety of statins in HF. Larger ongoing outcome studies (CORONA and GISSI-HF) should provide more definitive answers to question.

Immunoadsorption

Cardiac autoantibodies against cardiac cell proteins such as mitochondrial and contractile proteins, cardiac β₁-adrenergic receptors, and muscarinergic receptors may play a pathogenic role in IDCM, and their removal by immunoadsorption has been shown to improve cardiac function in this disorder [64]. Interestingly, such therapy in combination with subsequent intravenous immunoglobulin (IVIg) therapy was recently shown to decrease the numbers of activated leukocytes within the failing myocardium [65]. While IVIg has potent modulatory effects on the cytokine network (see below), no such effects have been demonstrated for immunoadsorption. Moreover, while immunoadsorption has been shown to remove autoantibodies against cardiac β_1-adrenergic receptors, we have recently shown that the beneficial effect on cardiac function by IVIg treatment in patients with IDCM is not due to neutralization of antireceptor autoantibodies. Thus, although similar, it is possible that these immunomodulatory treatment modalities may have different mechanisms of action with potential additive or even synergistic effects as a consequence.

Intravenous immunoglobulin

Therapy with IVIg has been evaluated in a wide range of immune-mediated disorders, such as Kawasaki syndrome, dermatomyositis, idiopathic thrombocytopenic purpura, and multiple sclerosis [66, 67]. Beneficial effects of IVIg have also been suggested in acute and peripartum cardiomyopathy [68, 69], and recently we demonstrated in a double-blind, placebo-controlled study that IVIg significantly enhanced LVEF by 5 EF% independent of the etiology of HF [40]. In contrast, in a recent study by McNamara *et al.* [70], they found no significant effect of IVIg compared with placebo on recent-onset IDCM, which may seem in conflict with our study. However, in the "IDCM study" there was a marked improvement in the study group as a whole (i.e., with or without IVIg), reflecting a spontaneous improvement in recent-onset IDCM. Moreover, it is noteworthy that the dosage schedule differs between the "IDCM" [70] and the "chronic HF" [40] study. Thus, while both studies gave induction therapy, maintenance therapy (monthly infusions (0.4 g/kg) for a total of 5 months) was only given in the HF study. Notably, in the latter study there was a gradual decline in N-terminal pro-atrial natriuretic peptide throughout the study with the most pronounced decline at the end of study [40]. Moreover, a recent follow-up study showed that most of the HF patients in the IVIg group had a decrease in LVEF 1 year after termination of the study (L. Gullestad and P. Aukrust, unpublished data). These data suggest that maintenance therapy is needed for an extended period of time as in other chronic inflammatory disorders.

Several nonmutually exclusive modes of action may be of importance for the clinical effects of IVIg in inflammatory disorders such as neutralization of microbial antigens and superantigens, Fc-receptor blockade, impairment of leukocyte adhesion to endothelial cells, and decreased apoptosis [71]. However, and probably most importantly, IVIg may modulate the cytokine network. In the chronic HF study [40] the improvement in LVEF in HF patients was correlated with a marked rise in the anti-inflammatory mediators IL-10, IL-1 receptor antagonist (IL-1Ra), and soluble TNF-Rs, accompanied by a slight decrease in TNFα and IL-1β, suggesting an anti-inflammatory net effect with potentially beneficial result on the myocardium. Finally, we have recently reported that IVIg therapy, but not placebo, may also downregulate chemokines and their corresponding receptors on peripheral blood mononuclear cells in HF patients, possibly contributing to the beneficial effect of IVIg in HF [10]. IVIg appears, therefore, to have a balanced and dual effect on the cytokine network with a downregulation of certain inflammatory mediators (e.g., IL-8 and IL-1) combined with an upregulation of anti-inflammatory mediators (e.g., IL-10 and IL-1Ra). In fact, enforcing the anti-inflammatory pathways might be as important as reducing the inflammatory cytokines. IL-10 may be a key component in this process by suppressing the production of several inflammatory cytokines such as TNFα, IL-6, and IL-1 [72], and by inhibiting chemotaxis at least partly by decreasing the production of IL-8 and other chemokines. IL-10 also has protective effects on the development of atherosclerosis and viral myocarditis in mice [73]. Furthermore, IL-1Ra has been found to protect against hepatic and cerebral ischemic injury in rats [74], and may prevent impairment of β-adrenergic responsiveness in rat cardiomyocytes exposed to activated macrophages [75].

Thalidomide

The sedative and antinausea drug thalidomide has been shown to have broad immunomodulatory and antioncogenic properties [76, 77]. Diseases such as erythema nodosum leprosum, rheumatoid arthritis, and cancer are currently being treated with thalidomide, although the mechanisms of action remain unclear [76, 77]. However, although thalidomide has been shown to have both anti-inflammatory and antioncogenic properties [77–80], the mechanisms of action of thalidomide in various disorders remain unclear and contradictory results have been reported concerning its effects on cytokine levels in vivo [81–83]. In a recent double-blind study, thalidomide (25 mg q.d. increasing to 200 mg q.d.) was tested in 56 patients with chronic HF and LVEF <40% on optimal conventional cardiovascular treatment [84]. Thalidomide treatment resulted in a significant increase in LVEF (∼7 EF units) along with a significant decrease in left ventricular end-diastolic volume and heart rate. This improvement in LVEF was accompanied by a decrease in matrix metalloproteinase-2 and in total neutrophil counts, while TNFα levels increased, suggesting both pro- and anti-inflammatory effects of thalidomide. These preliminary observations should therefore clearly be confirmed in a larger prospective study with morbidity and mortality as endpoints. Such studies should also more precisely try to define the optimal dosage as well as the mechanisms of action of this medication.

New therapeutic targets in HF

Recently, the plasticity of uncommitted stem cells has opened new perspectives in tissue regeneration, and such an approach has also been applied to restore cardiac function after MI. Interestingly, members of the TGF-β superfamily seem to promote differentiation of embryonic stem cells into cardiomyocytes together with other cytokines including chemokines and members of the TNF superfamily, and these cytokines could have a therapeutic potential as adjuvant in stem cell therapy.

We and others have demonstrated enhanced T-cell activation in chronic HF, potentially contributing to both systemic and myocardial inflammation. Intervention that inhibits this unwanted T-cell activity could represent a new treatment modality in HF. Thus, intervention that inhibits this unwanted T-cell activity could represent a new treatment modality in HF. By blocking the engagement of CD28 on T cells, a genetically constructed CTLA4Ig fusion protein prevents the delivery of the second costimulatory signal that is required for optimal T-cell activation [85]. Such an approach

to inhibit T-cell activation has demonstrated beneficial effects in animal models of autoimmune disease and allograft rejection [86], and CTLA4Ig was recently shown to improve signs and symptoms of disease activity in patients with rheumatoid arthritis [87]. It is tempting to hypothesize that such a therapeutic approach could also be beneficial in chronic HF. Moreover, based on the potential role of chemokines in the pathogenesis of HF, drugs targeting these mediators could be an interesting approach and, indeed, gene therapy with an MCP-1 antagonist was recently found to attenuate the development of ventricular remodeling in a mouse model for post-MI HF [88]. Also, IL-10 has been found to have protective effects on the development of viral myocarditis in mice [72], and IL-1 receptor antagonist may provide cardioprotection against ischemia–reperfusion injury in rat cardiomyocytes [89], underscoring a potential for other anti-inflammatory approaches than anti-TNF therapy in chronic HF. Future research in this area will have to more precisely identify the most important mechanisms and actors in the immunopathogenesis of chronic HF in order to develop better immunomodulating agents for this disorder.

Conclusions

Chronic HF appears to be accompanied not only by a rise in inflammatory cytokines, but also by an inadequate rise in anti-inflammatory mediators, resulting in a poorly regulated cytokine network. A sustained overexpression of these biologically active cytokines may contribute to progressive left ventricular remodeling and the syndrome of HF. While a specific anticytokine therapeutic approach so far has failed, recent studies of more general immunomodulating agents (i.e., pentoxyfylline, IVIg, and thalidomide) in HF patients clearly suggest a potential for such therapy in these patients in addition to "optimal" cardiovascular treatment regimens. However, the results from these small studies will have to be confirmed in larger placebo-controlled mortality studies. Further research in this area will also identify the crucial actors in the immunopathogenesis of chronic HF and help to develop more specific immunomodulating agents for HF.

References

1 Stewart S, MacIntyre K, MacLeod MMC, Bailey AM, Capwell S, McMurray JJ. Trends in hospitalization for heart failure in Scotland, 1990–1996. Eur Heart J 2001;22:209–17.

2 Cowie MR, Mosterd A, Wood DA *et al*. The epidemiology of heart failure. Eur Heart J 1997;18:208–25.

3 Aukrust P, Ueland T, Lien E *et al*. Cytokine network in congestive heart failure secondary to ischemic or idiopathic dilated cardiomyopathy. Am J Cardiol 1999;83:376–82.

4 Testa M, Yeh M, Lee P *et al*. Circulating levels of cytokines and their endogenous modulators in patients with mild to severe congestive heart failure due to coronary artery disease or hypertension. J Am Coll Cardiol 1996;28:964–71.

5 Torre-Amione G, Kapadia S, Benedict C, Oral H, Young JB, Mann DL. Proinflammatory cytokine levels in patients with depressed left ventricular ejection fraction: a report from the studies of left ventricular dysfunction (SOLVD). J Am Coll Cardiol 1996;27:1201–6.

6 Kawakami H, Shigematsu Y, Ohtsuka T. Increased circulating soluble form of Fas in patients with dilated cardiomyopathy. Jpn Circ J 1998;62:873–6.

7 Aukrust P, Ueland T, Muller F *et al*. Elevated circulating levels of C-C chemokines in patients with congestive heart failure. Circulation 1998;97:1136–43.

8 Damås JK, Gullestad L, Ueland T *et al*. CXC-chemokines, a new group of cytokines in congestive heart failure-possible role of platelets and monocytes. Cardiovasc Res 2000;45:428–36.

9 Kapadia S. Cytokines and heart failure. Cardiol Rev 1999;7:196–206.

10 Damås JK, Gullestad L, Aass H *et al*. Enhanced gene expression of chemokines and their corresponding receptors in mononuclear blood cells in chronic heart failure-modulatory effects of intravenous immunoglobulin. J Am Coll Cardiol 2001;38:187–93.

11 Deveaux B, Scholz D, Hirche A, Kløverkorn WP, Schaper J. Upregulation of cell adhesion molecules and the presence of low grade inflammation in human chronic heart failure. Eur Heart J 1997;18:470–9.

12 Damås JK, Eiken HG, Øie E *et al*. Myocardial expression of CC- and CXC-chemokines and their receptors in human end-stage heart failure. Cardiovasc Res 2000;47:778–87.

13 Seta Y, Shan K, Bozkurt B, Oral H, Mann DL. Basic mechanism in heart failure: the cytokine hypothesis. J Cardiac Failure 1996;2:243–49.

14 Deswal A, Petersen NJ, Feldman AM, Young JB, White BG, Mann DL. Cytokines and cytokine receptors in advanced heart failure. Circulation 2001;103:2055–9.

15 Ueland T, Kjekshus J, Froland SS *et al*. Plasma levels of soluble tumor necrosis factor receptor type I during the acute phase following complicated myocardial infarction predicts survival in high-risk patients. J Am Coll Cardiol 2005;46:2018–21.

16 Bozkurt B, Kribbs SB, Clubb FJ *et al*. Pathophysiologically relevant concentrations of tumor necrosis factor-alpha promote progressive dysfunction and remodelling in rats. Circulation 1998;97:1382–91.

17 Kubota T, McTernan CF, Frye CS *et al*. Dilated cardiomyopathy in transgenic mice with cardiac-specific overexpression of tumor necrosis factor-alpha. Circ Res 1997;81:627–35.

18 Finkel MS, Oddis CV, Jacob TD, Watkins SC, Hattler BG, Simmons RL. Negative inotropic effects of cytokines on the heart mediated by nitric oxide. Science 1992;257:387–9.

19 Yokoyama T, Vaca L, Rossen RD, Durante W, Hazarika P, Mann DL. Cellular basis for the negative inotropic effects of tumor necrosis factor-alpha in adult mammalian heart. J Clin Invest 1993;92:2303–12.

20 Krown KA, Page MT, Nguyen C *et al*. Tumor necrosis factor alpha-induced apoptosis in cardiac myocytes. J Clin Invest 1996;98:2854–65.

21 Mann DL, Lee-Jackson D, Yokoyama T. Tumor necrosis factor alpha and cardiac remodeling. Heart Fail 1995;11:166–76.

22 Hirota H, Chen J, Betz AK *et al*. Loss of gp130 cardiac muscle cell survival pathway is a critical event in the onset of heart failure during biomechanical stress. Cell 1999;97:189–98.

23 Geng Y, Wu Q, Muszynski M, Hansson GK, Libby P. Apoptosis of vascular smooth muscle cells induced by in vitro stimulation with interferon-gamma, tumor necrosis factor alpha, and interleukin-1b. Arterioscler Thromb Vasc Biol 1996;16:19–27.

24 Li YY, Feng YQ, Kadokami T *et al*. Myocardial extracellular matrix remodeling in transgenic mice overexpressing tumor necrosis factor alpha can be modulated by anti-tumor necrosis factor therapy. Proc Natl Acad Sci U S A 2000;23:12746–51.

25 Sasayama S, Okada M, Matsumori A. Chemokines and cardiovascular diseases. Cardiovasc Res 2000;45:267–9.

26 Kolattukudy PE, Quasch T, Berges S. Myocarditis induced by targeted expression of the MCP-1 gene in murine cardiac muscle. Am J Pathol 1998;152:101–11.

27 Cook DN, Beck MA, Coffman TM *et al*. Requirement of MIP-1 alpha for an inflammatory response to viral infection. Science 1995;269:1583–5.

28 Tachibana K, Hirota S, Ilzasa H *et al*. The chemokine receptor CXCR4 is essential for vascularization of the gastrointestinal tract. Nature 1998;393:524–5.

29 Kalra D, Sivasubramanian N, Mann DL. Angiotensin II induces tumor necrosis factor biosynthesis in the adult

mammalian heart through a protein kinase C-dependent pathway. Circulation 2002;105(18):2198–205.

30 Gullestad L, Aukrust P, Ueland T et al. Effect of high-versus low-dose angiotensin converting enzyme inhibition on cytokine levels in chronic heart failure. J Am Coll Cardiol 1999;34:2061–7.

31 Swedberg K, Held P, Kjekshus J, Rasmussen K, Ryden L, Wedel H. Effects of the early administration of enalapril on mortality in patients with acute myocardial infarction. Results of the Cooperative New Scandinavian Enalapril Survival Study II (CONSENSUS II). N Engl J Med 1992;327:678–84.

32 Maisel AS. Beneficial effects of metoprolol treatment in congestive heart failure. Reversal of sympathetic-induced alterations of immunological function. Circulation 1994;90:1774–80.

33 Maisel AS, Murray D, Lotz M, Rearden A, Irwin M, Michel MC. Propranolol treatment affects parameters of human immunity. Immunopharmacology 1991;22:157–64.

34 Haraguchi S, Good RA, Day NK. Immunosuppressive retroviral peptides: cAMP and cytokine patterns. Immunol Today 1995;16:595–603.

35 Ohtsuka T, Hamada M, Hiasa G et al. Effects of beta-blockers on circulating levels of inflammatory and anti-inflammatory cytokines in patients with dilated cardiomyopathy. J Am Coll Cardiol 2001;37:412–7.

36 Gullestad L, Ueland T, Brunsvig A et al. Effect of metoprolol on cytokine levels in chronic heart failure-a substudy in the Metoprolol Controlled-Release Randomized Intervention Trial in Heart failure (MERIT-HF trial). Am Heart J 2001;141:418–21.

37 Cleland JG, Daubert JC, Erdmann E et al., for the Cardiac Resynchronization-Heart Failure (CARE-HF) Study Investigators. The effect of cardiac resynchronization on morbidity and mortality in heart failure.[see comment]. N Engl J Med 2005;352:1539–49.

38 Boriani G, Regoli F, Saporito D et al. Neurohormones and inflammatory mediators in patients with heart failure undergoing cardiac resyncronization therapy: time courses and prediction of response. Peptides 2006;27:1776–86.

39 Bozkurt B, Torre-Amione G, Warren MS et al. Results of targeted anti-tumor necrosis factor therapy with etanercept (ENBREL) in patients with advanced heart failure. Circulation 2001;103:1044–7.

40 Gullestad L, Aass H, Fjeld JG et al. Effect of immunomodulating therapy with intravenous immunglobulin in chronic congestive heart failure. Circulation 2001;103:220–5.

41 Deswal A, Bozkurt B, Seta Y et al. Safety and efficacy of a soluble p75 tumor necrosis factor receptor (Enbrel, Etanercept) in patients with advanced heart failure. Circulation 1999;99:3224–6.

42 Mann DL, McMurray JJ, Packer M et al. Targeted anti-cytokine therapy in patients with chronic heart failure: results of the Randomized Etanercept Worldwide Evaluation (RENEWAL). Circulation 2004;109:1594–602.

43 Lisman KA, Stetson SJ, Koerner T et al. The role of tumor necrosis factor alpha in the treatment of congestive heart failure. Congest Heart Fail 2002;8:275–9.

44 Kadokami T, McTiernan CF, Kubota T et al. Effects of soluble TNF receptor treatment on lipopolysaccharide-induced myokardial cytokine expression. Am J Physiol 2001;280:H2281–91.

45 Lugering A, Schmidt M, Lugering N, Pauels HG, Domscke W. Infliximab induces apoptosis in myocytes from patients with chronic active Crohn's Disease by using caspase-dependent pathway. Gastroenterology 2001;121:1145–57.

46 Evans TJ, Moyes D, Carpenter A et al. Protective effect of 55- but not 75-kD soluble tumor necrosis factor receptor-immunoglobulin G fusion proteins in an animal model of gram-negative sepsis. J Exp Med 1994;180(6):2173–9.

47 Meldrum DR. Tumor necrosis factor in the heart. Am J Physiol 1998;274:R577–95.

48 Adamopoulos S, Parissis J, Karatzas D et al. Physical training modulates proinflammatory cytokines and the soluble Fas/soluble Fas ligand system in patients with chronic heart failure. J Am Coll Cardiol 2002;39:653–63.

49 Gielen S, Adams V, Linke A et al. Exercise training in chronic heart failure: correlation between reduced local inflammation and improved oxidative capacity in the skeletal muscle. Eur J Cardiovasc Prev Rehabil 2005;12:393–400.

50 Keith M, Geranmayegan A, Sole MJ et al. Increased oxidative stress in patients with congestive heart failure. J Am Coll Cardiol 1998;31:1352–6.

51 Keith ME, Jeejeebhoy KN, Langer A et al. A controlled trial of vitamin E supplementation in patients with congestive heart failure. Am J Clin Nutr 2001;73:219–24.

52 Nolan Y, Minogue A, Vereker E, Bolton AE, Campbell VA, Lynch MA. Attenuation of LPS-induced changes in synaptic activity in rat hippocampus by Vasogen's immune modulation therapy. Neuroimmunomodulation 2002;10:40–6.

53 Torre-Amione G, Sestier F, Radovancevic B, Young J. Effects of a novel immune modulation therapy in patients with advanced chronic heart failure: results of a randomized, controlled, phase II trial. J Am Coll Cardiol 2004;44:1181–6.

54 Sliwa K, Skudicky D, Candy G, Wisenbaugh T, Sareli P. Randomized investigation of effects of pentoxifylline on left ventricular performance in idiopathic dilated cardiomyopathy. Lancet 1998;351:1091–3.

55 Skudicky D, Bergemann A, Sliwa K, Candy G, Sareli P. Beneficial effects of pentoxifylline in patients with idiopathic dilated cardiomyopathy treated with angiotensin-converting enzyme inhibitors and carvedilol. Circulation 2001;103:1083–8.

56 Sliwa K, Woodiwiss A, Kone VN *et al.* Therapy of ischemic cardiomyopathy with the immunomodulating agent pentoxifylline: results of a randomized study. Circulation 2004;109:750–5.

57 Scandinavian Simvastatin Survival Study Group. Randomized trial of cholesterol lowering in 4444 patients with coronary artery disease: the Scandinavian Simvastatin Survival Study (4S). Lancet 1995;344:1383–9.

58 The Long-Term Intervention with Pravastatin in Ischemic Disease (LIPID) Study Group. Prevention of cardiovascular events and death with pravastatin in patients with coronary heart disease and a broad range of cholesterol levels. N Engl J Med 1998;339:1349–57.

59 Kwak B, Mulhaup F, Mylt S, Mach F. Statins as a newly recognized type of immunomodulator. Nat Med 2000;6:1399–402.

60 Takemoto M, Node K, Nakagami H *et al.* Statins as antioxidant therapy for preventing cardiac myocyte hypertrophy. J Clin Invest 2001;108:1429–37.

61 Sola S, Mir MQ, Rajagopalan S, Helmy T, Tandon N, Khan BV. Statin therapy is associated with improved cardiovascular outcomes and levels of inflammatory markers in patients with heart failure. J Card Fail 2005;11:607–12.

62 Horwich TB, Hamilton MA, Maclellan WR, Fonarow GC. Low serum total cholesterol is associated with marked increase in mortality in advanced heart failure. J Card Fail 2002;8:216–24.

63 Krum H, McMurray JJ. Statins and chronic heart failure: do we need a large scale outcome trial? J Am Coll Cardiol 2002;39:1567–73.

64 Muller J, Wallukat G, Dandel M *et al.* Immunoglobulin adsorption in patients with idiopathic dilated cardiomyopathy. Circulation 2000;101:285–391.

65 Staudt A, Schaper F, Stangl V *et al.* Immunohistological changes in dilated cardiomyopathy induced by immunoadsorption therapy and subsequent immunoglobulin substitution. Circulation 2001;103:2681–6.

66 Ballow M. Mechanism of action of intravenous immune serum globulin in autoimmune and inflammatory diseases. J Allergy Clin Immunol 1997;100:151–7.

67 Mobini N, Sarela A, Ahmed AR. Intravenous immunoglobulins in the therapy of autoimmune and systemic inflammatory disorders. Ann Allergy Asthma Immunol 1995;74:119–28.

68 McNamara DM, Rosenblum WD, Janosko KM *et al.* Intravenous immune globulin in the therapy of myocarditis and acute cardiomyopathy. Circulation 1997;95:2476–8.

69 Bozkurt B, Villaneuva FS, Holubkov R *et al.* Intravenous immune globulin in the therapy of peripartum cardiomyopathy. J Am Coll Cardiol 1999;34:177–80.

70 McNamara DM, Holubkov R, Starling RC *et al.* Controlled trial of intravenous immune globulin in recent-onset dilated cardiomyopathy. Circulation 2001;103:2254–9.

71 Viard I, Wehrli P, Schneider P *et al.* Inhibition of toxic necrolysis by blockade of CD95 with human intravenous immunoglobulin. Science 1998;282:490–3.

72 Nishio R, Matsumori A, Shioi T, Ishida H, Sasayama S. Treatment of experimental viral myocarditis with interleukin-10. Circulation 1999;100:1102–8.

73 Mallat Z, Besnard S, Duriez M *et al.* Protective role of interleukin-10 in atherosclerosis. Cir Res 1999;85:17–24.

74 Loddick SA, Rothwell NJ. Neuroprotective effects of human recombinant interleukin-1 receptor antagonist in focal cerebral ischaemia in the rat. J Cereb Blood Flow Metab 1996;16:932–40.

75 Ungureanu-Longrois D, Balligand J-L, Simmons WW *et al.* Induction of nitric oxide synthase activity by cytokines in ventricular myocytes is necessary but not sufficient to decrease contractile responsivness to β-adrenergic agonists. Circ Res 1995;77:494–502.

76 Jacobsen JM. Thalidomide: a remarkable comeback. Expert Opin Pharmacother 2000;1:849–63.

77 Adlard JW. Thalidomide in the treatment of cancer. Anticancer Drugs 2000;11:787–91.

78 Sampaio EP, Sarno EN, Galilly R, Cohn ZA, Kaplan G. Thalidomide selectively inhibits tumor necrosis factor a production by stimulated human monocytes. J Exp Med 1991;173:699–703.

79 Corral LG, Haslett PA, Muller GW *et al.* Differential cytokine modulation and T cell activation by two distinct classes of thalidomide analogues that are potent inhibitors of TNF-alpha. J Immunol 1999;163:380–6.

80 Keifer JA, Guttridge DC, Ashburner AP, Baldwin J. Inhibition of NF-kappaB activity by thalidomide through suppression of I kappaB kinase activity. J Biol Chem 2001;267:22382–7.

81 Zorat F, Shetty V, Dutt D. The clinical and biological effects of thalidomide in patients with myelodysplastic syndromes. Br J Haematol 2001;115:881–94.

82 Barlett JB, Michael A, Clarke IA *et al.* Phase I study to determine the safety, tolerability and immunostimulatory activity of thalidomide analogue CC-5013 in patients with metastatic malignant melanoma and other advanced cancers. Br J Cancer 2004;90:955–61.

83 Gelati M, Corsini E, Frigerio S *et al.* Effects of thalidomide on parameters involved in angiogenesis: an in vitro study. J Neurooncol 2003;64:193–201.

84 Gullestad L, Ueland T, Fjeld J *et al.* The effect of thalido-mide on cardiac remodeling in chronic heart failure: re-sults of a double-blind placebo-controlled study. Circu-lation 2005;112:3408–14.

85 Green JM. The B7/CD28/CTLA4 T-cell activation path-way. Implications for inflammatory lung disease [review] [53 refs]. Am J Respir Cell Mol Biol 2000;22(3): 261–4.

86 Salomon B, Bluestone JA. Complexities of CD28/B7: CTLA-4 costimulatory pathways in autoimmunity and transplantation [review] [163 refs]. Ann Rev Immunol 2001; 19:225–52.

87 Lee MS, Makkar RR. Stem-cell transplantation in myocar-dial infarction: a status report [see comment] [review] [80 refs]. Ann Intern Med 2004;140(9):729–37.

88 Hayashidani S, Tsutsui H, Shiomi T *et al.* Anti-monocyte chemoattractant protein-1 gene therapy attenuates left ventricular remodeling and failure after experimental my-ocardial infarction. Circulation 2003;108:2134–40.

89 Suzuki K, Murtuza B, Smolensky RT. Overexpression of interleukin-1 receptor antagonist provides cardioprotec-tion against ischemia–reperfusion injury associated with reduction in apoptosis. Circulation 2001;104(suppl I):I-308–13.

CHAPTER 11

Statins in atherosclerosis: role of immune regulation

Claire Arnaud & François Mach

Introduction

Atherosclerosis is a chronic inflammatory disease characterized by an important immunological activity and resulting essentially from hyperlipidemia, hypertension, and smoking diabetes [1]. These risk factors cause endothelial dysfunction that triggers leukocyte migration into the vessel wall, leading to the formation of an atherosclerotic plaque. The plaque is composed of a lipid core, surrounded by a fibrous cap that stabilizes the plaque and containing smooth muscle cells and collagen fibers. Immune cells, including macrophages, T cells, and mast cells, that populate the plaque produce cytokines, proteases, prothrombotic molecules, and vasoactive substances that maintain the inflammatory process [2]. Inflammation appears crucial in all stages of atherosclerosis, from the very initial phases through the progression and finally to the clinical complications.

The 3-hydroxy-3-methylglutaryl coenzyme A (HMG-CoA) reductase inhibitors, or statins, constitute the leading therapeutic to greatly reduce coronary morbidity and mortality in both primary and secondary intervention trials [3, 4]. Statins have revolutionized the treatment of hypercholesterolemia, since these drugs are the most efficient to reduce serum cholesterol levels. Initially shown to be effective in patients with substantially elevated cholesterol [5, 6], it has become increasingly apparent that the beneficial effects of statins in cardiovascular medicine cannot be ascribed solely to their lipid-lowering properties [7]. In particular, the inflammatory component of atherosclerosis seems to respond to statin-mediated effects that are independent of cholesterol reduction [8, 9]. By inhibit-

ing HMG-CoA reductase, statins block not only cholesterol synthesis but also those of many nonsteroidal isoprenoid compounds such as farnesyl pyrophosphate (FPP) and geranylgeranyl pyrophosphate (GGPP) [10]. Furthermore, several proteins, such as the small GTP-binding proteins Ras and Rho, need to be prenylated as a prerequisite to covalent attachment, subcellular localization, and intracellular trafficking of membrane-associated proteins [11, 12]. Members of the Ras and Rho GTPase family are major substrates for the posttranslational modification by isoprenylation and may be important targets for statins.

Clinical evidence of statins pleiotropic effects

Clinical data support some cholesterol-independent effects of statins. For example, the PROVE-IT trial showed that statin therapy decreases C-reactive protein (CRP) levels, in association with better clinical outcomes, regardless of cholesterol levels [13]. Furthermore, various studies have demonstrated a beneficial effect of statins in pathologies thought to be independent of cholesterol levels. Although there is no association between blood cholesterol levels and stroke [14], statins reduce the risk of stroke in patients with coronary artery disease [15–17]. Recent clinical trials also showed that statins markedly inhibit the number and volume of brain lesions in multiple sclerosis [18], and also exert modest but clinically apparent anti-inflammatory effects in rheumatoid arthritis [19]. In the same manner, the use of statins is associated with a 47% relative reduction in the risk of colorectal cancer in an observational study [20]. Finally, it has been shown that

Table 11.1 Key clinical trials where statins were shown to exert non-lipid-related effects.

Clinical trials	Initial disease	Statin treatment	Outcomes	References
PROVE-IT	Acute coronary syndromes	80 mg atorvastatin vs. 40 mg pravastatin	↓ CRP associated with better clinical outcomes, regardless of the resultant level of LDL cholesterol	[14]
REVERSAL	Documented coronary disease	80 mg atorvastatin vs. 40 mg pravastatin	↓ Rate of progression of atherosclerosis related to a great reduction in CRP levels	[24]
ASCOTT	Hypertension without high cholesterol levels	10 mg atorvastatin vs. placebo	↓ Fatal and nonfatal stroke, ↓ total cardiovascular events, ↓ total coronary events	[21]
CARDS	Type 2 diabetes without high cholesterol levels	10 mg atorvastatin vs. placebo	↓ Risk of cardiovascular disease events, including stroke	[22]
Heart Failure	Nonischemic heart failure	5–10 mg simvastatin vs. placebo	Improvement of cardiac function, neurohormonal imbalance, and symptoms associated with idiopathic dilated cardiomyopathy	[25]
TARA	Rheumatoid arthritis	40 mg atorvastatin vs. placebo	Modest but clinically apparent anti-inflammatory effects: ↓ CRP levels and erythrocyte sedimentation	[19]
Multiple sclerosis	Relapsing–remitting multiple sclerosis	80 mg simvastatin	↓ Number and volume of brain lesions	[18]
Colorectal cancer	Colorectal cancer		47% relative reduction in the risk of colorectal cancer after adjustment for other known risk factors	[20]

statins reduce cardiovascular events and stroke in normocholesterolemic patients with either hypertension [21] or diabetes [22].

All these observations confirm the speculation that statins might influence vascular biology also through nonlipid mechanisms [23] (Table 11.1). Recent evidence suggests that statins could modulate the immune response [23, 26–28] and supports the idea that the immunomodulatory actions of statins contribute to their beneficial effects in patients with atherosclerosis.

MHC-II expression

One of the first demonstration of an immune modulation by statins appears from clinical trials, which reported that statins therapy decreases mortality and rejection episodes in cardiac transplant recipients [29–31].

Major histocompatibilty complex class II (MHC-II) molecules, expressed on the surface of specialized cells, are directly involved in the activation of T lymphocytes and in the control of the immune response. Thus, reducing the availability or activation of MHC-II proteins is potential therapeutic strategies to promote immune tolerance and reduce rejection of transplanted organs. As a part of an exploration of possible interfaces between immune mechanisms and atherogenesis and to evaluate possible beneficial effects of statins independently of their well-known effects as lipid-lowering agents, we investigated in a previous study whether statins regulate both constitutive MHC-II expression in highly specialized antigen-presenting cells (APC) and inducible MHC-II expression by interferon-γ (IFN-γ) in primary culture of human endothelial cells and monocyte/macrophages. We reported that statins effectively repress the induced MHC-II protein and gene expression by IFN-γ, and thus act as direct repressors of MHC-II-mediated T-cell activation, whereas statins does not affect constitutive expression of MHC-II in APC, such as dendritic cells (DCs) and B lymphocytes. Furthermore, we showed that the repressive effect of statin on

MHC-II in human atheroma-associated cells occurred through a reduction of the inducible promoter IV of the transactivator CIITA [32], whereas more recent data indicate that statins also inhibit IFN-γ-inducible CIITA expression from the promoter I, indicating that statins are not selective for promoter IV [33]. All these effects of statins have been observed with the statins currently used in clinical medicine [32, 34], and other investigators have confirmed these findings in endothelial cells [35]. The fact that statin-induced repression of MHC-II also represses MHC-II-dependent activation of T lymphocytes indicates that statin is likely to have an immunosuppressive effect. This provides new evidence that could support the use of statins as immunomodulators in organ transplantation, as well as in diseases where aberrant expression of MHC-II is implicated, such as type 1 diabetes, multiple sclerosis, rheumatoid arthritis, and chronic inflammatory diseases like atherosclerosis. Further appropriated clinical trials are still required to confirm these findings.

Leukocyte adhesion and migration

Leukocyte adhesion to the vascular wall and subsequent migration into the tissue is central to the pathogenesis of autoimmune disease [36]. This complex process begins with the tethering of leukocytes to the endothelial cell surface and culminates in leukocyte infiltration into the vessel wall. Cell adhesion molecules play a central role in this process. In response to cholesterol accumulation in the intima, endothelial cells express leukocyte adhesion molecules, such as vascular cell adhesion molecule-1 (VCAM-1), that induces monocytes and T cells enter the arterial intima [37]. Recently, it has been reported that lovastatin reduces VCAM-1 expression by brain endothelial cells, resulting in a significant reduction in transendothelial-cell migration of monocytes [38]. In the case of intercellular adhesion molecule-1 (ICAM-1), numerous studies have shown that statins reduce both constitutive and induced expression of ICAM-1, which is also directly involved in leukocyte adhesion and diapedesis [36]. Furthermore, statins also selectively block the binding capacity of the integrin lymphocyte function-associated antigen-1 (LFA-1) to ICAM-1 [39]. LFA-1 is constitutively expressed in an inactive state on the surface of lymphocytes [40], and, in response to several stimuli, including the T-cell receptor (TCR) cross-linking with MHC-II complex, LFA-1 binds to ICAM-1 and provides a potent costimulatory signal for activated T cells [41]. The inhibitory effect of statins on LFA-1 is unrelated to the inhibition of HMG-CoA reductase, but occurs via the binding to a novel allosteric site within LFA-1, which blocks binding of LFA-1 to ICAM-1 and inhibits both lymphocyte adhesion and costimulation [39].

Once adherent, the leukocytes migrate through the vascular barrier into the intima in response to chemoattractant stimuli and this process requires external cues such as chemokines [42]. For example, it has been well described that monocyte chemoattractant protein-1 (MCP-1) and its receptor CCR2 play a key role in the initiation of atherosclerosis [43, 44]. Administration of a blocking of the interaction of RANTES with its receptor CCR5 attenuates atherogenesis in mice, indicating that, like MCP-1/CCR2, RANTES/CCR5 plays a crucial role in atherogenesis [45]. Other categories of chemokines, such as the CXC chemokines, may also participate in recruitment of leukocytes to atheroma [46, 47]. A very recent study supports the role of statins in the regulation of leukocyte trafficking since we have shown that statins downregulate expression of chemokine and chemokine receptors by human atheroma-associated cells, and that this effect could also be achieved by the use of geranylgeranyl transferase inhibitor [48].

T-cell immune response

Non-lipid-related functions of statins might implicate a regulation of many different inflammatory molecules, and beneficial effect of statins could also be due to the type of immune response they induce. In a murine model of autoimmune encephalomyelitis, atorvastatin induced a significant secretion of anti-inflammatory Th2 cytokines (interleukin (IL)-4, -5, and -10) and transforming growth factor (TGF)-β, and the phosphorylation (activation) of the transcription factor STAT6, which is involved in IL-4-dependent Th2 cell differentiation. On the contrary, phosphorylation of STAT4, which is involved in the proinflammatory Th1 cell differentiation, was reduced and secretion of Th1 cytokines (IL-2, IL-12, IFN-γ, and tumor necrosis factor (TNF)-α) was suppressed [33]. In a murine model of autoimmune retinal disease, it has been shown that lovastatin induced a reduction in T-cell proliferation and a decrease in IFN-γ production, whereas it had no effect on Th2 cytokine production [49]. These results have been confirmed in vitro, since lovastatin inhibits IFN-γ action in endothelial cell line [50]. Furthermore, in patient with no known cardiovascular disease, pravastatin reduced proinflammatory cytokine production [51], and in a recent study, it has been observed that whereas it has no effect on Th2 cell functions, atorvastatin can reduce Th1 development in patients with acute myocardial infarction (AMI) [52], suggesting that reduction of Th1 bias may be one of the mechanisms through which atorvastatin improves heart function after AMI. Taken together, these animal and human findings suggest that statins regulate Th1/Th2 imbalance both in vitro and in vivo. Thus, all these observations could explain the beneficial effect of statins in atherosclerosis, since it has been shown that the Th2 cytokines have antiatherogenic properties and their overexpression protects against atherosclerosis [53–55].

CD40–CD40L

Increasing evidence suggest a central role for the CD40–CD40L signaling pathway in the pathogenesis of atherosclerosis [56], and it has been shown that blocking CD40–CD40L interactions significantly prevents the development of atherosclerotic plaques and reduces already preestablished lesions [57, 58]. Moreover, CD40 signaling has been implicated in other chronic disorders such as rheumatoid arthritis, multiple sclerosis, and allograft rejection following organ transplantation [59]. CD40 signaling via an activation of vascular cells has been shown to induce inflammatory responses with expression of adhesion molecules and secretion of proinflammatory cytokines, chemokines, matrix metalloproteinases, and tissue factor [60]. Thus, in a recent study, we have investigated whether statins could regulate the expression of CD40 in vascular cells, and we have shown that statin therapy reduced CD40 expression and CD40-related activation of atheroma-associated cells in vitro, as well as in atherosclerotic lesions in situ in patients treated with statins [61].

The same results were also obtained by other investigators [33, 62, 63].

Moreover, CD40 acts as costimulatory molecule to enhance T-cell activation by DCs. DCs are APC with a unique ability to initiate a primary immune response. The activation of T cells by DCs requires the maturation of DCs with the upregulation of costimulatory molecules, such as CD40, and MHC-II molecules [64]. A recent study that demonstrates the colocalization of DC and T cells, as well as the expression of MHC-II and costimulatory molecules on DCs in atherosclerotic plaques, suggests that DCs initiate an antigen-specific immune response, contributing to the progression of atherosclerosis [65]. Yilmaz *et al.* recently showed that in contrast to nontreated DCs, statin-pretreated DCs exhibited an immature phenotype and a significant lower expression of the maturation-associated markers, CD40 and MHC-II molecules [66]. The authors also showed that statins significantly reduced the ability of cytokine-stimulated DC to induce T-cell proliferation. This effect of statins seems to be mediated through the inhibition of Rho geranylgeranylation. Together with observations of the reduced CD40 and MHC-II expression, these findings provide new mechanistic insight into the beneficial effects of statins as modulators of the immune system in atherosclerosis.

Conclusion

Statins are known to exert great beneficial effects by reducing cardiovascular morbidity and mortality in primary and secondary prevention. During the last decade, numerous in vivo and in vitro studies have described pleiotropic effects of statins, totally independent of their lipid-lowering effects. These cholesterol-independent properties of statins include improvement of endothelial function, stabilization of atherosclerotic plaques, inhibition of vascular smooth muscle cell proliferation as well as platelet aggregation, and reduction of vascular inflammation. Here, we focused on the immunomodulatory properties of statins, which include repression of MHC-II expression, blockage of LFA-1/ICAM-1 interaction, and inhibition of CD40–CD40L signaling (Figure 11.1). These observations are encouraging and raise the question of whether statins should be used as immunomodulators, not

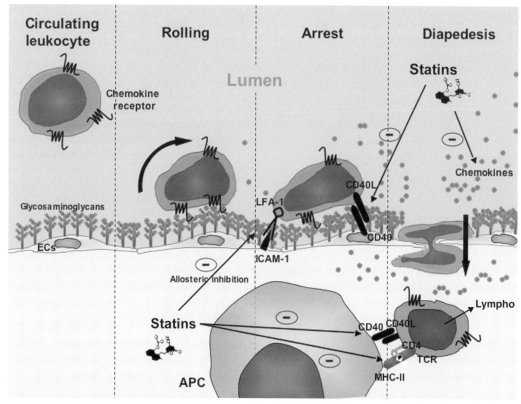

Figure 11.1 Statins immunomodulatory effects. HMG-CoA reductase inhibitor binds to a novel allosteric site within LFA-1, reducing LFA-1/ICAM-1 interaction and thus T-cell activation. Statins also decrease MHC-II, CD40, and CD40L expression. The sum of these pleiotropic effects of statins directs the immune response on the Th2 side and reduces inflammatory processes such as proinflammatory cytokine release and T-cell activation. APC, antigen-presenting cell; Ecs, endothelial cells; Lympho, lymphocytes.

only after transplantation, but also in autoimmune diseases such as type 1 diabetes, multiple sclerosis, rheumatoid arthritis, and also in chronic inflammatory diseases like atherosclerosis.

References

1 Lusis AJ. Atherosclerosis. Nature 2000;407(6801):233–41.

2 Hansson GK, Libby P. The immune response in atherosclerosis: a double-edged sword. Nat Rev Immunol 2006;6(7):508–19.

3 Maron DJ, Fazio S, Linton MF. Current perspectives on statins. Circulation 2000;101(2):207–13.

4 Vaughan CJ, Gotto AM, Jr, Basson CT. The evolving role of statins in the management of atherosclerosis. J Am Coll Cardiol 2000;35(1):1–10.

5 Pedersen TR, Kjekshus J, Berg K et al. Randomised trial of cholesterol lowering in 4444 patients with coronary heart disease: the Scandinavian Simvastatin Survival Study (4S). Lancet 1994;344:1383–9.

6 Shepherd J. Fibrates and statins in the treatment of hyperlipidaemia: an appraisal of their efficacy and safety. Eur Heart J 1995;16(1):5–13.

7 Palinski W. New evidence for beneficial effects of statins unrelated to lipid lowering. Arterioscler Thromb Vasc Biol 2001;21(1):3–5.

8 Downs JR, Clearfield M, Weis S et al. Primary prevention of acute coronary events with lovastatin in men and women with average cholesterol levels: results of AFCAPS/TexCAPS. Air Force/Texas Coronary Atherosclerosis Prevention Study. JAMA 1998;279(20): 1615–22.

9 The Long-Term Intervention with Pravastatin in Ischaemic Disease (LIPID) Study Group. Prevention of cardiovascular events and death with pravastatin in patients with coronary heart disease and a broad range of initial cholesterol levels. N Engl J Med 1998;339(19):1349–57.

10 Arnaud C, Braunersreuther V, Mach F. Toward immunomodulatory and anti-inflammatory properties of statins. Trends Cardiovasc Med 2005;15(6):202–6.

11 Van Aelst L, D'Souza-Schorey C. Rho GTPases and signaling networks. Genes Dev 1997;11(18):2295–322.

12 Hall A. Rho GTPases and the actin cytoskeleton. Science 1998;279(5350):509–14.

13 Ridker PM, Cannon CP, Morrow D et al. C-reactive protein levels and outcomes after statin therapy. N Engl J Med 2005;352(1):20–8.

14 Prospective Studies Collaboration. Cholesterol, diastolic blood pressure, and stroke: 13,000 strokes in 450,000 people in 45 prospective cohorts. Lancet 1995;346(8991–8992):1647–53.

15 Vaughan CJ, Delanty N, Basson CT. Statin therapy and stroke prevention. Curr Opin Cardiol 2001;16(4):219–24.

16 Schwartz GG, Olsson AG, Ezekowitz MD et al. Effects of atorvastatin on early recurrent ischemic events in acute coronary syndromes: the MIRACL study: a randomized controlled trial. JAMA 2001;285(13):1711–8.

17 Amarenco P, Labreuche J, Lavallee P, Touboul PJ. Statins in stroke prevention and carotid atherosclerosis: systematic review and up-to-date meta-analysis. Stroke 2004;35(12):2902–9.

18 Vollmer T, Key L, Durkalski V et al. Oral simvastatin treatment in relapsing-remitting multiple sclerosis. Lancet 2004;363(9421):1607–8.

19 McCarey DW, McInnes PI, Madhok R et al. Trial of Atorvastatin in Rheumatoid Arthritis (TARA): double-blind, randomised placebo-controlled trial. Lancet 2004;363(9426):2015–21.

20 Poynter JN, Gruber SB, Higgins PD et al. Statins and the risk of colorectal cancer. N Engl J Med 2005;352(21):2184–92.

21 Sever PS, Dahlof B, Poulter NR et al. Prevention of coronary and stroke events with atorvastatin in hypertensive patients who have average or lower-than-average cholesterol concentrations, in the Anglo-Scandinavian Cardiac Outcomes Trial–Lipid Lowering Arm (ASCOT-LLA): a multicentre randomised controlled trial. Lancet 2003;361(9364):1149–58.

22 Colhoun HM, Betteridge DJ, Durrington PN et al. Primary prevention of cardiovascular disease with atorvastatin in type 2 diabetes in the Collaborative Atorvastatin Diabetes Study (CARDS): multicentre randomised placebo-controlled trial. Lancet 2004;364(9435):685–96.

23 Vaughan CJ, Murphy MB, Buckley BM. Statins do more than just lower cholesterol. Lancet 1996;348(9034):1079–82.

24 Nissen SE, Tuzcu EM, Schoenhagen P et al. Statin therapy, LDL cholesterol, C-reactive protein, and coronary artery disease. N Engl J Med 2005;352(1):29–38.

25 Node K, Fujita M, Kitakaze M, Hori M, Liao JK. Short-term statin therapy improves cardiac function and symptoms in patients with idiopathic dilated cardiomyopathy. Circulation 2003;108(7):839–43.

26 Sherer Y, Shoenfeld Y. Immunomodulation for treatment and prevention of atherosclerosis. Autoimmun Rev 2002;1(1–2):21–7.

27 Steffens S, Mach F. Anti-inflammatory properties of statins. Semin Vasc Med 2004;4(4):417–22.

28 Gurevich VS, Shovman O, Slutzky L, Meroni PL, Shoenfeld Y. Statins and autoimmune diseases. Autoimmun Rev 2005;4(3):123–9.

29 Kobashigawa JA, Katznelson S, Laks H et al. Effect of pravastatin on outcomes after cardiac transplantation. N Engl J Med 1995;333(10):621–7.

30 Wenke K, Meiser B, Thiery J et al. Simvastatin reduces graft vessel disease and mortality after heart transplantation: a four-year randomized trial. Circulation 1997;96(5):1398–402.

31 Wenke K, Meiser B, Thiery J et al. Simvastatin initiated early after heart transplantation: 8-year prospective experience. Circulation 2003;107(1):93–7.

32 Kwak B, Mulhaupt F, Myit S, Mach F. Statins as a newly recognized type of immunomodulator. Nat Med 2000;6(12):1399–402.

33 Youssef S, Stuve O, Patarroyo JC et al. The HMG-CoA reductase inhibitor, atorvastatin, promotes a Th2 bias and reverses paralysis in central nervous system autoimmune disease. Nature 2002;420(6911):78–84.

34 Kwak B, Mulhaupt F, Veillard N, Pelli G, Mach F. The HMG-CoA reductase inhibitor simvastatin inhibits IFN-gamma induced MHC class II expression in human vascular endothelial cells. Swiss Med Wkly 2001;131(3–4):41–6.

35 Sadeghi MM, Tiglio A, Sadigh K et al. Inhibition of interferon-gamma-mediated microvascular endothelial cell major histocompatibility complex class II gene activation by HMG-CoA reductase inhibitors. Transplantation 2001;71(9):1262–8.

36 Greenwood J, Steinman L, Zamvil SS. Statin therapy and autoimmune disease: from protein prenylation to immunomodulation. Nat Rev Immunol 2006;6(5):358–70.

37 Cybulsky MI, Gimbrone MA, Jr. Endothelial expression of a mononuclear leukocyte adhesion molecule during atherogenesis. Science 1991;251(4995):788–91.

38 Prasad R, Giri S, Nath N, Singh I, Singh AK. Inhibition of phosphoinositide 3 kinase-Akt (protein kinase B)-nuclear factor-kappa B pathway by lovastatin limits endothelial-monocyte cell interaction. J Neurochem 2005;94(1):204–14.

39 Weitz-Schmidt G, Welzenbach K, Brinkmann V et al. Statins selectively inhibit leukocyte function antigen-1 by binding to a novel regulatory integrin site. Nat Med 2001;7(6):687–92.

40 Carlos TM, Harlan JM. Leukocyte-endothelial adhesion molecules. Blood 1994;84(7):2068–101.

41 Dustin ML, Springer TA. T-cell receptor cross-linking transiently stimulates adhesiveness through LFA-1. Nature 1989;341(6243):619–24.

42 Charo IF, Ransohoff RM. The many roles of chemokines and chemokine receptors in inflammation. N Engl J Med 2006;354(6):610–21.

43 Gu L, Okada Y, Clinton SK et al. Absence of monocyte chemoattractant protein-1 reduces atherosclerosis in low density lipoprotein receptor-deficient mice. Mol Cell 1998;2(2):275–81.

44 Boring L, Gosling J, Cleary M, Charo IF. Decreased lesion formation in CCR2–/– mice reveals a role for chemokines in the initiation of atherosclerosis. Nature 1998;394(6696):894–7.

45 Veillard NR, Kwak B, Pelli G et al. Antagonism of RANTES receptors reduces atherosclerotic plaque formation in mice. Circ Res 2004;94(2):253–61.

46 Mach F, Sauty A, Iarossi AS et al. Differential expression of three T lymphocyte-activating CXC chemokines by human atheroma-associated cells. J Clin Invest 1999;104(8):1041–50.

47 Haley KJ, Lilly CM, Yang JH et al. Overexpression of eotaxin and the CCR3 receptor in human atherosclerosis: using genomic technology to identify a potential novel pathway of vascular inflammation. Circulation 2000;102(18):2185–9.

48 Veillard NR, Braunersreuther V, Arnaud C et al. Simvastatin modulates chemokine and chemokine receptor expression by geranylgeranyl isoprenoid pathway in human endothelial cells and macrophages. Atherosclerosis 2006;188(1):51–8.

49 Gegg ME, Harry R, Hankey D et al. Suppression of autoimmune retinal disease by lovastatin does not require Th2 cytokine induction. J Immunol 2005;174(4):2327–35.

50 Chung HK, Lee IK, Kang H et al. Statin inhibits interferon-gamma-induced expression of intercellular adhesion molecule-1 (ICAM-1) in vascular endothelial and smooth muscle cells. Exp Mol Med 2002;34(6):451–61.

51 Rosenson RS, Tangney CC, Casey LC. Inhibition of proinflammatory cytokine production by pravastatin. Lancet 1999;353(9157):983–4.

52 Shimada K, Miyauchi K, Daida H. Early intervention with atorvastatin modulates TH1/TH2 imbalance in patients with acute coronary syndrome: from bedside to bench. Circulation 2004;109(18):e213–4; author reply e213–4.

53 Uyemura K, Demer LL, Castle SC et al. Cross-regulatory roles of interleukin (IL)-12 and IL-10 in atherosclerosis. J Clin Invest 1996;97(9):2130–8.

54 Mallat Z, Besnard S, Duriez M et al. Protective role of interleukin-10 in atherosclerosis. Circ Res 1999;85(8):e17–24.

55 Pinderski LJ, Fischbein MP, Subbanagounder G et al. Overexpression of interleukin-10 by activated T lymphocytes inhibits atherosclerosis in LDL receptor-deficient Mice by altering lymphocyte and macrophage phenotypes. Circ Res 2002;90(10):1064–71.

56 Schonbeck U, Libby P. The CD40/CD154 receptor/ligand dyad. Cell Mol Life Sci 2001;58(1):4–43.

57 Mach F, Schonbeck U, Sukhova GK, Atkinson E, Libby P. Reduction of atherosclerosis in mice by inhibition of CD40 signalling. Nature 1998;394(6689):200–3.

58 Lutgens E, Gorelik L, Daemen MJ et al. Requirement for CD154 in the progression of atherosclerosis. Nat Med 1999;5(11):1313–6.

59 Foy TM, Aruffo A, Bajorath J, Buhlmann JE, Noelle RJ. Immune regulation by CD40 and its ligand GP39. Annu Rev Immunol 1996;14:591–617.

60 Schonbeck U, Mach F, Libby P. CD154 (CD40 ligand). Int J Biochem Cell Biol 2000;32(7):687–93.

61 Mulhaupt F, Matter CM, Kwak BR et al. Statins (HMG-CoA reductase inhibitors) reduce CD40 expression in human vascular cells. Cardiovasc Res 2003;59(3):755–66.

62 Wagner AH, Gebauer M, Guldenzoph B, Hecker M. 3-hydroxy-3-methylglutaryl coenzyme A reductase-independent inhibition of CD40 expression by atorvastatin in human endothelial cells. Arterioscler Thromb Vasc Biol 2002;22(11):1784–9.

63 Schonbeck U, Gerdes N, Varo N et al. Oxidized low-density lipoprotein augments and 3-hydroxy-3-methylglutaryl coenzyme A reductase inhibitors limit CD40 and CD40L expression in human vascular cells. Circulation 2002;106(23):2888–93.

64 Banchereau J, Briere F, Caux C et al. Immunobiology of dendritic cells. Annu Rev Immunol 2000;18:767–811.

65 Bobryshev YV, Lord RS. Mapping of vascular dendritic cells in atherosclerotic arteries suggests their involvement in local immune-inflammatory reactions. Cardiovasc Res 1998;37(3):799–810.

66 Yilmaz A, Reiss C, Tantawi O et al. HMG-CoA reductase inhibitors suppress maturation of human dendritic cells: new implications for atherosclerosis. Atherosclerosis 2004;172(1):85–93.

CHAPTER 12

ACE inhibitors as immunomodulators: treatment of cardiovascular disease

Christina Grothusen & Bernhard Schieffer

Introduction

The involvement of the renin-angiotensin system (RAS) and its effector peptide angiotensin (ang) II in inflammation and immunomodulation was first established in arterial hypertension and renal dysfunction. Early observations demonstrated that ang II-induced renal hypertension results in necrotizing arteriolitis and infiltration of inflammatory cells in the kidney, providing evidence for "an immunological factor in the hypertensive vascular disease," as proposed by Olsen *et al.* in 1971 [1–3]. Until today, various experimental and clinical trials validated the importance of RAS-activation as a major mediator of proinflammatory reactions in the cardiovascular system in response to varying pathological conditions, including atherosclerosis, cancer, and rheumatoid arthritis [4–6]. In this chapter, we will review the current experimental and clinical data with a focus on the role of RAS-activation in atherosclerosis and the immunomodulatory potential of RAS-blockade by angiotensin-converting enzyme (ACE) inhibition in atherosclerotic cardiovascular disease.

RAS components

Under physiological conditions, the major task of the RAS is the regulation of electrolyte hemostasis, intravascular volume, and therefore blood pressure. Traditionally, the RAS-activation cascade contained the following steps (Figure 12.1a). In response to certain stimuli, renin is released from the kidney into the circulation, where it cleaves angiotensinogen which is primarily produced by the liver to ang I. Ang I is then converted to ang II by ACE. Due to the physiological direction of blood flow, this conversion primarily takes place in the lung, but as ACE is also expressed in other tissues, ang II may be locally generated, too. This local tissue RAS is expressed in a large variety of organs, including brain, heart, vasculature, kidney, and lung. The importance of local RAS-modulation has gained increasing attention, since (1) tissue ACE-inhibitors are seemingly more effective in the treatment of hypertensive patients and (2) patients with a relatively low systemic RAS-activity can nevertheless be treated effectively with RAS-inhibitors. Besides the cleavage through ACE, ang II may also be generated by tissue chymase, carboxypeptidase, cathepsin G, and tonin. Although ang II is considered to be the major effector peptide of the RAS, enzymes have been identified, which may produce other forms of ang, e.g., ang III and IV, which probably play an important role in the brain. These peptides are generated by activation of tissue endopeptidases or by ACE-2, a recently recognized ACE homologue. Ang II mediates more than 60 different reactions, including vasoconstriction, cardiac hypertrophy, and proliferation of vascular smooth muscle cells [6]. Although a number of different ang II receptor has been identified, two of these are considered as the major mediators of ang II effects.

1 Angiotensin II Type 1 (AT1) receptor
2 Angiotensin II Type 2 (AT2) receptor

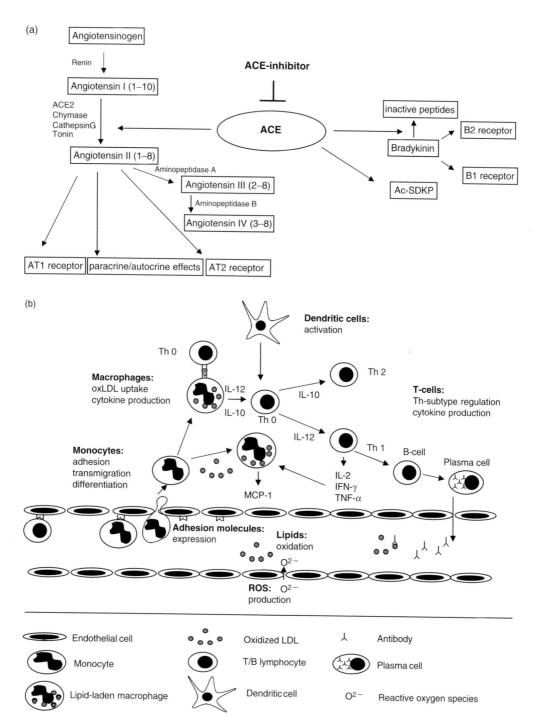

Figure 12.1 (a) *Signaling pathways of the angiotensin-converting enzyme (ACE)*. Angiotensinogen is cleaved to angiotensin (ang) I by renin. Formation of ang II predominantly involves ACE but may also happen via other peptides. Ang II activates the ang II receptors, mediates paracrine or autocrine effects or can be cleaved to other forms of ang. ACE hydrolyzes Ac-SDKP and bradykinin to inactive peptides. (b) *Renin-angiotensin system (RAS) mediated proinflammatory/immunomodulatory reactions in the vasculature*. The activated RAS mediates reactive oxygen species (ROS) formation, which results in lipid oxidation. Oxidized lipids are incorporated by monocytes and may serve as an autoantigen, which is processed and presented to T-lymphocytes. T-lymphocytes are activated in response to this contact and preferably differentiate into the Th1-subtype. T-lymphocyte activation may result in clonal expansion and activation of B-lymphocytes. B-lymphocyte may differentiate in plasma cells and secrete antibodies against oxidized lipids. RAS activation also mediates dendritic cell activation, which are involved in T-lymphocyte priming. In addition, RAS mediates leukocyte–endothelium interactions.

Both belong to the superfamily of G-Protein-coupled receptors. While there are still controversial data concerning the role of the AT2 receptor, the AT1 receptor mediates all the classical effects of ang II, including cell growth, proliferation, and vasoconstriction. It is expressed in various tissues, including vasculature, heart, lung, brain, liver, kidney, and adrenal gland. The AT2 receptor, on the other hand, seems to play a specific role during fetal development. After birth, its expression decreases, but increases again in case of acute tissue injury. The AT2-receptor mediates vasodilation, cell differentiation, and inhibits cell growth and apoptosis. Thus, the concept that the AT2-receptor may counteract the AT1-receptor effects has been developed in the past decade but still remains controversially discussed.

ACE signaling

The angiotensin-converting enzyme (ACE) is a metallopeptidase, which contains a zinc ion in the catalytically active site. It is not only responsible for the cleavage of ang I to ang II, but interacts with a number of different targets, such as bradykinin and N-acetyl-seryl-aspartyl-lysyl-proline (Ac-SDKP/goralatide) [7]. ACE exists as a somatic and a germinal form. The somatic form of ACE is abundantly expressed as an ectoenzyme on the surface of lung endothelial cells, although other types of endothelial cell, vascular smooth muscle cells (VSMCs), monocytes, T-lymphocytes, and adipocytes are also a source for ACE. In addition, ACE exists as a soluble form in blood plasma and other body fluids. In 1971, Yang et al. showed that ACE is identical with the kininase II. This finding linked the RAS with the kallikrein–kinin system as ACE hydrolyzes bradykinin to inactive fragments [8]. Bradykinin via its receptors B2 and in part B1 acts as a potent vasodilator, leading to the release of nitric oxide, prostacyclin, and the endothelium-derived hyperpolarizing factor [9]. Although activation of these receptors may profoundly contribute to the impact of ACE-blockade, as suggested by findings in B2 knock out mice, the experimental approach in mouse models remains difficult due to a differential expression pattern and strength of ang II mediated reactions [10]. As mentioned above, Ac-SDKP is another peptide degraded by

ACE, which has been identified as a stem cell regulator, acts proangiogenic, may modulate inflammatory cell infiltration after experimental myocardial infarction and reduces fibrosis in experimental ang II-induced hypertension [11–14]. The human homologue of ACE, ACE2 shares a 40% identity and 61% similarity with the "classical" ACE. ACE2 acts as a carboxypeptidase which may cleave ang I into ang II, ang 1–9, and ang 1–7 but does not directly hydrolyze bradykinin [15]. In contrast, ACE2 can remove the C terminus of the kinin metabolites, des-Arg kallidin and des-Arg bradykinin, which may lead to activation of the B1-receptor [16]. These reactions cannot be inhibited by ACE-inhibitors, such as lisinopril, captopril, or enalapril [17]. While ACE is expressed in a large variety of cells, ACE2 expression seems to be restricted to heart, kidney, and testis. In particular, ACE2 protein, as determined by immunohistochemistry can be found in coronary arterial and renal endothelium [15]. However, ACE2 has also been identified in the human gastrointestinal tract and in murine lungs. The function of ACE2 in the cardiovascular system remains a matter of debate. Experimental studies on knockout models showed differential results in regard of blood pressure regulation, while loss of ACE2 impairs heart function and seems to play a role in diabetic nephropathy [18].

Impact of RAS on immunomodulatory cells in atherosclerosis

Atherosclerosis is a chronic inflammatory cardiovascular disease characterized by the formation of so-called "plaques" in the arterial vascular wall. These lesions contain large amounts of inflammatory cells, e.g., macrophages, lymphocytes, dendritic cells, and mast cells. This observation led to the assumption that inflammatory/immunomodulatory processes may be major contributors to the onset, the progression and complications of this disease, which include myocardial infarction (MI), stroke, and sudden death. As reviewed by Medzhitov et al., the immune system exists of different but interacting mechanisms of response to antigen contact described as innate and adaptive immunity [19]. While the innate immunity is a rapidly reacting system of macrophages, dendritic cells, antimicrobial peptides, and the alternative complement pathway, activation and effective response of the adaptive immunity requires several days. This delay is due to the fact that adaptive immunity processes are driven by T- and B-lymphocytes, which can only be activated after antigen-presentation by components of the innate immunity and furthermore have to undergo clonal expansion. As mentioned above, macrophages, as part of the innate immunity, are abundantly present in atherosclerotic lesions and express pathogen-recognizing receptors, including scavenger and Toll-like receptors [20–23]. Activation of these receptors may result in endocytosis, apoptosis or nuclear factor (NF) kappa B activation, a transcription factor involved in the regulation of a large variety of inflammatory genes [23]. Although the role of microbial infection in the development of atherosclerosis remains controversially discussed, several studies throughout the years reported a correlation between infectious diseases, including tuberculosis, Chlamydia pneumoniae infection, and HIV as contributors to the severity of atherosclerosis [24–26]. However, the question remains, whether systemic infections are independently involved in the onset of atherosclerotic lesions or may only indirectly enhance the overall inflammatory host response. Nevertheless, macrophages have been identified as crucial components of the atherosclerotic plaque and are considered as major factors for the stability of the lesion. Large amounts of macrophages may weaken the plaque's ability to withstand arterial flow turbulences and thereby promote plaque rupture which may lead to thrombotic occlusion of the vessel or lesion growth [27]. Furthermore, macrophages play an essential role in the onset of atherosclerotic lesion formation. The early events in the development of an atherosclerotic lesion involve the invasion of modified lipoproteins into the vessel wall. In particular, oxidized low-density lipoprotein (oxLDL) seems to be of importance as its presence in the subendothelial space leads to transmigration of circulating monocytes, which then transform to macrophages and are able to incorporate oxLDL via scavenger receptors. Phagocytosis of oxLDL leads to a change of cell phenotype, upregulation of Toll-like receptor 4 expression, secretion of proinflammatory cytokines, and intensified re-

cruitment of lymphocytes, dendritic cells, or mast cells [28]. Thus, oxidized forms of LDL may represent pathogen patterns inducing activation of the effector cells of the innate immunity [29]. RAS components, including ang II and tissue ACE are both expressed by monocytes [30, 31]. Moreover, ACE and AT1-receptor expression is upregulated after differentiation of monocytes to tissue macrophages [32]. Ang II is also involved in lipoprotein oxidation by generation of reactive oxygen species (ROS) via the NAD(P)H oxidase or lipoxygenases and increases the uptake of modified LDL by macrophages via scavenger receptors [33, 34]. In addition, ang II regulates the uptake of oxidized LDL also in VSMCs and endothelial cells via the oxLDL receptor LOX-1 [35, 36]. Moreover, evidence has been gathered, that incorporation of oxLDL by macrophages may result in T-cell activation and specific antibody production. In this regard, oxLDL-reactive T-cells have been identified in human atherosclerotic plaques as well as circulating oxLDL antibodies, whose levels are elevated in patients with coronary artery disease (CAD) [37, 38]. T-lymphocytes just like macrophages are already found in early atherosclerotic lesions. They are mainly represented by the T helper (h) 1-subtype, secreting interferon (IFN)-γ, interleukin (IL)-2, and tumor necrosis factor (TNF)-α and -β [39]. Circulating Th1-cells are enhanced in patients suffering from acute coronary syndromes (ACS) [40]. Tissue ACE is found to co-localize with T-lymphocytes in human atherosclerotic plaques and ang II infusion results in an increase of IFN-γ, while IL-4 levels, a cytokine secreted by Th2-cells are reduced [41, 42]. Another experimental study performed in apoE mice, a murine model of atherosclerosis demonstrated, that splenocytes originating from mice with high ang II levels, secrete more IFN-γ, than animals with low ang II levels [43]. Moreover, ang II participates in T-cell activation via dendritic cell differentiation [44]. Balance of the Th-subtype is cross-regulated by IL-10 and IL-12. While IL-12 induces Th1-cell differentiation, IL-10 inhibits the release of IL-12 and thereby Th1-cell responses. Both cytokines are abundantly expressed in association with CD14 positive cells in human atherosclerotic lesions as compared to normal arteries. In addition, as demonstrated by Uyemura, monocytes secrete IL-10 and IL-12 in response to oxLDL stimulation.

However, IL-10 inhibits the LDL-induced release of IL-12, while neutralizing antibodies to IL-10 enhance IL-12 secretion [45]. Thus, high levels of IL-10 may be beneficial by reducing Th1-cell differentiation and thereby enhancing plaque stability, as the degree of macrophage and T-cell infiltration may determine the risk to rupture. These considerations are emphasized by clinical studies reporting significantly lower risks for patients with high levels of IL-10 for the re-occurrence of cardiovascular events [46]. In reverse, low levels of IL-10 are found in patients with ACS [47].

Detrimental interplay between cytokines and RAS in atherosclerosis

Ang II directly mediates inflammatory cell recruitment to the vascular wall by modifying leukocyte endothelium interactions. In this regard, ang II increases the endothelial expression of vascular adhesion molecule (VCAM)-1, intercellular adhesion molecule (ICAM)-1, P- and E-selectin, resulting in enhanced leukocyte adhesion in vivo [48]. Adhesion of leukocytes is also influenced by ang II via integrins, e.g., ß2 and alpha4-integrin, as reported by Alvarez *et al.* [48]. In addition, ang II regulates the expression of the monocyte chemoattracting protein (MCP)-1, a chemokine critically involved in atherosclerotic development and progression [49, 50]. MCP-1 is activated on human monocytes during transendothelial migration, but is also expressed by endothelial cells or VSMCs [51]. MCP-1 accelerates atherosclerosis in apoE-mice, while knock-out of the MCP-1 receptor CCR-2 leads to impaired monocyte migration and reduced Th1-cytokine response [52, 53]. The MCP-1 receptor CCR-2 on monocytes can be upregulated by ang II infusion [49], and as reviewed by Cheng *et al.*; ang II- and MCP-1-dependent inflammatory reactions are closely correlated [54]. Another cytokine modulating atherosclerosis is the proinflammatory IL-6. The IL-6 receptor consists of two subunits and is completely expressed only by hepatocytes and B-lymphocytes. Due to the existence of a soluble IL-6 receptor, it may also interact with other cells in the vasculature, including macrophages, lymphocytes, endothelial cells, and VSMCs. As reviewed by Rattazzi *et al.*, IL-6 mediates B-lymphocyte differentiation, co-stimulation of T-lymphocytes and thymocytes, proliferation of hematopoietic progenitor cells and the synthesis of acute-phase proteins by hepatocytes [55]. IL-6 is increased in patients with unstable angina or acute MI and serves as an independent risk marker for death and cardiovascular events [56–59]. Ang II upregulates IL-6 expression in macrophages and VSMCs in vitro [60, 61]. Furthermore, our group showed that IL-6 and ang II co-localize in the vulnerable shoulder region of human coronary plaques, while exogenous administration of IL-6 enhances the development of atherosclerotic lesions and leads to MCP-1 secretion from macrophages [61–63]. In contrast to these observations, knock-out of IL-6 in a murine model of atherosclerosis, leads to an increased lesion burden indicating a dual role for IL-6 in the development of atherosclerotic plaques [62]. IL-6 critically induces the synthesis of the acute-phase protein C-reactive protein (CRP) which is a strong independent risk factor for myocardial infarction [64]. As the major acute-phase reactant in humans, CRP is rapidly synthesized and secreted by hepatocytes in response to inflammatory stimuli, but is also expressed in human atherosclerotic lesions [65, 66]. CRP is directly involved in host defense processes. In this regard, CRP mediates the phagocytosis of its ligands, activates complement pathways and monocytes and increases endothelial cell sensitivity to T-cell cytotoxicity. CRP and IL-6 upregulate the AT1 receptor in vascular cells in vitro [67, 68]. Other proinflammatory cytokines regulated by ang II include the CC cytokine RANTES (Regulated on Activation normal T expressed and Secreted) and osteopontin. RANTES is a chemokine that selectively attracts T-lymphocytes, natural killer (NK) cells, monocytes, and eosinophils. It is strongly expressed in human transplant-associated atherosclerosis by macrophages, lymphocytes, myofibroblasts, and endothelial cells [69]. As demonstrated by Mateo *et al.*, using intravital microscopy, ang II-induced adhesion of leukocytes to the vascular endothelium critically involves RANTES [70]. Osteopontin, on the other hand, has recently been identified as an important contributor to atherogenesis [71]. Clinical trials, plasma levels of osteopontin are positively correlated with symptomatic carotid atherosclerotic lesions as well as the presence and extent of coronary artery disease (CAD) independent of other traditional risk factors [72, 73]. Osteopontin is expressed by VSMCs, macrophages, and T-lymphocytes and participates in T-cell differentiation by dendritic cell activation, inhibition of IL-10 production by macrophages and enhanced IFN-γ and Il-12 production [74, 75]. Although the exact mechanisms remain to be elucidated, interactions between the RAS and osteopontin have been reported and may involve ROS-sensitive signaling pathways. In this context, ang II upregulates osteopontin expression in rat cardiomyocytes and endothelial cells, while ang II infusion results in an attenuated atherosclerotic phenotype in osteopontin-deficient mice [76]. Ang II stimulation also upregulates the NF kappa B directly via activation of the AT1-receptor but also indirectly via ROS production in monocytes, neutrophils, cardiomyocytes, and VSMCs [60, 77–79].

ACE signaling and immunomodulation in cardiovascular disease

The kallikrein–kinin pathway as already described contributes to the immunomodulatory actions of the RAS. In this context, it was demonstrated that bradykinin exerts immunomodulatory features by triggering dendritic cells to produce IL-12, which—as mentioned above—modulates T-lymphocyte response into the direction of the Th1 subtype [80]. This immunomodulatory potential of bradykinin, however, may depend on the receptor—subtype, of which two have been identified so far, B1 and B2. While B2 is constitutively expressed, B1 is predominantly upregulated in case of tissue injury, treatment with interleukin-1 beta or TNF-α. The role of these receptors is currently under investigation in different pathophysiological settings, including diabetes and rheumatoid arthritis. The experimental data available so far, however, suggests a differential role for bradykinin receptors in inflammation [81]. The immunomodulatory effects of the RAS are summarized in Figure 12.1b.

ACE-inhibitors as immunomodulators in cardiovascular disease

ACE-inhibitors—a historical review

The first specific ACE-inhibitors isolated from snake venom were small peptides, which effectively reduced blood pressure, but had to be administered intravenously [82]. Cushman et al. developed the first orally available, nonpeptide ACE-inhibitor in 1977, while in 1981, ACE-inhibitors were finally available for the clinical treatment of hypertension [83]. ACE-inhibitors can be classified in three different chemical classes according to their zinc ligand, which also determines the strength of inhibition. In regard of pharmacokinetics, ACE-inhibitors differ in relation to half-life, potency, lipophilicity, and route of elimination. ACE-inhibitors competitively bind to ACE. As reviewed by Brown et al., short-term administration of ACE-inhibition leads to a decrease of endogenous ang II and aldosterone levels, while plasma renin activity and ang II increase. These effects, however, are only of contemporary nature in long-term treatment. A possible anti-atherosclerotic impact of ACE-inhibition was suggested soon after the clinical approval. In this regard, Mizuno et al. reported in 1985, that treatment with captopril in hypertensive subjects led to a significant decrease in circulating lipid peroxides. Thus, he speculated that ACE-inhibitors might be a future anti-atherosclerotic drug [84]. Others found a beneficial impact of ACE-inhibition on the peripheral blood flow in patients with hypertension and peripheral vascular disease, another form of atherosclerosis [85]. In 1992, Campbell et al. showed that ACE-inhibition ameliorates the extent of atherosclerotic lesions in a rabbit model. These early reports, however, attributed the benefit of this substance class mainly to the reduction of blood pressure and the attenuation of ang II mediated vascular remodeling processes.

ACE-inhibitors as anti-inflammatory drugs

The anti-inflammatory potential of ACE-inhibitors was first described in context with other pathophysiological entities, e.g., experimental granulomatous diseases and arthritis [86, 87]. In 1990, however, Rezkalla et al. reported that the ACE-inhibitor captopril reduced the inflammatory response of coxsackievirus-induced myocarditis [88] and only a few years later, Waltman showed that treatment with enalapril blunted the increase of leukocytes, lymphocytes, and neutrophils in a rat model of myocardial infarction and modulated antibody production [89]. Experimental studies followed, demonstrating that ACE-inhibition prevents the oxidation of LDL particles and their uptake by macrophages, leading to reduced foam cell formation [90, 91]. This effect may at least partially be due to a beneficial impact on the endothelial production of ROS [92]. In this regard, ACE-inhibition with ramipril results in enhanced nitric oxide (NO) bioavailability in patients with CAD via increased activity of the extracellular superoxide dismutase. Our group recently reported that ACE-blockade leads to a reduction of IL-6 and CRP-levels in patients with CAD and inhibits thromboxane-induced platelet aggregation. In addition, ACE-inhibition reduces arterial NF kappa B activation, osteopontin, endothelial VCAM-1, ICAM-1, and E-selectin expression as well as MCP-1 expression on VSMCs and macrophages in different models of atherosclerosis [93]. Subsequently, blockade of the ACE results in diminished postcapillary leukocyte adhesion and invasion in coronary arteries in experimental heart ischemia/reperfusion as well as decreased monocyte infiltration into atherosclerotic lesions independently of blood-pressure lowering [94, 95]. The immunomodulatory impact of ACE-inhibition has also been investigated in association with lymphocytes. In this context, ACE-blockade influences the Th1/Th2 cell balance by modulating IL-12, IL-10, and matrix metalloproteinases (MMP) levels as well as activity, suggesting a reduction of the Th1-cell subtype [96]. During the past years, cardiovascular scientists have gathered accumulating evidence for the active contribution of circulating hematopoietic progenitor cells to vascular regeneration and angiogenesis following ischemic events. Based on the clinical and experimental evidence so far, high levels of progenitor cells may be beneficial for the outcome of patients with ACS or MI. ACE-inhibitors may contribute to these effects by enhancing progenitor cell mobilization by specific cytokine modification, involving CD26/dipeptidylpeptidase IV (DPP IV) and SDF-1α/CXCR4 [97, 98].

ACE-inhibitors in clinical trials

Clinical trials have proven the benefit of ACE-inhibitors in different collectives of patients. The early clinical trials focused on the outcome of patients with left ventricular dysfunction after myocardial infarction or congestive heart failure, which demonstrated a significant reduction of mortality after treatment with ACE-inhibitor. These trials included the Cooperative North Scandinavian

Enalapril Survival Study (CONSENSUS), Studies on Left Ventricular Dysfunction (SOLVD), the Survival and Ventricular Enlargement (SAVE), and the Acute Infarction Ramipril Efficacy (AIRE) trials. The degree of LV dysfunction in the patients enrolled, however, did neither predict the future risk for cardiovascular events nor their prevention after treatment with ACE-inhibitors. Thus, it was speculated that ACE-blockade not only influences LV-remodeling, but may also possess anti-ischemic properties, as already suggested by experimental data. Thus, the first trials enrolling patients with CAD and preserved LV-function were conducted during the early nineties. As reviewed by van Gilst *et al.*, large clinical outcome trials have been conducted in this matter so far, including Heart Outcomes Prevention Evaluation (HOPE), the European Trial on Reduction of Cardiac Events with Perindopril in Stable Coronary Artery Disease (EUROPA), the Prevention of Events with Angiotensin-Converting-Enzyme inhibition trial (PEACE), and the Ischemia Management with Accupril post-bypass graft via inhibition of angiotensin-converting enzyme (IMAGE) trial [99]. One of the first major trials was HOPE, which enrolled patients with documented vascular disease or diabetes plus one other cardiovascular risk factor. After a mean follow-up of 5 years, the study was stopped because of a 13.5% risk reduction in the composite end point of cardiovascular death, MI and stroke after ramipril treatment. EUROPA and PEACE followed, both of which could document a significant risk reduction by ACE inhibition in patients with CAD. Another, still ongoing trial is IMAGINE, which investigates the effectiveness of quinapril in patients who have undergone cardiac bypass surgery. Besides these long-term trials, short intervention trials have been conducted, including CONSENSUS-II, the 4th International Study of Infarct Survival (ISIS-4), and the first Chinese Cardiac Study (CCS-1) [100]. These studies demonstrated that ACE-inhibition results in a post-MI risk reduction already within the first day of treatment. Although the impact of ACE-inhibitors on atherosclerotic lesion formation and content is well documented by experimental data, it still remains difficult to evaluate the underlying mechanisms in human patients. Although smaller clinical trials reported that ACE-inhibitors, especially those with a high tissue affinity, e.g., quinapril affect plaque growth after stent implantation, evidence for a direct interaction of ACE-inhibitors with atherosclerotic lesions is missing [101]. Moreover, the influence of these substances on blood pressure and, thus, blood flow turbulences may play a role even in the absence of a statistically significant impact.

Summary

Chronic RAS-activation mediates direct and indirect proinflammatory reactions within the cardiovascular system, and may thereby induce or amplify the onset and progression of atherosclerosis. Chronic ACE-inhibition in turn elicits effective anti-inflammatory and immunomodulatory effects, which were shown to be beneficial in the treatment of patients suffering from the clinical complications of atherosclerosis, including myocardial infarction, heart failure, and sudden cardiac death.

References

1 Olsen F. Type and course of the inflammatory cellular reaction in acute angiotensin-hypertensive vascular disease in rats. Acta Pathol Microbiol Scand [A] 1970;78(2):143–50.

2 Giese J. Acute hypertensive vascular disease. 1. Relation between blood pressure changes and vascular lesions in different forms of acute hypertension. Acta Pathol Microbiol Scand 1964;62:481–96.

3 Olsen F. Evidence for an immunological factor in the hypertensive vascular disease. Acta Pathol Microbiol Scand [A] 1971;79(1):22–6.

4 Cobankara V, Ozturk MA, Kiraz S et al. Renin and angiotensin-converting enzyme (ACE) as active components of the local synovial renin-angiotensin system in rheumatoid arthritis. Rheumatol Int May 2005;25(4):285–91.

5 Escobar E, Rodriguez-Reyna TS, Arrieta O, Sotelo J. Angiotensin II, cell proliferation and angiogenesis regulator: biologic and therapeutic implications in cancer. Curr Vasc Pharmacol October 2004;2(4):385–99.

6 Brasier AR, Recinos A, III, Eledrisi MS. Vascular inflammation and the renin-angiotensin system. Arterioscler Thromb Vasc Biol August 1, 2002;22(8):1257–66.

7 Fleming I. Signaling by the angiotensin-converting enzyme. Circ Res April 14, 2006;98(7):887–96.

8 Yang HY, Erdos EG, Levin Y. Characterization of a dipeptide hydrolase (kininase II: angiotensin I converting enzyme). J Pharmacol Exp Ther April 1971;177(1):291–300.

9 Busse R, Fleming I. Regulation of endothelium-derived vasoactive autacoid production by hemodynamic forces. Trends Pharmacol Sci January 2003;24(1):24–9.

10 Yang XP, Liu YH, Mehta D et al. Diminished cardioprotective response to inhibition of angiotensin-converting enzyme and angiotensin II type 1 receptor in B(2) kinin receptor gene knockout mice. Circ Res May 25, 2001;88(10):1072–9.

11 Rousseau A, Michaud A, Chauvet MT, Lenfant M, Corvol P. The hemoregulatory peptide N-acetyl-Ser-Asp-Lys-Pro is a natural and specific substrate of the N-terminal active site of human angiotensin-converting enzyme. J Biol Chem February 24, 1995;270(8):3656–61.

12 Wang D, Carretero OA, Yang XY et al. N-acetyl-seryl-aspartyl-lysyl-proline stimulates angiogenesis in vitro and in vivo. Am J Physiol Heart Circ Physiol November 2004;287(5):H2099–105.

13 Peng H, Carretero OA, Brigstock DR, Oja-Tebbe N, Rhaleb NE. Ac-SDKP reverses cardiac fibrosis in rats with renovascular hypertension. Hypertension December 2003;42(6):1164–70.

14 Yang F, Yang XP, Liu YH et al. Ac-SDKP reverses inflammation and fibrosis in rats with heart failure after myocardial infarction. Hypertension February 2004;43(2):229–36.

15 Donoghue M, Hsieh F, Baronas E et al. A novel angiotensin-converting enzyme-related carboxypeptidase (ACE2) converts angiotensin I to angiotensin 1-9. Circ Res September 1, 2000;87(5):E1–9.

16 Duka I, Kintsurashvili E, Gavras I, Johns C, Bresnahan M, Gavras H. Vasoactive potential of the b(1) bradykinin receptor in normotension and hypertension. Circ Res February 16, 2001;88(3):275–81.

17 Tipnis SR, Hooper NM, Hyde R, Karran E, Christie G, Turner AJ. A human homolog of angiotensin-converting enzyme. Cloning and functional expression as a captopril-insensitive carboxypeptidase. J Biol Chem October 27, 2000;275(43):33238–43.

18 Danilczyk U, Eriksson U, Oudit GY, Penninger JM. Physiological roles of angiotensin-converting enzyme 2. Cell Mol Life Sci November 2004;61(21):2714–9.

19 Medzhitov R, Janeway C, Jr. Innate immunity. N Engl J Med August 3, 2000;343(5):338–44.

20 Krieger M. The other side of scavenger receptors: pattern recognition for host defense. Curr Opin Lipidol October 1997;8(5):275–80.

21 Rhee SH, Hwang D. Murine Toll-like receptor 4 confers lipopolysaccharide responsiveness as determined by activation of NF kappa B and expression of the inducible cyclooxygenase. J Biol Chem November 3, 2000;275(44): 34035–40.

22 Edfeldt K, Swedenborg J, Hansson GK, Yan ZQ. Expression of Toll-like receptors in human atherosclerotic lesions: a possible pathway for plaque activation. Circulation March 12, 2002;105(10):1158–61.

23 Barnes PJ, Karin M. Nuclear factor-kappa B: a pivotal transcription factor in chronic inflammatory diseases. N Engl J Med April 10, 1997;336(15):1066–71.

24 Mussa FF, Chai H, Wang X, Yao Q, Lumsden AB, Chen C. Chlamydia pneumoniae and vascular disease: an update. J Vasc Surg June 2006;43(6):1301–7.

25 Sudano I, Spieker LE, Noll G, Corti R, Weber R, Luscher TF. Cardiovascular disease in HIV infection. Am Heart J June 2006;151(6):1147–55.

26 Leinonen M, Saikku P. Evidence for infectious agents in cardiovascular disease and atherosclerosis. Lancet Infect Dis January 2002;2(1):11–7.

27 Naghavi M, Libby P, Falk E et al. From vulnerable plaque to vulnerable patient: a call for new definitions and risk assessment strategies: Part I. Circulation October 7, 2003;108(14):1664–72.

28 Paoletti R, Gotto AM, Jr, Hajjar DP. Inflammation in atherosclerosis and implications for therapy. Circulation June 15, 2004;109(23 suppl 1):III20–6.

29 Xu XH, Shah PK, Faure E et al. Toll-like receptor-4 is expressed by macrophages in murine and human lipid-rich atherosclerotic plaques and upregulated by oxidized LDL. Circulation December 18, 2001;104(25): 3103–8.

30 Potter DD, Sobey CG, Tompkins PK, Rossen JD, Heistad DD. Evidence that macrophages in atherosclerotic lesions contain angiotensin II. Circulation August 25, 1998;98(8):800–7.

31 Ohishi M, Ueda M, Rakugi H et al. Enhanced expression of angiotensin-converting enzyme is associated with progression of coronary atherosclerosis in humans. J Hypertens November 1997;15(11):1295–302.

32 Okamura A, Rakugi H, Ohishi M et al. Upregulation of renin-angiotensin system during differentiation of monocytes to macrophages. J Hypertens April 1999;17(4):537–45.

33 Scheidegger KJ, Butler S, Witztum JL. Angiotensin II increases macrophage-mediated modification of low density lipoprotein via a lipoxygenase-dependent pathway. J Biol Chem August 22, 1997;272(34):21609–15.

34 Griendling KK, Minieri CA, Ollerenshaw JD, Alexander RW. Angiotensin II stimulates NADH and NADPH oxidase activity in cultured vascular smooth muscle cells. Circ Res June 1994;74(6):1141–8.

35 Li DY, Zhang YC, Philips MI, Sawamura T, Mehta JL. Upregulation of endothelial receptor for oxidized low-density lipoprotein (LOX-1) in cultured human coronary artery endothelial cells by angiotensin II type 1 receptor activation. Circ Res May 14, 1999;84(9):1043–9.

36 Limor R, Kaplan M, Sawamura T et al. Angiotensin II increases the expression of lectin-like oxidized low-density lipoprotein receptor-1 in human vascular smooth muscle cells via a lipoxygenase-dependent pathway. Am J Hypertens March 2005;18(3):299–307.

37 Toshima S, Hasegawa A, Kurabayashi M et al. Circulating oxidized low density lipoprotein levels. A biochemical risk marker for coronary heart disease. Arterioscler Thromb Vasc Biol October 2000;20(10):2243–7.

38 Zhou X, Robertson AK, Hjerpe C, Hansson GK. Adoptive transfer of CD4+ T cells reactive to modified low-density lipoprotein aggravates atherosclerosis. Arterioscler Thromb Vasc Biol April 2006;26(4):864–70.

39 Frostegard J, Ulfgren AK, Nyberg P et al. Cytokine expression in advanced human atherosclerotic plaques: dominance of pro-inflammatory (Th1) and macrophage-stimulating cytokines. Atherosclerosis July 1999;145(1):33–43.

40 Methe H, Brunner S, Wiegand D, Nabauer M, Koglin J, Edelman ER. Enhanced T-helper-1 lymphocyte activation patterns in acute coronary syndromes. J Am Coll Cardiol June 21, 2005;45(12):1939–45.

41 Diet F, Pratt RE, Berry GJ, Momose N, Gibbons GH, Dzau VJ. Increased accumulation of tissue ACE in human atherosclerotic coronary artery disease. Circulation December 1, 1996;94(11):2756–67.

42 Shao J, Nangaku M, Miyata T et al. Imbalance of T-cell subsets in angiotensin II-infused hypertensive rats with kidney injury. Hypertension July 2003;42(1):31–8.

43 Mazzolai L, Duchosal MA, Korber M et al. Endogenous angiotensin II induces atherosclerotic plaque vulnerability and elicits a Th1 response in ApoE−/− mice. Hypertension September 2004;44(3):277–82.

44 Nahmod KA, Vermeulen ME, Raiden S et al. Control of dendritic cell differentiation by angiotensin II. FASEB J March 2003;17(3):491–3.

45 Uyemura K, Demer LL, Castle SC et al. Cross-regulatory roles of interleukin (IL)-12 and IL-10 in atherosclerosis. J Clin Invest May 1, 1996;97(9):2130–8.

46 Kilic T, Ural D, Ural E et al. Relation between proinflammatory to anti-inflammatory cytokine ratios and long-term prognosis in patients with non-ST elevation acute coronary syndrome. Heart August 2006;92(8):1041–6.

47 Heeschen C, Dimmeler S, Hamm CW et al. Serum level of the antiinflammatory cytokine interleukin-10 is an important prognostic determinant in patients with acute coronary syndromes. Circulation April 29, 2003;107(16):2109–14.

48 Alvarez A, Cerda-Nicolas M, Naim Abu Nabah Y *et al.* Direct evidence of leukocyte adhesion in arterioles by angiotensin II. Blood July 15, 2004;104(2):402–8.

49 Ishibashi M, Hiasa K, Zhao Q *et al.* Critical role of monocyte chemoattractant protein-1 receptor CCR2 on monocytes in hypertension-induced vascular inflammation and remodeling. Circ Res May 14, 2004;94(9): 1203–10.

50 Ni W, Kitamoto S, Ishibashi M *et al.* Monocyte chemoattractant protein-1 is an essential inflammatory mediator in angiotensin II-induced progression of established atherosclerosis in hypercholesterolemic mice. Arterioscler Thromb Vasc Biol March 2004;24(3): 534–9.

51 Takahashi M, Masuyama J, Ikeda U *et al.* Induction of monocyte chemoattractant protein-1 synthesis in human monocytes during transendothelial migration in vitro. Circ Res May 1995;76(5):750–7.

52 Boring L, Gosling J, Chensue SW *et al.* Impaired monocyte migration and reduced type 1 (Th1) cytokine responses in C-C chemokine receptor 2 knockout mice. J Clin Invest November 15, 1997;100(10):2552–61.

53 Aiello RJ, Bourassa PA, Lindsey S *et al.* Monocyte chemoattractant protein-1 accelerates atherosclerosis in apolipoprotein E-deficient mice. Arterioscler Thromb Vasc Biol June 1999;19(6):1518–25.

54 Cheng ZJ, Vapaatalo H, Mervaala E. Angiotensin II and vascular inflammation. Med Sci Monit June 2005;11(6):RA194–205.

55 Rattazzi M, Puato M, Faggin E, Bertipaglia B, Zambon A, Pauletto P. C-reactive protein and interleukin-6 in vascular disease: culprits or passive bystanders? J Hypertens October 2003;21(10):1787–803.

56 Ridker PM, Hennekens CH, Buring JE, Rifai N. C-reactive protein and other markers of inflammation in the prediction of cardiovascular disease in women. N Engl J Med March 23, 2000;342(12):836–43.

57 Biasucci LM, Vitelli A, Liuzzo G *et al.* Elevated levels of interleukin-6 in unstable angina. Circulation September 1, 1996;94(5):874–7.

58 Ikeda U, Ohkawa F, Seino Y *et al.* Serum interleukin 6 levels become elevated in acute myocardial infarction. J Mol Cell Cardiol June 1992;24(6):579–84.

59 Ridker PM, Rifai N, Stampfer MJ, Hennekens CH. Plasma concentration of interleukin-6 and the risk of future myocardial infarction among apparently healthy men. Circulation April 18, 2000;101(15):1767–72.

60 Kranzhofer R, Schmidt J, Pfeiffer CA, Hagl S, Libby P, Kubler W. Angiotensin induces inflammatory activation of human vascular smooth muscle cells. Arterioscler Thromb Vasc Biol July 1999;19(7):1623–9.

61 Schieffer B, Schieffer E, Hilfiker-Kleiner D *et al.* Expression of angiotensin II and interleukin 6 in human coronary atherosclerotic plaques: potential implications for inflammation and plaque instability. Circulation March 28, 2000;101(12):1372–8.

62 Huber SA, Sakkinen P, Conze D, Hardin N, Tracy R. Interleukin-6 exacerbates early atherosclerosis in mice. Arterioscler Thromb Vasc Biol October 1999;19(10): 2364–7.

63 Biswas P, Delfanti F, Bernasconi S *et al.* Interleukin-6 induces monocyte chemotactic protein-1 in peripheral blood mononuclear cells and in the U937 cell line. Blood January 1, 1998;91(1):258–65.

64 Liang K, Sheu WH, Lee WL *et al.* Coronary artery disease progression is associated with C-reactive protein and conventional risk factors but not soluble CD40 ligand. Can J Cardiol June 2006;22(8):691–6.

65 Yasojima K, Schwab C, McGeer EG, McGeer PL. Generation of C-reactive protein and complement components in atherosclerotic plaques. Am J Pathol March 2001;158(3):1039–51.

66 Mortensen RF. C-reactive protein, inflammation, and innate immunity. Immunol Res 2001;24(2): 163–76.

67 Wassmann S, Stumpf M, Strehlow K *et al.* Interleukin-6 induces oxidative stress and endothelial dysfunction by overexpression of the angiotensin II type 1 receptor. Circ Res March 5, 2004;94(4):534–41.

68 Wang CH, Li SH, Weisel RD *et al.* C-reactive protein upregulates angiotensin type 1 receptors in vascular smooth muscle. Circulation April 8, 2003;107(13): 1783–90.

69 Pattison JM, Nelson PJ, Huie P, Sibley RK, Krensky AM. RANTES chemokine expression in transplant-associated accelerated atherosclerosis. J Heart Lung Transplant December 1996;15(12):1194–9.

70 Mateo T, Abu Nabah YN, Abu Taha M *et al.* Angiotensin II-induced mononuclear leukocyte interactions with arteriolar and venular endothelium are mediated by the release of different CC chemokines. J Immunol May 1, 2006;176(9):5577–86.

71 Matsui Y, Rittling SR, Okamoto H *et al.* Osteopontin deficiency attenuates atherosclerosis in female apolipoprotein E-deficient mice. Arterioscler Thromb Vasc Biol June 1, 2003;23(6):1029–34.

72 Golledge J, McCann M, Mangan S, Lam A, Karan M. Osteoprotegerin and osteopontin are expressed at high concentrations within symptomatic carotid atherosclerosis. Stroke July 2004;35(7):1636–41.

73 Ohmori R, Momiyama Y, Taniguchi H *et al.* Plasma osteopontin levels are associated with the presence and extent of coronary artery disease. Atherosclerosis October 2003;170(2):333–7.

74 Renkl AC, Wussler J, Ahrens T *et al.* Osteopontin functionally activates dendritic cells and induces their

differentiation toward a Th1-polarizing phenotype. Blood August 1, 2005;106(3):946–55.

75 Hirota S, Imakita M, Kohri K et al. Expression of osteopontin messenger RNA by macrophages in atherosclerotic plaques. A possible association with calcification. Am J Pathol October 1993;143(4):1003–8.

76 Bruemmer D, Collins AR, Noh G et al. Angiotensin II-accelerated atherosclerosis and aneurysm formation is attenuated in osteopontin-deficient mice. J Clin Invest November 2003;112(9):1318–31.

77 Kranzhofer R, Browatzki M, Schmidt J, Kubler W. Angiotensin II activates the proinflammatory transcription factor nuclear factor-kappa B in human monocytes. Biochem Biophys Res Commun April 21, 1999;257(3): 826–8.

78 Rouet-Benzineb P, Gontero B, Dreyfus P, Lafuma C. Angiotensin II induces nuclear factor-kappa B activation in cultured neonatal rat cardiomyocytes through protein kinase C signaling pathway. J Mol Cell Cardiol October 2000;32(10):1767–78.

79 El Bekay R, Alvarez M, Monteseirin J et al. Oxidative stress is a critical mediator of the angiotensin II signal in human neutrophils: involvement of mitogen-activated protein kinase, calcineurin, and the transcription factor NF-kappa B. Blood July 15, 2003;102(2):662–71.

80 Aliberti J, Viola JP, Vieira-de-Abreu A, Bozza PT, Sher A, Scharfstein J. Cutting edge: bradykinin induces IL-12 production by dendritic cells: a danger signal that drives Th1 polarization. J Immunol June 1, 2003;170(11): 5349–53.

81 Gama Landgraf R, Sirois P, Jancar S. Differential modulation of murine lung inflammation by bradykinin B1 and B2 selective receptor antagonists. Eur J Pharmacol January 26, 2003;460(1):75–83.

82 Gavras H, Brunner HR, Laragh JH, Sealey JE, Gavras I, Vukovich RA. An angiotensin converting-enzyme inhibitor to identify and treat vasoconstrictor and volume factors in hypertensive patients. N Engl J Med October 17, 1974;291(16):817–21.

83 Ondetti MA, Rubin B, Cushman DW. Design of specific inhibitors of angiotensin-converting enzyme: new class of orally active antihypertensive agents. Science April 22, 1977;196(4288):441–4.

84 Mizuno K, Gotoh M, Fukuchi S. Acute effect of captopril on serum lipid peroxides level in hypertensive patients. Tohoku J Exp Med May 1984;143(1):127–8.

85 Catalano M, Libretti A. Captopril for the treatment of patients with hypertension and peripheral vascular disease. Angiology May 1985;36(5):293–6.

86 Deepe GS, Jr, Taylor CL, Srivastava L, Bullock WE. Impairment of granulomatous inflammatory response to Histoplasma capsulatum by inhibitors of angiotensin-converting enzyme. Infect Immun May 1985;48(2):395–401.

87 Caspritz G, Alpermann HG, Schleyerbach R. Influence of the new angiotensin converting enzyme inhibitor ramipril on several models of acute inflammation and the adjuvant arthritis in the rat. Arzneimittelforschung November 1986;36(11):1605–8.

88 Rezkalla S, Kloner RA, Khatib G, Khatib R. Beneficial effects of captopril in acute coxsackievirus B3 murine myocarditis. Circulation March 1990;81(3):1039–46.

89 Waltman TJ, Harris TJ, Cesario D, Ziegler M, Maisel AS. Effects of enalapril on T and B cell function in rats after myocardial infarction. J Card Fail September 1995;1(4):293–302.

90 Kowala MC, Grove RI, Aberg G. Inhibitors of angiotensin converting enzyme decrease early atherosclerosis in hyperlipidemic hamsters. Fosinopril reduces plasma cholesterol and captopril inhibits macrophage-foam cell accumulation independently of blood pressure and plasma lipids. Atherosclerosis July 1994;108(1): 61–72.

91 Godfrey EG, Stewart J, Dargie HJ et al. Effects of ACE inhibitors on oxidation of human low density lipoprotein. Br J Clin Pharmacol January 1994;37(1):63–6.

92 Cominacini L, Pasini A, Garbin U et al. Zofenopril inhibits the expression of adhesion molecules on endothelial cells by reducing reactive oxygen species. Am J Hypertens October 2002;15(10, pt 1):891–5.

93 Hernandez-Presa M, Bustos C, Ortego M et al. Angiotensin-converting enzyme inhibition prevents arterial nuclear factor-kappa B activation, monocyte chemoattractant protein-1 expression, and macrophage infiltration in a rabbit model of early accelerated atherosclerosis. Circulation March 18, 1997;95(6): 1532–41.

94 Kupatt C, Habazettl H, Zahler S et al. ACE-inhibition prevents postischemic coronary leukocyte adhesion and leukocyte-dependent reperfusion injury. Cardiovasc Res December 1997;36(3):386–95.

95 Hayek T, Attias J, Coleman R et al. The angiotensin-converting enzyme inhibitor, fosinopril, and the angiotensin II receptor antagonist, losartan, inhibit LDL oxidation and attenuate atherosclerosis independent of lowering blood pressure in apolipoprotein E deficient mice. Cardiovasc Res December 1999;44(3):579–87.

96 Constantinescu CS, Goodman DB, Ventura ES. Captopril and lisinopril suppress production of interleukin-12 by human peripheral blood mononuclear cells. Immunol Lett May 1998;62(1):25–31.

97 Wang CH, Verma S, Hsieh IC et al. Enalapril increases ischemia-induced endothelial progenitor cell mobilization through manipulation of the CD26 system. J Mol Cell Cardiol July 2006;41(1):34–43.

98 Asahara T. ACE inhibitor raps CD26/dipeptidylpeptidase IV knuckles for cytokine EPC mobilization. J Mol Cell Cardiol July 2006;41(1):8–10.

99 van Gilst WH, Warnica JW, Baillot R *et al.* Angiotensin-converting enzyme inhibition in patients with coronary artery disease and preserved left ventricular function Ischemia Management with Accupril post-bypass graft via inhibition of angiotensin-converting enzyme (IMAGINE) compared with the other major trials in coronary artery disease. Am Heart J June 2006;151(6): 1240–6.

100 Sleight P. Angiotensin II and trials of cardiovascular outcomes. Am J Cardiol January 24, 2002;89(2A):11A–6A; discussion 6A–7A.

101 Okimoto T, Imazu M, Hayashi Y *et al.* Quinapril with high affinity to tissue angiotensin-converting enzyme reduces restenosis after percutaneous transcatheter coronary intervention. Cardiovasc Drugs Ther July 2001; 15(4):323–9.

CHAPTER 13

Treatment of heart failure by anticytokine therapies

Donna L. Vredevoe & Julia R. Gage

Inflammatory cytokines in HF

Inflammatory cytokines, particularly interleukin 6 (IL-6) and tumor necrosis factor (TNF) have been postulated to play a role in the pathophysiology of heart failure (HF) [1, 2]. Whereas these cytokines most likely provide a beneficial physiological response to short-term stress, chronically elevated levels of IL-6 and TNF have been postulated to contribute to cardiovascular disease [1]. Circulating levels of IL-6 [3–5] and TNF [6, 7] have been shown to be increased in patients with chronic HF. Expression of these cytokines has also been linked to disease severity [3, 8] and mortality [3, 9].

The exact source(s) of these cytokines and the stimulus that drives their production have not been identified. Our studies documented elevated levels of IL-6 production by peripheral blood mononuclear cells (PBMC) in patients with chronic HF compared to healthy control subjects [5], suggesting that these cells may contribute to the high systemic levels of IL-6 seen in these patients. We have also seen that PBMC from patients with chronic HF exposed to a T-cell stimulus produce significant amounts of TNF [10]. This finding suggests that T cells, in addition to myocytes [11] could be a source of TNF in these patients.

Effects of inflammatory cytokines in HF

IL-6 has been shown to play multiple roles in inflammation, including leukocyte activation and migration, transcriptional activation of acute-phase reactants, and resolution of the inflammatory process [12]. Given these multiple roles, it remains to be seen whether IL-6 is an active participant in the pathophysiology of HF or is simply a marker for the degree of inflammation in a given patient. Our studies have shown, however, that IL-6 expression by PBMC was correlated with natural killer (NK) cell dysfunction in patients with chronic HF [5]. Chronic IL-6 exposure may lead to NK-cell anergy by two possible mechanisms: down-regulation of cell-surface expression of the IL-6 receptor α subunit CD126 [13], and/or long-term induction of negative regulators of IL-6 signaling such as the suppressor of cytokine signaling (SOCS) family of proteins [14]. SOCS proteins are natural inhibitors of cytokine signaling involved in innate immunity and inflammatory diseases [15].

IL-6-mediated activation of SOCS proteins has been postulated to play a role in the progression of cardiac hypertrophy to heart failure [16]. IL-6 activates the JAK/STAT signal transduction pathway [17], which upregulates expression of SOCS proteins [18]. SOCS expression leads to decreases in STAT proteins, dampening IL-6 signal transduction. All of the components of IL-6 signaling and resolution are expressed in the heart [16]. In addition to IL-6-mediated signaling, the SOCS family of proteins regulates signaling by other members of the IL-6 family of cytokines, including cardiotrophin-1 (CT-1) [19]. IL-6-mediated SOCS proteins may cross-talk with other signaling systems [20]. A consequence of chronic production of SOCS may therefore be dampening of CT-1 function, leading to either maladaptive or beneficial cardiac responses [21].

Studies have demonstrated multiple roles for TNF in heart disease, including the promotion of left ventricular remodeling; nitric oxide production; down-regulation of cardiac motility; production of adhesion molecules; up-regulation of apoptosis in endothelial cells and myocytes; and development of dilated cardiomyopathy [22, 23]. In short-term, acute inflammatory responses TNF production is suppressed by cytokines such as IL-10 and transforming growth factor β. These anti-inflammatory cytokines appear to be decreased or inadequately produced in patients with congestive heart failure [24]. This observation highlights the complexity of the dysregulation of the cytokine network in HF patients, and suggests that blockade of one particular cytokine may not be an effective treatment for HF in general.

Anti-TNF therapies in HF

Although targeting of TNF would theoretically be a useful therapeutic strategy in patients with HF, clinical trails examining the effects of TNF antagonism have failed to demonstrate clinical benefit [25, 26]. Phase 1 and dose-finding trials of the soluble TNF receptor etanercept in HF patients were promising, with improvements in some clinical parameters (Table 13.1). However, effects of etanercept on clinical outcomes were similar to placebo in the larger, randomized, controlled RENAISSANCE

Table 13.1 Randomized, controlled clinical trials of TNF antagonists in patients with heart failure.

Treatment (Trial)	Reference	Treatment/dosage (No. patients enrolled)	Clinical outcomes	Treatment-related adverse events
Etanercept (RCT)	[27]	Placebo ($n = 6$) 1 mg/m^2 ($n = 2$) 4 mg/m^2 ($n = 2$) 10 mg/m^2 ($n = 2$)	Improvements in ejection fraction ($p = 0.03$), 6-min walk distance ($p = 0.01$), quality-of-life score ($p = 0.001$) in pts receiving 4 mg/m^2 and 10 mg/m^2	None
Etanercept (RCT)	[28]	Placebo ($n = 16$) 5 mg/m^2 ($n = 16$) 12 mg/m^2 ($n = 15$)	Improvements in LV ejection fraction ($p = 0.01$), LV end-diastolic volume ($p = 0.04$), LV end-systolic volume ($p = 0.02$) compared with placebo	None
Etanercept (RECOVER)	[29]	Placebo ($n = 373$) 25 mg QW ($n = 375$) 25 mg BIW ($n = 375$)	No improvements in rates of death or CHF hospitalization	None
Etanercept (RENAISSANCE)	[29]	Placebo ($n = 309$) 25 mg BIW ($n = 308$) 25 mg TIW ($n = 308$)	No improvements in rates of death or CHF hospitalization	None
Etanercept (RENEWAL) pooled analysis*	[29]	Placebo ($n = 682$) 25 mg BIW ($n = 683$) 25 mg BIW + TIW ($n = 991$)	No improvements in rates of death or CHF hospitalization	None
Infliximab (ATTACH)	[30]	Placebo ($n = 49$) 5 mg/kg ($n = 50$) 10 mg/kg ($n = 51$)	No clinical improvements in NYHA class, global assessment, or quality of life scores	Increased rates of hospitalization and death in pts treated with higher dose

RCT, randomized, controlled trial; LV, left ventricular; QW, once weekly; BIW, twice weekly; TIW, three times weekly; RECOVER, research into etanercept cytokine antagonism in ventricular dysfunction; RENAISSANCE, randomized etanercept North American strategy to study antagonism of cytokines; RENEWAL, randomized etanercept worldwide evaluation; ATTACH, anti-TNF therapy against congestive heart failure.
*Pooled analysis of data from RECOVER and RENAISSANCE trials.

and RECOVER trials [29]. The anti-TNF mono-clonal antibody infliximab also failed to improve clinical conditions in patients with HF, and high dosages were associated with an increased risk of adverse events in the ATTACH trial [30]. These un-expected results underscore the complexity of the role of cytokine dysregulation in patients with HF, and resulted in the early termination of several of the trials. These findings also suggest that TNF may not play an active role in the pathophysiology of chronic HF, but may be a marker of the inflamma-tion associated with the condition.

Despite the failure of TNF antagonists in trials of patients with HF, they have been shown to provide clinical benefit in patients with the chronic inflam-matory disease rheumatoid arthritis (RA) [31]. In-terestingly, this patient population is at increased risk of cardiovascular disease [32], which accounts for 35–50% of RA deaths [33]. In recent meet-ings of the European League Against Rheumatism (EULAR) and published studies, several investiga-tors reported decreased mortality due to cardio-vascular disease [34–38], congestive heart failure [39], and myocardial infarction [40] in RA patients treated with TNF antagonists. These results suggest that this anticytokine therapy can provide cardio-vascular benefit in particular patient populations.

Future strategies for cytokine-modulating therapies in HF

Two aspects of cytokine function may prohibit the use of specific anticytokine therapies: the fact that cytokines act within a network in any immune re-sponse, and the redundancy of the cytokine system. For example, sequestering of IL-6 may dampen in-flammation, but may also lead to downstream ad-verse events, such as defects in wound healing or in-appropriate pulmonary reactions to environmental antigens leading to increased risk of infections as the loss of IL-6 signaling may result in an inadequate immune response. The redundancy of pathogen-sensing components of the innate immune system has been associated with deleterious immune re-sponses to bacterial pathogens, leading to sepsis and inflammatory diseases [41]. Similar mecha-nisms may also play a role in the pathophysiology of HF.

Targeting of specific regulatory immune cells that produce cytokines may also not be technically fea-sible, as was recently demonstrated in a phase-1 trial of a therapy designed to stimulate regulatory T cells [42]. In this study, six healthy subjects expe-rienced a "cytokine storm" immediately following administration of a novel superagonist anti-CD28 monoclonal antibody. Th1, Th2, and inflamma-tory cytokines spiked within minutes of receipt of the T-cell stimulus, resulting in significant morbid-ity, including cardiovascular events, in all subjects. This detrimental systemic inflammatory response occurred in the absence of exposure to any pathogen or underlying disease, emphasizing the precarious balance of cytokine homeostasis, even in healthy people.

Despite the failures of TNF antagonists in the treatment of patients with HF, targeting of in-flammatory cytokines in general may still be a vi-able strategy. Broad-spectrum anti-inflammatory or immune-modulation therapies have recently been shown to provide clinical benefit in pa-tients with HF. Potential therapies include physi-cal training, vitamin E/antioxidants, pentoxifylline, statins, and intravenous immunoglobulins [43]. Preliminary studies of a novel immune-modulating therapy (Celacade) have shown that reduction of inflammatory cytokines in conjunction with pro-motion of anti-inflammatory cytokines reduced the risk of cardiac death and hospitalization of patients with severe HF [44].

Traditional therapies have also been shown to re-duce levels of inflammatory cytokines. We have seen that beta blocker and angiotensin converting en-zyme inhibitor therapies were associated with lower levels of TNF production by stimulated PBMC in patients with chronic HF [10]. Given the intricate cytokine balance in patients with HF, even incre-mental reductions in inflammatory cytokines may safely provide clinical benefit.

The timing of anticytokine therapy is another consideration in patients with chronic HF. Treat-ment of patients with significant pathology may be ineffective because too much damage has already been done. The targeting of patients who are at risk of developing chronic HF with prophylactic cytokine-modulating therapies may therefore be an appealing strategy as safer anticytokine therapies become available.

References

1 Mann DL. Stress-activated cytokines and the heart: from adaptation to maladaptation. Annu Rev Physiol 2003;65: 81–101.

2 Paulus WJ. Cytokines and heart failure. Heart Fail Monit 2000;1(2):50–6.

3 Deswal A, Bozkurt B, Seta Y et al. Safety and efficacy of a soluble P75 tumor necrosis factor receptor (Enbrel, etanercept) in patients with advanced heart failure. Circulation June 29, 1999;99(25):3224–6.

4 Torre-Amione G, Kapadia S, Benedict C, Oral H, Young JB, Mann DL. Proinflammatory cytokine levels in patients with depressed left ventricular ejection fraction: a report from the studies of left ventricular dysfunction (SOLVD). J Am Coll Cardiol April 1996;27(5):1201–6.

5 Vredevoe DL, Widawski M, Fonarow GC, Hamilton M, Martínez-Maza O, Gage JR. Interleukin-6 (IL-6) expression and natural killer (NK) cell dysfunction and anergy in heart failure. Am J Cardiol 2004;93:1007–11.

6 Levine B, Kalman J, Mayer L, Fillit HM, Packer M. Elevated circulating levels of tumor necrosis factor in severe chronic heart failure. N Engl J Med July 26, 1990;323(4): 236–41.

7 McMurray J, Abdullah I, Dargie HJ, Shapiro D. Increased concentrations of tumour necrosis factor in "cachectic" patients with severe chronic heart failure. Br Heart J November 1991;66(5):356–8.

8 Tsutamoto T, Hisanaga T, Wada A et al. Interleukin-6 spillover in the peripheral circulation increases with the severity of heart failure, and the high plasma level of interleukin-6 is an important prognostic predictor in patients with congestive heart failure. J Am Coll Cardiol February 1998;31(2):391–8.

9 Rauchhaus M, Doehner W, Francis DP et al. Plasma cytokine parameters and mortality in patients with chronic heart failure. Circulation December 19, 2000;102(25): 3060–7.

10 Gage JR, Fonarow G, Hamilton M, Widawski M, Martínez-Maza O, Vredevoe DL. Beta blocker and angiotensin-converting enzyme inhibitor therapy is associated with decreased Th1/Th2 cytokine ratios and inflammatory cytokine production in patients with chronic heart failure. Neuroimmunomodulation 2004;11(3): 173–80.

11 Doyama K, Fujiwara H, Fukumoto M et al. Tumour necrosis factor is expressed in cardiac tissues of patients with heart failure. Int J Cardiol June 1996;54(3):217–25.

12 Jones SA. Directing transition from innate to acquired immunity: defining a role for IL-6. J Immunol September 15, 2005;175(6):3463–8.

13 Zohlnhofer D, Graeve L, Rose-John S, Schooltink H, Dittrich E, Heinrich PC. The hepatic interleukin-6 receptor. Down-regulation of the interleukin-6 binding subunit (gp80) by its ligand. FEBS Lett July 20, 1992; 306(2–3):219–22.

14 Chen XP, Losman JA, Rothman P. SOCS proteins, regulators of intracellular signaling. Immunity September 2000;13(3):287–90.

15 Yoshimura A, Nishinakamura H, Matsumura Y, Hanada T. Negative regulation of cytokine signaling and immune responses by SOCS proteins. Arthritis Res Ther 2005; 7(3):100–10.

16 Terrell AM, Crisostomo PR, Wairiuko GM, Wang M, Morrell ED, Meldrum DR. JAK/STAT/SOCS signaling circuits and associated cytokine-mediated inflammation and hypertrophy in the heart. Shock September 2006;26(3):226–34.

17 Heinrich PC, Behrmann I, Muller-Newen G, Schaper F, Graeve L. Interleukin-6-type cytokine signalling through the gp130/JAK/STAT pathway. Biochem J September 1, 1998;334(pt 2):297–314.

18 Starr R, Willson TA, Viney EM et al. A family of cytokine-inducible inhibitors of signalling. Nature June 26, 1997;387(6636):917–21.

19 Hamanaka I, Saito Y, Yasukawa H et al. Induction of JAB/SOCS-1/SSI-1 and CIS3/SOCS-3/SSI-3 is involved in gp130 resistance in cardiovascular system in rat treated with cardiotrophin-1 in vivo. Circ Res April 13, 2001;88(7):727–32.

20 Piessevaux J, Lavens D, Montoye T et al. Functional cross-modulation between SOCS proteins can stimulate cytokine signalling. J Biol Chem September 6, 2006;281(44): 32953–66.

21 Freed DH, Cunnington RH, Dangerfield AL, Sutton JS, Dixon IM. Emerging evidence for the role of cardiotrophin-1 in cardiac repair in the infarcted heart. Cardiovasc Res March 1, 2005;65(4):782–92.

22 Ferrari R. The role of TNF in cardiovascular disease. Pharmacol Res August 1999;40(2):97–105.

23 Sharma R, Al-Nasser FO, Anker SD. The importance of tumor necrosis factor and lipoproteins in the pathogenesis of chronic heart failure. Heart Fail Monit 2001;2(2):42–7.

24 Aukrust P, Ueland T, Lien E et al. Cytokine network in congestive heart failure secondary to ischemic or idiopathic dilated cardiomyopathy. Am J Cardiol February 1, 1999;83(3):376–82.

25 Anker SD, Coats AJS. How to RECOVER from RENAISSANCE? The significance of the results of RECOVER, RENAISSANCE, RENEWAL and ATTACH. Int J Cardiol 2002;86:123–30.

26 Mann DL. Targeted anticytokine therapy and the failing heart. Am J Cardiol 2005;95(suppl):9C–16C.

27 Deswal A, Petersen NJ, Feldman AM, Young JB, White BG, Mann DL. Cytokines and cytokine receptors in advanced heart failure: an analysis of the cytokine database

from the Vesnarinone trial (VEST). Circulation April 24, 2001;103(16):2055–9.

28 Bozkurt B, Torre-Amione G, Warren MS *et al*. Results of targeted anti-tumor necrosis factor therapy with etanercept (ENBREL) in patients with advanced heart failure. Circulation February 27, 2001;103(8):1044–7.

29 Mann DL, McMurray JJ, Packer M *et al*. Targeted anti-cytokine therapy in patients with chronic heart failure: results of the randomized etanercept worldwide evaluation (RENEWAL). Circulation April 6, 2004;109(13): 1594–602.

30 Chung ES, Packer M, Lo KH, Fasanmade AA, Willerson JT, for the ATTACH Investigators. Randomized, double-blind, placebo-controlled, pilot trial of infliximab, a chimeric monoclonal antibody to tumor necrosis factor-α, in patients with moderate-to-severe heart failure. Results of the anti-TNF therapy against congestive heart failure (ATTACH) trial. Circulation 2003;107:3133–40.

31 Schwartzman S, Fleischmann R, Morgan GJ, Jr. Do anti-TNF agents have equal efficacy in patients with rheumatoid arthritis? Arthritis Res Ther 2004;6(suppl 2):S3–11.

32 Wolfe F, Michaud K. Heart failure in rheumatoid arthritis: rates, predictors, and the effect of anti-tumor necrosis factor therapy. Am J Med March 1, 2004;116(5):305–11.

33 Sarzi-Puttini P, Atzeni F, Shoenfeld Y, Ferraccioli G. TNF-α, rheumatoid arthritis, and heart failure: a rheumatological dilemma. Autoimmun Rev 2005;4:15361.

34 Haugeberg G, Dasgupta B, Gomez-Reino JJ *et al*. Mortality rate is reduced in RA patients treated with the TNF antagonists. Data from BIODASER. Ann Rheum Dis 2006;65(suppl II):318.

35 Kremer JM, Reed G, White B, Baumgartner S, Lin S. An analysis of risk factors and effect of treatment on the development of cardiovascular disease in patients with rheumatoid arthritis. Ann Rheum Dis 2006; 65(suppl II):307.

36 Michaud K, Wolfe F. Reduced mortality among RA patients treated with anti-TNF therapy and methotrexate. Ann Rheum Dis 2005;64(suppl III):87.

37 Turesson C, Jacobsson LTH, Nilsson J *et al*. Treatment with TNF-blockers is associated with reduced premature mortality in patients with rheumatoid arthritis. Ann Rheum Dis 2006;65(suppl II):506.

38 Wolfe F, Mitchell DM, Sibley JT *et al*. The mortality of rheumatoid arthritis. Arthritis Rheum 1994;37:481–94.

39 Michaud K, Mendelsohn AM, Wolfe F. Congestive heart failure in RA: rates, predictors and the effect of anti-TNF therapy. European League Against Rheumatism Congress; June 18–21, 2003; Lisbon, Portugal. Abstract OP0109.

40 Dixon WG, Watson KD, Lunt M, Hyrich KL, Silman AJ, Symmons DPM. Rates of myocardial infarction (MI) and cerebrovascular accident (CVA) are reduced in patients with rheumatoid arthritis (RA) treated with anti-TNF therapy compared to those treated with traditional DMARDs: results from the BSR Biologics Register. Ann Rheum Dis 2006;65(suppl II):109.

41 Abreu MT, Arditi M. Innate immunity and Toll-like receptors: clinical implications of basic science research. J Pediatr April 2004;144(4):421–9.

42 Suntharalingam G, Perry MR, Ward S *et al*. Cytokine storm in a phase 1 trial of the anti-CD28 monoclonal antibody TGN1412. N Engl J Med September 7, 2006;355(10):1018–28.

43 Gullestad L, Aukrust P. Review of trials in chronic heart failure showing broad-spectrum anti-inflammatory approaches. Am J Cardiol June 6, 2005;95(11A): 17C–23C.

44 Torre-Amione G, Sestier F, Radovancevic B, Young J. Broad modulation of tissue responses (immune activation) by Celacade may favorably influence pathologic processes associated with heart failure progression. Am J Cardiol June 6, 2005;95(11A):30C–37C.

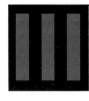

PART III

Immune dysfunction leading to heart dysfunction: induction or prevention by cardiotherapeutic drugs

CHAPTER 14

Pathogenesis of cardiovascular complications in the acquired immunodeficiency syndrome

Giuseppe Barbaro

Introduction

Studies published before the introduction of highly active antiretroviral therapy (HAART) have tracked the incidence and course of human immunodeficiency virus (HIV) infection in relation to both pediatric and adult cardiac illnesses [1]. These studies showed that subclinical echocardiographic abnormalities independently predict adverse outcomes and identify high-risk groups to target for early intervention and therapy. Understanding the effects of HAART on the cardiovascular system is only possible by understanding the effects of HIV co-infections first [2]. HAART is only available to a minority of HIV-infected individuals worldwide and studies published before the introduction of HAART remain globally applicable [3], especially in developing countries [4].

HIV-associated cardiomyopathy

HIV disease is recognized as an important cause of dilated cardiomyopathy, with an estimated annual incidence of 15.9/1000 before the introduction of HAART [5]. The importance of cardiac dysfunction is demonstrated by its effect on survival in acquired immunodeficiency syndrome (AIDS). Median survival to AIDS-related death is 101 days in patients with left ventricular dysfunction and 472 days in patients with a normal heart by echocardiography at a similar infection stage [5]. The unadjusted hazard ratio for death in HIV-associated cardiomyopathy compared to idiopathic cardiomyopathy is 4.0; the ratio adjusted after multivariate analysis is 5.86 [5]. The introduction of HAART regimens, by preventing opportunistic infections and reducing the incidence of myocarditis, has reduced the prevalence of HIV-associated cardiomyopathy by about 30% in developed countries [6, 7]. However, the median prevalence of HIV-associated cardiomyopathy is increasing in developing countries (about 32%), where the availability of HAART is scanty and greater is the pathogenetic impact of nutritional factors [4].

Pathologic features

Pathologic features of HIV-associated cardiomyopathy are similar to those observed in HIV-uninfected patients. At autopsy, the heart shape is modified, because of ventricular dilation and apical rounding. Heart weight is generally increased, owing to fibrosis and myocyte hypertrophy [8, 9]. On average, long-term survivors have significantly heavier hearts than those dying after a brief disease course. The epicardium is usually normal and coronary arteries do not show significant atherosclerosis. The myocardium is rather flabby and the ventricular wall usually collapses on section [8, 9]. On cut surface, the ventricles show an eccentric hypertrophy, that is, a mass increase with chamber volume enlargement. Although hypertrophy is demonstrated by the increase in cardiac weight, this is not always grossly evident owing to ventricular dilation; the free wall width may be normal, or even thinner than normal, as happens in short-term survivors. Endocardial fibrosis is a common finding, as well as mural thrombi, mainly located at the apex. Dilated cardiomyopathy can be associated with pericardial effusion or infective endocarditis, especially in intravenous drug abusers [8, 9]. On histology, myocytes show variable degrees of hypertrophy and degenerative changes, such as myofibril loss, causing hydropic changes within the myocardial cells. An increase in interstitial and endocardial fibrillar collagen is a constant feature in HIV-associated cardiomyopathy [8, 9].

Myocarditis

Myocarditis is still the best-studied cause of dilated cardiomyopathy in HIV disease. According to the author's clinical and pathologic experience, HIV-associated myocarditis may be defined as "a process characterized by a lymphocytic infiltrate of the myocardium with necrosis and/or degeneration of adjacent myocytes not typical of the ischemic damage associated with coronary artery disease in subjects infected by HIV with or without evidence of opportunistic infective agents" [10]. Myocarditis has been documented at autopsy in 40–52% of patients who died of AIDS before the introduction of HAART [8]. In the Gruppo Italiano per lo Studio Cardiologico dei pazienti affetti da AIDS (GISCA) autopsy series histological diagnosis of myocarditis was made in 30 of 82 patients (37%) with cardiac involvement [8]. Of 20 autopsy patients with dilated cardiomyopathy, 10 (83%) had active myocarditis at histological examination of myocardial tissue specimens [8].

Histological findings in HIV-infected patients with myocarditis do not substantially differ from those observed in HIV-uninfected patients. Lymphocytes, along with fewer macrophages, are distributed diffusely as single cells or in small clusters. Autopsy studies of AIDS patients dead of acute left ventricular dysfunction almost invariably show a marked inflammatory infiltrate [8]. However, mild and focal mononuclear infiltrates are frequently observed in hearts of AIDS patients, irrespective of the presence of cardiac symptoms [8]. The intracardiac conduction system is sometimes affected in AIDS patients, generally as a complication of myocarditis. Primary involvement of the conduction system is possible as a consequence of opportunistic infections, drug cardiotoxicity, or primary location of HIV-1 in the specific conduction tissue [8]. Histological examination of myocardium specimens at autopsy may show mononuclear infiltration of the intracardiac conduction tissue, which is frequently associated with vasculitis and fragmentation of the bundles with lobulation and fibrosis. These findings are generally associated with electrocardiographic conduction abnormalities (e.g., left anterior hemiblock, left bundle branch block, and first-degree atrioventricular block) [8]. In the GISCA autopsy series 5/12 patients (42%) with cardiomyopathy also had intracardiac conduction system alterations on histological examination. Two of them had lymphocytic infiltration of the conduction tissue as complication of active myocarditis, and the remaining three had fragmentation and fibromatous degeneration of the left bundle [8].

Nonviral myocarditis

The most common opportunistic infectious agent associated with myocarditis in AIDS is *Toxoplasma gondii*, observed as often as 12% in one autopsy series with deaths from AIDS between 1987 and 1991 [11]. There may be regional differences in the incidence of *Toxoplasma gondii* myocarditis, perhaps because the natural reservoir of organisms persists more easily in humid environments. Elevation of myocardial fraction of creatine kinase may commonly occur with myocardial toxoplasmosis. *Toxoplasma gondii* organisms can produce a gross pattern of patchy irregular white infiltrates in myocardium similar to non-Hodgkin's lymphoma. Microscopically, the myocardium shows scattered mixed inflammatory cell infiltrates with polymorphonuclear leukocytes, macrophages, and lymphocytes. *Toxoplasma gondii* can produce quite variable inflammation along with myocardial fiber necrosis. The three microscopic patterns of involvement by *Toxoplasma gondii* include acute diffuse myocarditis, focal myocarditis, and presence of organisms without significant inflammation or necrosis [9, 11]. In *Toxoplasma* myocarditis, true *Toxoplasma gondii* extracellular cysts, or pseudocysts within myocardial fibers, both of which contain the small 2-μ-sized bradyzoites, are often hard to find, even if inflammation is extensive. Immunohistochemical staining may reveal free tachyzoites, the organisms that are found outside of cysts. Otherwise, it is difficult with routine hematoxylin and eosin staining to distinguish these free tachyzoites from fragments of inflammatory cells or myocytes that have undergone necrosis within the areas of inflammation [9, 11].

Fungal opportunistic infections of the heart occur infrequently in HIV-infected patients. They are often incidental findings at autopsy, and cardiac involvement is probably the result of widespread dissemination, as exemplified by *Candida* sp. and by the fungi *Cryptococcus neoformans,Coccidioides immitis*, or *Histoplasma capsulatum* [8, 9, 11]. Fungal lesions are characterized grossly by the appearance of multiple small rounded white plaques. They may have a hemorrhagic border, particularly lesions caused by *Aspergillus* that can be angioinvasive. Microscopically, fungal lesions have variable inflammatory infiltrates and necrosis, and a specific diagnosis is made by identifying yeast forms or hyphae of specific organisms, aided by standard histological stains such as Gomori methenamine silver or periodic acid Schiff [8, 9, 11]. The near absence of an inflammatory infiltrate accompanying fungal organisms is a manifestation of immune system failure with progression of AIDS to a late stage when opportunistic infections are more likely to be widely disseminated to organs such as the heart [8, 9, 11].

Patients living in endemic areas for *Trypanosoma cruzi* may rarely develop a pronounced myocarditis [12, 13]. *Mycobacterium avium-complex* infection can be widely disseminated and involve the heart with microscopic lesions characterized by clusters of large macrophages filled with numerous acid-fast rod-shaped organisms [8, 9, 11].

Pneumocystis carinii can involve the heart in cases with widespread dissemination of this organism [11]. Grossly, the epicardium and cut surfaces of the myocardium may have a sandpaper-like quality due to the presence of multiple pinpoint foci of calcification. Microscopically, this calcification is not accompanied by significant inflammatory cell infiltrates, but there may be deposits of amorphous granular pink exudate similar to that seen in alveoli with *Pneumocystis carinii* pneumonia [9, 11]. The cysts may be difficult to recognize, even with Gomori methenamine silver stain, and diagnosis is aided by immunohistochemical staining [9, 11].

Viral myocarditis

Histology and immunohistochemistry rarely detect the presence of viruses in the myocardium [8]. However, in situ hybridization or polymerase chain reaction studies reveal a high frequency of either cytomegalovirus or HIV-1 or both, in AIDS patients with lymphocytic myocarditis and severe left ventricular dysfunction [8, 14]. These data support the hypothesis that, at least in a subset of patients, HIV-1 has a pathogenetic action and possibly influences the clinical evolution toward dilated cardiomyopathy.

Herskowitz *et al.* detected a positive hybridization signal for HIV-1 in endomyocardial biopsy specimens from 15 of 37 patients (40%) with left ventricular dysfunction. Histological and immuno-histological techniques documented that most of these patients had myocarditis [14]. HIV-1 nucleic acid sequences were detected at autopsy by in situ DNA hybridization in 35% of the GISCA patients with cardiac involvement; 86% of them had active myocarditis at histological examination. Among patients with myocarditis, coinfection with coxsackievirus B3 was documented in 32%, with Epstein-Barr virus in 8%, and with cytomegalovirus in 4% [8]. In autopsy biopsy samples, myocytes with a positive hybridization signal were sparse, usually only one to four cells per section [8]. Although about 70% of patients with positive hybridization signals had active myocarditis at histological examination, most myocytes with positive hybridization signal were not surrounded by inflammatory cells [8]. In the GISCA autopsy series, HIV-1 was documented by in situ hybridization in 83% of patients with myocarditis [8].

Coinfection with other viruses seems to have an important etiopathogenetic role. The GISCA autopsy records show that 83% of patients with myocarditis and 50% of those with dilated cardiomyopathy were coinfected with cardiotropic viruses (usually, coxsackievirus B3 and cytomegalovirus) [8]. Herskowitz *et al.* used in situ hybridization to detect myocardial cytomegalovirus infection in 48% of HIV-infected patients with myocarditis and left ventricular dysfunction who underwent endomyocardial biopsy [14]. Bowles *et al.* used polymerase chain reaction and found that 42% of HIV-infected patients with cardiomyopathy had cytomegalovirus or adenovirus in the myocardial tissue [15]. Some patients with adenovirus coinfection had congestive heart failure but not myocarditis, suggesting that the virus may be virulent without associated inflammatory response [15].

Myocardial cytokine expression

Myocardial dendritic cells may play a role in the interaction between HIV-1 and the cardiac myocyte and in the activation of cytotoxic cytokines [16]. It has been demonstrated that HIV-1 invades the myocardium through endothelial cells by micropinocytosis and infects perivascular macrophages, which produce additional virus and cytokines, such as tumor necrosis factor-(TNF) alpha [17]. The virus produces cardiomyocyte apoptosis either by signaling through CCR3, CCR5 or CXCR4, by entry into cardiomyocytes (after binding to ganglioside GM1), or through TNF-alpha [17, 18]. It is also possible that HIV-1-associated protein gp 120 (envelope glycoprotein) may induce myocyte apoptosis through a mitochondrion-controlled pathway by activation of inflammatory cytokines (e.g., TNF-alpha) [18].

In HIV infection, dendritic cells can initiate the primary immunologic response and present the antigen to T-lymphocytes. The interaction between dendritic cells and T-lymphocytes, particularly CD8 cells, could promote a local elevation in the multifunctional cytokine TNF-alpha, which can also be produced and secreted by infected macrophages [17]. TNF-alpha produces a negative inotropic effect by altering intracellular calcium homeostasis, possibly by inducing nitric oxide (NO) synthesis, which also reduces myocyte contractility. Kan et al. demonstrated that HIV gp120 enhances NO production by cardiac myocytes through p38 MAP kinase-mediated NK-kB activation [19]. Myocarditis and dilated cardiomyopathy are associated with markedly elevated cytokine production, but the elevations may be highly localized within the myocardium, making peripheral cytokine levels uninformative [16]. When myocardial biopsies from patients with HIV-associated cardiomyopathy are compared to samples from patients with idiopathic dilated cardiomyopathy, the former stain more intensely for both TNF-alpha and inducible nitric oxide synthase (iNOS). Staining is particularly intense in samples from patients with a myocardial viral infection and correlates with CD4 count, independently of antiretroviral treatment [16]. Staining is also more intense in samples from patients with HIV-associated cardiomyopathy coinfected with coxsackievirus B3, cytomegalovirus, Epstein-Barr virus or adenovirus [16]. Moreover, staining for iNOS is more intense in samples from patients coinfected with HIV-1 and coxsackievirus B3 or cytomegalovirus than in samples from patients with idiopathic dilated cardiomyopathy and myocardial infection with coxsackievirus B3 or who had adenovirus infection alone [16]. In patients with HIV-associated dilated cardiomyopathy and more intense iNOS staining, the survival rate was significantly lower: those whose samples stained more than 1 optical density unit had a hazard ratio of mortality of 2.57 [16]. Survival in HIV-infected patients with less intense staining was not significantly different from survival in patients with idiopathic dilated cardiomyopathy [16].

HIV-infected patients with encephalopathy are more likely to die of congestive heart failure than are those without encephalopathy (hazard ratio: 3.4) [20, 21]. Cardiomyopathy and encephalopathy may both be traceable to the effects of HIV-1 reservoir cells in the myocardium and the cerebral cortex [22]. These cells may hold HIV-1 on their surfaces for extended time periods even after antiretroviral treatment, and they may chronically release cytotoxic cytokines (TNF-alpha, interleukin-1, interleukin-6, interleukin-10), which contribute to progressive and late tissue damage in both systems [22]. Since the reservoir cells are not affected by treatment, the effect is independent of whether the patients receive HAART.

Autoimmunity as a contributor to HIV-associated cardiomyopathy

Cardiac-specific autoantibodies (anti-alpha-myosin autoantibodies) are more common in HIV-infected patients with dilated cardiomyopathy than in HIV-infected patients with healthy hearts. Currie et al. reported that HIV-infected patients were more likely to have specific cardiac autoantibodies than were HIV-uninfected controls [23]. Those with echocardiographic evidence of left ventricular dysfunction were particularly likely to have cardiac autoantibodies, supporting the theory that cardiac autoimmunity plays a role in the pathogenesis of HIV-associated cardiomyopathy and suggesting that cardiac autoantibodies could be used as markers of left ventricular dysfunction in HIV-infected patients with previously normal echocardiographic findings [23]. In addition, monthly intravenous immunoglobulin in

HIV-infected pediatric patients minimizes left ventricular dysfunction, increases left ventricular wall thickness, and reduces peak left ventricular wall stress, suggesting that both impaired myocardial growth and left ventricular dysfunction may be immunologically mediated [24]. These effects may be the result of immunoglobulins inhibiting cardiac autoantibodies by competing for Fc receptors, or they could be the result of immunoglobulins dampening the secretion or effects of cytokines and cellular growth factors [24]. These findings suggest that immunomodulatory therapy might be helpful in HIV-infected patients with declining left ventricular function, although further study of this possible therapy is needed.

Nutritional deficiencies as a factor in left ventricular dysfunction

Nutritional deficiencies are common in HIV infection and may contribute to ventricular dysfunction independently of HAART. Malabsorption and diarrhea can both lead to trace element deficiencies which have been directly or indirectly associated with cardiomyopathy [25, 26]. Selenium, as a component of glutathione peroxidase, is involved in the antioxidant response in cells and tissues. Selenium deficiency is associated with congestive cardiomyopathy and skeletal-muscle disorders. Furthermore, low levels of selenium or other micronutrients may be responsible for the cardiotoxic effects of coxsackievirus B3 and for the ability of these viruses to enhance the toxic effects of zidovudine on skeletal muscle [27]; both findings may be relevant to selenium-related ventricular dysfunction [26, 27]. Selenium replacement may reverse cardiomyopathy and restore left ventricular function in selenium-deficient patients [25, 26, 28]. HIV infection may also be associated with altered levels of vitamin B_{12}, carnitine, growth hormone, and thyroid hormone, all of which have been associated with left ventricular dysfunction [25, 26].

Autonomic dysfunction as a factor in left ventricular dysfunction

There is the evidence that an altered autonomic function is present in HIV-infected patients [29, 30]. In a previous study, autonomic dysfunction in HIV-infected patients was assessed by a significant decrease of the corrected coefficients of electro-cardiographic R–R interval variation (CVc) compared to healthy controls [31]. CVc correlated significantly with CD4 count and with the values of hepatic, plasmatic, lymphocyte, and erythrocyte concentrations of reduced glutathione and with erythrocyte malonyldialdehyde levels as expression of increased lipoperoxidation [31]. This correlation was more evident in patients coinfected with hepatitis C virus (HCV) where the lipoperoxidation process and the production of free radicals of the oxygen are enhanced by the inflammatory process induced by HIV/HCV coinfection [31]. According to this study, the autonomic dysfunction in HIV-infected patients may be expression of a reduced response to the oxidative stress related to HIV infection because of a systemic depletion of reduced glutathione associated with the state of immunodeficiency [31].

Left ventricular asynergy may develop due to regional differences in the distribution of cardiac sympathetic nerve endings, even in the context of acute myocarditis. In fact, an alteration of catecholamine dynamics (or autonomic function) has been associated with a transient extensive akinesis of the apical and mid portions of the left ventricle with hypercontraction of the basal segment (*takotsubo*-like dysfunction) in an HIV-infected patient with cytomegalovirus myocarditis [32].

Left ventricular dysfunction caused by drug cardiotoxicity

Studies of transgenic mice suggest that zidovudine is associated with diffuse destruction of cardiac mitochondrial ultrastructure and inhibition of mitochondrial DNA replication [33, 34]. This mitochondrial dysfunction may result in lactic acidosis, which could also contribute to myocardial cell dysfunction. However, in a study of infants born to HIV-infected mothers followed from birth to age 5, perinatal exposure to zidovudine was not found to be associated with acute or chronic abnormalities in left ventricular structure or function [35]. Other nucleoside reverse transcriptase inhibitors, such as didanosine, zalcitabine, or lamivudine, do not seem to either promote or prevent dilated cardiomyopathy. In AIDS patients with Kaposi's sarcoma, reversible cardiac dysfunction was associated with prolonged, high-dose therapy with interferon alpha [36]. High-dose interferon alpha treatment is not associated with myocardial dysfunction in other patient populations, so it has been proposed that it may have a synergistic effect with HIV-1 infection [36]. Doxorubicin (adriamycin), which is used to treat AIDS-associated Kaposi's sarcoma and non-Hodgkin's lymphoma, has a dose-related effect on dilated cardiomyopathy [37], as does foscarnet sodium when used to treat cytomegalovirus esophagitis [38]. The principal cardiovascular actions/interactions of common HIV therapies are reported in Table 14.1.

HIV infection, opportunistic infections, and vascular disease

Endothelial dysfunction

Endothelial dysfunction and injury have been described in HIV infection [39]. Circulating markers of endothelial activation, such as soluble adhesion molecules and procoagulant proteins, are elaborated in HIV infection. HIV-1 may enter endothelium via CD4 or galactosyl-ceramide receptors [39]. Other possible mechanisms of entry include chemokine receptors [40]. Endothelium isolated from the brain of HIV-infected subjects strongly expresses both CCR3 and CXCR4 HIV-1 coreceptors, whereas coronary endothelium strongly expresses CXCR4 and CCR2A coreceptors [40]. CCR5 is expressed at a lower level in both types of endothelium [40]. The fact that CCR3 is more common in brain endothelium than in coronary endothelium could be significant in light of the different susceptibilities of heart and brain to HIV-1 invasion. Endothelial activation in HIV-1 infection may also be caused by cytokines (e.g., TNF-alpha) secreted in response to mononuclear or adventitial cell activation by the virus, or may be a direct effect of the secreted HIV-1-associated proteins gp 120 and tat (transactivator of viral replication) on endothelium with possible induction of apoptosis process [18]. Opportunistic agents, such as cytomegalovirus, as well as human herpes virus-8 (a virus that is involved in the development of AIDS-associated Kaposi's sarcoma), frequently co-infect HIV-infected patients and may contribute to the development of endothelial damage. In spite of all these observations, the clinical consequences of HIV-1 and opportunistic agents on endothelial function has not been elucidated yet.

Vasculitis

A wide range of inflammatory vascular diseases including polyarteritis nodosa, Henoch–Schonlein purpura, and drug-induced hypersensitivity vasculitis may develop in HIV-infected individuals. Kawasaki-like syndrome [41, 42] and Takayasu's arteritis [43] have also been described. The course of vascular disease may be accelerated in HIV-infected patients because of atherogenesis stimulated by HIV-infected monocyte-macrophages, possibly via altered leukocyte adhesion or arteritis [42, 44].

The incidence of vasculitis (excluding adverse drug reactions) in HIV infection is estimated to be about 1% [42, 44]. Some HIV-infected patients have a clinical presentation resembling systemic lupus erythematosus including vasculitis, arthralgias, myalgias, and autoimmune phenomena with a low titer positive antinuclear antibody, coagulopathy with lupus anticoagulant, hemolytic anemia, and thrombocytopenic purpura [42, 44]. Hypergammaglobulinemia from polyclonal B-cell activation may be present, but often diminishes in the late stages of AIDS. Specific autoantibodies to double-stranded DNA, Sm antigen, RNP antigen, SSA, SSB, and other histones may be found in a majority of HIV-infected persons, but their significance is unclear [42, 44].

HIV infection and coronary arteries

The association between viral infection (cytomegalovirus or HIV-1 itself) and coronary artery lesions is not clear. HIV-1 sequences have been detected by in situ hybridization in the coronary vessels of an HIV-infected patient who died from acute myocardial infarction [45]. Potential mechanisms through which HIV-1 may damage coronary arteries include activation of cytokines and cell-adhesion molecules and alteration of major-histocompatibility-complex class I molecules on the surface of smooth-muscle cells [45]. It is possible also that HIV-1-associated protein gp 120 may induce smooth-muscle cell apoptosis through a mitochondrion-controlled pathway by activation of inflammatory cytokines [18].

Pericardial effusion

The prevalence of pericardial effusion in asymptomatic HIV-infected patients has been estimated

Table 14.1 Cardiovascular actions/interactions of common HIV therapies [1].

Class	Drugs	Cardiac drug interactions	Cardiac side effects
Antiretroviral			
(A) Nucleoside reverse transcriptase inhibitors (RTI)	Abacavir (Ziagen), zidovudine (AZT, Retrovir)	Dipyridamole	Lactic acidosis (rare), hypotension, skeletal muscle myopathy, (mitochondrial dysfunction hypothesized, but not seen clinically)
(B) Nucleotide RTI	Tenofovir (Viread)		
(C) Non-nucleoside RTI	Delavirdine (Rescriptor), Efavirenz (Sustiva), Nevirapine (Viramune)	Warfarin (class interaction), calcium channel blockers, beta-blockers, quinidine, steroids, theophylline	Delavirdine can cause serious toxic effects if given with antiarrhythmic drugs and myocardial ischemia if given with vasoconstrictors
(D) Protease inhibitors	Amprenavir (Agenerase), indinavir (Crixivan), nelfinavir (Viracept), ritonavir (Norvir), saquinavir (Invirase, Fortovase), Atazanavir (Reyataz)	All are metabolized by cytochrome p-450 and interact with: sildenafil, amiodarone, lidocaine, quinadine, warfarin, statins. Calcium channel blockers, beta-blockers (1.5–3× increase), prednisone, quinine, theophylline (decrease concentrations)	Implicated in premature atherosclerosis, dyslipidemia, insulin resistance, and lipodystrophy/lipoatrophy
Anti-infective			
(A) Antibiotics	Erythromycin, clarithromycin	Cytochrome p-450 metabolism and drug interactions	Orthostatic hypotension, ventricular tachycardia, bradycardia, QT prolongation
	Rifampicin	Reduces therapeutic effect of digoxin by induction of intestinal P-glycoprotein	Orthostatic hypotension, QT prolongation
	Trimethoprim/ sulfamethoxazole (Bactrim)	Increases warfarin effects	
(B) Antifungal agents	Amphotericin B	Digoxin toxicity	Hypertension, renal failure, hypokalemia, thrombophlebitis, angioedema, dilated cardiomyopathy, arrhythmias
	Ketoconazole, itraconazole	Cytochrome p-450 metabolism and drug interactions—increases levels of sildenafil, warfarin, "statins," nifedipine, digoxin	
(C) Antiviral agents	Foscarnet, Ganciclovir	Zidovudine	Reversible cardiac failure (dose-related effect), electrolyte abnormalities, ventricular tachycardia (QT prolongation), hypotension

(Continued)

Table 14.1 (Continued)

Class	Drugs	Cardiac drug interactions	Cardiac side effects
(D) Antiparasitic	Pentamidine (intravenous)		Hypotension, arrhythmias (Torsade de pointes, ventricular tachycardia), hyperglycemia, hypoglycemia, sudden death. *Note:* Contraindicated if baseline QTc > 0.48
Chemotherapy agents	Vincristine, doxorubicin (Adriamycin)	Decrease digoxin level	Arrhythmias, myocardial infarction, dilated cardiomyopathy (dose-related effect), autonomic neuropathy
	Recombinant interferon-alpha		Hypertension, hypotension, dilated cardiomyopathy, ventricular and supraventricular arrhythmias, atrioventricular block
	Interleukin-2		Hypotension, arrhythmias, myocardial infarction, cardiac failure, capillary leak, thyroid alterations

at 11% before the introduction of HAART [46]. According to some retrospective data, the prevalence of pericardial effusion in HIV-infected patients is reduced by about 30–35% after the introduction of HAART, with a trend similar to that observed for HIV-associated cardiomyopathy [6, 7]. HIV infection should be included in the differential diagnosis of unexplained pericardial effusion or tamponade. Pericardial effusion in HIV disease may be related to opportunistic infections (e.g., *Mycobacterium tuberculosis*, *Mycobacterium avium-complex* infection) or to malignancy (e.g., non-Hodgkin lymphoma), but most often a clear etiology is not found. The effusion may be part of a generalized serous effusive process also involving pleural and peritoneal surfaces. This "*capillary leak*" syndrome is likely related to enhanced cytokine expression (e.g., TNF-alpha) in the later stages of HIV disease and correlates with the immunodeficiency state of the patient [46, 47].

Endocarditis

The prevalence of infective endocarditis did not vary in HIV-infected patients who use intravenous drugs after the introduction of HAART even in the developed countries, being similar to that observed in HIV-uninfected intravenous drug addicts [5]. Estimates of infective endocarditis prevalence vary

from 6.3% to 34% of HIV-infected patients who use intravenous drugs independently of HAART [8]. Among intravenous drug addicts, the tricuspid valve is most frequently affected and the most frequent agents are *Staphylococcus aureus* (>75% of cases), *Streptococcus pneumoniae*, *Haemophilus influenzae*, *Candida albicans*, *Aspergillus fumigatus*, and *Cryptococcus neoformans* [8]. Avirulent bacteria, as the HACEK group (*Haemophilus* species, *Actinobacillus actinomycetemcomitans*, *Cardiobacterium hominis*, *Eikenella corrodens*, and *Kingella kingae*), which are often part of the endogenous flora of the mouth, can cause endocarditis in HIV-infected patients [9]. Vegetations may form on the tricuspid or pulmonary valves with resultant pulmonary embolism and consequent septic pulmonary infarcts which appear as multiple opacities on chest radiograms. Systemic emboli often involve coronary arteries, spleen, bowel, extremities, and central nervous system. Cardiac rhythm alterations (i.e, atrioventricular block) may suggest the presence of an abscess in proximity to the atrioventricular node. Peripheral pulses should be examined for signs of embolic occlusion or pulsating mass suggesting mycotic aneurysm. Mycotic aneurysms may occur in the intracranial arteries potentially leading to intracranial hemorrhage [48]. Patients with HIV infection generally have similar presentations and survival (85% versus 93%) from infective endocarditis as those without HIV. However, patients with late-stage HIV disease have about 30% higher mortality with endocarditis than asymptomatic HIV-infected patients, which may be related to the degree of immunodeficiency [49]. Nonbacterial thrombotic endocarditis, also known as marantic endocarditis, had a prevalence of 3–5% in AIDS patients, mostly in patients with HIV-wasting syndrome, before the introduction of HAART [8]. Friable endocardial vegetations, affecting predominantly the left-sided valves, consisting of platelets within a fibrin mesh with few inflammatory cells characterize it. Marantic endocarditis is now more frequently observed in developing countries with a high incidence (about 10–15%) and mortality for systemic embolization [4].

HIV-associated pulmonary hypertension

The incidence of HIV-associated pulmonary hypertension has been estimated in 1/200, much higher than 1/200,000 found in the general population and it increased after the introduction of HAART [50, 51]. The histopathology of HIV-associated pulmonary hypertension is similar to that of primary pulmonary hypertension. The most common alteration in HIV-associated pulmonary hypertension is the plexogenic pulmonary arteriopathy, while thrombotic pulmonary arteriopathy and pulmonary veno-occlusive disease are more rare histologic findings [50, 51]. This observation may suggest that similar etiopathogenetic mechanisms are at the basis of both HIV-associated pulmonary hypertension and primary pulmonary hypertension. A key pathogenetic role is played by pulmonary dendritic cells which are not sensitive to HAART and may hold HIV-1 on their surfaces for extended time periods [50, 51]. The infection of these cells by HIV-1 causes a chronic release of cytotoxic cytokines (e.g., endothelin-1, interleukin-6, interleukin-1 beta, and TNF-alpha) contributing to vascular plexogenic lesions and progressive tissue damage, independently of opportunistic infections, stage of HIV disease, and HAART regimens [50, 51]. Activation of alpha-1 receptors and genetic factors (increased frequency of HLA-DR6 and DR52) have also been hypothesized in the pathogenesis of HIV-associated pulmonary hypertension [50, 51].

Cardiac involvement in AIDS-associated neoplasms

The prevalence of cardiac Kaposi's sarcoma in AIDS patients ranges from 12% to 28% in retrospective autopsy studies performed in the pre-HAART era [8]. Cardiac involvement with Kaposi's sarcoma usually occurs when widespread visceral organ involvement is present. The lesions are typically less than 1 cm in size and may be pericardial or, less frequently, myocardial, and are only rarely associated with obstruction, dysfunction, morbidity, or mortality. Microscopically, there are atypical spindle cells lining slit-like vascular spaces [8]. Non-Hodgkin lymphoma involving the heart is infrequent in AIDS [8]. Most are high-grade B-cell (small non-cleaved) Burkitt-like lymphomas, with the rest classified as diffuse large B cell lymphomas (in the REAL classification). Lymphomatous lesions may appear grossly as either discreet localized or more diffuse nodular to polypoid masses [8, 52, 54]. Most involve the pericardium with variable myocardial infiltration [8, 52, 54]. There is little or no accompanying inflammation and necrosis. The prognosis of patients with HIV-associated cardiac lymphoma is generally poor because of widespread organ involvement, although some patients treated with combination chemotherapy have experienced clinical remission [55]. The introduction of HAART led to a reduction by about 50% in the overall incidence of cardiac involvement by Kaposi's sarcoma and non-Hodgkin lymphomas. The fall may be attributable to the improved immunologic state of the patients and the prevention of opportunistic infections (human herpes virus-8 and Epstein-Barr virus) known to play an etiologic role in these neoplasms. On the contrary, an increased prevalence of cardiac involvement of AIDS-associated tumors may be observed in developing countries in relation to the scanty availability of HAART [4].

HAART-associated lipodystrophy and metabolic syndrome

The introduction of HAART has significantly modified the course of HIV disease, with longer survival and improved quality of life in HIV-infected subjects. However, HAART regimens, especially those including protease inhibitors (PI) have shown to cause in a high proportion of HIV-infected patients somatic (lipodystrophy/lipoatrophy) and metabolic (dyslipidemia, insulin-resistance) changes that in the general population are associated with an increased risk of cardiovascular disease, producing an intriguing clinical scenery.

HIV-associated lipodystrophy or lipoatrophy, unreported before the introduction of HAART, was first described in 1998 [56]. It is characterized by the presence of a dorsocervical fat pad (also known as *buffalo hump*), increased abdominal girth and breast size, lipoatrophy of subcutaneous fat of the face, buttocks and limbs, and prominence of veins on the limbs. The overall prevalence of at least one physical abnormality is thought to be about 50% in otherwise healthy HIV-infected patients receiving HAART, although reported rates range from 18% to 83% [57, 58]. Differences in rates might be influenced by age, sex, the type and duration of antiretroviral therapy, and the lack of an objective and validated case definition [57, 58]. As in genetic lipodystrophy syndromes [59], fat redistribution may precede the development of metabolic complications in HIV-infected patients receiving HAART. Among HIV-infected patients with lipodystrophy, increased serum total and low-density lipoprotein cholesterol and triglyceride levels have been observed in about 70%, whereas insulin resistance (elevated C-peptide and insulin) and type 2 diabetes mellitus have been observed in 8% to 10% [57, 58]. The severity of these metabolic abnormalities increases with increasing severity of lipodystrophy, and they are associated with a raised risk of cardiovascular events: approximately 1.4 cardiac events per 1000 years of therapy according to the Framingham score [58].

The pathogenesis of HAART-associated lipodystrophy and metabolic syndrome is complex and a number of factors are involved, including direct effects of HAART on lipid metabolism, endothelial and adipocyte cell function, and mitochondria [3] (Figure 14.1).

Molecular mechanisms

PI-associated lipodystrophy and metabolic alterations

PI target the catalytic region of HIV-1 protease. This region is homologous with regions of two human proteins that regulate lipid metabolism: cytoplasmic retinoic-acid binding protein-1 (CRABP-1) and low-density lipoprotein-receptor-related protein (LRP) [56, 60]. It has been hypothesized, although without strong experimental support, that this homology may allow PI to interfere with these proteins, which may be the cause of the metabolic and somatic alterations that develop in PI-treated patients [56, 60]. The hypothesis is that PI inhibit CRABP-1-modified and cytochrome P450-3A-mediated synthesis of cis-9-retinoic acid and peroxisome proliferator-activated receptor type-gamma heterodimer. The inhibition increases the rate of apoptosis of adipocytes and reduces the rate at which pre-adipocytes differentiate into adipocytes, with the final effect of reducing triglyceride storage and increasing lipid release. PI-binding to LRP would impair hepatic chylomicron uptake and endothelial triglyceride clearance, resulting in hyperlipidemia and insulin resistance [56, 60].

Ultrastructural analysis of adipocytes in PI-induced lipodystrophy reveals changes including disruption of cell membranes, fragmented cytoplasmic rims, irregular cell outlines, and eventually fat droplets laying free in the connective tissue, with macrophages around them. Many adipocytes show variable compartmentalization of fat droplets with decrease in cell size and abundant, mitochondria-rich cytoplasm. These findings suggest that HAART-associated lipodystrophy may be the result of adipocyte remodeling involving variable combinations of apoptosis, defective lipogenesis, and increased metabolic activity in different adipose areas of the body [60].

Some data indicate that PI-associated dyslipidemia may be caused, at least in part, either by PI-mediated inhibition of proteasome activity and accumulation of the active portion of sterol regulatory element-binding protein (SREBP)-1c in liver cells and adipocytes [61], or by apo-CIII polymorphisms in HIV-infected patients [62]. Bonnet *et al.* have described a two to threefold increase in apo-E and apo C-III, essentially recovered as associated to apo-B-containing lipoparticles [63]. In this study, multivariate analysis revealed that, among the investigated parameters, apo C-III was the only parameter strongly associated with the occurrence of lipodystrophy [63]. Sequence homologies have been described between HIV-1 protease and human

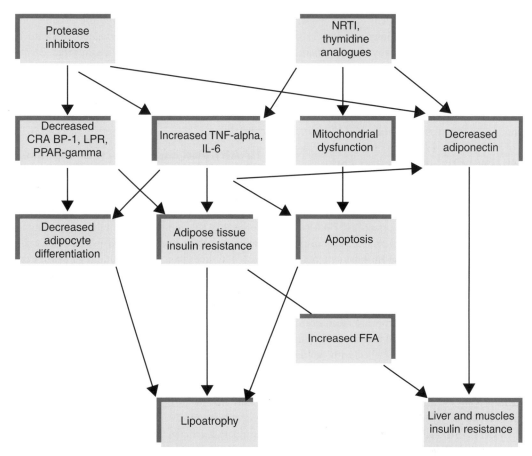

Figure 14.1 A hypothetical scheme of the mechanisms responsible for lipodystrophy and insulin resistance in HAART-associated metabolic syndrome [3]. Protease inhibitors are responsible for a decrease in cytoplasmic retinoic-acid binding protein 1 (CRABP-1) in low-density lipoprotein-receptor-related protein (LPR) and in peroxisome proliferator activated receptor-type gamma (PPAR-gamma). Nucleoside reverse transcriptase inhibitors (NRTI), and thymidine analogues, are responsible for mitochondrial dysfunction as demonstrated by a decrease in subcutaneous adipose tissue mitochondrial DNA content. Both phenomena are responsible for a decreased differentiation of adipocytes, increased levels of free fatty acids (FFA) and lipoatrophy. The increased levels of inflammatory cytokines, such as tumor necrosis factor-alpha (TNF-alpha) and interleukin-6 (IL-6) may further contribute in development of lipodystrophy. TNF-alpha activates 11-beta-hydroxysteroid dehydrogenase type-1, which converts inactive cortisone to active cortisol, resulting in increased lipid accumulation in adipocytes and insulin resistance. HAART drugs and inflammatory cytokines are associated with a decrease in adiponectin. The levels of adiponectin and adiponectin-to-leptin ratio correlate positively with insulin resistance in HIV-infected patients with HAART-associated metabolic syndrome.

site-1 protease (S1P), which activates SREBP-1c and SREBP-2 pathways. A polymorphism in the S1P/SREBP-1c gene confers a difference in risk for development of an increase in total cholesterol with PI-therapy. This suggests the presence of a genetic predisposition to hyperlipoproteinemia in PI-treated patients [64]. There is also evidence that PI directly inhibit the uptake of glucose in insulin-sensitive tissues, such as fat and skeletal muscle, by selectively inhibiting the glucose transporter Glut4 [65].

TNF-alpha and lipodystrophy

The relationship between the degree of insulin resistance and levels of soluble type-2-TNF-alpha receptor suggests that an inflammatory stimulus may contribute to the development of HIV-associated lipodystrophy [66]. TNF-alpha activates 11-beta-hydroxysteroid dehydrogenase type-1, which converts inactive cortisone to active cortisol. The activity of this enzyme is higher in visceral fat compared to subcutaneous fat. Visceral fat is able to locally produce cortisol which could act inside adipocytes and increase lipid accumulation [67].

Mitochondrial dysfunction and lipodystrophy

There is evidence for nucleoside-induced mitochondrial dysfunction in HIV-infected patients treated with nucleoside-containing HAART because lipodystrophy with peripheral fat wasting is associated with a decrease in subcutaneous adipose tissue mitochondrial DNA content [68]. Disrupted pools of nucleotide precursors and inhibition of DNA pol-gamma by specific nucleoside reverse transcriptase inhibitors are mechanistically important in mitochondrial toxicity [69]. This effect has been especially described with the use of stavudine and was correlated with the length of exposure to this drug [70]. HAART regimens with didanosine plus stavudine are more likely to produce a greater increase in serum lactate and lipodystrophy than therapies based on zidovudine plus lamivudine within the first year of therapy [68]. Substitution of stavudine with abacavir or zidovudine improves mitochondrial indices and fat apoptosis in the setting of lipoatrophy [71].

Adipocytokines and lipodystrophy

Adipocytes secrete a range of adipocytokines which control insulin sensitivity [72]. There is evidence that an adipocytokine, adiponectin, a protein product of the apM1 gene, which is expressed exclusively in adipocytes, plays a role in development of HIV-associated lipodystrophy as well as in congenital and acquired lipodystrophies in non-HIV infected subjects [73]. In vitro and animal studies and cross-sectional studies in humans have shown that adiponectin is inversely correlated with features of HAART-associated metabolic syndrome. This syndrome has recently been linked to a quantitative trait locus on chromosome 3q27, the location of the apM1 gene [72, 74, 75]. These studies have shown

that both adiponectin levels and the adiponectin-to-leptin ratio are positively correlated with features of HAART-associated metabolic syndrome [72, 74, 75]. According to these studies, this ratio could be used to predict insulin sensitivity and potential cardiovascular risk in HIV-infected patients receiving HAART.

HAART and cardiovascular disease

HAART-associated endothelial dysfunction

In vitro data reported by Fiala *et al.* suggest that some HAART regimens, such as those including zidovudine, some non-nucleoside reverse transcriptase inhibitors (e.g., efavirenz) and PI disrupt endothelial cell junctions and cytoskeleton actin of the endothelial cells leading to endothelial dysfunction [76]. These findings are in agreement with those previously reported in vivo by Stein *et al.* [77] and in vitro by Zhong *et al.* [78]. In particular, Zhong *et al.* demonstrated that ritonavir at concentrations near clinical plasma levels is able to directly cause endothelial mitochondrial DNA damage and cell death mainly through necrosis pathway but not through apoptosis [78]. Chai *et al.* investigated and compared the effects of PI on isolated porcine arteries and observed a reduced endothelial NO synthase expression and increased levels of superoxide anion as expression of increased endothelial oxidative stress [79]. The HIV-1 entry inhibitor TAK-799 is an antagonist for the chemokine receptors CCR5 and CXCR3, which are expressed on leucocytes, especially T-helper-1 cells, and these receptors may be involved in recruitment of these cells to atherosclerotic vascular lesions [80]. In low-density lipoprotein receptor-deficient mice treated with TAK-799, the number of T cells in the atherosclerotic plaque was reduced by 95%, concurrently with a 98% reduction in the relative interferon-gamma area [80]. According to this study, TAK-779 not only suppresses HIV-1 entry via blockade of CCR5 but also attenuates atherosclerotic lesion formation by blocking the influx of T-helper-1 in the atherosclerotic plaque [80]. Since TAK-799 impairs atherogenesis, treatment with TAK-799 could beneficial for young HIV-infected patients facing lifelong HAART regimens.

HAART-associated vasculitis

Drug-induced hypersensitivity vasculitis is common in HIV-infected patients receiving HAART [42, 44]. The vasculitis associated with drug reactions typically involves small vessels and has a lymphocytic or leukocytoclastic histopathology. The pathologic mechanisms include T-cell recognition of haptenated proteins or the deposition of immune complexes in blood-vessel walls [42, 44]. Medical practitioners need to be especially aware of abacavir hypersensitivity reactions because of the potential for fatal outcomes. Hypersensitivity reactions of this type should always be considered as a possible etiology for a vasculitic syndrome in an HIV-infected patient [42, 44].

HAART-associated coagulation disorders

HIV-infected patients receiving HAART, especially those with fat redistribution and insulin resistance, might develop coagulation abnormalities, including increased levels of fibrinogen, D-dimer, plasminogen activator inhibitor-1, and tissue-type plasminogen activator antigen, or deficiency of protein S [81, 82]. For instance, protein S deficiency has been reported in up to 73% of HIV-infected men [81, 82]. These abnormalities have been associated with thromboses involving veins and arteries and seem to be related to HAART regimens that include PI [83]. Thrombocytosis has been reported in 9% of patients receiving HAART, with cardiovascular complications in up to 25% of cases [84].

HAART-associated arterial hypertension and coronary artery disease

The prevalence of arterial hypertension in HIV disease has been estimated to be about 20–25% before the introduction of HAART [85]. Arterial hypertension, even in agreement with the Adult Treatment Panel-III guidelines [86], is currently considered part of HAART-associated metabolic syndrome [87]. It appears to be related to PI-induced lipodystrophy [88] and metabolic disorders, especially to elevated fasting triglyceride and insulin resistance [87, 89]. HIV-infected patients receiving HAART with preexisting additional risk factors (e.g., hypertension, diabetes, or increased plasma homocysteine levels) might be at raised risk of developing coronary artery disease because of accelerated atherosclerosis. Conflicting data exist, however, on the relationship between HAART and the incidence of acute coronary syndromes, such as unstable angina or myocardial infarction, among HIV-infected patients receiving PI-containing HAART [90–94]. Differences in the study design, selection of the patients, and statistical analyses might explain this disparity. However, longer exposure to HAART and/or PI seem to increase the risk of myocardial infarction. The results of the Data Collection on Adverse Events of Anti-HIV Drugs study showed that HAART therapy is associated with a 26% relative risk increase in the rate of myocardial infarction per year of HAART exposure [92].

HAART-associated peripheral vascular disease

Also, the issue of surrogate markers of subclinical atherosclerosis has been addressed. A study was performed on a cohort of 168 HIV-infected patients to measure the intima-media thickness (IMT) and assess indirectly the cardiovascular risk. In this population a high prevalence of atherosclerotic plaques within the femoral or carotid arteries was observed, but their presence was not associated with the use of PI [95]. Similar results were reported also by Hsue et al. [96] and by Currier et al. [97] in case–control studies suggesting that traditional risk factors may contribute to atherosclerosis in HIV-infected patients independently of PI exposure. Alonso-Villaverde et al. reported that HIV-infected patients with subclinical atherosclerosis have a higher circulating levels of monocyte chemoattractant protein-1 (MCP-1), especially of the allele MCP-1-2518G, compared to patients without atherosclerotic lesions, independently of HAART regimen [98]. Different results were reported by Maggi et al. who observed a higher than expected prevalence of premature carotid lesions in PI-treated patients compared to PI-naive patients [99]. Similar results have been reported in a study by Jerico et al. in 68 HIV-infected patients [100]. These authors conclude stating that HAART should be considered a strong, independent predictor for the development of subclinical atherosclerosis in HIV-infected patients, regardless of known major cardiovascular risk factors and atherogenic

metabolic abnormalities induced by this therapy
[100]. The impact of individual measures to reduce the cardiovascular risk and the progression of
atherosclerosis has been addressed by Thiebaut *et al.*
[101]. According to these authors, the increased use
of lipid-lowering agents, of PI-free HAART regimes
and the reduction of smoking may decrease the
IMT in HIV-infected patients over time [101]. In
spite of these different results, markers of subclinical atherosclerosis should be carefully assessed in
HIV-infected patients receiving HAART, especially
in those with lipodystrophy [102].

Conclusions

Cardiac and pulmonary complications of HIV disease are generally late manifestations and may be
related to prolonged effects of immunosuppression
and a complex interplay of mediator effects from
opportunistic infections, viral infections, autoimmune response to viral infection, drug-related cardiotoxicity, nutritional deficiencies, and prolonged
immunosuppression. HAART has significantly reduced in developed countries the prevalence of
HIV-associated cardiomyopathy which heavily influenced the prognosis of HIV-infected patients
in the pre-HAART period. However, HAART-
associated metabolic syndrome is an increasingly
recognized clinical entity. The atherogenic effects
of PI-including HAART may synergistically promote the acceleration of coronary and cerebrovascular disease and increase the risk of death from
myocardial infarction and stroke even in young
HIV-infected people. A better understanding of the
molecular mechanisms responsible for this syndrome will lead to the discovery of new drugs that
will reduce the cardiovascular risk in HIV-infected
patients receiving HAART.

References

1 Barbaro G. Cardiovascular manifestations of HIV infection. Circulation 2002;106:1420–5.
2 Barbaro G. Pathogenesis of HIV-associated heart disease. AIDS 2003;17(S1):S12–20.
3 Barbaro G. Reviewing the cardiovascular complications
of HIV infection after the introduction of highly active antiretroviral therapy. Curr Drug Targets Cardiovasc
Haematol Disord 2005;5:337–43.
4 Nzuobontane D, Blackett KN, Kuaban C. Cardiac
involvement in HIV-infected people in Yaounde,
Cameroon. Postgrad Med J 2002;78:678–81.
5 Barbarini G, Barbaro G. Incidence of the involvement
of the cardiovascular system in HIV infection. AIDS
2003;17(S1):S46–50.
6 Bijl M, Dieleman JP, Simoons M, Van Der Ende ME.
Low prevalence of cardiac abnormalities in an HIV-
seropositive population on antiretroviral combination
therapy. J AIDS 2001;27:318–20.
7 Torre D, Pugliese A, Orofino G. Effect of highly active
antiretroviral therapy on ischemic cardiovascular disease in patients with HIV-1 infection. Clin Infect Dis
2002;35(5):631–2.
8 Barbaro G, Di Lorenzo G, Grisorio B, Barbarini G, for the
Gruppo Italiano per lo Studio Cardiologico dei pazienti
affetti da AIDS investigators. Cardiac involvement in the
acquired immunodeficiency syndrome. A multicenter
clinical-pathological study. AIDS Res Hum Retroviruses
1998;14:1071–7.
9 Klatt EC. Cardiovascular pathology in AIDS. Adv Cardiol 2003;40:23–48.
10 Barbaro G. HIV-associated myocarditis. Heart Failure
Clin 2005;1:439–48.
11 Klatt EC, Nichols L, Noguchi TT. Emerging patterns of
heart disease in human immunodeficiency virus infection. Hum Pathol 1994;118:884–90.
12 Oddo D, Casanova M, Acuna G, Ballesteros J, Morales
B. Acute Chagas' disease (Trypanosomiasis amaericana)
in acquired immunodeficiency syndrome: report of two
cases. Hum Pathol 1992;23:41–4.
13 Sartori AM, Lopes MH, Benvenuti LA *et al.* Reacti-
vation of Chagas' disease in a human immunodeficiency virus-infected patient leading to severe heart
disease with a late positive direct microscopic examination of the blood. Am J Trop Med Hyg 1998;59:784–
6.
14 Herskowitz A, Tzyy-Choou W, Willoughby SB *et al.* Myocarditis and cardiotropic viral infection associated with
severe left ventricular dysfunction in late-stage infection
with human immunodeficiency virus. J Am Coll Cardiol
1994;24:1025–32.
15 Bowles NE, Kearney DL, Ni J *et al.* The detection of
viral genomes by polymerase chain reaction in the myocardium of pediatric patients with advanced HIV disease. J Am Coll Cardiol 1999;34:857–65.
16 Barbaro G, Di Lorenzo G, Soldini M *et al.* The intensity
of myocardial expression of inducible nitric oxide synthase influences the clinical course of human immunodeficiency virus-associated cardiomyopathy. Circulation
1999;100:633–9.
17 Fiala M, Popik W, Qiao JH *et al.* HIV-1 induces cardiomyopathy by cardiomyocyte invasion and gp120, tat

and cytokine signaling. Cardiovasc Toxicol 2004;4:97–107.

18 Twu C, Liu QN, Popik W *et al.* Cardiomyocytes undergo apoptosis in human immunodeficiency virus cardiomyopathy through mitochondrion and death receptor-controlled pathways. Proc Natl Acad Sci U S A 2002;99:14386–91.

19 Kan H, Xie Z, Finkel MS. HIV gp120 enhances NO production by cardiac myocytes through p38 MAP kinase-mediated NK-kB activation. Am J Physiol 2000;279:138–43.

20 Cooper ER, Hanson C, Diaz C *et al.* Encephalopathy and progression of human immunodeficiency virus disease in a cohort of children with perinatally acquired human immunodeficiency virus infection. J Pediatr 1998;132:808–12.

21 Lipshultz SE, Easley KA, Orav EJ *et al.* Left ventricular structure and function in children infected with human immunodeficiency virus. The Prospective P²C² HIV Multicenter Study. Circulation 1998;97:1246–56.

22 Fiala M, Rhodes RH, Shapshak P *et al.* Regulation of HIV-1 infection in astrocytes: expression of Nef, TNF-alpha and IL-6 in enhanced coculture of astrocytes with macrophages. J Neurovirol 1996;2:158–66.

23 Currie PF, Goldman JH, Caforio AL *et al.* Cardiac autoimmunity in HIV related heart muscle disease. Heart 1998;79:599–604.

24 Lipshultz SE, Easley KA, Orav EJ *et al.* Cardiac dysfunction and mortality in HIV-infected children. The Prospective P²C² HIV Multicenter Study. Circulation 2000;102:1542–8.

25 Miller TL, Orav EJ, Colan SD, Lipshultz SE. Nutritional status and cardiac mass and function in children infected with the human immunodeficiency virus. Am J Clin Nutr 1997;66:660–4.

26 Hoffman M, Lipshultz SE, Miller TL. Malnutrition and cardiac abnormalities in the HIV-infected patients. In: Miller TL, Gorbach S, eds. Nutritional aspects of HIV infection. Arnold, London, 1999:33–9.

27 Beck MA, Kolbeck PC, Shi Q, Rohr LH, Morris VC, Levander OA. Increased virulence of a human enterovirus (coxackievirus B3) in selenium-deficient mice. J Infect Dis 1994;170:351–7.

28 Chariot P, Perchet H, Monnet I. Dilated cardiomyopathy in HIV-infected patients. N Engl J Med 1999;340:732 (letter).

29 Shahmanesh M, Bradbeer CS, Edwards A, Smith SE. Autonomic dysfunction in patients with human immunodeficiency virus infection. Int J STD AIDS 1991;2:419–23.

30 Gluck T, Degenhardt E, Scholmerich J, Lang B, Grossman J, Straub RH. Autonomic neuropathy in patients with HIV: course, impact of disease stage, and medication. Clin Auton Res 2000;10:17–22.

31 Barbaro G, Di Lorenzo G, Soldini M *et al.* Vagal system impairment in human immunodeficiency virus-positive patients with chronic hepatitis C: does glutathione deficiency have a pathogenetic role? Scand J Gastroenterol 1997;32:1261–6.

32 Barbaro G, Pellicelli A, Barbarini G, Akashi YI. Takotsubo-like left ventricular dysfunction in HIV-infected patient. Curr HIV Res 2006;4:239–41.

33 Lewis W, Simpson JF, Meyer RR. Cardiac mitochondrial DNA polymerase gamma is inhibited competitively and noncompetitively by phosphorylated zidovudine. Circ Res 1994;74:344–8.

34 Lewis W, Grupp IL, Grupp G *et al.* Cardiac dysfunction in the HIV-1 transgenic mouse treated with zidovudine. Lab Invest 2000;80:187–97.

35 Lipshultz SE, Easley KA, Orav EJ *et al.* Absence of cardiac toxicity of zidovudine in infants. N Engl J Med 2000;343:759–66.

36 Sonnenblick EH, Rosin A. Cardiotoxicity of interferon: a review of 44 cases. Chest 1991;99:557–61.

37 Bristow MR, Mason JW, Billingham ME, Daniels JR. Doxorubicin cardiomyopathy: evaluation by phonocardiography, endomyocardial biopsy and cardiac catheterization. Ann Intern Med 1978;88:168–75.

38 Brown DL, Sather S, Cheitlin MD. Reversible cardiac dysfunction associated with foscarnet therapy for cytomegalovirus esophagitis in an AIDS patient. Am Heart J 1993;125:1439–41.

39 Chi D, Henry J, Kelley J, Thorpe R, Smith JK, Krishnaswamy G. The effect of HIV infection on endothelial function. Endothelium 2000;7:223–42.

40 Berger O, Gan X, Gujuluva C *et al.* CXC and CC chemokine receptors on coronary and brain endothelia. Mol Med 1999;5:795–805.

41 Johnson RM, Little JR, Storch GA. Kawasaki-like syndromes associated with human immonodeficiency virus infection. Clin Infect Dis 2001;32:1628–34.

42 Johnson RM, Barbarini G, Barbaro G. Kawasaki-like syndromes and other vasculitic syndromes in HIV-infected patients. AIDS 2003;17(S1):S77–82.

43 Shingadia D, Das L, Klein-Gitelman N, Chadwick E. Takayasu's arteritis in a human immunodeficiency virus-infected adolescent. Clin Infect Dis 1999;29:458–9.

44 Barbaro G. Vasculitic syndromes in HIV-infected patients. Adv Cardiol 2003;40:185–96.

45 Barbaro G, Barbarini G, Pellicelli AM. HIV-associated coronary arteritis in a patient with fatal myocardial infarction. N Engl J Med 2001;344:1799–800.

46 Heidenreich PA, Eisenberg MJ, Kee LL *et al.* Pericardial effusion in AIDS. Incidence and survival. Circulation 1995;92:3229–34.

47 Barbaro G, Fisher SD, Lipshultz SE. Pathogenesis of HIV-associated cardiovascular complications. Lancet Infect Dis 2001;1:115–24.

48 Barbaro G, Fisher SD, Giancaspro G, Lipshultz SE. HIV-associated cardiovascular complications: a new challenge for emergency physicians. Am J Emerg Med 2001;19:566–74.

49 Nahass RG, Weinstein MP, Bartels J, Gocke DJ. Infective endocarditis in intravenous drug users: a comparison of human immunodeficiency virus type 1-negative and -positive patients. J Infect Dis 1990;162:967–70.

50 Pellicelli A, Barbaro G, Palmieri F et al. Primary pulmonary hypertension in HIV disease: a systematic review. Angiology 2001;52:31–41.

51 Barbaro G. Reviewing the clinical aspects of HIV-associated pulmonary hypertension. J Respir Dis 2004;25:289–93.

52 Duong M, Dubois C, Buisson M et al. Non-Hodgkin's lymphoma of the heart in patients infected with human immunodeficiency virus. Clin Cardiol 1997;20:497–502.

53 Sanna P, Bertoni F, Zucca E et al. Cardiac involvement in HIV-related non Hodgkin lymphoma: a case report and short review of the literature. Ann Hematol 1998;77:75–8.

54 Sanna P, Bertoni F, Zucca E et al. Cardiac involvement in HIV-related non-Hodgkin's lymphoma: a case report and short review of the literature. Ann Hematol 1998;77(1–2):75–8.

55 Dal Maso L, Serraino D, Franceschi S. Epidemiology of HIV-associated malignancies. Cancer Treat Res 2001;104:1–18.

56 Carr A, Samaras K, Burton S et al. A syndrome of peripheral lipodystrophy, hyperlipidaemia and insulin resistance in patients receiving HIV protease inhibitors. AIDS 1998;12:F51–8.

57 Carr A. HIV lipodystrophy: risk factors, pathogenesis, diagnosis and management. AIDS 2003;17(S1):S141–8.

58 Grinspoon S, Carr A. Cardiovascular risk and body-fat abnormalities in HIV-infected adults. N Engl J Med 2005;352:48–62.

59 Garg A. Acquired in inherited lipodystrophies. N Engl J Med 2005;350:1220–34.

60 Carr A, Samaras K, Chisholm DJ, Cooper DA. Pathogenesis of HIV-1 protease inhibitor-associated peripheral lipodystrophy, hyperlipidaemia, and insulin resistance. Lancet 1998;351:1881–3.

61 Mooser V, Carr A. Antiretroviral therapy-associated hyperlipidemia in HIV disease. Curr Opin Lipidol 2001;12:313–9.

62 Fauvel J, Bonnet E, Ruidavets JB et al. An interaction between apo C-III variants and protease inhibitors contributes to high triglyceride/low HDL levels in treated HIV patients. AIDS 2001;15:2397–406.

63 Bonnet E, Ruidavets JB, Tuech J et al. Apoprotein C-III and E-containing lipoparticles are markedly increased in HIV-infected patients treated with protease inhibitors: association with the development of lipodystrophy. J Clin Endocrinol Metab 2001;86:296–302.

64 Caron M, Auclair M, Sterlingot H, Kornprobst M, Capeau J. Some HIV protease inhibitors alter lamin A/C maturation and stability, SREBP-1 nuclear localization and adipocyte differentiation. AIDS 2003;17:2437–44.

65 Murata H, Hruz PW, Mueckler M. The mechanism of insulin resistance caused by HIV protease inhibitor therapy. J Biol Chem 2000;275:20251–4.

66 Myarcik DC, McNurlan MA, Steigbigel RT, Fuhrer J, Gelato MC. Association of severe insulin resistance with body loss and limb fat and elevated serum tumor necrosis factor receptor levels in HIV lipodystrophy. J AIDS 2000;25:312–21.

67 Gougeon ML, Penicaud L, Fromenty B, Leclercq P, Viard JP, Capeau J. Adipocytes targets and actors in the pathogenesis of HIV-associated lipodystrophy and metabolic alterations. Antivir Ther 2004;9:161–77.

68 Caron M, Auclair M, Lagathu C et al. The HIV-1 nucleoside reverse transcriptase inhibitors stavudine and zidovudine alter adipocyte function in vitro. AIDS 2004;18:2127–36.

69 Lewis W, Kohler J, Hosseini S et al. Antiretroviral nucleosides, deoxynucleotide carrier and mitochondrial DNA: evidence supporting the DNA pol-gamma hypothesis. AIDS 2006;20:675–84.

70 Seminari E, Tinelli C, Minoli L et al. Evaluation of the risk factors associated with lipodystrophy development in a cohort of HIV-positive patients. Antivir Ther 2002;7:175–80.

71 McComsey GA, Paulsen D, Lonergan JT et al. Improvements in lipoatrophy, mitochondrial DNA levels and fat apoptosis after replacing stavudine with abacavir or zidovudine. AIDS 2005;19:15–23.

72 Vigouroux C, Maachi M, Nguyen TH et al. Serum adipocytokines are related to lipodystrophy and metabolic disorders in HIV-infected men under antiretroviral therapy. AIDS 2003;17:1503–11.

73 Haque WA, Shimomura I, Matsuzawa Y, Garg A. Serum adiponectin and leptin levels in patients with lipodystrophies. J Clin Endocrinol Metab 2002;87(5):2395–98.

74 Addy CL, Gavrila A, Tsiodras S, Brodovicz B, Karchmer AW, Mantzoros CS. Hypoadiponectinemia is associated with insulin resistance, hypertriglyceridemia, and fat redistribution in human immunodeficiency virus-infected patients treated with highly active antiretroviral therapy. J Clin Endocrinol Metab 2003;88:627–36.

75 Kosmiski L, Kuritzkes D, Lichtenstein K, Eckel R. Adipocyte-derived hormone levels in HIV lipodystrophy. Antivir Ther 2003;8:9–15.

76 Fiala M, Murphy T, MacDougall J et al. HAART drugs induces mitochondrial damage and intercellular gaps ans gp120 causes apoptosis. Cardiovasc Toxicol 2005;4: 327–37.

77 Stein JH, Klein MA, Bellehumeur JL et al. Use of human immunodeficiency virus-1 protease inhibitors is associated with atherogenic lipoprotein changes and endothelial dysfunction. Circulation 2001;104:257–62.

78 Zhong DS, Lu XH, Conklin BS et al. HIV protease ritonavir induces cytotoxicity of human endothelial cells. Arterioscler Thromb Vasc Biol 2002;22:1560–6.

79 Chai H, Yang H, Yan S et al. Effects of 5 HIV protease inhibitors on vasomotor function and superoxide anion production in porcine coronary arteries. J AIDS 2005;40:12–9.

80 van Wanrooij EJ, Happe H, Hauer AD et al. HIV entry inhibitor TAK-779 attenuates atherogenesis in low-density lipoprotein receptor-deficient mice. Arterioscler Thromb Vasc Biol 2005;25:2642–7.

81 Hadigan C, Meigs JB, Rabe J et al. Increased PAI-1 and tPA antigen levels are reduced with metformin therapy in HIV-infected patients with fat redistribution and insulin resistance. J Clin Endocrinol Metab 2001;86:939–43.

82 Witz M, Lehmann J, Korzets Z. Acute brachial artery thrombosis as the initial manifestations of human immunodeficiency virus infection. Am J Hematol 2000;64:137–9.

83 Sullivan PS, Dworkin MS, Jones JL, Hooper WC. Epidemiology of thrombosis in HIV-infected individuals. The Adult/Adolescent Spectrum of HIV Disease Project. AIDS 2000;14:321–4.

84 Miguez-Burbano MJ, Burbano X, Rodriguez A, Lecusay R, Rodriguez N, Shor-Posner G. Development of thrombocytosis in HIV+ drug users: impact of antiretroviral therapy. Platelets 2002;13:183–5.

85 Aoun S, Ramos E. Hypertension in the HIV-infected patient. Curr Hyperten Rep 2000;2:478–81.

86 National Cholesterol Education Program (NCEP) Expert Panel on Detection EaToHBCiAATPI. Third Report of the national Cholesterol Education Program (NCEP) Expert Panel on Detection, Evaluation, and Treatment of High Blood Cholesterol in Adults (Adult Treatment Panel III) final report. Circulation 2002;106:3143–421.

87 Gazzaruso C, Bruno R, Garzaniti A et al. Hypertension among HIV patients: prevalence and relationship to insulin resistance and metabolic syndrome. J Hypertens 2003;21:1377–82.

88 Crane H, Van Rompaey S, Kitahata M. Antiretroviral medications associated with elevated blood pressure among patients receiving highly active antiretroviral therapy. AIDS 2006;20:1019–26.

89 Sattler FR, Qian D, Louie S et al. Elevated blood pressure in subjects with lipodystrophy. AIDS 2001;15:2001–10.

90 Barbaro G, Di Lorenzo G, Cirelli A et al. An open-label, prospective, observational study of the incidence of coronary artery disease in patients with HIV receiving highly active antiretroviral therapy. Clin Ther 2003;25:2405–18.

91 Bozzette SA, Ake CF, Tam HK, Chang SW, Louis TA. Cardiovascular and cerebrovascular events in patients treated for human immunodeficiency virus infection. N Engl J Med 2003;348(8):702–10.

92 Friis-Moller N, Weber R, Reiss P et al. Cardiovascular risk factors in HIV patients-association with antiretroviral therapy. Results from DAD study. AIDS 2003;17: 1179–93.

93 Holmberg SD, Moorman AC, Williamson JM et al. Protease inhibitors and cardiovascular outcomes in patients with HIV-1. Lancet 2002;360:1747–8.

94 Mary-Krause M, Cotte L, Simon A, Partisani M, Costagliola D, for the Clinical Epidemiology Group from the French Hospital Database. Increased risk of myocardial infarction with duration of protease inhibitor therapy in HIV-infected men. AIDS 2003;17:2479–86.

95 Depairon M, Chessex S, Sudre P et al. Premature atherosclerosis in HIV-infected individuals: focus on protease inhibitor therapy. AIDS 2001;15:329–34.

96 Hsue PY, Lo JC, Franklin A et al. Progression of atherosclerosis as assessed by carotid intima-media thickness in patients with HIV infection. Circulation 2004;109:1603–8.

97 Currier JS, Kendall MA, Zackin R et al. Carotid artery intima-media thickness and HIV infection: traditional risk factors overshadow impact of protease inhibitor exposure. AIDS 2005;19:927–33.

98 Alonso-Villaverde C, Coll B, Parra S et al. Atherosclerosis in patients infected with HIV is influenced by a mutant monocyte chemoattractant protein-1 allele. Circulation 2004;110:2204–9.

99 Maggi P, Serio G, Epifani G et al. Premature lesions of the carotid vessels in HIV-1-infected patients treated with protease inhibitors. AIDS 2000;14:F123–8.

100 Jerico C, Knobel H, Calvo N et al. Subclinical carotid atherosclerosis in HIV-infected patients: role of combination antiretroviral therapy. Stroke 2006;37:812–7.

101 Thiebaut R, Aurillac-Lavignole V, Bonnet F et al. Change in atherosclerosis progression in HIV-infected patients: ANRS Aquitane Cohort, 1999–2004. AIDS 2005;19:729–31.

102 Volberding P, Murphy R, Barbaro G et al. The Pavia Consensus Statement. AIDS 2003;17(S1):S170–9.

CHAPTER 15

Cytokines and T cell-mediated responses in autoimmune myocarditis

Jin Zhang

Introduction

Myocarditis and dilated cardiomyopathy are often associated with an autoimmune process in which cardiac myosin is a major autoantigen in both human and murine virus-induced myocarditis. Myocarditis is an inflammatory disease of the heart that is characterized by a cellular infiltrate in the myocardium, and dilated cardiomyopathy is a chronic heart muscle disease characterized by ventricular hypertrophy. The pathomechanisms of autoimmune myocarditis are very complex, in which cardiac myosin fragments, proper dendritic cells, and autoreactive T cells are the three major elements in initiating and promoting the inflammation. This chapter reviews current experimental rodent models, a serial of cytokines and immune cell players during autoimmune myocarditis as well as potential therapeutic targets for it.

Experimental autoimmune myocarditis

Experimental autoimmune myocarditis (EAM) has been used as a model for human myocarditis in relation to the autoimmune mechanism and proved to be a T cell-mediated autoimmune disease. Three distinct murine models exist in the literature. The first model involves infecting mice with Coxsackie virus B3 (CVB3) to study the induction and effector phases of myocarditis [1, 2]. CVB3-induced myocarditis closely resembles the course of human myocarditis, which is believed to be initiated by viral infection. Despite differences in susceptibility to CVB3-induced myocarditis between mouse strains, and probably some mechanistic differences as well, a number of common features are evident. The severity of inflammation correlates with increased tissue-specific expression of interleukin (IL)-1β and IL-18 [3]. The inflammatory infiltrate is focal and mixed, comprised largely of macrophages, neutrophils, and CD4[+] and CD8[+] T lymphocytes. The CD4[+] T helper 1 (Th1) cells provide help for activation of autoimmune CD8[+] T cells. The later autoimmune phase of the disease is dependent on CD8[+] T cells [4].

The second model is cardiac myosin-induced EAM. In this model, cardiac myosin heavy chain or the relevant peptide emulsified in Freund's complete adjuvant is injected subcutaneously into mice [5]. Immunizing mice with purified myosin in adjuvant induces severe myocarditis that resembles the late stage disease caused by viral infection. The immune responses, histological changes, and genetic susceptibilities observed in EAM closely parallel those of CVB3-induced myocarditis.

A third model of autoimmune myocarditis was developed by Grabie and colleagues. The model involves adoptive transfer of ovalbumin peptide-specific TCR transgenic CD8[+] T cells into a C57/BL6 mouse line named CMy-mOva (cardiac myocyte restricted membrane-bound ovalbumin) engineered to express membrane-bound ovalbumin exclusively in cardiac myocytes [6]. A limitation of the myosin-induced EAM model is that CD8[+] T-cell responses, fundamental in the immune response to viruses, may not be efficiently induced by immunization with exogenous protein antigens, which are preferentially processed by the class II MHC pathway of antigen presentation. In contrast, the CMy-mOva model of myocarditis permits investigation of pathogenicity of uniform populations of CD8$^+$ T cells specific for a single antigen expressed in the myocardium.

The involvement of T cells and cytokines in EAM

T cells are involved in most adaptive immune responses, including cell-mediated responses and T cell-dependent antibody responses. Cytokines are important in controlling T cells responsive to self-antigens and are critical in shifting the immune response toward a Th1 or a T-helper 2 (Th2) pattern. Recent evidence suggests that both B and T cells are involved in polarized cytokine production [7]. CD4$^+$ and CD8$^+$ T cells as well as natural killer and dendritic cells may also be involved in production of polarizing cytokines. The Th1 response shifts the cytokine profile toward delayed hypersensitivity, macrophage activation, and a proinflammatory T-cell response associated with interferon gamma (IFN-γ) and IL-12, whereas the Th2 response is associated with B-cell activation and humoral immunity, and IL-4, -5, -10, and IgE production. IL-12 has been shown to induce the differentiation of Th1 autoreactive T cells and to enhance autoimmune disease in certain animal models [8]. Th1 cells secrete IL-2 and IFN-γ that suppress Th2 responses, whereas Th2 cells secrete IL-4 and IL-10 that inhibit Th1 responses [9].

Th1/Th2 cell involvement in myocarditis

Previous studies suggest that Th1 cytokines are involved in the initiation and progression of EAM, whereas Th2 cytokines are associated with the remission. Fuse and colleagues used Lewis rats immunized with cardiac myosin. Serum levels of Th1 cytokines, IFN-γ, and IL-2 significantly increased in the acute phase and immediately decreased in the early recovery phase. On the other hand, serum levels of Th2 cytokine, IL-10 significantly increased in the early recovery phase [10].

Another rat study also supports that Th1 and Th2 cytokines are produced at different stages of EAM and modulate the inflammation and the course of EAM. Antigen (Ag) primed Ag presenting cells or macrophages interact with Th1 cells to produce IL-2 and subsequent IFN-γ, which further activates macrophages in the myocardium. Consequently, tumor necrosis factor alpha (TNF-α) and inducible nitric oxide synthase (iNOS) may cause tissue damage to myocardium. The study also suggests that TGF-β and Th2 cytokine IL-10 help inhibit inflammation [11].

There are other mechanisms by which Th1 cells may be specialized to coordinate the complex effector cell interactions of a destructive immune response in autoimmune myocarditis. Th1 cells mediate more destructive myocarditis than Th2 cells. Strikingly, the Th1-mediated inflammation was comprised primarily of CD8$^+$ T cells and macrophages, suggesting a specialized recruitment function for Th1 cells. Studies showed that Th1 and Th2 subsets had polarized secretion of certain CC-chemokines, including macrophage inflammatory protein-1 alpha (MIP-1α) and RANTES, which have selective recruitment properties on effector cells. Th1 cell secreted factors were up to 1000-fold more potent in mediating cytotoxic effector CD8$^+$ T-cell recruitment compared to Th2 cell secreted factors, and this advantage was partially mediated by their specialized MIP-1α secretion [12].

Cytokine orchestras during EAM

IL-12 and IFN-γ positively regulate each other and Th1 responses, which are believed to cause tissue damage in autoimmune diseases. IL-12 mediates proinflammatory effect primarily through the activation of signal transducer and activator of transcription 4 (STAT4) and subsequent production of IFN-γ. Both IL-12Rβ1-deficient mice and STAT4-deficient mice were resistant to the induction of myocarditis. Treatment with exogenous IL-12 exacerbated disease. Although IL-12 mediates disease by induction/expansion of Th1-type cells, IFN-γ production from these cells limits disease progression due to its ability to control the expansion of activated T lymphocytes. Therefore, IL-12/IFN-γ is a double-edged sword for the development of autoimmune myocarditis [13, 14]. Research also shows that IL-2 and IFN-γ mRNA are expressed in the myocardium of rats with EAM. In addition, IL-12 and IL-2 synergistically enhance the expansion of cardiac myosin-specific Th1 lymphocytes and play an important role in the development of autoimmune myocarditis in rats [15].

Other immune cells involved in immunopathology of EAM

Dendritic cells (DCs) readily migrate from bone marrow into the heart, and cardiac tissue may be constitutively rich in DCs. DC activation is an essential part of innate immune responses and is induced by Toll-like receptor (TLR) and cytokine signaling. Adoptive transfer of cardiac-antigen (myosin peptide)-pulsed DCs can cause T cell-mediated myocarditis in mice [16, 17]. TLRs or IL-1 receptors are required to activate the DCs so they can initiate myocarditis in this model. Li and colleagues induced protection against EAM in Lewis rats by administration of S2-16 peptide in incomplete Freund's adjuvant (IFA). Purified DCs from S2-16: IFA-treated rats promoted S2-16-reactive CD4+ T cells to produce increased IL-10 and reduced IFN-γ. In addition, adoptive transfer of IL-10-producing DCs from S2-16: IFA-treated rats also induced protection to EAM in recipient rats. These studies demonstrated DCs and key cytokines, such as IL-10 and IL-12, regulated the fate of T cells in myocarditis development in the Lewis rat [18].

Infiltration of monocytes and T cells is known to be an essential trigger for the progression of EAM in rats. Monocyte chemotactic protein-1 (MCP-1) and granulocyte-macrophage colony-stimulating factor (GM-CSF) were shown to mediate the migration of monocytes and T cells into inflammatory sites and to proliferate monocytes. The MCP-1 and GM-CSF mRNA levels were positively correlated with TNF-α, IL-1β, and IL-6 mRNA levels in the same lesion of EAM. They also demonstrated that serum MCP-1 concentrations were increased during the active stage of EAM, and were correlated with MCP-1 mRNA levels in the myocardium of each rat. Therefore, elevated MCP-1 and GM-CSF may associate with the migration and proliferation of monocytes/macrophages in EAM [19].

Therapeutic targets of autoimmune myocarditis

Th1/Th2 modulator

Hepatocyte growth factor (HGF) plays a role in cell protection, antiapoptosis, antifibrosis, and angiogenesis. Futamatsu's group examined the influence of HGF on T cells and the effects of HGF therapy in acute myocarditis. Lewis rats were immunized on Day 0 with cardiac myosin to establish EAM. Human HGF gene with hemagglutinating virus of the Japan-envelope vector was injected directly into the myocardium on Day 0 or on Day 14 (two groups of treated rats). At the end of Day 21, myocarditis-affected areas were smaller in the treated rats than in control rats. Cardiac function in the treated rats was markedly improved. HGF suppressed T-cell proliferation and production of IFN-γ and increased production of IL-4 and IL-10 secreted from CD4+ T cells in vitro. Additionally, HGF reduced apoptosis in cardiomyocytes. Therefore, HGF reduced the severity of EAM via inducing Th2 cytokines and suppressing apoptosis of cardiomyocytes [20].

Peroxisome proliferator-activated receptor gamma ligand (PPAR γ), which is a member of nuclear hormone receptor superfamily, has been known to affect not only glucose homeostasis but also immune responses, by regulating the Th1/Th2 balance. In a rat EAM model, cardiac dysfunction and remodeling were inhibited in PPAR γ activator-treated rats. Heart weight/body weight ratio and the degree of inflammation and fibrosis were significantly lower in PPAR γ activator-treated EAM rats. The mRNA levels of macrophage inflammatory protein-1alpha (MIP-1α), which plays an important role in the recruitment of inflammatory cells in the early stage of EAM, were upregulated in the heart of EAM rats, but not in the heart of PPAR γ activator-treated EAM rats. Furthermore, the treatment with PPAR γ activator decreased the expression levels of proinflammatory cytokine (TNFα and IL-1β) genes and Th1 cytokine (IFN-γ) genes, and increased the expression levels of Th2 cytokine (IL-4) gene. PPAR γ ligands may have beneficial effects on myocarditis by inhibiting MIP-1α expression and modulating the Th1/Th2 balance [21].

Other examples include suramin and fluvastatin. Suramin, a growth factor blocker, suppressed myocardial inflammation in EAM by increasing the number of Th2 and reducing transforming growth factor beta (TGF-β) expression in the heart [22]. Fluvastatin, a hydroxymethylglutaryl coenzyme A reductase inhibitor, ameliorated EAM by inhibiting T-cell responses and suppressing Th1-type and inflammatory cytokines via inactivation of nuclear factor-kappa B in rats [23].

Macrophage migration inhibitory factor blockade

Macrophage migration inhibitory factor (MIF) is a cytokine that plays a critical role in the regulation of macrophage effector functions and T-cell activation. MIF blockade decreased the expression of vascular cell adhesion molecule 1, TNF-α, and IL-1β and the migration of T cells and macrophages in the EAM heart. These results demonstrate an important role of MIF in the pathogenesis of EAM and suggest that MIF blockade may be a promising new strategy for the treatment of myocarditis [24].

TNF-α blockade

Tyrphostins AG-556 was previously shown to reduce TNF-α production and its end-organ cytotoxicity, thus proving beneficial in animal models of septic shock and experimental autoimmune encephalomyelitis. AG-556 administered daily for 21 days from the day of EAM induction in rats, significantly reduced the severity of myocarditis. Similarly, AG-556 administered for an additional 10 days after myosin immunization (when signs of inflammation are already present) attenuated the progression of myocarditis. TNF-α and IFN-γ production by in vitro sensitized splenocytes from AG-556-treated rats was significantly diminished as compared with control cells from EAM animals. Therefore, AG-556 may represent a novel strategy of ameliorating the progression of myocarditis without non-selectively compromising the immune system [25].

Blockade of T-cell activation

CD28 is a transmembrane molecule-evenly distributed at T-cell surface. Co-ligation of T-cell receptor/CD3 and CD28 promotes T-cell proliferation, IL-2 production, and cell survival. Inducible costimulator (ICOS) is a member of the CD28 family. Blockade of T-cell activation through ICOS suppressed expression of cytokines including IFN-γ, IL-4, IL-6, IL-10, IL-1β, and TNF-α and inhibited

T-cell proliferation in vitro, suggesting ICOS may be an effective target for treating myocarditis [26].

Conclusion

The study of Th1/Th2 cytokines in EAM is an important aspect for understanding human autoimmune myocarditis. Further studies of human autoimmune myocarditis will be warranted as well as investigation of the cytokine profiles in the heart, circulation and lymphoid tissues. Because development of the different stages or types of autoimmune myocarditis is dependent on various factors, it is difficult to attribute the disease to a single entity. This creates challenges for therapeutic application, which will deserve continuous effort to be better.

References

1 Wolfgram LJ, Beisel KW, Herskowitz A *et al.* Variations in the susceptibility to coxsackievirus B3-induced myocarditis among different strains of mice. J Immunol 1986;136:1846–52.

2 Huber SA, Lodge PA. Coxsackievirus B-3 myocarditis in Balb/c mice. Evidence for autoimmunity to myocyte antigens. Am J Pathol 1984;116:21–9.

3 Fairweather D, Yusung S, Frisancho S *et al.* IL-12 receptor beta 1 and Toll-like receptor 4 increase IL-1 beta- and IL-18-associated myocarditis and coxsackievirus replication. J Immunol 2003;170:4731–7.

4 Huber SA, Sartini D, Exley M. Vγ4+ T cells promote autoimmune CD8+ cytolytic T-lymphocyte activation in coxsackievirus B3-induced myocarditis in mice: role for CD4+ Th1 cells. J Virol 2002;76:10785–90.

5 Cihakova D, Sharma RB, Fairweather D *et al.* Animal models for autoimmune myocarditis and autoimmune thyroiditis. Methods Mol Med 2004;102:175–93.

6 Grabie N, Delfs MW, Westrich JR *et al.* IL-12 is required for differentiation of pathogenic CD8+ T cell effectors that cause myocarditis. J Clin Invest 2003;111:671–80.

7 Harris DP, Haynes L, Sayles PC *et al.* Reciprocal regulation of polarized cytokine production by effector B and T cells. Nat Immunol 2000;1:475–82.

8 Seder R, Gazzinelli AP, Sher A *et al.* IL-12 acts directly on CD4+ T cells to enhance priming for IFN-γ production and diminishes IL-4 inhibition of such priming. Proc Natl Acad Sci 1993;90:10188–92.

9 Paul WE, Seder RA. Lymphocyte responses and cytokines. Cell 1994;76:241–51.

10 Fuse K, Kodama M, Ito M *et al.* Polarity of helper T cell subsets represents disease nature and clinical course of

experimental autoimmune myocarditis in rats. Clin Exp Immunol 2003;134:403–8.

11 Kihara I, Izumi T, Shibata A *et al.* Characterization of cytokine and iNOS mRNA expression in situ during the course of experimental autoimmune myocarditis in rats. J Mol Cell Cardiol 1997;29:491–502.

12 Song HK, Noorchashm H, Lin TH *et al.* Specialized CC-chemokine secretion by Th1 cells in destructive autoimmune myocarditis. J Autoimmun 2003;21:295–303.

13 Eriksson U, Kurrer MO, Sebald W *et al.* Dual role of the IL-12/IFN-gamma axis in the development of autoimmune myocarditis: induction by IL-12 and protection by IFN-gamma. J Immunol 2001;167:5464–9.

14 Afanasyeva M, Wang Y, Kaya Z *et al.* Interleukin-12 receptor/STAT4 signaling is required for the development of autoimmune myocarditis in mice by an interferon-gamma-independent pathway. Circulation 2001;104:3145–51.

15 Okura Y, Takeda K, Honda S *et al.* Recombinant murine interleukin-12 facilitates induction of cardiac myosin-specific type 1 helper T cells in rats. Circ Res 1998;82:1035–42.

16 Eriksson U, Ricci R, Hunziker L *et al.* Dendritic cell-induced autoimmune heart failure requires cooperation between adaptive and innate immunity. Nat Med 2003;9:1484–90.

17 Eriksson U, Kurrer MO, Sonderegger I *et al.* Activation of dendritic cells through the interleukin 1 receptor 1 is critical for the induction of autoimmune myocarditis. J Exp Med 2003;197:323–31.

18 Li Y, Heuser JS, Kosanke SD *et al.* Protection against experimental autoimmune myocarditis is mediated by interleukin-10-producing T cells that are controlled by dendritic cells. Am J Pathol 2005;167:5–15.

19 Kobayashi Y, Kubo A, Iwano M *et al.* Levels of MCP-1 and GM-CSF mRNA correlated with inflammatory cytokines mRNA levels in experimental autoimmune myocarditis in rats. Autoimmunity 2002;35:97–104.

20 Futamatsu H, Suzuki J, Mizuno S *et al.* Hepatocyte growth factor ameliorates the progression of experimental autoimmune myocarditis: a potential role for induction of T helper 2 cytokines. Circ Res 2005;96:823–30.

21 Hasegawa H, Takano H, Zou Y *et al.* Pioglitazone, a peroxisome proliferator-activated receptor gamma activator, ameliorates experimental autoimmune myocarditis by modulating Th1/Th2 balance. J Mol Cell Cardiol 2005;38:257–65.

22 Shiono T, Kodama M, Hanawa H *et al.* Suppression of myocardial inflammation using suramin, a growth factor blocker. Circ J 2002;66:385–9.

23 Azuma RW, Suzuki J, Ogawa M *et al.* HMG-CoA reductase inhibitor attenuates experimental autoimmune myocarditis through inhibition of T cell activation. Cardiovasc Res 2004;64:412–20.

24 Matsui Y, Okamoto H, Jia N *et al.* Blockade of macrophage migration inhibitory factor ameliorates experimental autoimmune myocarditis. J Mol Cell Cardiol 2004;37:557–66.

25 George J, Barshack I, Goldberg I *et al.* The effect of early and late treatment with the tyrphostin AG-556 on the progression of experimental autoimmune myocarditis. Exp Mol Pathol 2004;76:234–41.

26 Futamatsu H, Suzuki J, Kosuge H *et al.* Attenuation of experimental autoimmune myocarditis by blocking activated T cells through inducible costimulatory molecule pathway. Cardiovasc Res 2003;59:95–104.

CHAPTER 16

Drugs of abuse: accentuation of immunomodulation of viral myocarditis

Oana Madalina Petrescu & James P. Morgan

Introduction

The recreational use of legal and illegal drugs of abuse has become increasingly common among the general population, and especially among those infected with the human immunodeficiency virus (HIV). Several of these drugs have been associated with detrimental effect on immunity and increased susceptibility to a variety of infections. There have also been numerous clinical reports and experimental studies that have demonstrated the potential of several abused drugs to induce myocarditis. Myocarditis is an inflammatory disease of the myocardium with cardiac dysfunction most commonly caused by viral infections. Since both the myopathic viruses and drugs of abuse produce cardiac toxicity, it is conceivable that the concomitant exposure of both will enhance cardiac damage and dysfunction.

A variety of viruses are implicated in myocarditis, including coxsackie virus (CV), cytomegalovirus (CMV), influenza viruses, poliovirus, echo, adenovirus, Epstein-Barr virus (EBV), herpes simplex virus, and many others [1, 2]. Recently, there has been growing evidence of myocarditis among HIV-seropositive patients [3]. Myocarditis may be due either to the HIV virus directly or from resultant-induced immune dysfunction, facilitating infectivity of a concomitant myopathic pathogen. Myocarditis is a multifaceted process, involving initial viral invasion of the myocardium, which then triggers an immune response, resulting in heart pathology. It is characterized by myocardial inflammation

and necrosis in the acute stages, followed by myocardial necrosis, inflammation, fibrosis, calcification, and dilatation in the chronic stages [1, 4]. The pathogenesis of viral myocarditis is founded on a disruption in the balance of the immune milieu between the virus and host immunity.

There are several mechanisms through which these drugs may worsen myocarditis. One mechanism may be mediated through the induction of a hypercatecholamine state, which is known to produce cardiomyopathy. Alternatively or concomitantly, the drugs' immunomodulatory effect may negatively impact the virus/host immune response balance. If the effect leads to an insufficient or suppressed host immune response, increased viral cytotoxicity ensues along with suboptimal recognition and clearance of infected cells. Conversely, the drugs' effect may stimulate too strong an immune response, resulting in immunopathology.

This chapter will review the existing data on the cardiotoxic effect and immunomodulatory properties of several drugs and their potential mechanisms of exacerbating viral myocarditis. The drugs discussed include: cocaine, methamphetamines (MA), amphetamine derivatives, heroin, alcohol, cocaethylene, and clozapine.

Cocaine

Cocaine abuse remains a significant health hazard in the United States [5]. It is estimated that up to 30 million Americans have used cocaine, and approximately 5 million people use it on a regular basis [6]. Particularly throughout the history of HIV epidemic, researchers have observed a strong association between cocaine abuse and the risk of HIV infection [7, 8]. Cocaine abuse is accompanied by a high risk of adverse effects on the cardiovascular system, including myocardial ischemia and infarction, arrhythmia and sudden death, hypertension, aortic dissection, accelerated atherosclerosis, cardiomyopathy, and myocarditis [9].

Evidence for cocaine-induced myocarditis has been demonstrated by several investigators. Virmani et al. [10] reported an incidence of myocarditis of 20% among individuals who abused cocaine. The cellular infiltrate consisted predominantly of lymphocytes and macrophages and occasional eosinophils, and myocyte necrosis was found in all of the hearts. Peng et al. [11] studied endomyocardial biopsies from seven patients who abused cocaine and demonstrated multifocal myocyte necrosis in five cases and infiltrates consisting of mononuclear cells surrounding necrotic myocytes in two cases. Tazelaar et al. [12] noted the presence of myocardial contraction bands in 93% of patients and proposed that cocaine induces a hypercatecholaminemic state that contributes to contraction band necrosis through calcium homeostasis disruption and provides the anatomic pathways for lethal arrhythmias.

These results suggest a toxic mechanism related to catecholamine excess induced by cocaine abuse. It is well known that cocaine blocks the reuptake of catecholamines at the presynaptic level in the central and peripheral nervous system and increases the release of catecholamines from both central and peripheral stores [6, 13]. Several studies have demonstrated the rise in catecholamines with cocaine [6, 13]. Nahas et al. [14] demonstrated that cocaine increased plasma adrenaline, dopamine, and noradrenaline in squirrel monkeys and rats. Karch et al. [15] noted a rise in catecholamine levels in patients with cocaine cardiotoxicity. Chiueh and Kopin reported that cocaine caused a significant release of norepinephrine and epinephrine from the rat adrenal medulla [16].

The pattern of myocardial damage noted with cocaine resembles that of catecholamine-related myocarditis. Catecholamines have been demonstrated to cause myocarditis in animal models [17–22], in patients with pheochromocytoma [23–26], and in patients given large amounts of pressor agents to treat shock states [26–28].

A range of mechanisms have been proposed to explain the morphological and functional myocardial damages seen with catecholamine myocarditis. Major hypotheses include a relative cardiac hypoxemia due to increased cardiac work and demand [29, 30] and coronary arterial vasoconstriction and spasm causing endocardiac ischemia [22, 31]. This theory is supported by findings that alpha-receptor blockade has been shown to inhibit both coronary vasoconstriction and myocyte injury by norepinephrine [19].

Another hypothesis is related to catecholamine-induced calcium transport into myocytes, resulting in intracellular calcium overload [32, 33], which may lead to ATP hydrolysis or/and increased production of free fatty acids and lysophospholipids, causing myocardial injury. Support for this theory has been demonstrated by Opie et al. [33] as their study demonstrated that lowering calcium concentration in the perfusate and use of calcium antagonists reduced the extent of injury by catecholamines. Other metabolic effects resulting from catecholamine excess and inducing injury have been related to depletion of potassium [34] and of intracellular magnesium, which is essential for ATP-dependent enzymatic processes [35, 36]. Another hypothesis is injury from catecholamine-induced oxidative stress through formation of free radicals and adrenochromes, oxidation products of catecholamines [37–39]. Injury through hypercontraction of myofilaments with formation of contraction bands and disorganization and fragmentation of myofibrils has been demonstrated, attributed to adrenaline-induced violent muscle contractions [40, 41]. Other postulations are related to free fatty acid toxicity [42, 43] and platelet aggregation with microvascular obstruction [44–46].

Since both viruses and cocaine independently cause myocarditis, it is reasonable to hypothesize that the combination of the two heightens the cardiotoxic effects. Cocaine as a cardiotoxic agent can hypothetically potentiate an underlying viral myocarditis through its enhancing effect on catecholamine state.

The enhancement of virus myocarditis by cocaine through catecholamine-related injury was nicely demonstrated by Wang *et al.* [47]. In this study, mice were inoculated with encephalomyocarditis virus (EMCV) and then infused various doses of cocaine or saline. EMCS is a picornavirus biologically similar to CV, which causes severe myocarditis in experimental animals. The investigators observed that the severity of myocarditis in EMCS-infected mice treated with cocaine increased significantly compared to those without cocaine infusion. The incidence of inflammatory cell infiltration and myocardial necrosis was higher in the infected mice exposed to cocaine. The mortality of myocarditis mice treated with cocaine increased significantly from EMCV mice alone. The rising rate correlated to the dose of cocaine infused, and reached 51.4% in the 50 mg/kg cocaine/EMCV group compared with 22% in EMCV alone group. Cocaine exposure significantly increased NE concentration. Notedly, reduction of catecholamines resulted in an improvement in myocarditis. The treatment with propanolol on cocaine/EMCV mice significantly reduced the effects of cocaine on mortality and severity of myocarditis. Adrenalectomy also led to reduction of mortality and severity of myocardial toxicity to the level of controls.

The authors attributed the exacerbation of viral myocarditis by cocaine to elevated levels of catecholamines. They theorized that the high catecholamine state directly induces myocardial necrosis and inflammatory infiltration, and likely enhances the cytotoxicity of the virus by causing vessel spasm and ischemia, thus lessening a structural barrier to cellular penetration of the virus. Their results substantiate that cocaine's detrimental effects are in large mediated by the hypercatecholamine state induced myocardio-toxicity.

The potentiating effect of catecholamines on viral myocarditis and its improvement with beta-adrenergic agents has been documented. Wang *et al.* [48] investigated the effect of epinephrine and propanolol on the progression of viral myocarditis in EMCV infected mice and found that epinephrine increased the severity of inflammatory cell infiltration and myocardial necrosis that was induced by EMCV. Treatment with propanolol significantly decreased the mortality and the severity of myocarditis in the EMCV-inoculated mice. Tominaga *et al.* [49] showed that carteolol had a favorable effect on dilated cardiomyopathy induced by EMCV and

Nishio *et al.* [50] reported that carvedilol improved the survival of mice infected with EMCV.

The ameliorating effect of beta-blockers on viral myocarditis exacerbated by cocaine and adrenalin further substantiates the postulation that catecholamines play a significant role in promoting progression of viral myocarditis.

Another mechanism for cocaine's heightened effect on the progression of viral myocarditis may be related to its effect on cytokine balance. Cocaine has been demonstrated to increase several immunomodulatory cytokines including IL-10 [48], TNF-α [51, 52], IL-6 [52], natural killer (NK) cells [53], all of which have been demonstrated to contribute to myocardial damage and dysfunction, and facilitate progression of viral myocarditis [54–64]. These proinflammatory cytokines have also been implicated in HIV pathogenesis. Investigators have found that TNF-α stimulate HIV replication in PBMC cultures [65]. Augmentation of HIV-1 proliferation has been demonstrated with TNF-α [66–71] and IL-1 [70]. Peterson *et al.* [72] reported that cocaine enhances the levels of transforming growth factor-β (TGF- β) in human peripheral blood mc (PBMC), which participates in augmentation of viral replication since the viral proliferation was subsequently inhibited by TGF-β blockade. The authors concluded that TGF-β may stimulate viral replication either directly or via an interactive effect with cytokines already established to enhance HIV replication.

Thus, it is very reasonable to assume that cocaine accentuates the immunomodulation produced by the inciting viral myocardial infection through cytokine imbalance.

The immune dysregulation provoked by cocaine may affect the myocarditis by increasing the virus myocardial infectivity at differing levels or by altering the autoimmune response to yield an injurious effect on the myocardium.

In his study of *Propanolol ameliorates and epinephrine exacerbates progression of acute and chronic viral myocarditis*, Wang *et al.* [48] also measured the levels of TNF-α, IL-6, and IL-10 and noted they were markedly enhanced by epinephrine in the EMCV infected mice and then significantly attenuated after treatment of propanolol. This effect suggests that catecholamines through beta-receptor activation may play a significant immunomodulatory role. This effect illustrates the intricate relationship between catecholamines and cytokines in their negative immunomodulatory effect on viral myocarditis.

Cocaine has been shown to promote progression of viral myocarditis through its immunomodulatory effect. Sepulveda et al. [73] investigated the effect of cocaine on Coxsackie B3 (CVB3) induced myocarditis during murine AIDS and showed that it greatly exacerbated the pathogenesis of CVB3 myocarditis. Histopathology revealed greater amount and severity of myocardial lesions compared to murine AIDS and CVB3 without cocaine. In their model, the Th-1 response was decreased in the CVB3 mice infected with the murine retrovirus, whereas the Th-2 response was enhanced, with increased humoral response. The increased Th-2 response is known to be a mechanism in viral myocarditis, resulting from generation of anti-myocyte antibodies. This shift, favoring Th2 cells has been observed in human and in murine AIDS [74,75]. The authors attributed cocaine's enhancing effect to additional shifting of Th1 to Th2 immune response.

In addition, cocaine's enhancing effect on neuroendocrine hormones such as ACTH and corticosterone may amplify the dysregulation and exacerbation of an underlying viral myocarditis. Corticosterones are known to be immunosuppressive [76, 77]. Cocaine's induction of corticosterones were observed in Sepulveda et al.'s study [73]. Moldow and Fischman noted an induction of ACTH and corticosterone in plasma after intraperitoneal administration of cocaine [78].

Overall, all the mechanisms through with cocaine enhances the progression of viral myocarditis including the resultant hypercatecholamines, the cytokine imbalance, and the neurohormonal effects are likely intricately interconnected and all playing a role in the overall effect.

Methamphetamine

MA is a derivative of amphetamine and is also known as speed, crank, go, crystal, meth, ICE, or poor man's cocaine. MA as a recreational drug has become more widespread and its use has become highly related to HIV infection and progression to AIDS [79]. Similar to cocaine, MA inhibits the re-uptake and promotes the release of NE at adrenergic nerve endings in the peripheral and central nervous system [80, 81]. In addition, it prevents the metabolism of NE and causes tissue sensitization to catecholamines.

MA has been reported in the literature to lead to several cardiovascular complications including arrhythmias, myocardial ischemia, hypertension, tachycardia, myocardial rupture, aortic dissection as well as myocarditis and cardiomyopathy [82–87].

The MA-induced lesions noted in myocarditis and cardiomyopathy are similar to those previously reported in patients who abuse cocaine, or those administered epinephrine and NE, and in patients who die of pheochromocytoma. Zalis et al. [88] reported myocardial necrosis and subendocardial hemorrhage. Kaiho and Ishiyama [89] noted necrotic myocytes with myoglobin loss and mitochondrial swelling in their ultrastructural and immunohistochemistry staining. They observed time-dependent myocardial changes. In the early exposure stage (14 day) chronic MA-induced myocarditis type changes including multiple foci of myocytic degeneration and necrosis whereas chronic exposure (56 days) led to cardiomyopathy. He et al. [90] confirmed the investigated effect of MA injection on rat hearts and noted that relevance of time to development of cardiotoxicity. After 14 days, heart examination demonstrated changes consistent with myocarditis including foci of myocytic necrosis and degeneration as well as contraction bands. After 54 days, the myocyte necrosis and degeneration has become more extensive, with interspersed cellular infiltrates and contraction bands, as well as fibrotic changes.

MA-induced myocarditis and cardiomyopathy has been documented in humans after chronic methamphetamine abuse. Smith et al. [86] reported a case of this in a woman patient who had used oral dextroamphetamine for almost 12 years on a regular basis. Autopsy of the heart revealed foci of myocytic necrosis, lymphocytic infiltration, interstitial edema, and spotty fibrosis. The coronary arteries were not atherosclerotic. Tanaka et al. [91] reported a similar case of a male patient who abused intravenous methamphetamine for approximately 28 years. Microscopic examination of the heart revealed foci of myocytic necrosis, lymphocytic infiltration, and areas of hypertrophy and fibrosis.

Hong *et al.* [92] described two cases of cardiomyopathy associated with crystal MA smoking. At autopsy, one patient had patchy interstitial fibrosis and myocardial ischemia, while the coronary arteries were free of atherosclerosis. Rajs and Falconer [93] studied the hearts of 25 IV drug users who died suddenly after MA misuse. Autopsy of the heart revealed foci of myocytic necrosis, contraction bands, hemorrhage, and fibrosis.

The mechanism of MA-induced cardiotoxicity is multifactorial, and related to its sympathomimetic, immunomodulatory, and oxidative inducing properties. The sympathomimetic effect is likely a predominant factor involved in the cardiovascular effect. NE has been reported to be enhanced with MA abuse [94] and propanolol has been noted to antagonize the NE augmentation due to MA [95].

Catecholamine-induced hypoxia and chronic ischemia likely contributes to the cardiotoxic effect of MA, as indicated by the similarity of lesions to those caused by coronary artery ligation. Since the coronary arteries were noted to be nonobstructive in many of these patients, it is plausible that ischemia resulted from the increased myocardial oxygen demand coupled with vasospasm, both due to the hyperadrenergic state induced by amphetamine. Amphetamine-provoked ischemia and myocardial infarction has been described in the literature. Packe *et al.* [96] and Veenstra *et al.* [97] reported the cases of young, previously healthy males who developed chest pain shortly after amphetamine abuse. Although ECGs were consistent with myocardial infarction, the coronary arteriography revealed normal coronary system in all patients.

MA-induced hypercatecholamines can cause cardiotoxicity through increasing the overall level of oxidative stress. Wagner *et al.*'s study noted the production of oxygen-free radicals via autooxidation of catecholamines or their degradation by monoamine oxygenase [81]. Yu *et al.* [98] demonstrated that MA exposure heightened the levels of lipid peroxides in the liver of uninfected and retrovirus-infected mice. These data suggest the potential of MA to cause heart dysfunction through increasing the overall oxidative stress.

MA may damage myocytes directly. Welder [99] and He [100] reported myotoxicity in culture systems devoid of catecholamines. MA can also directly affect cardiac myocytes through augmentation of intracellular Ca^{2+} concentration. The elevated intracellular calcium has been shown to inhibit myosin synthesis and damages the microtubular and actin structural components of cardiomyocytes [101–104].

In addition, amphetamine has been described in the literature to have immunomodulation properties. Yu *et al.* [98] evaluated the immune function alteration due to chronic MA use in normal and retrovirus-infected mice. They found that MA greatly enhanced levels of TNF-α and suppressed Th1 cytokine production, while increasing Th2 cytokine secretion, all of which are known to promote HIV replication and infection [74, 75]. This particular immune effect resembles that of cocaine, as demonstrated by Sepulveda *et al.* [73]. In an in vitro study, MA exposure decreased IL-2 production by T-lymphocytes and suppressed B-lymphocyte proliferation [105]. Iwasa *et al.* demonstrated that rats administered MA-induced thymic and splenic lymphocytes death by apoptosis [106]. Lee *et al.* showed that MA markedly increases the DNA binding activities of redox responsive transcription factors including AP-1 and NF-κB, which increase lipid peroxides and upregulate gene expression for TNF-α [107]. Yu *et al.* [108] investigated the effect of chronic MA exposure on retrovirus-infected mice. Although the TH1 cytokines already reduced by murine AIDS were not further lessened by MA, TNF-α, and lipid peroxides were noted to be increased. Since both oxidative stress and TNF-α have been implicated in cardiotoxicity and exacerbation of viral myocarditis [61, 63, 64, 69], these data suggest that MA contributes to heart disease and progression of viral myocarditis.

Another immunomodulatory effect of MA, shared with cocaine, is the activation of pituitary–adrenal system and the production of increased corticosterone levels [109, 110]. This effect is known to confer an immunosuppressive effect.

Although till date there is limited direct experimental data demonstrating the effect of MA to exacerbate viral myocarditis, MA's effect on raising catecholamines, oxidative stress, and inducing myocarditis coupled with its potent immunomodulatory actions suggest definite potential in augmenting viral cardiotoxicity.

Amphetamine derivatives: MDMA, MDEA, MDA

Amphetamine derivatives such as MDMA (3,4-methylenedioxymethyl-amphvetamine), MDEA (3,4-methylenedioxyethy-amphetamine), and MDA (3,4-methylenedioxyamphetamine) have become widely used recreational drugs. Although their effect on the heart has not been widely studied, toxic myocarditis has been reported by several investigators. Milroy et al. [111] studied the postmortem pathology in seven young white males whose deaths were associated with MDMA or MDEA. Histological analysis revealed changes consistent with myocarditis in five of the seven cases, including contraction band necrosis, myocyte necrosis with surrounding neutrophil, and macrophage inflammatory response. Badon et al. [112] studied the effect of binge administration of MDMA on the heart and the cardiovascular system in rats. They noted that, compared to saline treated controls, MDMA binge produced toxic myocarditis, consisting of multiple foci of inflammation with and without necrosis in both ventricles. The inflammatory infiltrate was predominantly lymphocytic. The degree of cardiac toxicity was proportional to the dosage administered. Jacobs [113] analyzed the hearts of six young people who died suddenly after the chronic abuse of derived amphetamines. In three cases, histopathology revealed dispersed areas of myocyte necrosis with and without influx of granulocytes. The areas of necrosis were randomly distributed and not confined to an area supplied by a specific branch of a coronary artery and the coronary arteries were patent.

One of the mechanisms implicated in MDMA, MDEA, and MDA's induction of myocarditis may be related to its sympathomimetic properties, especially as the pattern of cardiac toxicity resemble those produced by cocaine, MA, and catecholamine-induced myocarditis. Similarly to cocaine and MA, the MA derivatives are known to increase the levels of catecholamines [114]. Experimental work in rats has shown that MDMA potentiates the actions of NE on cardiac muscle [115, 116]. MDMA was documented to inhibit the synaptosomal uptake of NE [117]. Hence, the actions of MDMA resemble those of cocaine and amphetamine/MA.

Similar to cocaine and amphetamine, the MA derivatives have been reported to exert immunomodulation properties. Connor et al. showed that MDMA alters concavalin A-induced Th1- and Th2-type cytokine production and suppresses LPS-induced secretion of TNF-α from diluted whole blood cultures [118]. Experimental studies in rats demonstrated that acute MDMA administration generated a suppression of mitogen-stimulated lymphocyte proliferation and a reduction in circulating lymphocytes [119]. In an in vivo study, whereas in controls LPS challenge produced an increase in circulating TNF-α and IL-1β, MDMA administration significantly impaired secretion following an in vivo LPS challenge [120].

These data suggest the possibility of these drugs to possess immunotoxic properties, which may enhance susceptibility to infections. In addition, the myocarditis generated by these derived amphetamines resemble the pattern of the other sympathomimetic agents.

Thus, although not yet directly investigated, the MA derivatives' immunomodulatory properties coupled with their cardiotoxic effect render them as strong potentials in exacerbating viral myocarditis.

Alcohol

Prolonged and marked consumption of alcohol is known to result in a marked attenuation of host immunity and an increased susceptibility to infection. Alcohol is commonly abused among HIV (+). Lefevre et al. reported that HIV seropositive patients are 82% more likely to consume alcohol compared to the general population [121].

Alcohol is an established cardiotoxin, and can result in myocarditis and cardiomyopathy. Furthermore, alcohol is well known to have immunomodulation properties, which have been documented to significantly exacerbate HIV infection. Alcohol-induced immune dysregulation has been found to result from increased production of proinflammatory cytokines implicated as stimulators of the HIV replication process and responsible for reduction of T-cell response to mitogens, suppression of NK cells function and reduction of granulocyte migration, and macrophage phagocytic activity [122, 123]. Alcohol has also been shown to alter the immune function directly through its action on immunocompetent cells [124, 125], cytokine balance [126], monocytic function [127], or indirectly through alteration of various neuroendocrine hormones [128], and neurotransmitters [129] which regulate the immune system. In a study performed by the Multicenter AIDS Cohort, 209 bisexual and homosexual alcoholics became HIV seropositive within 6 months after initiation of the study, compared to a control group of bisexual/homosexual men who did not become infected in the same time period [130].

Alcohol was observed to affect the balance of Th1/Th2 cytokine release profile, inhibiting Th1 cytokine production and further activating Th2 cells during murine AIDS, further supporting the concept that alcoholics may be predisposed to accelerated immune-dysfunction during HIV infection [131, 132]. Chronic Etoh was demonstrated to act in a synergistic fashion with retrovirus infection to exacerbate elevation of IL-6 and TNF-α [123, 133, 134]. These cytokines are known to be implicated in myocardial dysfunction and in exacerbating viral myocarditis [58, 59, 61, 63, 64]. Furthermore, the hypothalamic–pituitary–adrenal (HPA) axis is disturbed in alcoholics [135]. These data serve to confirm that alcohol has potential to alter host immunity to retroviral infection and accelerate onset of AIDS.

Alcohol consumption was reported to accentuate myocarditis during murine AIDS through its immunomodulatory effects. Sepulveda et al. [136] demonstrated that excessive and prolonged consumption of alcohol accentuated CVB3 cardiotoxicity during murine AIDS. The mice co-infected with retrovirus and CVB3 and treated with alcohol exhibited more severe myocarditis compared to the same group without alcohol. This correlated with the degree of suppression of Th1 cells and with enhancement of Th2 cytokine secretion. This shift of Th1/Th2 known to be caused by HIV virus is further promoted by alcohol, thereby promoting conditions that favor opportunistic viral infection that cause cardiac pathology. The authors postulated two mechanisms for the exacerbation of cardiac pathology produced by alcohol. One possibility may be related to infection with CVB3, leading to synthesis of antibodies to pathogen that cross-react with cardiac myosin, inducing myocarditis. Another possibility may be related to CVB3-induced myocardial damage, with concomitant release of myosin by the myocyte cells, which may be engulfed by dendritic cells thus activating autoreactive T cells.

Cocaethylene

Cocaine and alcohol are often abused in combination for a more prolonged euphoria, especially among HIV seropositive individuals [137]. The combination of the two drugs is more toxic than either drug alone [138] and there have been several medical reports on sudden cardiac death resulting from combined alcohol and cocaine abuse [139]. Cocaethylene is a pharmacological metabolite of cocaine, which is generated in the liver by trans-esterification of cocaine with ethanol [140]. Cocaethylene has immunomodulatory properties. Stein showed that prolonged and excessive abuse of cocaine in combination with alcohol produces marked alteration of host immunity and increased susceptibility to HIV infection [137].

The immunomodulatory effect of cocaethylene has been documented to result in exacerbation of myocarditis in HIV seropositive subjects. Liu et al. [141] showed that cocaethylene administration exacerbated CVB3 and CMV cardiomyopathy during murine AIDS. The severity of myocarditis was more remarkable with the addition to cocaethylene. This effect has been documented with cocaine [73]. Their data showed that the basis of their results is due to enhanced shifting of cytokine balance through suppression of Th1 response and enhancement of Th2 response, an immunomodulatory phenomenon known to be mediated by HIV, facilitating more pronounced CVB3- or CMV-induced myocarditis. Furthermore, the data showed that cocaethylene significantly increased oxidative stress, indicated by the increased lipid peroxides in the liver of retrovirus and CMV-infected mice. This mechanism may be playing a role in promoting viral myocarditis since there is strong evidence for the adverse role of oxidative stress in heart failure in animals and humans [142, 143].

Clozapine

Clozapine is an atypical antipsychotic agent, which is considered to be superior to the typical antipsychotic drugs and is used to treat refractory schizophrenia [144–147]. Clozapine's mechanism of action is mediated through its effects at dopamine receptors, and additionally antagonizes adrenergic, cholinergic, histaminergic, and serotoninergic receptors [148].

Clozapine has been significantly linked with the occurrence of myocarditis and cardiomyopathy. There have been several case reports documenting the incidence of myocarditis in association with use of clozapine [145, 146,149–153]. Necropsy results among them demonstrated lymphocytic infiltrates with myocytolysis [149, 152], eosinophilic infiltrates [154], and mixed infiltrates [149, 152, 155].

One mechanism implicated in the production of myocarditis is related to the hypercatecholamine state generated by clozapine. Several studies have shown that clozapine results in marked increases in NE levels in animal models [156–158] and in patients [159–162]. Malek *et al.*'s study [158] demonstrated the contributory role of catecholamines in clozapine-induced myocarditis. Their results confirmed the prior findings that clozapine induces myocarditis in a dose-related fashion and noted that clozapine stimulates a marked rise in serum catecholamines, which correlated with the severity of myocarditis. The histopathology was similar to prior studies, including cardiac necrosis and cellular infiltration. In addition, they found that propanolol reduced the cardiotoxic effect of clozapine, as previously demonstrated with cocaine [47] and with catecholamines [48]. This data supports the hypothesis that the hyperadrenergic state created by clozapine promotes the myocarditis.

Moreover, clozapine has immunomodulatory properties, which may disturb the host immune response and increase susceptibility to infection. Clozapine treatment was shown to increase plasma levels of cytokines and cytokine receptors that are pivotal immune mediators. There are consistent reports on increases in plasma levels of TNF-α, soluble TNF-receptor p55 (TNF-Rp55), TNF-Rp75, and soluble interleukin-2 receptor [163, 164]. In an in vitro study, clozapine-induced PBMC proliferation and secretion of IL-6, sIL-2r, and serum IgG levels [165]. Clozapine was also shown to increase the serum concentration of endogenous anti-inflammatory agents such as IL-1RA [166]. These immunomodulatory effects, especially the

increased TNF-α and IL-6, which are known to cause heart damage and mediate exacerbation of viral myocarditis, may contribute to promoting progression of viral myocarditis.

These data raise the possibility of clozapine, through its disturbing effect of the immune system and enhancing effect on catecholamines, to exacerbate viral myocarditis.

Opiates

Opiates make up a collection of drugs that include opium, morphine, and heroin. It is now widely recognized that opiates are immunomodulatory and enhance susceptibility to various infectious agents in both humans and animals. Opiate users have been observed to be at higher risk for infections, including pulmonary disease, endocarditis, hepatitis, sexually transmitted diseases, skeletal infections, cellulitis, and HIV [167–169]. Approximately 30% of patients with AIDS have a history of opiate drug [170].

Opiate drug abusers become highly susceptible to HIV not only because of contaminated shared needles, associated malnutrition with weight loss but also because of associated immunosuppression. Opioids have been implicated as co-factors in the immunopathogenesis of HIV [171–174]. Studies have shown that opiates markedly affect immune responses, both in vivo and in vitro. Morphine and methadone was shown to activate and enhance HIV replication in human immune cells [175, 176].

Opiates's immunomodulatory effects have been shown to be exerted through direct and indirect actions. Opiates directly affects the immune system through opioid receptors on immune cells. In vitro studies of immune cells have shown reduced receptor-mediated phagocytosis, chemotaxis, and cytokine and chemokine production [174, 177–181]. Immunosuppression has been observed through increasing the production of immunosuppressive cytokines such as transforming growth factor β (TGF-β) [182, 183] and through suppression of NK cells [184]. Opiates have been demonstrated to also alter the HPA axis and increases the serum levels of glucocorticoid and corticosterone, which are known to suppress several immune parameters and increase susceptibility to infection [185, 186]. The opioid immunomodulatory effect has been demonstrated to be reversed with opioid receptor antagonists such as naltrexone [175, 187] and methylnaltrexone [170].

Opiates have been shown to increase susceptibility to HIV infection. Animal studies demonstrated that morphine treatment results in sustained elevation of CD4/CD8 cells and heroin addicts have increased CD4/T cells. CD4 cells are known to be target cells for HIV, which could result in more targets for HIV to infect, altering the immune status and facilitating susceptibility to infection.

These data provide evidence for opiates' immunomodulatory effect and thus their potential to potentiate a variety of infections. It seems reasonable to postulate that opiates would likely promote progression of viral myocarditis as well via its immunomodulatory properties. However, further studies regarding this direct effect are necessary.

References

1 Kearney MT, Cotton JM, Richardson PJ, Shah AM. Viral myocarditis and dilated cardiomyopathy: mechanisms, manifestations, and management. Postgrad Med J 2001;77(903):4–10.

2 Barbaro G, Di Lorenzo G, Grisorio B, Barbarini G. Incidence of dilated cardiomyopathy and detection of HIV in myocardial cells of HIV-positive patients. Gruppo Italiano per lo Studio Cardiologico dei Pazienti Affetti da AIDS. N Engl J Med 1998;339(16):1093–9.

3 Larrat EP, Zierler S, Mayer K. Cocaine use and heterosexual exposure to human immunodeficiency virus. Epidemiology 1994;5(4):398–403.

4 Burian J, Buser P, Eriksson U. Myocarditis: the immunologist's view on pathogenesis and treatment. Swiss Med Wkly 2005;135(25–26):359–64.

5 Chen Y. Cocaine and catecholamine enhance inflammatory cell retention in coronary circulation of mice by upregulation of adhesion molecules. Am J Physiol Heart Circ Physiol 2005;288(5):2323–31.

6 Kloner RA, Hale S, Alker K, Rezkalla S. The effects of acute and chronic cocaine use on the heart. Circulation 1992;85(2):407–19.

7 Larrat EP, Zierler S. Entangled epidemics: cocaine use and HIV disease. J Psychoactive Drugs 1993;25(3): 207–21.

8 Soodini G, Morgan JP. Can cocaine abuse exacerbate the cardiac toxicity of human immunodeficiency virus? Clin Cardiol 2001;24(3):177–81.

9 Rump AF, Theisohn M, Klaus W. The pathophysiology of cocaine cardiotoxicity. Forensic Sci Int 1995;71(2): 103–15.

10 Virmani R, Robinowitz M, Smialek JE, Smyth DF. Cardiovascular effects of cocaine: an autopsy study of 40 patients. Am Heart J 1988;115(5):1068–76.

11 Peng SK, French WJ, Pelikan PC. Direct cocaine cardiotoxicity demonstrated by endomyocardial biopsy. Arch Pathol Lab Med 1989;113(8):842–5.

12 Tazelaar HD, Karch SB, Stephens BG, Billingham ME. Cocaine and the Heart. Human Pathology 1987;18:195–199.

13 Trouve R, Nahas GG, Manger WM, Vinyard C, Goldberg S. Interactions of nimodipine and cocaine on endogenous catecholamines in the squirrel monkey. Proc Soc Exp Biol Med 1990;193(3):171–5.

14 Nahas G, Trouve R, Manger WM, Vinyard C, Goldberg S. Cocaine toxicity and endogenous catecholamines. 1988:457–462.

15 Karch SB, Billingham, ME. The Pathology and Etiology of Cocaine-Induced Heart Disease. Arch Pathol Lab Med 1988;112:225–230.

16 Chiueh CC, Kopin IJ. Centrally mediated release by cocaine of endogenous epinephrine and norepinephrine from the sympathoadrenal medullary system of unanesthetized rats. J Pharmacol Exp Ther 1978;205(1):148–54.

17 Rump AF, Klaus W. Evidence for norepinephrine cardiotoxicity mediated by superoxide anion radicals in isolated rabbit hearts. Naunyn Schmiedebergs Arch Pharmacol 1994;349(3):295–300.

18 Noda M, Kawano O, Uchida O, Sawabe T, Saito G. Myocarditis induced by sympathomimetic amines. I. Jpn Circ J 1970;34(1):7–12.

19 Downing SE, Chen V. Myocardial injury following endogenous catecholamine release in rabbits. J Mol Cell Cardiol 1985;17(4):377–87.

20 Wexler BC, Judd JT, Kittinger GW. Myocardial necrosis induced by isoproterenol in rats. Changes in serum protein, lipoprotein, lipids and glucose during active necrosis and repair in arteriosclerotic and nonarteriosclerotic animals. Angiology 1968;19(12):665–82.

21 Maling HM, Highman B, Thompson EC. Some similar effects after large doses of catecholamines and myocardial infarction in dogs. Am J Cardiol 1960;5:628–33.

22 Handforth CP. Isoproterenol-induced myocardial infarction in animals. Arch Pathol 1962;73:161–5.

23 Van Vliet PD, Burchell HB, Titus JL. Focal myocarditis associated with pheochromocytoma. N Engl J Med 1966;274(20):1102–8.

24 Watkins DB. Pheochromocytoma: a review of the literature. J Chronic Dis 1957;6(5):510–27.

25 Kline IK. Myocardial alterations associated with pheochromocytomas. Am J Pathol 1961;38:539–51.

26 Szakacs JE, Cannon A. ʟ-Norepinephrine myocarditis. Am J Clin Pathol 1958;30(5):425–34.

27 Szakacs JE, Mehlman B. Pathologic changes induced by 1-norepineprine: quantitative aspects. Am J Cardiol 1960;5:619–27.

28 Haft JI. Cardiovascular injury induced by sympathetic catecholamines. Progress Cardiovasc Dis 1974; XVIII(1):73–85.

29 Rona G, Zsoter T, Chappel C, Gaudry R. Myocardial lesions, circulatory and electrocardiographic changes produced by isoproterenol in the dog. Rev Can Biol 1959;18(1):83–94.

30 Rona G, Kahn DS, Chappel CI. Studies on infarct-like myocardial necrosis produced by isoproterenol: a review. Rev Can Biol 1963;22:241–55.

31 Simons M, Downing SE. Coronary vasoconstriction and catecholamine cardiomyopathy. Am Heart J 1985;109(2):297–304.

32 Tritthart H, Volkmann R, Weiss R, Fleckenstein A. Calcium-mediated action potentials in mammalian myocardium. Alteration of membrane response as induced by changes of Cae or by promoters and inhibitors of transmembrane Ca inflow. Naunyn Schmiedebergs Arch Pharmacol 1973;280(3):239-52.

33 Opie LH, Walpoth B, Barsacchi R. Calcium and catecholamines: relevance to cardiomyopathies and significance in therapeutic strategies. J Mol Cell Cardiol 1985;17(suppl 2):21–34.

34 Raab W. Myocardial electrolyte derangement: crucial feature of pluricausal, so-called coronary, heart disease (dysionic cardiopathy). Ann N Y Acad Sci 1969;147(17):627–86.

35 Lehr D. Tissue electrolyte alteration in disseminated myocardial necrosis. Ann N Y Acad Sci 1969;156(1):344–78.

36 Lehr D, Chau R, Kaplan J. Prevention of experimental myocardial necrosis by electrolyte solutions. Recent Adv Stud Cardiac Struct Metab 1972;1:684–98.

37 Yates JC, Beamish RE, Dhalla NS. Ventricular dysfunction and necrosis produced by adrenochrome metabolite of epinephrine: relation to pathogenesis of catecholamine cardiomyopathy. Am Heart J 1981;102(2):210–21.

38 Yates JC, Dhalla NS. Induction of necrosis and failure in the isolated perfused rat heart with oxidized isoproterenol. J Mol Cell Cardiol 1975;7(11):807–16.

39 Dhalla NS, Yates JC, Lee SL, Singh A. Functional and subcellular changes in the isolated rat heart perfused with oxidized isoproterenol. J Mol Cell Cardiol 1978;10(1):31–41.

40 Csapo Z, Dusek J, Rona G. Early alterations of the cardiac muscle cells in isoproterenol-induced necrosis. Arch Pathol 1972;93(4):356–65.

41 Downing SE, Lee JC. Effects of insulin on experimental catecholamine cardiomyopathy. Am J Pathol 1978;93(2):339–52.

42 Norkin SA, Griffith E, Dubin IN, Czernobilsky B. Effect Of Albumin And Fatty Acids On Cellular Growth In Vitro. Arch Pathol 1965;80:273–7.

43 Hoak JC, Connor WE, Eckstein JW, Warner ED. Fatty Acid-Induced Thrombosis And Death: Mechanisms And Prevention. J Lab Clin Med 1964;63:791–800.

44 Kammermeier H, Ober M. Essential contribution of thrombocytes to the occurrence of catecholamine-induced cardiac necroses. J Mol Cell Cardiol 1985; 17(4):371–6.

45 Haft JI, Gershengorn K, Kranz PD, Oestreicher R. Protection against epinephrine-induced myocardial necrosis by drugs that inhibit platelet aggregation. Am J Cardiol 1972;30(8):838–43.

46 Haft JI, Kranz PD, Albert FJ, Fani K. Intravascular platelet aggregation in the heart induced by norepinephrine. Microscopic studies. Circulation 1972;46(4):698–708.

47 Wang JF, Zhang J, Min JY et al. Cocaine enhances myocarditis induced by encephalomyocarditis virus in murine model. Am J Physiol Heart Circ Physiol 2002;282(3):H956–63.

48 Wang JF, Meissner A. Malek, S et al. Propranolol ameliorates and epinephrine exacerbates progression of acute and chronic viral myocarditis. Am J Physiol Heart Circ Physiol 2005;289(4):H1577–83.

49 Tominaga M, Matsumori A, Okada I, Yamada T, Kawai C. Beta-blocker treatment of dilated cardiomyopathy. Beneficial effect of carteolol in mice. Circulation 1991;83(6):2021–8.

50 Nishio R, Shioi T, Sasayama S, Matsumori A. Carvedilol increases the production of interleukin-12 and interferon-gamma and improves the survival of mice infected with the encephalomyocarditis virus. J Am Coll Cardiol 2003;41(2):340–5.

51 Wang JF, Ren X, DeAngelis J et al. Differential patterns of cocaine-induced organ toxicity in murine heart versus liver. Exp Biol Med (Maywood) 2001;226(1):52–60.

52 Wang Y, Huang DS, Watson RR. In vivo and in vitro cocaine modulation on production of cytokines in C57BL/6 mice. Life Sci 1994;54(6):401–11.

53 Van Dyke C, Stesin A, Jones R, Chuntharapai A, Seaman W. Cocaine increases natural killer cell activity. J Clin Invest 1986;77(4):1387–90.

54 Raymond RJ, Dehmer GJ, Theoharides TC, Deliargyris EN. Elevated interleukin-6 levels in patients with asymptomatic left ventricular systolic dysfunction. Am Heart J 2001;141(3):435–8.

55 Tsutamoto T, Hisanaga T, Wada A et al. Interleukin-6 spillover in the peripheral circulation increases with the

severity of heart failure, and the high plasma level of interleukin-6 is an important prognostic predictor in patients with congestive heart failure. J Am Coll Cardiol 1998;31(2):391–8.

56 Birks EJ, Yacoub MH. The role of nitric oxide and cytokines in heart failure. Coron Artery Dis 1997;8(6):389–402.

57 Kubota T, Miyagishima M, Alvarez RJ et al. Expression of proinflammatory cytokines in the failing human heart: comparison of recent-onset and end-stage congestive heart failure. J Heart Lung Transplant 2000;19(9):819–24.

58 Deng MC, Erren M, Lutgen A et al. Interleukin-6 correlates with hemodynamic impairment during dobutamine administration in chronic heart failure. Int J Cardiol 1996;57(2):129–34.

59 Tanaka T, Kanda T, McManus BM et al. Overexpression of interleukin-6 aggravates viral myocarditis: impaired increase in tumor necrosis factor-alpha. J Mol Cell Cardiol 2001;33(9):1627–35.

60 Matsumori A, Yamada T, Kawai C. Immunomodulating therapy in viral myocarditis: effects of tumour necrosis factor, interleukin 2 and anti-interleukin-2 receptor antibody in an animal model. Eur Heart J 1991;12(suppl D):203–5.

61 Yamada T, Matsumori A, Sasayama S. Therapeutic effect of anti-tumor necrosis factor-alpha antibody on the murine model of viral myocarditis induced by encephalomyocarditis virus. Circulation 1994;89(2):846–51.

62 Young LH, Joag SV, Zheng LM et al. Perforin-mediated myocardial damage in acute myocarditis. Lancet 1990;336(8722):1019–21.

63 Huber SA, Sartini D. Roles of tumor necrosis factor alpha (TNF-alpha) and the p55 TNF receptor in CD1d induction and coxsackievirus B3-induced myocarditis. J Virol 2005;79(5):2659–65.

64 Lane JR, Neumann DA, Lafond-Walker A, Herskowitz A, Rose NR. Role of IL-1 and tumor necrosis factor in coxsackie virus-induced autoimmune myocarditis. J Immunol 1993;151(3):1682–90.

65 Vyakarnam A, McKeating J, Meager A, Beverley PC. Tumour necrosis factors (alpha, beta) induced by HIV-1 in peripheral blood mononuclear cells potentiate virus replication. Aids 1990;4(1):21–7.

66 Clouse KA, Powell D, Washington I et al. Monokine regulation of human immunodeficiency virus-1 expression in a chronically infected human T cell clone. J Immunol 1989;142(2):431–8.

67 Israel N, Hazan U, Alcami J et al. Tumor necrosis factor stimulates transcription of HIV-1 in human T lymphocytes, independently and synergistically with mitogens. J Immunol 1989;143(12):3956–60.

68 Folks TM, Clouse KA, Justement J et al. Tumor necrosis factor alpha induces expression of human immunodeficiency virus in a chronically infected T-cell clone. Proc Natl Acad Sci U S A 1989;86(7):2365–8.

69 Matsuyama T, Hamamoto Y, Soma G, Mizuno D, Yamamoto N, Kobayashi N. Cytocidal effect of tumor necrosis factor on cells chronically infected with human immunodeficiency virus (HIV): enhancement of HIV replication. J Virol 1989;63(6):2504–9.

70 Kobayashi N, Hamamoto Y, Koyanagi Y, Chen IS, Yamamoto N. Effect of interleukin-1 on the augmentation of human immunodeficiency virus gene expression. Biochem Biophys Res Commun 1989;165(2):715–21.

71 Matsuyama T, Yoshiyama H, Hamamoto Y et al. Enhancement of HIV replication and giant cell formation by tumor necrosis factor. AIDS Res Hum Retroviruses 1989;5(2):139–46.

72 Peterson PK, Gekker G, Chao CC, Schut R, Molitor TW, Balfour HH, Jr. Cocaine potentiates HIV-1 replication in human peripheral blood mononuclear cell cocultures. Involvement of transforming growth factor-beta. J Immunol 1991;146(1):81–4.

73 Sepulveda RT, Jiang S, Beischel J, Bellamy WT, Watson RR. Cocaine injection and coxsackievirus B3 infection increase heart disease during murine AIDS. J Acquir Immune Defic Syndr 2000;25 Suppl 1:S19–26.

74 Shearer GM, Clerici M. Abnormalities of immune regulation in human immunodeficiency virus infection. Pediatr Res 1993;33(suppl 1):S71–4; discussion S74–5.

75 Clerici M, Sarin A, Coffman RL et al. Type 1/type 2 cytokine modulation of T-cell programmed cell death as a model for human immunodeficiency virus pathogenesis. Proc Natl Acad Sci U S A 1994;91(25):11811–5.

76 Munck A, Guyre PM, Holbrook NJ. Physiological functions of glucocorticoids in stress and their relation to pharmacological actions. Endocr Rev 1984;5(1):25–44.

77 Watzl B, Watson RR. Immunomodulation by cocaine—a neuroendocrine mediated response. Life Sci 1990;46(19):1319–29.

78 Moldow RL, Fischman AJ. Cocaine induced secretion of ACTH, beta-endorphin, and corticosterone. Peptides 1987;8(5):819–22.

79 Rotheram-Borus MJ, Luna GC, Marotta T, Kelly H. Going nowhere fast: methamphetamine use and HIV infection. NIDA Res Monogr 1994;143:155–82.

80 Ruth JA, Grunewald GL, Rutledge CO. Conformationally defined adrenergic agents. III: The importance of compartmentation in the release of norepinephrine from rat atria by endo- and exo-2-methylaminobenzobicyclo-[2.2.2]octene, conformationally defined analogs of methamphetamine. J Pharmacol Exp Ther 1978; 204(3):615–24.

81 Wagner GC, Ricaurte GA, Seiden, LS, Schuster CR, Miller RJ, Westley J. Long-lasting depletions of striatal dopamine and loss of dopamine uptake sites following repeated administration of methamphetamine. Brain Res 1980;181(1):151–60.

82 Varner KJ, Ogden BA, Delcarpio J, Meleg-Smith S. Cardiovascular responses elicited by the "binge" administration of methamphetamine. J Pharmacol Exp Ther 2002;301(1):152–9.

83 Derlet RW, Horowitz BZ. Cardiotoxic drugs. Emerg Med Clin North Am 1995;13(4):771–91.

84 Citron BP, Halpern M, McCarron M *et al*. Necrotizing angiitis associated with drug abuse. N Engl J Med 1970;283(19):1003–11.

85 Swalwell CI, Davis GG. Methamphetamine as a risk factor for acute aortic dissection. J Forensic Sci 1999;44(1):23–6.

86 Smith HJ, Roche AH, Jausch MF, Herdson PB. Cardiomyopathy associated with amphetamine administration. Am Heart J 1976;91(6):792–7.

87 Kalant H, Kalant OJ. Death in amphetamine users: causes and rates. Can Med Assoc J 1975;112(3):299–304.

88 Zalis EG, Lundberg GD, Knutson RA. The pathophysiology of acute amphetamine poisoning with pathologic correlation. J Pharmacol Exp Ther 1967;158(1):115–27.

89 Kaiho M, Ishiyama I. Morphological study of acute myocardial lesions experimentally induced by methamphetamine. Nippon Hoigaku Zasshi 1989;43(6):460–8.

90 He SY, Matoba R, Fujitani N, Sodesaki K, Onishi S. Cardiac muscle lesions associated with chronic administration of methamphetamine in rats. Am J Forensic Med Pathol 1996;17(2):155–62.

91 Tanaka Y, Nishi T, Chin M *et al*. A case of hypertrophic cardiomyopathy associated with amphetamine abuse. Nippon Naika Gakkai Zasshi 1989;78(7):944–8.

92 Hong R, Matsuyama E, Nur K. Cardiomyopathy associated with the smoking of crystal methamphetamine. JAMA 1991;265(9):1152–4.

93 Rajs J, Falconer B. Cardiac lesions in intravenous drug addicts. Forensic Sci Int 1979;13(3):193–209.

94 Uchima E, Ogura Y, Hiraga Y, Shikata I. Relationship between methamphetamine toxicity and catecholamine levels in heart and brain of mice. Nippon Hoigaku Zasshi 1983;37(3):198–208.

95 Erdo SL, Kiss B, Rosdy B, Szporny L, In vivo interaction between amphetamine and beta-adrenoceptor blockers: effects on the release of norepinephrine from mouse heart. Pharmacol Res Commun 1982;14(7):613–9.

96 Packe GE, Garton MJ, Jennings K. Acute myocardial infarction caused by intravenous amphetamine abuse. Br Heart J 1990;64(1):23–4.

97 Veenstra J, van der Wieken LR, Schuilenburg RM. Myocardial infarct following use of amphetamine derivatives. Ned Tijdschr Geneeskd 1990;134(23):1150–1.

98 Yu Q, Zhang D, Walston M, Zhang J, Liu Y, Watson RR. Chronic methamphetamine exposure alters immune function in normal and retrovirus-infected mice. Int Immunopharmacol 2002;2(7):951–62.

99 Welder AA. A primary culture system of postnatal rat heart cells for the study of cocaine and methamphetamine toxicity. Toxicol Lett 1992;60(2):183–96.

100 He SY. Methamphetamine-induced toxicity in cultured adult rat cardiomyocytes. Nippon Hoigaku Zasshi 1995;49(3):175–86.

101 Salomon R. The effect of amphetamines on culture myotubes: selective inhibition of protein synthesis. Life Sci 1978;23(19):1941–9.

102 Guo JX, Jacobson SL, Brown DL. Rearrangement of tubulin, actin, and myosin in cultured ventricular cardiomyocytes of the adult rat. Cell Motil Cytoskeleton 1986;6(3):291–304.

103 Keith C, DiPaola M, Maxfield FR, Shelanski ML. Microinjection of Ca++-calmodulin causes a localized depolymerization of microtubules. J Cell Biol 1983;97(6):1918–24.

104 Schliwa M, Euteneuer U, Bulinski JC, Izant JG. Calcium lability of cytoplasmic microtubules and its modulation by microtubule-associated proteins. Proc Natl Acad Sci U S A 1981;78(2):1037–41.

105 House RV, Thomas PT, Bhargava HN. Comparison of immune functional parameters following in vitro exposure to natural and synthetic amphetamines. Immunopharmacol Immunotoxicol 1994;16(1):1–21.

106 Iwasa M, Maeno Y, Inoue H, Koyama H, Matoba R. Induction of apoptotic cell death in rat thymus and spleen after a bolus injection of methamphetamine. Int J Legal Med 1996;109(1):23–8.

107 Lee YW, Hennig B, Yao J, Toborek M. Methamphetamine induces AP-1 and NF-kappaB binding and transactivation in human brain endothelial cells. J Neurosci Res 2001;66(4):583–91.

108 Yu Q, Montes S, Larson DF, Watson RR. Effects of chronic methamphetamine exposure on heart function in uninfected and retrovirus-infected mice. Life Sci 2002;71(8):953–65.

109 Swerdlow NR, Koob GF, Cador M, Lorang M, Hauger RL. Pituitary-adrenal axis responses to acute amphetamine in the rat. Pharmacol Biochem Behav 1993;45(3):629–37.

110 Knych ET, Eisenberg RM. Effect of amphetamine on plasma corticosterone in the conscious rat. Neuroendocrinology 1979;29(2):110–8.

111 Milroy CM, Clark JC, Forrest AR. Pathology of deaths associated with "ecstasy" and "eve" misuse. J Clin Pathol 1996;49(2):149–53.

112 Badon LA, Hicks A, Lord K, Ogden BA, Meleg-Smith S. Varner KJ. Changes in cardiovascular responsiveness and cardiotoxicity elicited during binge administration of Ecstasy. J Pharmacol Exp Ther 2002;302(3):898–907.

113 Jacobs W. Fatal amphetamine-associated cardiotoxicity and its medicolegal implications. Am J Forensic Med Pathol 2006;27(2):156–60.

114 Ferdinand KC. Substance abuse and hypertension. J Clin Hypertens (Greenwich) 2000;2(1):37–40.

115 Al-Sahli W, Ahmad H, Kheradmand F, Connolly C, Docherty JR. Effects of methylenedioxymethamphetamine on noradrenaline-evoked contractions of rat right ventricle and small mesenteric artery. Eur J Pharmacol 2001;422(1-3):169–74.

116 Cleary L, Buber R, Docherty JR. Effects of amphetamine derivatives and cathinone on noradrenaline-evoked contractions of rat right ventricle. Eur J Pharmacol 2002;451(3):303–8.

117 Steele TD, Nichols DE, Yim GK. Stereochemical effects of 3,4-methylenedioxymethamphetamine (MDMA) and related amphetamine derivatives on inhibition of uptake of [3H]monoamines into synaptosomes from different regions of rat brain. Biochem Pharmacol 1987;36(14):2297–303.

118 Connor TJ, Kelly JP, Leonard BE. An assessment of the acute effects of the serotonin releasers methylenedioxymethamphetamine, methylenedioxyamphetamine and fenfluramine on immunity in rats. Immunopharmacology 2000;46(3):223–35.

119 Connor TJ, McNamara MG, Finn D et al. Acute 3,4-methylenedioxymethamphetamine(MDMA) administration produces a rapid and sustained suppression of immune function in the rat. Immunopharmacology 1998;38(3):253–60.

120 Connor TJ, Kelly JP, McGee M, Leonard BE. Methylenedioxymethamphetamine (MDMA; Ecstasy) suppresses IL-1beta and TNF-alpha secretion following an in vivo lipopolysaccharide challenge. Life Sci 2000;67(13):1601–12.

121 Lefevre F, O'Leary B, Moran M et al. Alcohol consumption among HIV-infected patients. J Gen Intern Med 1995;10(8):458–60.

122 Wang Y, Watson RR. Chronic ethanol consumption prior to retrovirus infection alters cytokine production by thymocytes during murine AIDS. Alcohol 1994; 11(5):361–5.

123 Wang Y, Watson RR. Chronic ethanol consumption before retrovirus infection is a cofactor in the development of immune dysfunction during murine AIDS. Alcohol Clin Exp Res 1994;18(4):976–81.

124 Jerrells TR, Sibley D. Effects of ethanol on cellular immunity to facultative intracellular bacteria. Alcohol Clin Exp Res 1995;19(1):11–6.

125 Lopez MC, Watzl B, Colombo LL, Watson RR. Alterations in mouse Peyer's patch lymphocyte phenotype after ethanol consumption. Alcohol 1997;14(2):107–10.

126 Ahluwalia B, Wesley B, Adeyiga O, Smith DM, Da-Silva A, Rajguru S. Alcohol modulates cytokine secretion and synthesis in human fetus: an in vivo and in vitro study. Alcohol 2000;21(3):207–13.

127 Chen H, George I, Sperber K. Effect of ethanol on monocytic function in human immunodeficiency virus type 1 infection. Clin Diagn Lab Immunol 1998;5(6):790–8.

128 Doll R. Epidemiological evidence of the effects of behaviour and the environment on the risk of human cancer. Recent Results Cancer Res 1998;154:3–21.

129 De Witte P. The role of neurotransmitters in alcohol dependence: animal research. Alcohol Alcohol Suppl 1996;1:13–6.

130 Penkower L, Dew MA, Kingsley L et al. Behavioral, health and psychosocial factors and risk for HIV infection among sexually active homosexual men: the Multicenter AIDS Cohort Study. Am J Public Health 1991;81(2):194–6.

131 Wang JY, Liang B, Watson RR. Alcohol consumption alters cytokine release during murine AIDS. Alcohol 1997;14(2):155–9.

132 Cohen DA. Alcohol abuse as a possible cofactor in the progression of acquired immune deficiency syndrome: do Th1 and Th2 helper T cells subsets play a role. In: Watson RR, ed. *Alcohol Drugs of Abuse and Immunomodulation*. CRC Press, Boca Raton 1995:2113–228.

133 Wang Y, Huang DS, Giger PT, Watson RR. Ethanol-induced modulation of cytokine production by splenocytes during murine retrovirus infection causing murine AIDS. Alcohol Clin Exp Res 1993;17(5):1035–9.

134 Wang Y, Huang DS, Giger PT, Watson RR. Dietary ethanol-induced modification of cytokine release induced by LP-BM5 retrovirus causing murine AIDS. Alcohol Clin Exp Res 1993;17:1035–1040.

135 Wang YW. The role of alcohol on endocrine-immune interactions. In: Watson RR, ed. *Drugs of Abuse and Immunomodulation*. CRC Press, Boca Raton 1995:203–28.

136 Sepulveda RT, Jiang S, Besselsen DG, Watson RR, Alcohol consumption during murine acquired immunodeficiency syndrome accentuates heart pathology due to coxsackievirus. Alcohol Alcohol 2002;37(2):157–63.

137 Stein MD. Medical consequences of substance abuse. Psychiatr Clin North Am 1999;22(2):351–70.

138 Uszenski RT, Gillis RA, Schaer GL, Analouei AR, Kuhn FE. Additive myocardial depressant effects of cocaine and ethanol. Am Heart J 1992;124(5):1276–83.

139 Hearn WL, Flynn DD, Hime GW *et al.* Cocaethylene: a unique cocaine metabolite displays high affinity for the dopamine transporter. J Neurochem 1991;56(2):698–701.

140 Dean RA, Harper ET, Dumaual N, Stoeckel DA, Bosron WF. Effects of ethanol on cocaine metabolism: formation of cocaethylene and norcocaethylene. Toxicol Appl Pharmacol 1992;117(1):1–8.

141 Liu Y, Montes S, Zhang D *et al.* Cocaethylene and heart disease during murine AIDS. Int Immunopharmacol 2002;2(1):139–50.

142 Dhalla AK, Hill MF, Singal PK. Role of oxidative stress in transition of hypertrophy to heart failure. J Am Coll Cardiol 1996;28(2):506–14.

143 Ghatak A, Brar MJ, Agarwal A *et al.* Oxy free radical system in heart failure and therapeutic role of oral vitamin E. Int J Cardiol 1996;57(2):119–27.

144 Conley RR. Optimizing treatment with clozapine. J Clin Psychiatry 1998;59(suppl 3):44–8.

145 Kakar P, Millar-Craig M, Kamaruddin H, Burn S, Loganathan S. Clozapine induced myocarditis: A rare but fatal complication. Intl J Cardiol 2006;112(2): e5–6.

146 Merrill DB, Dec GW, Goff DC. Adverse cardiac effects associated with clozapine. J Clin Psychopharmacol 2005;25(1):32–41.

147 Green AI, Tohen M, Patel JK *et al.* Clozapine in the treatment of refractory psychotic mania. Am J Psychiatry 2000;157(6):982–6.

148 Owens DG. Adverse effects of antipsychotic agents. Do newer agents offer advantages? Drugs 1996;51(6):895–930.

149 Hagg S, Spigset O, Bate A, Soderstrom TG. Myocarditis related to clozapine treatment. J Clin Psychopharmacol 2001;21(4):382–8.

150 Merrill DB, Ahmari SE, Bradford JM, Lieberman JA. Myocarditis during clozapine treatment. Am J Psychiatry 2006;163(2):204–8.

151 Tanner MA, Culling W. Clozapine associated dilated cardiomyopathy. Postgrad Med J 2003;79(933):412–3.

152 Killian JG, Kerr K, Lawrence C, Celermajer DS. Myocarditis and cardiomyopathy associated with clozapine. Lancet 1999;354(9193):1841–5.

153 Bandelow B, Degner D, Kreusch U, Ruther E. Myocarditis under therapy with clozapine. Schizophr Res 1995;17(3):293–4.

154 Jensen VE, Gotzsche O. Allergic myocarditis in clozapine treatment. Ugeskr Laeger 1994;156(28):4151–2.

155 La Grenade L, Graham D, Trontell A. Myocarditis and cardiomyopathy associated with clozapine use in the United States. N Engl J Med 2001;345(3):224–5.

156 Baldessarini, RJ, Huston-Lyons D, Campbell A, Marsh E, Cohen BM. Do central antiadrenergic actions contribute to the atypical properties of clozapine? Br J Psychiatry Suppl 1992(17): p. 12-6.

157 Gross G, Schumann HJ. Enhancement of noradrenaline release from rat cerebral cortex by neuroleptic drugs. Naunyn Schmiedebergs Arch Pharmacol 1980; 315(2):103–9.

158 Malek S *et al. Animal Model of Clozapine-Induced Myocarditis: Role of Elevated Catecholamines.* 2006, Personal Communication.

159 Breier A, Buchanan RW, Waltrip RW, 2nd, Listwak S, Holmes C, Goldstein DS. The effect of clozapine on plasma norepinephrine: relationship to clinical efficacy. Neuropsychopharmacology 1994;10(1): 1–7.

160 Pickar D, Owen RR, Litman RE, Konicki E, Gutierrez R, Rapaport MH. Clinical and biologic response to clozapine in patients with schizophrenia. Crossover comparison with fluphenazine. Arch Gen Psychiatry 1992;49(5):345–53.

161 Ackenheil M. Clozapine—pharmacokinetic investigations and biochemical effects in man. Psychopharmacology (Berl) 1989;99(suppl):S32–7.

162 Green AI, Alam MY, Sobieraj JT *et al.* Clozapine response and plasma catecholamines and their metabolites. Psychiatry Res 1993;46(2):139–49.

163 Pollmacher T, Hinze-Selch D, Mullington J. Effects of clozapine on plasma cytokine and soluble cytokine receptor levels. J Clin Psychopharmacol 1996;16(5):403–9.

164 Pollmacher T, Fenzel T, Mullington J, Hinze-Selch D. The influence of clozapine treatment on plasma granulocyte colony-stimulating (G-CSF) levels. Pharmacopsychiatry 1997;30(4):118–21.

165 Song C, Lin A, Kenis, G., Bosmans, E., Maes, M. Immunosuppressive effects of clozapine and haloperidol: enhanced production of the interleukin-1 receptor antagonist. Schizophr Res 2000;42:157–164.

166 Maes M, Bosmans E, Kenis G, De Jong R, Smith RS, Meltzer HY. In vivo immunomodulatory effects of clozapine in schizophrenia. Schizophr Res 1997;26(2–3): 221–5.

167 Friedman H, Newton C, Klein TW. Microbial infections, immunomodulation, and drugs of abuse. Clin Microbiol Rev 2003;16(2):209–19.

168 Almirall J, Bolibar I, Balanzo X, Gonzalez CA. Risk factors for community-acquired pneumonia in adults: a population-based case-control study. Eur Respir J 1999;13(2):349–55.

169 Haverkos HW, Curran JW. The current outbreak of Kaposi's sarcoma and opportunistic infections. CA Cancer J Clin 1982;32(6):330–9.

170 Ho WZ, Guo CJ, Yuan CS, Douglas SD, Moss J. Methylnaltrexone antagonizes opioid-mediated enhancement of HIV infection of human blood

mononuclear phagocytes. J Pharmacol Exp Ther 2003;307(3):1158–62.

171 Donahoe RM, Vlahov D. Opiates as potential cofactors in progression of HIV-1 infections to AIDS. J Neuroimmunol 1998;83(1–2):77–87.

172 Alcabes P, Friedland G. Injection drug use and human immunodeficiency virus infection. Clin Infect Dis 1995;20(6):1467–79.

173 Risdahl JM, Khanna KV, Peterson PK, Molitor TW. Opiates and infection. J Neuroimmunol 1998;83(1–2): 4–18.

174 McCarthy L, Wetzel M, Sliker JK, Eisenstein TK, Rogers TJ. Opioids, opioid receptors, and the immune response. Drug Alcohol Depend 2001;62(2):111–23.

175 Li Y, Wang X, Tian S, Guo CJ, Douglas SD, Ho WZ. Methadone enhances human immunodeficiency virus infection of human immune cells. J Infect Dis 2002;185(1):118–22.

176 Peterson PK, Sharp BM, Gekker G, Portoghese PS, Sannerud K, Balfour HH, Jr. Morphine promotes the growth of HIV-1 in human peripheral blood mononuclear cell cocultures. AIDS 1990;4(9):869–73.

177 Szabo I, Rojavin M, Bussiere JL, Eisenstein TK, Adler MW, Rogers TJ. Suppression of peritoneal macrophage phagocytosis of Candida albicans by opioids. J Pharmacol Exp Ther 1993;267(2):703–6.

178 Grimm MC, Ben-Baruch A, Taub DD *et al.* Opiates transdeactivate chemokine receptors: delta and mu opiate receptor-mediated heterologous desensitization. J Exp Med 1998;188(2):317–25.

179 Belkowski SM, Alicea C, Eisenstein TK, Adler MW, Rogers TJ. Inhibition of interleukin-1 and tumor necrosis factor-alpha synthesis following treatment of macrophages with the kappa opioid agonist U50, 488H. J Pharmacol Exp Ther 1995;273(3):1491–6.

180 Chao CC, Molitor TW, Close K, Hu S, Peterson PK. Morphine inhibits the release of tumor necrosis factor in human peripheral blood mononuclear cell cultures. Int J Immunopharmacol 1993;15(3):447–53.

181 Alicea C, Belkowski S, Eisenstein TK, Adler MW, Rogers TJ. Inhibition of primary murine macrophage cytokine production in vitro following treatment with the kappa-opioid agonist U50,488H. J Neuroimmunol 1996;64(1):83–90.

182 Peng X, Cebra JJ, Adler MW *et al.* Morphine inhibits mucosal antibody responses and TGF-beta mRNA in gut-associated lymphoid tissue following oral cholera toxin in mice. J Immunol 2001;167(7):3677–81.

183 Chao CC, Hu S, Molitor TW *et al.* Morphine potentiates transforming growth factor-beta release from human peripheral blood mononuclear cell cultures. J Pharmacol Exp Ther 1992;262(1):19–24.

184 Mellon RD, Bayer BM. Evidence for central opioid receptors in the immunomodulatory effects of morphine: review of potential mechanism(s) of action. J Neuroimmunol 1998;83(1–2):19–28.

185 Allolio B, Schulte HM, Deuss U, Kallabis D, Hamel E, Winkelman W. Effect of oral morphine and naloxone on pituitary–adrenal response in man induced by human corticotropin-releasing hormone. Acta Endocrinol (Copenh) 1987;114(4):509–14.

186 Boumpas DT, Chrousos GP, Wilder RL, Cupps TR, Balow JE. Glucocorticoid therapy for immune-mediated diseases: basic and clinical correlates. Ann Intern Med 1993;119(12):1198–208.

187 Guo CJ, Li Y, Tian S, Wang X, Douglas SD, Ho WZ. Morphine enhances HIV infection of human blood mononuclear phagocytes through modulation of beta-chemokines and CCR5 receptor. J Investig Med 2002;50(6):435–42.

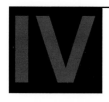

PART IV

Immune dysfunction leading to heart disease: induction by pathogens

CHAPTER 17

Osteopontin: the link between the immune system and cardiac remodeling

Samira Najmaii, Qianli Yu & Douglas F. Larson

Background

Cardiac fibroblasts

Cardiac fibroblasts are recognized as the cell types primarily responsible for homeostatic maintenance of ECM in normal hearts and represent 90% of all non-myocyte cells in the heart [1, 2]. Fibroblasts play an important role in synthesis, organization, turnover, and transmission of signals in the ECM. In the event of an injury or overload this homeostatic balance is tipped and stimulated cardiac fibroblasts start the process of cardiac remodeling and fibrosis.

Cardiac fibrosis is a result of increased synthesis of collagen types I and III and equally as important in the reduction in collagen degradation. Collagen synthesis and degradation is mainly regulated by cardiac fibroblasts. Fibroblasts up-regulate the synthesis of collagen in the presence of tissue growth factor, TGF-β, also have the capacity to down-regulate the synthesis by releasing collagen-degradation enzymes known as metalloproteinases (MMPs). A number of metalloproteinases, MMP1-8 and 13, have been identified each with specific targets [3, 4]. The regulatory mechanism controlling the activity of MMPs is defined as the activity of inhibitory enzymes known as tissue inhibitors of metalloproteinases (TIMPs). In the heart a decrease in the activity of MMP-1 and MMP-4 is as a result of increased activity of TIMP-1. In vitro experiments have shown that angiotensin II (Ang II), up-regulated upon cardiac injury, increases cardiac fibroblast-mediated collagen type I and type III synthesis, inhibits MMP-1 activity, and increases the concentration of TIMP-1 [5, 6].

Collagen is the most abundant extracellular matrix protein in the heart and as a structural protein it encompasses the cardiac myocytes and plays a vital role in contractility. Among the 18 subtypes of collagen, five (types I, III, IV, V, and VI) have been identified to play a role in myocardium and among these collagen types I and III are known to be the most abundant in the heart. Collagen type I is a stiff protein whereas collagen type III is an elastic protein [7, 8].

Post-translational collagen modification

Collagen synthesis in the heart is regulated by cardiac fibroblasts, which express mRNAs for type I and type III collagens and MMP-1, the key enzyme for interstitial collagen degradation. In the fibroblasts, pro-collagen is synthesized and converted into collagen molecules by collagen peptidases. Collagen molecules are then released into extracellular space, where their lysine and hydroxylysine residues are oxidized into reactive aldehyde derivatives by the enzyme lysyl oxidase (LOX). The aldehyde derivatives spontaneously form specific covalent cross-links between two chains of collagen molecules that polymerize to form collagen fibrils. The covalent cross-links contribute to fibril strength and increase their resistance to degradation by extracellular collagenases. These fibrillar collagen networks are a major contributing factor to myocardial stiffness [9, 10].

Metalloproteinase proteins are a large family of zinc-dependent enzymes that are categorized into five subgroups based on the specific targeted activities. Among these subgroups, gelatinases consisting of MMP-2 and MMP-9 are of special interest due to their activity against basement membrane components, collagen types IV and V. MMP-2 is a specific marker of cardiac remodeling and fibrosis. We believe that up-regulation of MMP-2 in cardiac remodeling and fibrosis is as a result of a compensatory mechanism. In heart tissues it has been proposed that increased levels of MMP-2 activities allow for proliferation and migration of cardiac fibroblasts in the ECM by breaking down the gelatinase. Furthermore, MMP-2 activities may control the overproduction of collagen in the event of a pro-fibrotic event [11, 12].

Plasma TIMP-1 levels correlate with markers of LV diastolic filling and predictive of LV dysfunction, and potentially a noninvasive marker of fibrosis [5]. There is a relationship between the activity of MMP1/TIMP1 and the TH1/TH2 network in physiological conditions [13]. In the event of fibrosis, a cell-mediated pro-inflammatory event, there is a defined balance of MMP and TIMP, in particular, TIMP-1 and MMP-1, activities. As fibrosis occurs, there is an up-regulation of TGF-β release, which results in increased production of collagen and TIMP-1 activity [14].

Collagen cross-linking, mediated by LOX and LOX-like proteins (LOXLs), is another important factor in regulating the extracellular matrix. LOX and LOXLs, mainly LOXL-3 in the myocardium, are copper-containing extracellular enzymes that oxidize and deaminate lysine and hydroxylysine residues into aldehyde groups [15]. These reactive aldehydes form covalent cross-links between adjacent chains strengthening the collagen fibrils and the collagen network. Lysyl oxidase (LOX1) is a key enzyme transforming the soluble collagen into insoluble form. The up-regulation of LOX1 is closely linked to up-regulation of TGF-β which is responsible for stimulating the collagen synthesis by fibroblasts and cardiac myocytes, resulting in fibrosis [3, 16–18]. Production of LOXL3 is also up-regulated as a coenzyme to LOX1 and it works as an intrinsic enzyme activator of LOX1 [15].

Matricellular proteins

As we had discussed earlier, fibroblasts are the key cells regulating and maintaining the homeostasis of the ECM. Matricellular proteins also known as signaling proteins play an important role in communicating with the external environment and fibroblasts triggering changes in ECM. Among these, signaling proteins are thrombospondins and osteopontin.

Thrombospondins

Thrombospondins (TSP) are a family of secreted glycoproteins that participate in cell-to-matrix communication. Within this family, the role of TSP-1 and TSP-2 in left ventricular hypertrophy has been studied extensively. Biological properties of TSP-1 and TSP-2 appear to be similar; however, there are some major structural differences between the two. One of the established functions of TSP-1 and TSP-2 is to proteolytically process latent TGF-β to an active form. Active TGF-β, on the other hand, has a profound effect on the ECM through the induction of collagen expression and synthesis, specifically collagen types I and III (the most abundant collagens in the heart). TSP-1 and TSP-2 also bind to a specific domain on the MMPs, resulting in their decreased activity. Myocardial TSP-2, more than TSP-1, appears to play a vital role in cardiac remodeling and left ventricular hypertrophy and it also has been shown to play a stronger role in regulating the MMP-2 activities [19–21].

Osteopontin

Osteopontin (OPN), also described as early T-lymphocyte activator-1 (Eta-1), is an extracellular matrix protein with a wide range of functions. It was originally thought to be a major sialylated noncollagenous matrix protein of the bone primarily synthesized by osteoblasts, regulated by preosteoblasts, and released into osteoids where it was further incorporated into the bone matrix [22]. In later studies OPN showed a widespread participation in tissue remodeling and inflammation of myocardium, kidney, lymph node, joint, and malignant tissues. The participation of OPN in these tissue types has manifested diseases such as rheumatoid arthritis [23], diabetes mellitus [14], atherosclerosis [24], lung disease [25], joint malignant tissues [26, 27], and myocardial injuries [3, 28].

Recently, there has been a great interest in OPN playing a key role in cardiac fibrosis in Ang II-induced cardiac hypertrophy [28–30]. Weber *et al.* showed that the OPN levels were increased in relation to Ang II infusion and collagen cross-linking was up-regulated, resulting in hypertrophy and myocardial stiffness [31]. In the study done by Matsui *et al.*, there was a significant decrease in cardiac fibrosis in OPN−/− mice treated with Ang II infusion in comparison with control groups, emphasizing the significance of the role OPN plays in cardiac fibrosis [32]. The results showed an increased left ventricular dilation of the heart and decreased myocardial stiffness. Therefore, OPN appears to be a pivotal factor in cardiac ECM remodeling.

OPN is a single-chain polypeptide ECM protein with a molecular mass of approximately 41,500 Daltons [33]. A molecule of OPN, depicted in Figure 17.1, consists of approximately eight α-helix and six β-sheets connected together via reverse turns and the carboxyl and amino-terminals functioning as the cell's binding sites [34]. Other features of the molecule include: two heparin binding sites and one hydroxyapatite binding site also known as calcium binding site [35]. One heparin binding site is located adjacent to the RGD motif and one near the carboxy-terminal [36, 37]. There are also three thrombin cleavage sites in a molecule of OPN. One cleavage site is the Arg-Gly bound in the RGD tripeptide and the other two cleavage sites are the Arg-Ser located at residues 153 to 154 and 157 to 158 [38, 39]. However, the main cleavage site is at residues 153 to 154.

OPN is a highly acidic glycoprotein containing the adhesive motif Arg-Glycine-Aspartate (RGD) [34, 36]. It is through this motif (RGD) where OPN can engage multiple cell surface receptors. The receptors specific for OPN have been identified as $\alpha_v\beta_3$, $\alpha_v\beta_1$, and $\alpha_v\beta_5$ integrins, $\alpha_v\beta_3$ being the most important receptor for adhesion and migration [40]. Among others it has been known that OPN can interact with other receptors such as α_4, α_5, α_8, α_9, and CD44 [38]. Adhesion and migration of OPN is dependent on the interaction of RGD with these receptors, activating cellular signaling pathways and therefore allowing cell–matrix and possibly cell–cell interaction [40].

OPN and immune function

One other interesting feature of OPN is its ability not to only behave as a matrix protein but also as a cytokine [41]. In a normal state, high levels of OPN are only expressed in kidney, bone, and epithelial lining of some tissues [42, 43]. The up-regulation of OPN is only noted in a pro-inflammatory response where T lymphocytes and macrophages are activated, invading synoviocytes, and articular chondrocytes for tissue repair [44]. OPN plays a role in wound healing by regulating cell adhesion, migration, and proliferation [45].

It has been well documented that OPN functions as a pro-inflammatory cytokine and chemokine initiating a cell-mediated immunity and therefore, plays a central role in initiating a Th1-mediated immune response [43, 46, 47]. From this basis it has also been referred to as early T-lymphocyte activator-1 (Eta-1) [48]. In the initiation of an

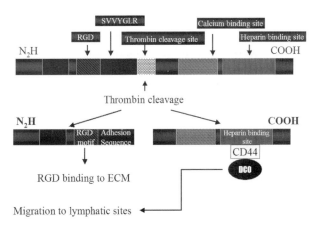

Figure 17.1 Osteopontin molecule.

insult, dendritic cells are the primary cells that differentiate into DC1 and DC2 and further drive the differentiation of T lymphocytes into Th1 and Th2 subtypes [38, 49]. OPN has been shown to induce migration and activation of dendritic cells, polarizing them into Th1-promoting effector DCs [46, 50, 51]. As OPN activates the immune response, a chain of reactions unfolds, creating a domino effect.

Furthermore, in a pro-inflammatory response, triggered by Ang II, high levels of OPN are released and induce the secretion of IL-12 by macrophages [43, 52]. This is accomplished by thrombin, an anticoagulant factor released in a pro-inflammatory response. Thrombin cleaves OPN at thrombin cleavage site (residues Arg153-Ser154) making RGD motif more accessible to $\alpha_v\beta_3$ integrins on macrophages and fibroblasts promoting activation of chemotaxins and, therefore, stimulation and expression of IL-12 cytokine [43]. The C-terminal domain, on the other hand, can interact with CD44 receptors on naïve DC, allowing for migration of these cells to lymphatic sites, polarization of lymphocytes to a Th1, and activation of M1 pathway.

T lymphocytes communicate with cardiac fibroblasts and initiate a response through the release of cytokines and proteins [53, 54]. We believe OPN is one of the key proteins involved in this communication and variations in the release of OPN by the Th1 and Th2 lymphocytes may present an avenue for explaining the differences in the remodeling process in the two subgroups. OPN is mainly expressed in Th1 lymphocytes, but Th2 lymphocytes, as a result of an anti-inflammatory response, also release OPN. Glucocorticoids are among a few stimulants that can interact with OPN, resulting in an anti-inflammatory response. The outcome of an anti-inflammatory response is activation of Th2 and M2 macrophage-type response. M2 macrophages follow a different metabolic pathway than M1 macrophages resulting in a reduction in NO synthesis by iNOS [55].

OPN and cardiac remodeling

There has been a great deal of research done to gain a better understanding of the myocardial stiffness in relation to Ang II induction and OPN up-regulation. Ang II resulted in a significant and dose-dependent increase in collagen synthesis and a significant decrease in MMP1 activity. Increase in collagen synthesis was explained by increased expression of TGFβ-1 and further up-regulation of OPN mRNA expression. OPN also has the potential to bind to the $\alpha_v\beta_3$ integrins receptors on the surface of fibroblasts via its RGD binding site, promoting fibroblast binding to collagen. OPN, in the presence of transglutaminase (TG), interacts with both fibronectin and collagen, forming a heat-stable complex and catalyzing the covalent cross-linking of these proteins. Furthermore, OPN is a substrate of TG, a biological glue for cartilage–cartilage interfaces, therefore could be an essential component of the "glue" and function as an adhesive protein.

In cardiac hypertrophy there is an increase in the ratio of cardiac fibroblast and ECM relative to that of myocytes, which results in progressive fibrosis and ventricular dysfunction [27, 31, 43]. The OPN expression in the heart is an important factor in controlling cardiac fibroblast growth and adhesion to the extracellular matrix, and as importantly collagen gel contraction. OPN can potentially regulate cell differentiation and function by activating cell signaling pathways and gene expression through an RGD motif [30, 56]. Fibroblast changes that occur during cardiac hypertrophy and the promoters of these changes have not been completely characterized. However, OPN released by lymphocytes is a promising regulatory protein that could possibly regulate the gene expression of cardiac fibroblasts by interacting with $\alpha_v\beta_3$ integrins on cardiac fibroblasts [39, 57].

Increased expression and activity of MMPs, specifically MMP-2 and MMP-9, have also been demonstrated in human, rat, and porcine hearts during the remodeling process following MI. One hypothesis has been that pro-inflammatory cytokines such as interleukin-1β and tumor necrosis factor-α are increased in the heart following MI and play a role in increasing MMP-2 and MMP-9 expression and activities [58]. Other studies, done on different fibroblast cell lines, have proposed that up-regulation of MMP-2 activity is mediated through TGF-β [4, 59]. We suggest a third mediator, OPN, as the promoter of MMP-2 activity. It has been well documented that OPN is a potent stimulator of both MMP-2 and MMP-9 activity in mammary gland, lung, and liver tissues among other cell types and is a key marker of fibrosis

[43, 57, 60, 61]. Activation of MMP-2 and MMP-9 by OPN is mediated through two distinct ikappabalpha/ikappabalpha kinase (IKK) signaling pathways [62]. In a recent study, OPN-treated aortas showed a twofold increase in MMP-2 levels, enhancing vascular healing by reducing calcification and thus maintaining luminal integrity [63].

Conclusion

Remodeling of the heart as a response to insult is a very complex and multipathway process. A series of events in response to multiple cytokines and regulatory protein results in proliferation and migration of cardiac fibroblasts, increased collagen synthesis, and rearrangement of ECM. As we mentioned earlier, cardiac remodeling results in an imbalance between the ECM, cardiac fibroblast, and myocytes.

In the event of an injury, cardiac overload, or Ang II release, the immune system is activated and cytokines are released resulting in a shift to a Th1 cell-mediated pro-inflammatory phenotype. Cytokine and regulatory protein profiles of Th1 lymphocytes are the key mediators of fibrosis. Among these cytokines and regulatory proteins, OPN has been of interest to us since it is released by T lymphocytes and is up-regulated in response to injury and Ang II release.

One key factor that leads us to believe that OPN released by Th1 subgroups is involved in signaling cardiac fibroblasts is its up-regulation and release by these subgroups. Therefore, it can be considered as a mediator of the communication between T lymphocytes and cardiac fibroblasts.

Two very important events in fibrosis are the proliferation and migration of cardiac fibroblasts and collagen synthesis. Previous studies strongly suggest that OPN plays a key role in cardiac remodeling. Changes in ECM occur as a response to inflammation and OPN is an integral part of this acute response. Not only is it involved in polarization of T lymphocytes to Th1 subgroups but it also has the potential to communicate with cardiac fibroblasts, which are the key cells in ECM-mediating changes.

References

1 Marijianowski MM, Teeling P, Mann J, Becker AE. Dilated cardiomyopathy is associated with an increase in the type I/type III collagen ratio: a quantitative assessment. J Am Coll Cardiol May 1995;25(6):1263–72.

2 Noh YH, Matsuda K, Hong YK et al. An N-terminal 80 kDa recombinant fragment of human thrombospondin-2 inhibits vascular endothelial growth factor induced endothelial cell migration in vitro and tumor growth and angiogenesis in vivo. J Invest Dermatol December 2003;121(6):1536–43.

3 Gray MO, Long CS, Kalinyak JE, Li HT, Karliner JS. Angiotensin II stimulates cardiac myocyte hypertrophy via paracrine release of TGF-beta 1 and endothelin-1 from fibroblasts. Cardiovasc Res November 1998;40(2):352–63.

4 Saed GM, Zhang W, Diamond MP. Effect of hypoxia on stimulatory effect of TGF-beta 1 on MMP-2 and MMP-9 activities in mouse fibroblasts. J Soc Gynecol Investig November 2000;7(6):348–54.

5 Lindsay MM, Maxwell P, Dunn FG. TIMP-1: a marker of left ventricular diastolic dysfunction and fibrosis in hypertension. Hypertension August 2002;40(2):136–41.

6 Li YY, McTiernan CF, Feldman AM. Proinflammatory cytokines regulate tissue inhibitors of metalloproteinases and disintegrin metalloproteinase in cardiac cells. Cardiovasc Res April 1999;42(1):162–72.

7 McClain PE. Characterization of cardiac muscle collagen. Molecular heterogeneity. J Biol Chem April 10, 1974;249(7):2303–11.

8 Bishop JE, Greenbaum R, Gibson DG, Yacoub M, Laurent GJ. Enhanced deposition of predominantly type I collagen in myocardial disease. J Mol Cell Cardiol October 1990;22(10):1157–65.

9 Yu Z, Schneider C, Boeglin WE, Brash AR. Human and mouse eLOX3 have distinct substrate specificities: implications for their linkage with lipoxygenases in skin. Arch Biochem Biophys 2006 Nov 15;455(2):188–96.Epub 2006 Sep 25.

10 Yu Z, Schneider C, Boeglin WE, Brash AR. Mutations associated with a congenital form of ichthyosis (NCIE) inactivate the epidermal lipoxygenases 12R-LOX and eLOX3. Biochim Biophys Acta 2005 Jan 5; 1686 3:238–47.

11 Briest W, Holzl A, Rassler B et al. Cardiac remodeling after long term norepinephrine treatment in rats. Cardiovasc Res November 2001;52(2):265–73.

12 Takahashi N, Calderone A, Izzo NJ, Jr, Maki TM, Marsh JD, Colucci WS. Hypertrophic stimuli induce transforming growth factor-beta 1 expression in rat ventricular myocytes. J Clin Invest October 1994;94(4):1470–6.

13 Contasta I, Berghella AM, Pellegrini P, Del BT, Casciani CA, Adorno D. Relationships between the activity of MMP1/TIMP1 enzymes and the TH1/TH2 cytokine network. Cancer Biother Radiopharm December 1999;14(6):465–75.

14 Chua CC, Chua BH, Zhao ZY, Krebs C, Diglio C, Perrin E. Effect of growth factors on collagen metabolism in

cultured human heart fibroblasts. Connect Tissue Res 1991;26(4):271–81.

15 Jourdan-Le SC, Tomsche A, Ujfalusi A, Jia L, Csiszar K. Central nervous system, uterus, heart, and leukocyte expression of the LOXL3 gene, encoding a novel lysyl oxidase-like protein. Genomics June 1, 2001;74(2): 211–8.

16 kiyama-Uchida Y, Ashizawa N, Ohtsuru A et al. Nore-pinephrine enhances fibrosis mediated by TGF-beta in cardiac fibroblasts. Hypertension August 2002;40(2): 148–54.

17 Rajalalitha P, Vali S. Molecular pathogenesis of oral sub-mucous fibrosis—a collagen metabolic disorder. J Oral Pathol Med July 2005;34(6):321–8.

18 Trivedy C, Warnakulasuriya KA, Hazarey VK, Tavassoli M, Sommer P, Johnson NW. The upregulation of lysyl oxidase in oral submucous fibrosis and squamous cell carcinoma. J Oral Pathol Med July 1999;28(6):246–51.

19 Adams JC, Lawler J. The thrombospondins. Int J Biochem Cell Biol June 2004;36(6):961–8.

20 Carron JA, Hiscott P, Hagan S, Sheridan CM, Magee R, Gallagher JA. Cultured human retinal pigment epithe-lial cells differentially express thrombospondin-1, -2, -3, and -4. Int J Biochem Cell Biol November 2000; 32(11–12):1137–42.

21 Streit M, Riccardi L, Velasco P et al. Thrombospondin-2: a potent endogenous inhibitor of tumor growth and angiogenesis. Proc Natl Acad Sci U S A December 21, 1999;96(26):14888–93.

22 Ozawa H, Amizuka N. Structure and function of bone cells. Nippon Rinsho September 1994;52(9):2246–54.

23 Kennedy JH, Henrion D, Wassef M, Shanahan CM, Bloch G, Tedgui A. Osteopontin expression and calcium content in human aortic valves. J Thorac Cardiovasc Surg August 2000;120(2):427.

24 Golledge J, McCann M, Mangan S, Lam A, Karan M. Os-teoprotegerin and osteopontin are expressed at high con-centrations within symptomatic carotid atherosclerosis. Stroke July 2004;35(7):1636–41.

25 Sahai A, Malladi P, Pan X et al. Obese and diabetic db/db mice develop marked liver fibrosis in a model of nonalco-holic steatohepatitis: role of short-form leptin receptors and osteopontin. Am J Physiol Gastrointest Liver Physiol November 2004;287(5):G1035–43.

26 Martin I, Jakob M, Schafer D, Dick W, Spagnoli G, Heberer M. Quantitative analysis of gene expression in human articular cartilage from normal and osteoarthritic joints. Osteoarthritis Cartilage February 2001;9(2): 112–8.

27 Ohtsuki T, Furuya S, Yamada T et al. Gene expression of noncollagenous bone matrix proteins in the limb joints and intervertebral disks of the twy mouse. Calcif Tissue Int August 1998;63(2):167–72.

28 Collins AR, Schnee J, Wang W et al. Osteopontin modu-lates angiotensin II-induced fibrosis in the intact murine heart. J Am Coll Cardiol May 5, 2004;43(9):1698–705.

29 Mochida S, Hashimoto M, Matsui A et al. Genetic poly-morphims in promoter region of osteopontin gene may be a marker reflecting hepatitis activity in chronic hep-atitis C patients. Biochem Biophys Res Commun January 23, 2004;313(4):1079–85.

30 Shai SY, Harpf AE, Ross RS. Integrins and the my-ocardium. Genet Eng (N Y) 2002;24:87–105.

31 Weber KT, Sun Y, Guarda E et al. Myocardial fibrosis in hypertensive heart disease: an overview of potential reg-ulatory mechanisms. Eur Heart J May 1995;16(suppl C): 24–8.

32 Matsui Y, Jia N, Okamoto H et al. Role of osteopontin in cardiac fibrosis and remodeling in angiotensin II-induced cardiac hypertrophy. Hypertension June 2004;43(6): 1195–201.

33 Franzen A, Heinegard D. Isolation and characterization of two sialoproteins present only in bone calcified matrix. Biochem J December 15, 1985;232(3):715–24.

34 Prince CW. Secondary structure predictions for rat os-teopontin. Connect Tissue Res 1989;21(1–4):15–20.

35 Singh K, Deonarine D, Shanmugam V et al. Calcium-binding properties of osteopontin derived from non-osteogenic sources. J Biochem (Tokyo) November 1993; 114(5):702–7.

36 Hultenby K, Reinholt FP, Norgard M, Oldberg A, Wen-del M, Heinegard D. Distribution and synthesis of bone sialoprotein in metaphyseal bone of young rats show a distinctly different pattern from that of osteopontin. Eur J Cell Biol April 1994;63(2):230–9.

37 Oldberg A, Franzen A, Heinegard D. Cloning and se-quence analysis of rat bone sialoprotein (osteopontin) cDNA reveals an Arg-Gly-Asp cell-binding sequence. Proc Natl Acad Sci U S A December 1986;83(23):8819–23.

38 van der Heijden FL, Wierenga EA, Bos JD, Kapsenberg ML. High frequency of IL-4-producing CD4+ allergen-specific T lymphocytes in atopic dermatitis lesional skin. J Invest Dermatol September 1991;97(3):389–94.

39 Graf K, Neuss M, Stawowy P, Hsueh WA, Fleck E, Law RE. Angiotensin II and alpha(v)beta(3) integrin expression in rat neonatal cardiac fibroblasts. Hypertension April 2000;35(4):978–84.

40 Liaw L, Skinner MP, Raines EW et al. The adhesive and migratory effects of osteopontin are mediated via distinct cell surface integrins. Role of alpha v beta 3 in smooth muscle cell migration to osteopontin in vitro. J Clin Invest February 1995;95(2):713–24.

41 Patarca R, Saavedra RA, Cantor H. Molecular and cellular basis of genetic resistance to bacterial infection: the role of the early T-lymphocyte activation-1/osteopontin gene. Crit Rev Immunol 1993;13(3–4):225–46.

42 Brown LF, Berse B, Van de WL *et al.* Expression and distribution of osteopontin in human tissues: widespread association with luminal epithelial surfaces. Mol Biol Cell October 1992;3(10):1169–80.

43 Mishra BB, Poulter LW, Janossy G, James DG. The distribution of lymphoid and macrophage like cell subsets of sarcoid and Kveim granulomata: possible mechanism of negative PPD reaction in sarcoidosis. Clin Exp Immunol December 1983;54(3):705–15.

44 Denhardt DT, Noda M, O'Regan AW, Pavlin D, Berman JS. Osteopontin as a means to cope with environmental insults: regulation of inflammation, tissue remodeling, and cell survival. J Clin Invest May 2001;107(9): 1055–61.

45 Kyriakides TR, Bornstein P. Matricellular proteins as modulators of wound healing and the foreign body response. Thromb Haemost December 2003;90(6):986–92.

46 O'Regan A, Berman JS. Osteopontin: a key cytokine in cell-mediated and granulomatous inflammation. Int J Exp Pathol December 2000;81(6):373–90.

47 O'Regan AW, Chupp GL, Lowry JA, Goetschkes M, Mulligan N, Berman JS. Osteopontin is associated with T cells in sarcoid granulomas and has T cell adhesive and cytokine-like properties in vitro. J Immunol January 15, 1999;162(2):1024–31.

48 Ashkar S, Weber GF, Panoutsakopoulou V *et al.* Eta-1 (osteopontin): an early component of type-1 (cell-mediated) immunity. Science February 4, 2000;287(5454):860–4.

49 de MA, Medrano GA, Villarreal A, Sodi-Pallares D. Protective effect of glucose–insulin–potassium solutions in myocardial damage caused by emetine. Arch Inst Cardiol Mex July 1975;45(4):469–86.

50 Renkl AC, Wussler J, Ahrens T *et al.* Osteopontin functionally activates dendritic cells and induces their differentiation toward a Th1-polarizing phenotype. Blood August 1, 2005;106(3):946–55.

51 Denhardt DT, Giachelli CM, Rittling SR. Role of osteopontin in cellular signaling and toxicant injury. Annu Rev Pharmacol Toxicol 2001;41:723–49.

52 de Jong EC, Smits HH, Kapsenberg ML. Dendritic cell-mediated T cell polarization. Springer Semin Immunopathol January 2005;26(3):289–307.

53 Marchalonis JJ, Schluter SF, Sepulveda RT, Watson RR, Larson DF. Immunomodulation by immunopeptides and autoantibodies in aging, autoimmunity, and infection. Ann N Y Acad Sci December 2005;1057:247–59.

54 Fujii T, Onohara N, Maruyama Y *et al.* Galpha12/13-mediated production of reactive oxygen species is critical for angiotensin receptor-induced NFAT activation in cardiac fibroblasts. J Biol Chem June 17, 2005;280(24): 23041–7.

55 Singh K, Balligand JL, Fischer TA, Smith TW, Kelly RA. Glucocorticoids increase osteopontin expression in cardiac myocytes and microvascular endothelial cells. Role in regulation of inducible nitric oxide synthase. J Biol Chem November 24, 1995;270(47):28471–8.

56 Giachelli CM, Liaw L, Murry CE, Schwartz SM, Almeida M. Osteopontin expression in cardiovascular diseases. Ann N Y Acad Sci April 21, 1995;760:109–26.

57 Vogt M, Motz WH, Schwartzkopf B, Strauer BE. Pathophysiology and clinical aspects of hypertensive hypertrophy. Eur Heart J July 1993;14(suppl D):2–7.

58 Xie Z, Singh M, Siwik DA, Joyner WL, Singh K. Osteopontin inhibits interleukin-1beta-stimulated increases in matrix metalloproteinase activity in adult rat cardiac fibroblasts: role of protein kinase C-zeta. J Biol Chem December 5, 2003;278(49):48546–52.

59 Norman JT, Clark IM, Garcia PL. Hypoxia promotes fibrogenesis in human renal fibroblasts. Kidney Int December 2000;58(6):2351–66.

60 Yuki N, Hayashi N, Kasahara A *et al.* Pretreatment viral load and response to prolonged interferon-alpha course for chronic hepatitis C. J Hepatol April 1995;22(4): 457–63.

61 Yuki N, Hayashi N, Hagiwara H *et al.* IgG and IgM core antibodies and viral replication in hepatitis C virus carriers. J Hepatol July 1994;21(1):110–4.

62 Rangaswami H, Bulbule A, Kundu GC. Nuclear factor-inducing kinase plays a crucial role in osteopontin-induced MAPK/IkappaBalpha kinase-dependent nuclear factor kappaB-mediated promatrix metalloproteinase-9 activation. J Biol Chem September 10, 2004;279(37): 38921–35.

63 Nemir M, DeVouge MW, Mukherjee BB. Normal rat kidney cells secrete both phosphorylated and nonphosphorylated forms of osteopontin showing different physiological properties. J Biol Chem October 25, 1989; 264(30):18202–8.

CHAPTER 18

Inflammatory immune activation in heart failure patients: therapeutic implications

Mohammad Abraham Kazemizadeh Gol &
Mohsen Araghi-Niknam

Introduction

Heart failure (HF) can arise from several initial causes including the following: (1) hypertension, (2) viral infection, (3) myocardial infarction (MI), or (4) genetic muscular abnormalities. Each of these insults causes cardiac muscle to be weakened. Other nearby cardiac muscle is required to compensate for the muscle loss and work harder in order to maintain a proper ejection fraction. Eventually these compensatory responses cause heart muscle to become overworked and weakened, which causes HF to progress. This idea, that overworking heart muscle causes heart failure to progress, is supported by the Studies of Left Ventricular Dysfunction (SOLVD) trial. This trial suggested that increasing heart contractility had a worse prognosis than a systemic adaptation to the heart problem [1]. It has also been shown that inotropic drugs are associated with increased mortality [2]. This could be a result of overworking the heart. Therefore, instead of focusing on the heart alone in order to better understand heart failure and create new treatments, many researchers address the problem as a systemic problem instead of a problem of the pump alone [3]. Heart failure is now being looked at from a neurohormonal and immunological prospective. The neurohormonal research has provided promising drugs such as B-blockers and ACE inhibitors [2]. The immunological research is showing promise with anti-inflammatory drugs and treatments.

Heart failure and the immune system

HF apparently causes an activation of the immune system. Raised levels of immunologic inflammatory factors such as tumor necrosis factor α, interleukin (IL) 1-β, IL-6, monocyte chemoattractant peptide (MCP)-1, IL-8, and macrophage inflammatory protein (MIP)-1α have been observed. Anti-inflammatory factors such as IL-1 receptor antagonist (IL-1Ra), IL-4, IL-10, and soluble tumor necrosis factor receptors, are apparently not produced at an increased level, therefore, HF leads to an increase in inflammation [3–8]. Increased immunological activity is also seen in circulating leukocytes, which produce increased levels of protein and mRNA [3, 9, 10]. This increased immunological activity and inflammation seems to influence contractility, increase hypertrophy, and increase apoptosis; therefore contributing to myocardial remodeling and HF.

TNFα trial

TNFα has been suggested as a possible target to repress immune activation in heart failure. TNFα and IL-6 have been shown to be upregulated in myocardium and in the circulation of heart failure patients, and their expression correlates with the progression of heart disease. Both TNFα and IL-6 are also known to contribute to the inflammatory response. In a series of three clinical studies, a recombinant soluble TNF receptor fusion protein (etanercept) was used to inhibit TNFα's activity as a possible treatment for inflammation [11]. These studies (RENAISSANCE, RECOVER, ATTACH) unfortunately did not show positive results and were therefore discontinued [12, 13]. It is possible that these disappointing clinical results arise from the redundancy of the immune system. A selective treatment like etanercept may be too specific to limit the inflammatory response [3]. Future studies need to be done to better characterize other factors involved in the inflammatory response and how they relate to HF. Also, studies involving less selective anti-inflammatory treatments need to be done. It is likely that a less selective inhibition of the inflammatory response would have more effective results.

Current cardiovascular drugs and the inflammatory response

Several recent studies have shown the possibility that some current cardiovascular drugs can affect the inflammatory response. Recent in vitro and animal studies have shown that neurohormones such as Angiotensin II and Noradrenalin can increase inflammatory cytokine levels. These studies also show that cardiovascular drugs such as ACE-inhibitors and β-blockers can have the opposite effect, decreasing inflammation [14–16]. Enalapril, an ACE-inhibitor, has been shown to decrease the expression of IL-6, an inflammatory cytokine. This in turn slows HF down by decreasing hypertrophy. Selective Angiotensin II blockers have also been shown to have similar effects as enalapril. Although metroprolol, a β1-selective blocker, showed no significant effect on cytokine levels, carvedilol, a less selective β-blocker lowered plasma IL-6 levels. It is possible that metroprolol was too selective of a β-blocker to produce the desired inhibition of IL-6 production [3]. Although there is preliminary data on several of the current medications, clinical studies need to be performed to better characterize the effects of conventional cardiovascular drugs on the inflammatory response to HF in humans. Studies also need to be done to determine whether the beneficial effects of these drugs are actually due to additionally inhibiting the inflammatory response, and therefore

treating HF directly through their original intended use and indirectly by inhibiting the immune response as opposed to treating the, original problem (i.e., hypertension) and therefore decreasing inflammation.

Inflammatory activity of the serum in HF patients

Hoare *et al.* conducted a study on the serum of end-stage heart failure to determine if it had the ability to activate proinflammatory pathways in vascular endothelial cells. Specifically, serum from end-stage heart failure patients was added to cultured endothelial cells. The cultured cells were then observed to determine if the NFκB pathway was activated and inflammatory gene expression began. The study showed that the serum was able to activate the NFκB pathway in vascular endothelial cells. However, the NFκB pathway was not always efficiently activated suggesting a functional amount of anti-inflammatory factors as well as the proinflammatory factors in the serum. The specific factor in the serum that activates the NFκB pathway is unknown. Although TNFα is upregulated in HF and is also known to be a strong inducer of the NFκB pathway, it seems unlikely to be causing this activation for the following reasons: (1) NFκB pathway activation was similar regardless of the serum TNFα levels; (2) although TNFα levels are upregulated in HF, soluble TNFα receptors are also upregulated. It is possible that the soluble TNFα receptors inhibit TNFα to the point where it is not an effective activator. Also, the etanercept experiments seemed to suggest that TNFα may not be an effective inflammation factor to regulate in HF, and therefore may only have minimal inflammatory effects in HF patients. More studies need to be done to determine what serum factors are responsible for the increased NFκB pathway activation in vascular endothelial cells [17].

Possible treatments

There are several possible treatments to HF. One possibility involves tissue regeneration via uncommitted stem cells and adjuvant treatment. The tumor necrosis factor (TNF)-β superfamily seems to stimulate stem cells to develop into cardiomyocytes. Members of this superfamily could be used to help stimulate regrowth via stem cell therapy [3].

Another possibility involves increasing anti-inflammatory factors such as IL-10 and IL-1Ra. Currently in HF, inflammatory factors are more expressed than anti-inflammatory factors. Increasing anti-inflammatory factors to a sufficient level could inhibit the inflammatory response. This type of inhibition would be less selective than the anti TNFα drug etanercept, and might therefore be more effective.

A third treatment is IVIG therapy. The intervention in myocarditis and acute cardiomyopathy (IMAC) trail treated a group of 62 patients with recent-onset cardiomyopathy with high-dose IVIG or a placebo for two consecutive days. The change in LVEF was observed at 6 months. Surprisingly, patients who were given the placebo had a mean change in LVEP from 0.23 to 0.42. Because of this large change in LVEP in the placebo group, there was no change isolated to the IVIG treatment. However, other studies have shown significant increases in LVEF and increases in anti-inflammatory factors in response to IVIG treatment. In one trial a group of 40 ischemic and nonischemic patients with LVEF below 0.40 were treated with IVIG monthly for 6 months. The mean LVEF was observed to increase from 0.26 to 0.31. There was also an increase in several anti-inflammatory factors including IL-10, soluble IL-1 receptors, and soluble TNF receptors [2]. The other was a placebo-controlled study that showed a significant increase in LVEF in 5% of HF patients regardless of the etiology [3, 18]. The exact mechanism that IVIG works through is unknown, but it is thought that IVIG may supplement a natural anti-inflammatory response of γ-globulin. More specifically, IVIG treatment is thought to influence inflammation in the following ways: (1) neutralize microbial antigens and superantigens, (2) form an Fc-receptor blockade, (3) decrease apoptosis, (4) inhibit adhesion of leukocytes to endothelial cells, (5) downregulate inflammatory cytokines, and (6) upregulate anti-inflammatory cytokines. However, IVIG treatment was not shown to inhibit complement in HF. Therefore, it seems likely that dual treatment of IVIG and a complement inhibitor would be more effective in HF patients [3].

A fourth treatment is Immunoadsorption, which involves removing specific antibodies from a patient's blood. A small study on 34 HF patients showed promising results. The patients were given five consecutive days of immunoadsorption to remove anti-β1-adrenoceptor antibodies. Before the treatment the LVEF was 0.22, after the treatment the average LVEF raised to 0.38. There were also improvements in systolic and end-diastolic volumes. Additionally, after 3 months anti-β1-adrenoceptor antibodies were not detectable in the patients' blood. Although these results are promising, more studies need to be done to confirm them.

A fifth treatment is immune-modulation therapy (IMT). This involves removing blood from the patient and inducing apoptosis ex vivo via oxidative stress. The cells are then administered to the patient intramuscularly. The immune system responds to the presence of the apoptotic cells by increasing expression of anti-inflammatory factors.

Conclusion

Several studies have shown that HF is accompanied by an inflammatory response. It seems likely that this response is responsible for some of the adverse effects associated with HF. Although TNFα repression alone had disappointing results, it is still likely that repressing the immune response in HF can be helpful. Further studies involving less selective immune inhibition, inhibiting different inflammatory factors, increasing anti-inflammatory factors, better characterizing the anti-inflammatory/ inflammatory affects of conventional medications, and better characterizing inflammatory pathways such as the NFκB pathway in HF will likely provide more effective treatments for HF patients.

References

1 The SOLVD Investigators. Effect of enalapril on mortality and the development of heart failure in asymptomatic patients with reduced left ventricular ejection fractions. N Engl J Med 1992 Sep 3;327(10):685–91.

2 Torre-Amione G. Immune activation in chronic heart failure. Am J Cardiol June 6, 2005;95(11A):3C–8C; discussion 38C–40C.

3 Aukrust P, Gullestad L, Ueland T, Damas J, Yndestad A. Inflammatory and anti-inflammatory cytokines in

chronic heart failure: potential therapeutic implications. Ann Med 2005;37(2):74–85.

4 Aukrust P, Ueland T, Lien E *et al.* Cytokine network in congestive heart failure secondary to ischemic or idiopathic dilated cardiomyopathy. Am J Cardiol 1999;83:376–82.

5 Aukrust P, Ueland T, Müller F *et al.* Elevated circulating levels of C-C chemokines in patients with congestive heart failure. Circulation 1998;97:1136–43.

6 Damås JK, Gullestad L, Ueland T *et al.* CXC-chemokines, a new group of cytokines in congestive heart failure—possible role of platelets and monocytes. Cardiovasc Res 2000;45:428–36.

7 Testa M, Yeh M, Lee P *et al.* Circulating levels of cytokines and their endogenous modulators in patients with mild to severe congestive heart failure due to coronary artery disease or hypertension. J Am Coll Cardiol 1996;28: 964–71.

8 Torre-Amione G, Kapadia S, Benedict C, Oral H, Young JB, Mann DL. Proinflammatory cytokine levels in patients with depressed left ventricular ejection fraction: a report from the studies of left ventricular dysfunction (SOLVD). J Am Coll Cardiol 1996;27:1201–6.

9 Damås JK, Gullestad L, Aass H *et al.* Enhanced gene expression of chemokines and their corresponding receptors in mononuclear blood cells in chronic heart failure—modulatory effect of intravenous immunoglobulin. J Am Coll Cardiol 2001;38:187–93.

10 Yndestad A, Holm AM, Müller F *et al.* Enhanced expression of inflammatory cytokines and activation markers in T-cells from patients with chronic heart failure. Cardiovasc Res 2003;60:141–6.

11 Bozkurt B, Torre-Amione G, Warren MS *et al.* Results of targeted anti-tumor necrosis factor therapy with etanercept (ENBREL) in patients with advanced heart failure. Circulation 2001;103:1044–7.

12 Mann DL, McMurray JJV, Packer M *et al.* Targeted anticytokine therapy in patients with chronic heart failure: results of the randomized etanercept worldwide evaluation (RENEWAL). Circulation 2004;109:1594–602.

13 Chung ES, Packer M, Lo KH, Fasanmade AA, Willerson JT. Randomized, double-blind, placebo-controlled, pilot trial of infliximab, a chimeric monoclonal antibody to tumor necrosis factor-alpha, in patients with moderate to severe heart failure: results of the anti-TNF therapy against congestive heart failure (ATTACH) trial. Circulation 2003;107:3133–40.

14 Sano M, Fukuda K, Kodama H *et al.* Interleukin-6 family of cytokines mediate angiotensin II-induced cardiac hypertrophy in rodent cardiomyocytes. J Biol Chem 2000;275:29717–23.

15 Prabhu SD, Chandrasekar B, Murray DR, Freeman GL. Beta-adrenergic blockade in developing heart failure: effects on myocardial inflammatory cytokines, nitric oxide, and remodeling. Circulation 2000;101:2103–9.

16 Wei GC, Sirois MG, Qu R, Liu P, Rouleau JL. Subacute and chronic effects of quinapril on cardiac cytokine expression, remodeling, and function after myocardial infarction in the rat. J Cardiovasc Pharmacol 2002;39:842–50

17 Hoare G, Birks E, Bowles C, Marczin N, Yacoub M. In vitro endothelial cell activation and inflammatory responses in end stage heart failure. J Appl Physiol 2006 Nov;101(5);1466–73. Epub 2006 Jul 6.

18 Gullestad L, Aass H, Fjeld JG *et al.* Immunomodulating therapy with intravenous immunoglobulin in patients with chronic heart failure. Circulation 2001;103: 220–5.

CHAPTER 19

Role of innate immune dysregulation in diabetic heart failure

Betsy B. Dokken & Paul F. McDonagh

Introduction

Diabetes is a prime risk factor for cardiovascular disease. Vascular disorders include retinopathy and nephropathy, peripheral vascular disease, stroke, and coronary artery disease. Diabetes also affects the heart muscle, causing both systolic and diastolic heart failure. The etiology of this excess cardiovascular morbidity and mortality is not completely clear. Evidence suggests that although hyperglycemia, the hallmark of diabetes, contributes to myocardial damage after ischemic events, it is clearly not the only factor, since both pre-diabetes (with blood glucose levels only slightly above normal) and the presence of the metabolic syndrome, even in normoglycemic patients, increase the risk of most types of cardiovascular disease [1–4].

Due to the multifactorial nature of the diabetic state as well as the comorbidities commonly associated with it, the relationship between diabetes and heart disease is profoundly complex. Diabetes is typically associated with multiple metabolic and physiologic abnormalities, such as dyslipidemia, hypertension, and overweight or obesity, each of which have interdependent effects on the cardiovascular system and on the heart. Type 2 diabetes, by far the most common type, is associated with a higher prevalence and incidence of heart failure [5] than is found in the non-diabetic population. In addition, the prevalence of diabetes is increasing among heart failure patients much faster than in the general population. Between 1989 and 1999, while the prevalence of diabetes increased by 54%, among patients with heart failure diabetes prevalence increased by an alarming 360% [6]. De Groote *et al.* found that out of 1248 European patients with both diabetes and left ventricular dysfunction, the etiology of heart failure included an ischemic component in 58% and the remainder had non-ischemic cardiomyopathy [7]. Diabetic cardiomyopathy can be defined as myocardial disease in patients with diabetes that cannot be attributed to any other known cardiovascular disease, such as hypertension or coronary artery disease [8]. In clinical practice, it is often difficult to dissect the pathophysiologic processes that cause heart failure in diabetic patients. Due to the structural and functional changes that occur in diabetic cardiomyopathy, patients with diabetes are vulnerable to heart failure, even early in the course of their disease. Patients with diabetes are more likely than their non-diabetic counterparts to develop heart failure after an ischemic event, and this is likely due to the preexisting left ventricular dysfunction [9] present in these patients. For these reasons, it is difficult to discuss ischemic heart failure and diabetic cardiomyopathy as if they were mutually exclusive conditions.

Activation of the innate immune system is known to play a role in the development and progression of heart failure [10]; a role that appears to be enhanced in diabetic patients [11]. Diabetes has long been considered a state of chronic, low-level inflammation [12], and there is some evidence to suggest that this immune activation may actually be a precursor for the diabetic and pre-diabetic states, and ultimately the factor that initially increases cardiovascular risk in these disease processes [13]. This review will focus on diabetic heart failure, both ischemic and non-ischemic, and will review the experimental and clinical data supporting a role for innate immune dysregulation, or inflammation, in these burgeoning health problems.

Heart failure

Chronic heart failure is a complex clinical syndrome that can result from any structural or functional cardiac disorder that impairs the ability of the ventricle to fill with or eject blood [14]. Systolic heart failure arises from any condition that compromises the contractility of the heart, and is defined as a left ventricular ejection fraction of less than 45%. Diastolic dysfunction interferes with the heart's ability to relax and fill with blood and is typically diagnosed by Doppler echocardiography and/or cardiac catheterization [15]. In patients with diabetes, chronic heart failure either may have an ischemic or non-ischemic etiology or may have components of both types of disease. Diabetic cardiomyopathy is a distinct entity, initially characterized by diastolic dysfunction, which may not be clinically apparent unless (or until) it is associated with hypertension and/or with myocardial ischemia. When diabetic cardiomyopathy does become apparent, it is likely to present with severe clinical manifestations [16].

Inflammation and the metabolic syndrome

The metabolic syndrome is a constellation of risk factors characterized by abdominal obesity, insulin resistance (with or without glucose abnormalities), elevated blood pressure, atherogenic dyslipidemia, and pro-thrombotic and pro-inflammatory states [17]. Large epidemiological studies support a relationship between the metabolic syndrome and the development of atherosclerosis and cardiovascular disease [18–20]. The metabolic syndrome is central to the relationship between diabetes and cardiovascular risk, because 75–80% of people with type 2 diabetes also meet the diagnostic criteria for the metabolic syndrome [21]. In addition, normoglycemic people with the metabolic syndrome are likely to develop future glycemic abnormalities [22].

In 1995, McNulty *et al.* reported that hyperinsulinemia in insulin-resistant subjects inhibited normal myocardial protein degradation [23]. Subsequently, Phillips *et al.* reported that in normoglycemic subjects with blood pressures in the high-normal range, insulin sensitivity was conversely associated with left ventricular mass, suggesting that left ventricular hypertrophy in type 2 diabetes is most likely related to the insulin-resistant state rather than to hyperglycemia [24]. Recent evidence suggests that there may be cross-talk between the molecular pathways involved in both inflammation and insulin signaling, and this cross-talk may provide clues to the strong relationship between insulin-resistant states (such as the metabolic syndrome and type 2 diabetes), inflammation, and cardiovascular disease [25]. Specifically, researchers have found a reduced production of the potent vasodilator nitric oxide (NO) and an increased secretion of the vasoconstrictor and growth factor endothelin-1 in subjects with the metabolic syndrome, and these abnormalities enhance both vasoconstriction and the release of pro-inflammatory cytokines [26]. Recently, Pickup and Mattock [27] found a relationship between serum sialic acid, a marker of activated innate immunity [12], strongly predictive of type 2 diabetes in 128 patients from the United Kingdom who were followed for a mean of 12.8 years. In addition to predicting type 2 diabetes, this marker of low-grade inflammation also predicted cardiovascular mortality. This relationship was found to be independent of other known risk factors for CVD, including preexisting CVD [27]. These observations have led investigators to suspect a common, unknown antecedent [28] and to consider immune dysregulation as one candidate for this precursor [27].

Inflammation and obesity

Given that up to 90% of diabetic patients have type 2 diabetes, and that 85–90% of people with type 2 diabetes are overweight or obese, the effects of obesity are critical to the overall health effects of diabetes. Like insulin resistance, obesity is independently associated with an increased activation of the innate immune system. One explanation for the relationship between obesity and chronic inflammation is the evidence of signaling molecules that are simultaneously involved in immune system function and energy balance [29]. For example, obesity is associated with increased levels of a number of adipokines (cytokines released from adipose tissue) including tumor necrosis factor-α(TNF-α), interleukin 1β(IL-1β), interleukin 6 (IL-6), and plasminogen activator inhibitor 1 (PAI-1), all linked to the inflammatory response [30]. The levels of these pro-inflammatory cytokines typically increase as fat mass increases, however, one exception is the adipokine adiponectin, which has anti-inflammatory properties, and is decreased in obese subjects [31], exacerbating the chronic inflammatory nature of obesity. In addition to their endocrine properties, these locally produced cytokines have been found to possess autocrine/paracrine properties that can influence neighboring tissues as well as the entire organism. In fact, Mazurek *et al.* found that epicardial fat produces higher levels of several inflammatory mediators (such as TNF-α, IL-1, and IL-6) than can be detected systemically in high-risk cardiac patients, and therefore that plasma inflammatory biomarkers did not adequately reflect local tissue inflammation. In addition, the levels of these inflammatory markers from epicardial adipose tissue were not decreased by systemic anti-inflammatory therapies such as statins or modulators of the renin–angiotensin system (RAS) [32]. These data suggest that excess fat around the heart may enhance inflammatory damage in the myocardium, and that current systemic therapies to mitigate this damage may not have the expected beneficial effect on the heart.

Systemically, excess adiposity is associated with lipotoxicity, due to the chronic elevation of plasma free fatty acids (FFA). FFA are potent signaling molecules, and high levels of FFA associated with obesity, hyperglycemia and/or the metabolic syndrome are toxic not only to skeletal muscle, but to the myocardium as well [33]. One potential mechanism by which FFA contributes to cardiovascular toxicity is through the activation of innate immune inflammatory pathways upstream of the nuclear transcription factor NF-kappa B. Activation of this molecular signaling pathway causes endothelial dysfunction by upregulating the transcription of adhesion molecules VCAM-1 and ICAM-1. In addition, this pathway also activates genes encoding chemoattractant factors and inflammatory cytokines that promote the attachment and extravasation of monocytes and macrophages into vessel walls, a key step in the process of atherosclerosis [26].

Inflammation and hyperglycemia

In addition to the associated disease states that contribute to heart disease in diabetic patients, it appears that diabetes alone causes heart failure. Even well-controlled patients early in the disease process have been found to have preexisting subclinical left ventricular dysfunction. At least two different epidemiological studies found the prevalence of asymptomatic diastolic dysfunction in patients with type 2 diabetes to be between 52 and 60%, despite meeting clinical criteria for acceptable glycemic control [34, 35]. Left ventricular diastolic dysfunction, characterized by impaired early diastolic filling, prolonged isovolumetric relaxation, and increased atrial filling, has even been demonstrated in young patients with type 1 diabetes [36] who were neither obese nor insulin-resistant. Findings of the Strong Heart Study, the first large, comprehensive comparison of left ventricular structure and function between diabetic and non-diabetic subjects, support a strong relationship between diabetes, heart failure, and inflammation. In this clinical investigation, the presence of type 2 diabetes was associated with left ventricular enlargement and decreased myocardial function in both men and women. In addition, the extent and frequency of diastolic dysfunction was directly proportional to the hemoglobin A_{1c}(HbA$_{1c}$) level, which is the standard clinical measurement of glycemic control in diabetic patients [37]. In the United Kingdom Prospective Diabetes Study (UKPDS), every 1% increase in the HbA$_{1c}$ was associated with a 12% increase in heart failure [38]. Thus, the more glycemic control deteriorated, the higher the likelihood that ventricular function would be impaired. Palmiere *et al.* also found a strong correlation between left ventricular hypertrophy and markers of chronic inflammation in patients with type 2 diabetes. In 1299 adults with type 2 diabetes, those with left ventricular hypertrophy had higher levels of fibrinogen and C-reactive protein (both markers of chronic inflammation) and urinary albumin (a marker of microangiopathy and endothelial dysfunction), independent of traditional cardiovascular risk factors. Moreover, fibrinogen and C-reactive protein levels were independently and significantly higher in subjects with left ventricular hypertrophy among those without pathologic albuminuria, suggesting that the association between cardiac hypertrophy and low-grade inflammation may precede development of the vascular dysfunction [39]. Taken together, these data suggest that hyperglycemia, even mild or transient, plays an important role in the development of immune-mediated diabetic cardiomyopathy.

There are a number of mechanisms by which hyperglycemia can contribute to the development and progression of diabetic heart failure. Diastolic dysfunction in diabetic cardiomyopathy is thought to be due to myocellular hypertrophy and myocardial fibrosis. In addition, defects in calcium transportation, myocardial contractile protein collagen formation, and fatty acid metabolism have been demonstrated [16]. In the laboratory, there is evidence that cardiac efficiency is decreased in diabetes due to increased fatty acid utilization [40]. It is thought that increased fatty acid utilization leads to an increased production of reactive oxygen species (ROS) and mitochondrial uncoupling [40]. The increase in oxidative stress in diabetic hearts has been found to decrease nitric oxide levels, worsen endothelial function, and induce myocardial inflammation through stimulation of inflammatory mediators [41].

In 2001, Brownlee [42] published an integrating paradigm of the biochemical and molecular biological mechanisms for hyperglycemia-induced vascular damage. He presented convincing evidence that four main molecular mechanisms are responsible for the development of diabetes complications: overactivation of protein kinase C (PKC), increased formation of advanced glycation end products (AGEs), increased polyol pathway activity, and increased flux through the hexosamine pathway. In addition, he demonstrates how all of these pathways can be tied together by a single process—the overproduction of superoxide radicals by the mitochondrial electron-transport chain [42], which in turn creates excessive oxidative stress.

Oxidative stress occurs when the cellular production of ROS exceeds the capacity of anti-oxidant defenses within cells. A number of studies have demonstrated chronic oxidative stress in diabetic humans and animals, purportedly related to the excessive metabolism of substrates present in this physiologic state [43], as well as to the mitochondrial dysfunction associated with insulin resistance [44]. For example, plasma levels of hydroperoxides (ROS) are higher in subjects with type 2 diabetes compared to nondiabetic subjects, and these levels are inversely correlated with the degree of metabolic control [43]. ROS are generated not only from intracellular processes, but also from activated leukocytes. Hokama et al. found that the expression of adhesion proteins on the surface of polymorphonuclear leukocytes (PMNs) was significantly increased in diabetes [45]. Freedman and Hatchell [46] found that stimulated PMNs from diabetic animals generated superoxide radical, at significantly higher rates, than did those from normal animals [46]. Under ischemic conditions, Hokama et al. found that leukocyte accumulation during reperfusion was enhanced in the diabetic coronary microcirculation [45]. The excess chronic oxidative stress produced in the hyperglycemic state by intracellular sources as well as the additional acute stress mediated by accumulated PMNs may largely explain the mechanism of increased oxidative injury associated with ischemic heart disease in diabetes.

Myocardial interstitial fibrosis, a key feature of diabetic cardiomyopathy, is associated with hyperglycemia-induced overactivity of protein kinase C (PKC) [47]. Overactivation of PKC has been implicated as one of the mechanisms behind the vascular complications of diabetes, via hyperglycemia-induced overproduction of diacylglycerol (DAG) [42], and vascular dysfunction is ameliorated in diabetic rats by inhibition of PKC [48]. High glucose-dependent PKC signaling has been demonstrated to increase ROS production in cultured aortic endothelial cells, smooth muscle cells, and renal mesangial cells [49, 50]. Elevations of both DAG and PKC activity have been found in the aorta and heart of hyperglycemic diabetic rats. After a 2-week period of hyperglycemia, the normalization of blood glucose levels for up to 3 weeks with islet cell transplants in STZ-induced diabetic BB rats reversed the biochemical changes in the heart, but not in the aorta. These results suggest that PKC activity and DAG level may be persistently activated in the macrovascular tissues from diabetic animals and indicate a possible role for these biochemical parameters in the development of diabetic chronic vascular complications [51]. In chronic heart failure, myocardial fibrosis is caused by impaired remodeling of the extracellular matrix [52]. Activation of PKC in the kidney has been found to increase TGF-β production by mesangial cells. This pro-inflammatory cytokine acts to increase extracellular matrix protein synthesis through a mechanism that does not require active protein kinase C [53], thus creating a positive feedback cycle that perpetuates the inflammatory state. These data suggest that overactivation of protein kinase C in diabetes could contribute to myocardial fibrosis by stimulating TGF-β production and activity, demonstrating another link between hyperglycemia, inflammation, and the pathophysiology of chronic heart failure.

Another mechanism that explains the intimate association between hyperglycemia and myocardial damage is the accumulation of advanced glycosylation end products (AGEs) in the myocardium [54]. AGEs are the products of nonenzymatic glycation and the oxidation of proteins and lipids. Although these products develop under normoglycemic conditions (driven by oxidative stress), the rate of production and accumulation is greatly enhanced by diabetes, due to the excess availability of substrate. The receptor for AGE (RAGE) transduces signals that mediate the effects of AGEs on a wide variety of processes. AGEs, after binding to RAGE, cause the expression and activation of pro-inflammatory molecules as well as the activation of NF-kappa B. As discussed earlier, the activation of this transcription factor is a key step in the expression and induction of inflammatory cytokines [55] such as TNF-α, IL-1 and IL-6. Environments rich in RAGE ligands, such as diabetes, promote extended cell surface expression of these receptors, and lead to a spiral of RAGE-dependent cellular damage [56]. The generation of AGEs and the activation of RAGE, which augment inflammatory processes, provide a feedback loop for the sustained oxidant stress, further generation of AGEs, and the chronic inflammation associated with diabetes and heart failure.

An addition to PKC activation and the accumulation of AGEs, another mechanism by which hyper-glycemia promotes immune-mediated myocardial injury is through activation of the polyol (aldose reductase) pathway. The polyol pathway is an alternate pathway for glucose metabolism that is overactive in the hyperglycemic state. In this pathway, glucose is reduced to sorbitol by the enzyme aldose reductase using NADPH as a cofactor, and sorbitol is subsequently converted to fructose. Sorbitol accumulation causes osmotic stress, and is directly toxic to a variety of tissues [57]. The fructose that is generated is converted into fructose-3-phosphate, which generates 3-deoxyglucosone, a central precursor to the generation of several potent AGEs [55] that activate the RAGE pathway and contribute to inflammatory tissue damage. In addition, excess flux through this pathway increases intracellular oxidative stress, both by the production of oxygen radicals and by the consumption of anti-oxidant defenses. The oxidation of NADPH to NADP+ by aldose reductase generates free radicals [58], and since NADPH is required for the regeneration of the potent intracellular antioxidant glutathione, the consumption of NADPH by the polyol pathway could induce or exacerbate oxidative stress [42]. The oxidation of sorbitol to fructose is coupled with the reduction of NAD+ to NADH, creating an increased cytosolic NADH/NAD+ ratio [58]. This alteration in the intracellular redox state can decrease the availability of tetrahydrobiopterin (BH_4), an essential cofactor for the synthesis of nitric oxide from L-arginine by nitric oxide synthase (NOS) [59]. BH_4 depletion leads to an "uncoupling" of NOS, resulting in the production of increased superoxide radicals rather than NO [60]. Chung *et al.* demonstrated that the polyol pathway is the major source of diabetes-induced oxidative stress in lens of the eye and the nerve [61]. Both the accumulation of metabolites from the polyol pathway as well as the concomitant increase in oxidative stress have been implicated in the development of multiple diabetes-related complications [62], including myocardial ischemia [63].

In addition to playing an indirect role in the inflammatory nature of diabetic heart disease, high concentrations of glucose have also been found to directly activate pro-inflammatory pathways. The JAK signaling pathway plays a key role in a variety of biological activities, including cell growth, differentiation, apoptosis, and inflammation [64]. In human non-failing myocytes, high glucose allows angiotensin II to activate JAK2 (growth-related) signaling, whereas in failing myocytes, hyperglycemia alone is able to induce angiotensin II generation, which in turn activates JAK2 via enhanced oxidative stress [65]. Activation of JAK2 and its downstream signaling elements is associated with enhanced myocardial ischemia [66] and could be one mechanism by which hyperglycemia increases the extent of myocardial damage in diabetes.

Diabetic blood is also pro-inflammatory, and can provide clues to the excessive cardiovascular morbidity and mortality associated with this disease. Using the total white blood cell count as a marker of inflammation, investigators found that chronic inflammation is associated with both macro and microvascular complications in Chinese patients with type 2 diabetes [67]. Enhanced leukocyte-mediated inflammation is found in the coronary microcirculation of diabetic animals [45] and enhanced

platelet–neutrophil conjugation, a marker of cell–cell adhesion and activation, is present in plasma from diabetic women [68].

In summary, growing evidence demonstrates an intimate relationship between diabetes, heart failure, and inflammation (Figure 19.1). Inflammatory cytokines and other markers of active innate immunity are elevated in diabetes and the metabolic syndrome. Markers of low-grade inflammation are predictive of type 2 diabetes, and of cardiovascular mortality, which suggests that the inflammatory response precedes these disease states. One explanation for these findings might be obesity, a condition that commonly accompanies type 2 diabetes, and is independently associated with high levels of inflammatory cytokines. Once diabetes develops, it is clear that glycemic control is critical to optimizing cardiovascular outcomes, and that inflammation also plays a role in the morbidity and mortality

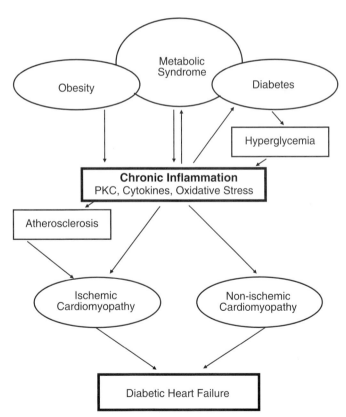

Figure 19.1 Chronic inflammation is an underlying condition associated with obesity and diabetes and may also exacerbate the diabetic state and the metabolic syndrome. In turn, chronic inflammation may contribute to atherosclerosis, and directly to cardiomyopathy through both ischemic and nonischemic mechanisms, thus providing a link between inflammation and diabetic heart failure.

associated with hyperglycemia. Given the extreme burden of diabetes and heart failure, further investigations that focus on the relationships between these disease states, are warranted, as well as effective interventions to improve outcomes in these patients.

Acknowledgments

The authors wish to acknowledge the support of NIH funding through NIHLB grants 58859 and HL07249.

References

1 Muhlestein JB, Anderson JL, Horne BD *et al*. Effect of fasting glucose levels on mortality rate in patients with and without diabetes mellitus and coronary artery disease undergoing percutaneous coronary intervention. Am Heart J 2003;146:351–8.

2 Nielson C, Lange T. Blood glucose and heart failure in nondiabetic patients. Diabetes Care 2005;28:607–11.

3 The DECODE Study Group. Glucose tolerance and mortality: comparison of WHO and American Diabetic Association diagnostic criteria. Lancet 1999;354:617–21.

4 Thrainsdottir IS, Aspelund T, Thorgeirsson G *et al*. The association between glucose abnormalities and heart failure in the population-based Reykjavík study. Diabetes Care 2005;28:612–6.

5 Nichols GA, Hillier TA, Erbey JR, Brown JB. Congestive heart failure in type 2 diabetes: prevalence, incidence, and risk factors. Diabetes Care 2001;24:1614–9.

6 Kamalesh M, Nair G. Dirproportionate increase in prevalence of diabetes among patients with congestive heart failure due to systolic dysfunction. Int J Cardiol 2005;90:125–7.

7 De Groote P, Lamblin N, Mouquet F *et al*. Impact of diabetes mellitus on long-term survival in patients with congestive heart failure. Eur Heart J 2004;25:656–62.

8 Marwick TH. Diabetic heart disease. Heart 2006;92:296–300.

9 Bell DS. Heart failure: the frequent, forgotten and often fatal complication of diabetes. Diabetes Care 2003;26:2433–41.

10 Anker SD, von Haehling S. Inflammatory mediators in chronic heart failure: an overview. Heart 2004;90:464–70.

11 Matsumoto K, Sera Y, Abe Y, Ueki Y, Tominaga T, Miyake S. Inflammation and insulin resistance are independently related to all-cause of death and cardiovascular events in Japanese patients with type 2 diabetes mellitus. Atherosclerosis 2003;169:317–21.

12 Pickup JC, Mattock MB, Chusney GD, Burt D. NIDDM as a disease of the innate immune system: association of acute-phase reactants and interleukin-6 with metabolic syndrome X. Diabetologia 1997;40:1286–92.

13 Festa A, D'Agostino R, Jr, Howard G, Mykkänen L, Tracy RP, Haffner SM. Chronic subclinical inflammation as part of the insulin resistance syndrome: the insulin resistance atherosclerosis study (IRAS). Circulation 2000;102:42–7.

14 Hunt SA, Baker DW, Chin MH *et al*. ACC/AHA Guidelines for the evaluation and management of chronic heart failure in the adult: executive summary: a report of the American College of Cardiology/American Heart Association Task Force on practice guidelines (Committee to revise the 1995 guidelines for the evaluation and management of heart failure). Circulation 2001;104:2996–3007.

15 Gutierrez C, Blanchard DG. Diastolic heart failure: challenges of diagnosis and treatment. Am Fam Physician 2004;69:2609–16.

16 Bell DS. Diabetic cardiomyopathy. A unique entity or a complication of coronary artery disease? Diabetes Care 2003;18:5708–14.

17 Executive summary of the Third Report of the National Cholesterol Education Program (NCEP) Expert Panel on Detection, Evaluation, and Treatment of High Blood Cholesterol in Adults (Adult Treatment Panel III). JAMA 2001;285:2486–97.

18 Hu FB, Stampfer MJ, Haffner SM, Solomon CG, Willett WC, Manson JE. Elevated risk of cardiovascular disease prior to clinical diagnosis of type 2 diabetes. Diabetes Care 2002;25:1129–34.

19 Rutter MK, Meigs JB, Sullivan LM, D'Agostina RB, Wilson PWF. C-reactive protein, the metabolic syndrome, and prediction of cardiovascular events in the Framingham offspring study. Circulation 2004;110:380–5.

20 Sundström J, Risérus U, Byberg L, Zethelius B, Lithell H, Lind L. Clinical value of the metabolic syndrome for long term prediction of total and cardiovascular mortality: prospective, population based cohort study. BMJ 332, 878-882.

21 Lemieux I, Almeëras N, MaurieËge P *et al*. Prevalence of "hypertriglyceridemic waist" in men who participated in the Queëbec Health Survey: association with atherogenic and diabetogenic metabolic risk factors. Can J Cardiol 2002;18:725–732.

22 Kahn HS, Valdez R. Metabolic risks identified by the combination of enlarged waist and elevated triacylglycerol concentration. Am J Clin Nutr 2003;78:928–34.

23 McNulty PH, Luard RJ, Deckelbaum LI, Zaret BL, Young LH. Hyperinsulinemia inhibits myocardial protein degradation in patients with cardiovascular disease and insulin resistance. Circulation 1995;92:2151–6.

24 Phillips RA, Krakoff LR, Dunaif A, Finegood DT, Gorlin R, Shimabukuro S. Relation among left ventricular mass, insulin resistance, and blood pressure in nonobese subjects. J Clin Endocrinol Metab 1998;83:4284–8.

25 Kim J, Koh KK, Quon MJ. The union of vascular and metabolic actions of insulin in sickness and in health. Arterioscler Thromb Vasc Biol 2005;46: 1978–85.

26 Koh KK, Han SH, Quon MJ. Inflammatory markers and the metabolic syndrome. J Am Coll Cardiol 2005;46: 1978–85.

27 Pickup JC, Mattock MB. Activation of the innate immune system as a predictor of cardiovascular mortality in type 2 diabetes mellitus. Diabet Med 2003;20:723–6.

28 Jarrett RJ, Shipley MJ. Type 2 (non-insulin-dependent) diabetes mellitus and cardiovascular disease: putative association via common antecedents; further evidence from the Whitehall study. Diabetalogia 1998;31:737–40.

29 Fernandez-Real JM, Ricart W. Insulin resistance and chronic cardiovascular inflammatory syndrome. Endoc Rev 2003;24:278–301.

30 Trayhurn P, Wood IS. Signalling role of adipose tissue: adipokines and inflammation in obesity. Biochem Soc Trans 2005;33:1078–81.

31 Arita Y, Kihara S, Ouchi N et al. Paradoxical decrease of an adipose-specific protein, adiponectin, in obesity. Biochem Biophys Res Commun 1999;257:79–83.

32 Mazurek T, Zhang L, Zalewski A et al. Human epicardial adipose tissue is a source of inflammatory mediators. Circulation 2003;108:2460–6.

33 Young ME, McNulty P, Taegtmeyer H. Adaptation and maladaptation of the heart in diabetes. Part II: Potential mechanisms. Circulation 2002;105:1861–70.

34 Poirier P, Bogaty P, Garneau C, Marois L, Dumesnil JG. Diastolic dysfunction in normotensive men with well-controlled type 2 diabetes: importance of maneuvers in echocardiographic screening for preclinical diabetic cardiomyopathy. Diabetes Care 2001;24:5–10.

35 Redfield MM, Jcobsen SJ, Burnett JC, Mahoney DW, Bailey KR, Rodeheffer RJ. Burden of systolic and diastolic ventricular dysfunction in the community. JAMA 2003;289:194–202.

36 Schannwell CM, Schneppenheim M, Perings S, Plehn G, Strauer BE. Left ventricular diastolic dysfunction as an early manifestation of diabetic cardiomyopathy. Cardiology 2002;98:33–9.

37 Devereux RB, Roman MJ, Paranicas M et al. Impact of diabetes on cardiac structure and function: the strong heart study. Circulation 2000;101:2271–6.

38 Stratton IM, Adler AI, Neil HAW et al. Association of glycaemia with macrovascular and microvascular complications of type 2 diabetes (UKPDS 35): prospective observational study. BMJ 2000;321:405–12.

39 Palmiere V, Tracy RP, Roman MJ et al. Relation of left ventricular hypertrophy to inflammation and albuminuria in adults with type 2 diabetes. Diabetes Care 2003;26: 2764–9.

40 Boudina S, Abel ED. Mitochondrial uncoupling: a key contributor to reduced cardiac efficiency in diabetes. Physiology 2005;21:250–8.

41 Szabo C. PARP as a drug target for the therapy of diabetic cardiovascular dysfunction. Drug News Perspectives 2002;15:197–205.

42 Brownlee M. Biochemistry and molecular cell biology of diabetic complications. Nature 2001;414:813–20.

43 Nourooz-Zadeh J, Rahimi A, Tajaddini-Sarmadi J et al. Relationships between plasma measures of oxidative stress and metabolic control in NIDDM. Diabetologia 1997;40:647–53.

44 Petersen KF, Dufour S, Befroy D, Garcia R, Shulman GI. Impaired mitochondrial activity in the insulin-resistant offspring of patients with type 2 diabetes. N Engl J Med 2004;350:664–71.

45 Hokama J, Ritter LS, Davis-Gorman G, Cimetta AD, Copeland JG, McDonagh PF. Diabetes enhances leukocyte accumulation in the coronary microcirculation early in reperfusion following ischemia. J Diabetes Complications 2000;14(2):96–107.

46 Freedman SF, Hatchell DL. Enhanced superoxide radical production by stimulated polymorphonuclear leukocytes in a cat model of diabetes. Exp Eye Res 1992;55: 767–73.

47 Wakasaki H, Koya D, Schoen FJ et al. Targeted overexpression of protein kinase C beta2 isoform in myocardium causes cardiomyopathy. Proc Natl Acad Sci 1997;94: 9320–5.

48 Ishii H, Jirousek MR, Koya D et al. Amelioration of vascular dysfunction in diabetic rats by an oral PKC beta inhibitor. Science 1996;272:728–731.

49 Inoguchi T, Sonta T, Tsubouchi H et al. Protein kinase C-dependent increase in reactive oxygen species (ROS) production in vascular tissues of diabetes: role of vascular NAD(P)H oxidase. JASN 2003;14:S227–32.

50 Lyle AN, Griendling KK. Modulation of vascular smooth muscle signaling by reactive oxygen species. Physiology 2006;21:269–80.

51 Inoguchi T, Battan R, Handler E, Sportsman JR, Heath W, King GL. Preferential elevation of protein kinase C isoform beta II and diacylglycerol levels in the aorta and heart of diabetic rats: differential reversibility to glycemic control by islet cell transplantation. Proc Natl Acad Sci 1992;89:11059–63.

52 Weber KT, Brilla CG, Campbell SE, Zhou G, Matsubara L, Guarda E. Pathologic hypertrophy with fibrosis: the structural basis for myocardial failure. Blood Press 1992;1:75–85.

53 Craven PA, Studer RK, Negrete H, DeRubertis FR. Protein kinase C in diabetic nephropathy. J Diabetes Complications 1995;9:241–5.

54 Bauters C, Lamblin N, McFadden EP, Van Bell E, Millaire A, DeGroote P. Influence of diabetes mellitus on heart failure risk and outcome. Cardiovas Diabetol 2003;2: 1–16.

55 Yan SF, Ramasamy R, Naka Y, Schmidt AM. Glycation, inflammation, and RAGE: a scaffold for the macrovascular complications of diabetes and beyond. Circ Res 2003;93:1159–69.

56 Schmidt AM, Yan SD, Yan SF, Stern DM. The multiligand receptor RAGE as a progression factor amplifying immune and inflammatory responses. J Clin Invest 2001;108:949–55.

57 Chandra D, Jackson EB, Ramana1 KV, Kelley R, Srivastava1 SK, Bhatnagar A. Nitric oxide prevents aldose reductase activation and sorbitol accumulation during diabetes. Invest Ophthalmol Vis Sci 1981: 314–26.

58 Honing MLH, Morrison PJ, Banga JD, Stroes ESG, Rabelink TJ. Nitric oxide availability in diabetes mellitus. Diabetes/Metabolism Rev 1998;14:241–9.

59 Cai H, Harrison DG. Endothelial dysfunction in cardiovascular diseases: the role of oxidant stress. Circ Res 2000;87:840–4.

60 Consentino F, Katusic Z. Tetrahydrobiopterin and dysfunction of endothelial nitric oxide synthase in coronary arteries. Circulation 1995;91:139–44.

61 Chung SM, Ho ECM, Lam KSK, Chung SK. Contribution of polyol pathway to diabetes-induced oxidative stress. JASN 2003;14:S233–6.

62 Yabe-Nishimura C. Aldose reductase in glucose toxicity: a potential target for the prevention of diabetic complications. Pharmacol Rev 1998;50:21–34.

63 Williamson JR, Chang K, Frangos M et al. Hyperglycemic pseudohypoxia and diabetic complications. Diabetes 1993;42:801–13.

64 Ni C, Hsieh H, Chao Y, Wang DL. Interleukin-6-induced JAK2/STAT3 signaling pathway in endothelial cells is suppressed by hemodynamic flow. Am J Physiol 2004;287:C771–80.

65 Modesti A, Bertolozzi I, Gamberi T et al. Hyperglycemia activates JAK2 signaling pathway in human failing myocytes via angiotensin II-mediated oxidative stress. Diabetes 2005;54:294–401.

66 Hwang JC, Shaw S, Kaneko M, Redd H, Marrero MB, Ramasamy R. Aldose reductase pathway mediates JAK-STAT signaling: a novel axis in myocardial ischemic injury. FASEB J 2005;19:795–7.

67 Tong PC, Lee KF, So WY et al. White blood cell count is associated with macro- and microvascular complications in Chinese patients with type 2 diabetes. Diabetes Care 2004; 27:216–22.

68 Tuttle HA, Davis-Gorman G, Goldman S, Copeland JG, McDonagh PF. Platelet–neutrophil conjugate formation is increased in diabetic women with cardiovascular disease. Cardiovasc Diabetol 2003;2:1–16.

CHAPTER 20

Tolerance in heart transplantation: current and future role

Kimberly Gandy, Jos Domen & Jack Copeland

Introduction

Cardiac transplantation has become an effective therapy for the treatment of end-stage heart disease when alternative medical therapies have been exhausted. At present, patients that undergo transplantation need to be placed on medications that will suppress their immune system. In turn, they need to take a variety of other medications that help reduce or prevent the complications associated with immune suppression. The resultant scenario for the recipient and treatment team, therefore, continues to be complicated. A possible solution to this problem rests in a phenomenon called transplantation tolerance. For a clinician, tolerance is characterized by a scenario in which a recipient accepts an organ from a genetically disparate donor without the need for immunosuppression. For an immunologist, tolerance is characterized by a scenario in which a recipient demonstrates no immunological reactivity to donor tissue in the presence of preserved immunological reactivity to third-party antigens. Ideally, these two scenarios would be one and the same. In reality, we realize that these scenarios may not be. We are well aware of situations in which, by gross analysis, a recipient appears to have accepted an allogeneic organ, only to find out years later that there has been chronic immunological damage to the organ at a clinically undetectable level. Similarly, we may find that an immunological assay may be suggestive of rejection in the face of what appears to be functional and histological tolerance. The former can be explained by the inability of our monitoring methods to detect subclinical levels of rejection. The latter can be explained by the inability of our clinical assays to fully appreciate the symphony that is the immune system; though some components of the immune system may be programmed to react against the allogeneic stimulus, other components may provide counterbalance by suppressing such reactivity. In recognition of this latter issue, a more accurate definition of tolerance would be one that refers to the lack of destructive immunological activity to the graft in the presence of an otherwise immunocompetent host [1, 2].

Tolerance induction in organ transplantation has been a goal as elusive in its attainment as it is tantalizing in its offerings. For the last 50 years, investigators and clinicians alike have seen the light of this offering, only to see such hopes lost in the tribulations of clinical reality. At the heart of these failures is the understanding that as we become more sophisticated in our ability to evaluate the immune system, so does our realization of the many layers of sophistication intrinsic to the immune system itself. As we gain understanding of one layer of the immune system and identify a way of subverting it, another layer emerges. In this chapter, efforts to achieve experimental and clinical transplantation tolerance will be reviewed.

Need for tolerance

Cardiac transplantation is an effective form of therapy. The majority of patients that receive heart transplantation have dramatic improvements in their quality and duration of life. Though the 1-year graft survival exceeds 80% in most centers and the 5-year survival is around 70%, the 10-year survival

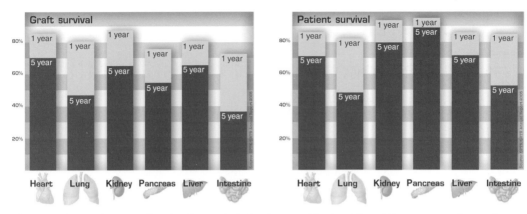

Figure 20.1 One- and 5-year graft and patient survival of patients receiving heart, lung, kidney, pancreas, liver, and intestinal transplantation.

sometimes falls to less than 40% (Figure 20.1). The causes of death are multifactorial, but most still relate to complications associated with suppression of the immune system. Some patients die from loss of graft function, most often thought to be the result of our inability to fully suppress the immune system's propensity to react against the tissues of the donor. Though retransplantation is offered as a form of therapy to increasing numbers of patients, the disproportionate ratio of available organs to recipients in need limits the ability to offer retransplantation. For instance, at the end of 2004, there were 3237 patients on the waiting list for cardiac transplantation. In the same year, 1973 hearts were recovered from donors, resulting in 1961 transplants [3]. The need far outstrips the supply. Still other patients die from complications associated with immunosuppression, namely infection and cancer. There are also other morbidities associated with immunosuppression that are not always fatal when considered alone, but which dramatically decrease the quality of life: diabetes, hypertension, osteoporosis, cataracts, fluid retention, and hair loss, to name a few. The ability to establish a method of tolerance induction should reduce these complications.

Even so, the risk–benefit ratio of tolerance induction regimens needs to be considered [4]. Transplantation has now reached a level of success that can provide survival and an acceptable level of complications for a great number of organ recipients. Most tolerance induction regimens carry some risk of associated complications. The most reliable methods could significantly increase potential complications at the onset. The decision then becomes one of determining if the potential complications encountered at the outset are worth the potential benefits in the long term.

Definition of tolerance

Tolerance can be defined in a variety of ways. In its most general immunological sense, it represents a lack of immunological reactivity to a defined set of transplantation antigens in the presence of preserved immunological reactivity to third-party antigens. A critical issue then becomes that of the definition of immunological activity. In initial immunological studies, immune reactivity was defined by an end organ effect. In skin transplantation, it was represented by visible rejection of the graft. In renal transplantation, it was recognized by a lack of urine output or an increase in the patient's creatinine. In cardiac transplantation, it was recognized by a decrease in graft function, often recognized by echocardiography. Eventually, histological diagnoses of rejection were defined. Rejection was defined by lymphocytic infiltrates or antibody deposition [5]. The classification devised by Billingham has stood the test of time. Though the histological grading system was somewhat modified [6], current systems are more reminiscent of her initial grading system. Ongoing efforts focus on defining tolerance and rejection through gene expression profiles, which can be determined in a noninvasive fashion [7]. There are, however, no assays, experimental or clinical that predict rejection as well as histological evaluation of a transplanted graft.

Mechanisms of tolerance induction

Experimentally, there have been multiple methods of tolerance induction. One of the first successful efforts toward tolerance induction was designed in the 1950s in the lab of Peter Medawar. In a large number of highly organized experiments, Medawar, Brent, and Billingham infused a variety of cellular extracts into recipients [8–11]. They found that a certain percentage of these recipients were subsequently tolerant of donor-specific organ grafts. Tolerance appeared to correlate most closely with those regimens that resulted in hematopoietic chimerism. They were awarded the Nobel Prize for this work in 1960. Ironically, this work actually had its origin in experimental work performed for a vastly different purpose. Peter Medawar had been asked to design a series of experiments to determine which twin cattle were fertile. It was known that a large percentage of nonidentical twin cattle were infertile, a condition that was known as a "freemartin." Medawar assumed that the cattle that were born of the same zygote would accept grafts from each other, and those that were not would reject these grafts. After performing a series of skin grafts, it was determined that the number of grafts accepted was far greater than that which could be explained by monozygotic twinning [12]. It was through collaborative reference to the work of Owen [13], and Lilie [14] that the answer to the mystery was discerned. It became clear that these cattle had exchanged hematopoietic cells *in utero* and indeed were hematopoietic chimeras, allowing them to be tolerant of the antigens of their twin and accept the organ graft.

When evaluating laboratory protocols, it is apparent that the literature is replete with "tolerance induction" protocols. There are many model systems in rodents that cannot be translated to clinical scenarios. The test of time has shown that only those systems tested in the high responder rodent systems seem to have correlative value in other animal or mammalian systems. Recognizing the distinct range of reactivity in rodent systems, rat systems have even been divided into those evaluating low responder systems and those evaluating high responder systems. Some strains of rats are known to have a vigorous response to alloantigens (for instance, Lewis rats). Others are known to have a low response to alloantigens (ACI rats). As an example, for the most part, only systems evaluated in high responder rat systems have realistic hope of having clinical applicability. An experimental tolerance protocol is only as rigorous as the system in which it is tested. We do know, however, that if one selects the most rigorous of systems, the results can have very close correlation with clinical scenarios. For instance, syngeneic hematopoietic engraftment studies in mice seem to have close correlates with human engraftment studies, even on a cell dosage basis [15]. It remains to be seen if the allogeneic systems will have similar correlates.

Experimental systems have evaluated the different methods of tolerance induction for decades now. One line of thought attempted to divide tolerance induction methods into central and peripheral (Figure 20.2).

Central tolerance

Clonal deletion is the main principle upon which central tolerance is founded. Clonal deletion involves the deletion of specific T-cell clones in the thymus during ontogeny. In normal ontogeny, the design is for the most self-reactive T-cell clones to be deleted after they have been presented with self-peptide in the context of self-MHC, a phenomenon which prevents rampant autoimmune disease. This maturational process initially takes place in the thymus and is divided into two major steps: positive and negative selection [16–18]. The first step of thymic maturation involves positive selection, a process that occurs when a thymocyte or developing T-cell encounters, and responds to, thymic stroma with self-MHC. The second stage of selection is termed negative selection. The most popular theory posits the differential negative selection of cells based on TCR affinity for peptide: those cells which have a high affinity for self-peptide are negatively selected or deleted whereas those with low or intermediate affinity for peptide are positively selected [19]. Some tolerance induction methods aim to capitalize on this selection process. If allopeptide in the context of self-MHC is presented to T-cell clones that develop in the thymus, they are similarly

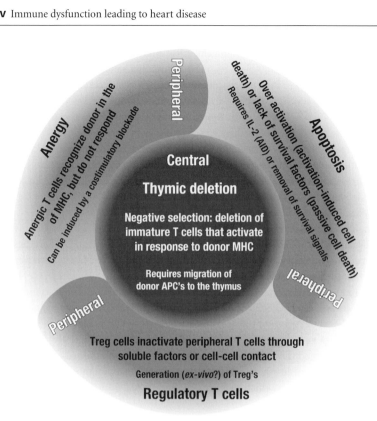

Figure 20.2 Mechanisms of tolerance induction.

deleted, resulting in a loss of the T-cell clone with high affinity for alloreactive peptide or antigen. For this mechanism to be operational, antigen must make it to the thymus for presentation. Systemic injection of many cellular antigens is sufficient for this process to take place. There have been numerous model systems, however, which have attempted to optimize this with direct intrathymic injection of antigen. Most translational systems focus on systemic delivery of antigens to the thymus, secondary to the attempted minimization of morbidity.

An important principle in clonal deletion is the need for cells that are positively selected but are reactive to self-peptide to be "anergized," or made nonreactive. Anergy is thought to result from a variety of mechanisms, though these mechanisms are apparently still not well understood. One can see, however, that a breakdown in the anergic properties of such selected T cells will result in autoimmunity. The corollary then for tolerance induction strategies is that a breakdown in the anergic properties of positively selected alloreactive T cells will result in a breakdown in tolerance.

Peripheral tolerance

From the above description, it can be seen that the central tolerance induction mechanisms are not infallible, and that there is a need for additional layers of regulation to prevent autoimmunity. Anergy is not necessarily a permanent state. It can be reversed by both lack of exposure to antigen [20] as well as by cytokines [21–23]. Similarly, not all antigens are likely presented in the thymus. There are some anatomical sites that are effectively immunologically privileged, that is, sites to which T cells and antigen presenting cells normally have no access. When such barriers are broken in disease or trauma, autoimmunity would most certainly ensue without peripheral mechanisms of tolerance induction in place. Accordingly, there are multiple methods present peripherally to aid the achievement of tolerance.

Regulatory cells

The presence of regulatory cells has been a controversial subject, accompanied by a significant amount of immunological emotion. In the 1980s and 1990s, there was much discussion of cells known as "suppressor cells." There were definitely cell populations that persisted in the periphery, be it in lymph node, peripheral blood, or bone marrow that appeared to have the ability to suppress immune function. It was in the characterization of these cells that the debate ensued. Over time, the word suppressor cell seemed to take on a rather dubious distinction, and the word has almost vanished from the literature [24]. However, regulatory cell-types continued to emerge. The cells known as the VETO cells were characterized in the lab of Judith Thomas [25] and thought to be active in tolerance induction regimens in nonhuman primates. Another cell-type that can regulate aspects of allorecognition are known as facilitator cells [26, 27]. Facilitator cells were initially recognized by their ability to enhance engraftment of hematopoietic cells across allogeneic barriers. Most recently, the emphasis has been on Treg's or T regulatory cells. These cells are known to suppress immune responses in the periphery, and are studied in a wide variety of tolerance models [28].

Re-programming

In the 1990s, it was determined that T cells needed more than one cell surface signal to undergo effective activation. The concept of costimulation emerged [29–31] in which cells needed not only a signal through the T Cell Receptor, but also a signal through another cell surface receptor. These receptors were termed "costimulatory molecules." The "signal one, signal two" hypothesis emerged to describe the fact that T cell need two signals for effective activation [32]. Stimulation through the TCR in the absence of signaling through the costimulatory molecule could lead to anergy or even deletion. Efforts were then made to block these costimulatory molecules with antibodies or other agonists, efforts that even extended to the clinic. In mice, simultaneous blockade of the CTLA4-IG and CD40-CD154 pathways resulted in tolerance induction [33]. This principle was subsequently evaluated in a nonhuman primate model with what appeared initially as similar results [34]. Long-term evaluation, however, revealed that these nonhuman primates were not tolerant [35]. Subsequently, a variety of costimulatory molecules were identified and the signal

one-signal two hypothesis seemed to grow into the signal one-signal multiple [32].

Peripheral deletion

Still other efforts simply try to eliminate as many T cells as possible, the assumption being that a majority of the T cells deleted will be the alloreactive ones [36–38]. Anti-thymocyte globulin (ATG), antilymphocyte globulin (ALG) [39, 40], a variety of antibodies directed against the CD3 molecule (OKT3, CD3 immunotoxin), costimulatory molecules such as CD154 and most recently Campath-1 (alemtuzumab), an antibody directed against CD52 have been used. None of these deletional strategies alone appears to be capable of inducing tolerance clinically (see section on clinical tolerance). These are nonselective processes, and full deletion of T-cell clones would result in dire immune incompetence. A similar principle of mass deletion is encountered with total lymphoid irradiation (TLI) that aims to delete peripheral T cells with irradiation [41]. Finally, there continues to be evidence that peripheral deletion can occur through mechanisms other than antibody mediated depletion and TLI. Selection may occur via deletion of T cells after presentation of antigen on peripheral dendritic cells as opposed to the thymic stromal counterparts [42, 43].

Cytokine milieu

Finally, it appears that the cytokine environment around T cells can greatly affect their behavior [44, 45]. A paradigm termed TH-1/Th-2 emerged. Cells were characterized as TH-1 or TH-2 depending on their expressed cytokine profile. A significant number of tolerance induction strategies aimed to bias the immune system to TH-2 expression, providing for a more tolerogenic environment in which T cells were present [46, 47].

Clinical protocols

Most clinical tolerance induction protocols involve transplantation of organs other than hearts. This is in large part secondary to the severe repercussions of cardiac rejection. The potential for support of a patient with a failing kidney is manifest as dialysis. The potential for support of a failing heart refractory to medical management involves device implantation, a procedure that has much greater attendant morbidity. In addition, a majority of the clinical studies that are currently performed, and protocols that are being developed are aimed at achieving tolerance for LRD-derived organs. The use of LRD-derived organs greatly reduces the time constraints on hematopoietic reconstitution and solid organ transplant, facilitating protocol development and pretransplant testing. However, to enable any protocol for use with cadaveric organs, which represent the majority of all transplants, including all heart transplants, protocols will have to be adapted to accommodate hematopoietic transplantation simultaneously with or subsequent to, organ transplantation. Several recent reports on successful tolerance induced by hematopoietic cell transplantation after the initial solid organ transplant indicate that it should be possible to develop protocols suitable for cadaveric donors [48–50].

Though the data to be discussed below involves renal transplantation, it is likely that protocols that are successful in renal transplantation can be adapted to heart transplantation. In experimental models there appears to be a hierarchy with respect to the difficulty with which certain organs are rejected [51, 52]. Whereas liver appears to be on the most favorable end of the spectrum, skin transplants appear to be one of the least favorable. Clinical data seems consistent with this observation. Kidney and heart transplantation appear to be in the middle of this spectrum, and experimental data has suggested that protocols that result in acceptance of transplanted allogeneic kidneys will likely result in acceptance of transplanted allogeneic hearts.

Withdrawal of immunosuppression after conventional protocols

For over three decades, there have been anecdotal reports of patients that were removed from immunosuppressants without detectable damage to their transplant grafts [53–56]. Most of these reports have involved renal transplants. A system emerged in which patients were classified as high responders or low responders based upon their response to withdrawal of immunosuppressants. Some of these patients have eventually lost their grafts or been found to be undergoing rejection. Through retrospective analysis, it has been difficult to determine which patients would be able to persist with low levels of immunosuppression on a long-term basis. Recently, 10 patients that were withdrawn from immunosuppressive drugs were followed long-term to determine the results of such withdrawal [57]. This was the first study to follow these patients over a significant period of time. It continued to be difficult to determine parameters that would be predictive of long-term tolerance. There were, however, several factors that appeared to be correlative: a slow withdrawal of immunosuppression (in most of the cases studied here through incompliance), a young organ donor age and a low PRA. Anti-donor class II antibodies were present in two of the "operational tolerant" patients. It is interesting, however, that one of the first patients that was withdrawn from immunosuppression [54] was most recently analyzed at a later point in time and found to be microchimeric for donor transplantation antigens [58], presumptively from birth or previous transfusion. It is possible that a situation similar to this is found in many of the other noninfusional reported cases of tolerance induction.

Tolerance through pharmacology

Several approaches have been tested that can potentially induce tolerance through manipulation of the immune cells present, rather than through infusion of cells. These approaches typically use depleting or blocking monoclonal antibodies to prevent the immune system from mounting a successful rejection of the graft. While graft survival can be demonstrated in experimental systems, none of these approaches result in sustained and reproducible induction of tolerance.

Costimulatory blockade

As discussed earlier in the Mechanisms of Tolerance section, blocking of co-stimulatory T-cell receptors such as CD28-CD80/CD86 or CD154-CD40 can result in T-cell anergy rather than activation. Both pathways have been targeted in clinical trials aimed at inducing tolerance. Trials testing the CD154-specific antibody have been halted due to thromboembolic events, possibly due to its expression on platelets [38, 59]. Several agents that target the CD28 pathway do not show obvious toxicity, and are being tested in trials. Costimulatory blockers are increasingly studied as primary maintenance drugs rather than tolerance-induction drugs [38].

Peripheral T-cell depletion

A second strategy that has been tested in clinical trials focuses on depletion of peripheral T cells using depleting antibodies directed against epitopes such as CD3 and CD52. The use of Campath or alemtuzumab (anti-CD52) results in severe T-cell depletion. However, several trials testing this antibody clinically in a renal transplant setting have failed to achieve tolerance, not even when combined with deoxyspergualin, a drug inhibitory for monocytes and macrophages [60, 61]. Antibodies to CD3 are not believed to clear T cells effectively from the lymph nodes and spleen, limiting its use in tolerance induction [59]. Polyclonal anti-lymphocyte sera have shown some promise [62], but have not resulted in tolerance.

Tolerance through cellular therapy

Tolerance induction through hematopoietic infusion may proceed through multiple mechanisms, and the mechanisms may be dependent on the amount of donor-specific hematopoietic engraftment achieved. The amount of donor-specific engraftment is, in turn, dependent on multiple factors: the donor antigen infused, the amount of donor antigen, the preconditioning regimen, and the postconditioning regimen.

In the late 1980s, there was a series of studies, a majority originating from Pittsburgh that demonstrated that some recipients of liver transplants that appeared to be tolerant of their organ grafts were chimeric in reference to their hematopoietic cells [63, 64]. These studies spurred a dramatic resurgence in the interest in tolerance induction after hematopoietic infusion.

Total lymphoid irradiation

Dr Samuel Strober has persistently sought tolerance induction with the use of TLI and lymphocyte infusion. A series of studies by Slavin *et al.* [65–67] set the groundwork for the future work and Dr Strober has been persistent in his search for translational ap-

plication of these principles for decades. His studies have progressed from rodent studies [67, 68], to studies in dogs [69], to studies in nonhuman primates. Original studies utilized a long period of TLI preconditioning prior to organ transplant. When it became clear that translational application would be limited by the necessity of such pretreatment, further protocols were designed in the rodent that did not require such time consuming preconditioning. There have been two significant clinical reports from this group. The first reports on three patients that have become tolerant with this preconditioning regimen [56, 70]. The second report describes four patients, two of which were withdrawn from immunosuppression [41]. Both experienced acute rejection at 5 months. Though this rejection was responsive to therapy, both patients now remain on immunosuppressive therapy.

Mixed chimerism

The laboratory of David Sachs has long been in pursuit of tolerance through infusion of hematopoietic cells. Original studies demonstrated donor specific tolerance in mixed hematopoietic chimeras after the infusion of combinations of donor and recipient bone marrow, using various combinations of T-cell depletion to give donor or recipient engraftment advantage [71]. Over time, as it appeared that full hematopoietic chimeras would be immunoincompetent, this laboratory moved to sublethal preconditioning regimens. They pursued a systematic line of experimentation that progressed from miniature swine [72, 73], and nonhuman primate [74, 75], to clinical trials [76–78]. The results in HLA identical transplantation were promising. This led to a progression toward haploidentical transplantation. These results were less promising. Of the three patients receiving renal transplantation, one experienced antibody mediated rejection resulting in graft loss. One of the remaining two experienced a humoral rejection episode that was successfully treated with anti-rejection medications.

Hematopoietic reconstitution

There are those that feel that it is only through full donor-derived reconstitution that reliable and permanent tolerance will be achieved [79]. The tolerance that is achieved with full donor-derived reconstitution is reliable, persistent, stable to challenge, and experimentally inducible in all animal strains tested. There are others that believe that the complications associated with full donor-derived reconstitution are too great and that mixed chimera's are a better avenue to explore [80]. It is also possible that the complications associated with full donor-derived reconstitution can be overcome with developments to enhance immune competence. For instance, recently, cellular populations have been identified that transiently help prevent fungal and bacterial infections in the neutropenic period surrounding stem cell transplantation and chemotherapy [81, 82] and can do so in a non-MHC restricted fashion [83]. The human homologues of these cells exist and appear to have the same functional properties in experimental systems [84]. Component therapy may offer the promise of reliable tolerance induction regimens with preserved immune competence.

Incomplete tolerance

A variety of terms have been used to describe incomplete states of tolerance. The terms Prope tolerance [85] or minimal immune suppression tolerance (MIST) [86] have been coined to describe situation in which patients can be partially withdrawn from their immunosuppressants without evidence of graft rejection. Another term that has been coined is "metastable" tolerance. The time between withdrawal of immunosuppression, and rejection of an allogeneic organ transplant can be fairly long, suggesting the existence of a "metastable" state of tolerance [87]. One reason for loss of tolerance in some situations may be that cross-reactivity with viral or other infectious agents may stimulate the alloimmune response (reviewed in [88]).

The fact that the scientific community has now acquiesced to allowing scenarios that do not correspond with our heretofore-proposed definitions of tolerance to be classified as tolerance is in some sense a nod to the difficulty encountered in this search for tolerance. A half-century later, realizing that nature can reproducibly induce tolerance on a daily basis to allow for each of us to breathe, we as clinicians and scientists cannot induce tolerance. Many investigators have spent their lives in search of this tolerance. While Prope tolerance indeed is a capitulation to the forces that have prevented us from finding absolute tolerance, it is also recognition of the fact that we have successfully and frequently partially averted the immune system.

Myocardial rescue

An alternative method of transplantation that may prove useful in the treatment of heart failure involves "cellular therapy." By this, we refer to the infusion of cells in the absence of organ transplantation in the hopes of obtaining some form of myocardial rescue [89, 90]. Studies have been ongoing for some time. Some original studies focused on the use of skeletal myoblasts, e.g. [91]. More recently, studies have focused on the use of bone marrow preparations. Though interest originally focused on the capacity of hematopoietic stem cells for the regenerative capacity [92], subsequent studies seem to suggest that this regenerative capacity is not confined to hematopoietic stem cells [93]. The capacity most likely rests within other cellular populations within bone marrow, though the mechanisms by which these cells confer myocardial rescue is entirely unclear. One promising theory rests within the ability of bone marrow cells to release substances that may enhance remodeling [90].

A critical issue for the optimal clinical application of myocardial rescue through cellular therapy will be the source of the cells. Currently, the source for many of these cells is autologous BM. Immunologically, the ideal scenario would be to utilize autologous cells as opposed to those from an allogeneic donor. Hypothetically, however, the individual's own bone marrow may not be the optimal source of myocardial rescue potential. One could imagine that the rescue potential between different individuals bone marrow may be vastly different, in part explaining the inability of a patient's own bone marrow to have induced rescue and therefore prevent the development of the disease. As such, attempts will be made to find a universal donor type of cell for infusion, something that could be produced in a much larger scale and be readily available. Candidates for such an approach could potentially be derived both from adult stem cells such as mesenchymal stem cells and embryonic stem cells [94, 95]. Such a source, however, might encounter the problems associated with allorejection, and thus tolerance induction would help enable this type of approach.

Summary

In the end, there will most likely be a convergence of transplant therapies for the heart. It is our bias that many of these therapies will be dependent on cellular transplantation. Ideally, we will eventually be able to determine which cardiomyopathies will be amenable to rescue with cellular therapy. Those patients with cardiomyopathies that are not candidates for cellular therapy may be candidates for cardiac transplantation. Tolerance induction has the potential to significantly enhance both modes of therapy. At present, the most promising tolerance induction strategies involve hematopoietic infusion, be it those that result in full donor-derived reconstitution or partial chimerism. There will likely be developments in each of these areas that are unpredictable. The ideal tolerance induction regimen will likely be found only through parallel and persistent exploration of each of these paths.

References

1 Suthanthiran M. Transplantation tolerance: fooling mother nature. Proc Natl Acad Sci U S A 1996;93(22): 12072–5.

2 Kirk AD. Immunosuppression without immunosuppression? How to be a tolerant individual in a dangerous world. Transpl Infect Dis 1999;1(1):65–75.

3 HHS/HRSA/HSB/DOT, OPTN/SRTR Annual Report 1995–2004. 2005. http://www.hrsa.gov.

4 Kirk AD. Ethics in the quest for transplant tolerance. Transplantation 2004;77(6):947–51.

5 Billingham ME, Cary NR, Hammond ME et al. A working formulation for the standardization of nomenclature in the diagnosis of heart and lung rejection: Heart Rejection Study Group. The International Society for Heart Transplantation. J Heart Transplant 1990;9(6): 587–93.

6 Stewart S, Winters GL, Fishbein MC et al. Revision of the 1990 working formulation for the standardization of nomenclature in the diagnosis of heart rejection. J Heart Lung Transplant 2005;24(11):1710–20.

7 Deng MC, Eisen HJ, Mehra MR et al. Noninvasive discrimination of rejection in cardiac allograft recipients using gene expression profiling. Am J Transplant 2006;6(1):150–60.

8 Billingham RE, Brent L, Medawar PB. Quantitative studies of tissue transplantation immunity III. Proc R Soc Lond B Biol Sci 1956;239:357–414.

9 Billingham RE, Brent L. Quantitative studies of tissue transplantation immunity IV. Proc R Soc Lond B Biol Sci 1959;46:78.

10 Brent L, Brooks CG, Medawar PB. Transplantation tolerance. Br Med Bull 1976;32(2):101.

11 Billingham RE, Brent L, Medawar PB. Actively acquired tolerance of foreign cells. Nature 1953;172(4379):603–6.

12 Anderson A, Billingham R, Lampkin G, Medawar PB. Use of skin grafting to distinguish between monozygotic and dizygotic twin cattle. Heredity 1951;5:379–97.

13 Owen RD. Immunogenetic consequences of vascular anastomoses between bovine twins. Science 1945;102: 400–1.

14 Lilie FR. The theory of the free-martin. Science 1916;43: 611–3.

15 Domen J, Weissman IL. Self-renewal, differentiation or death: regulation and manipulation of hematopoietic stem cell fate. Mol Med Today 1999;5(5):201–8.

16 Webb SR, Sprent J. Induction of neonatal tolerance to Mlsa antigens by CD8+ T cells. Science 1990;248(4963):1643–6.

17 Blackman M, Kappler J, Marrack P. The role of the T cell receptor in positive and negative selection of developing T cells. Science 1990; 248(4961):1335–41.

18 von Boehmer H, Kisielow P. Self-nonself discrimination by T cells. Science 1990;248(4961):1369–73.

19 Ashton-Rickardt PG, Bandeira A, Delaney JR et al. Evidence for a differential avidity model of T cell selection in the thymus. Cell 1994;76(4):651–63.

20 Ramsdell F, Fowlkes BJ. Maintenance of in vivo tolerance by persistence of antigen. Science 1992;257(5073):1130–4.

21 Jenkins MK, Chen CA, Jung G, Mueller DL, Schwartz RH. Inhibition of antigen-specific proliferation of type 1 murine T cell clones after stimulation with immobilized anti-CD3 monoclonal antibody. J Immunol 1990;144(1):16–22.

22 Beverly B, Kang SM, Lenardo MJ, Schwartz RH. Reversal of in vitro T cell clonal anergy by IL-2 stimulation. Int Immunol 1992;4(6):661–71.

23 Boussiotis VA, Barber DL, Nakarai T et al. Prevention of T cell anergy by signaling through the gamma c chain of the IL-2 receptor. Science 1994;266(5187): 1039–42.

24 Green DR, Webb DR. Saying the 'S' word in public. Immunol Today 1993;14(11):523–5.

25 George JF, Thomas JM. The molecular mechanisms of veto mediated regulation of alloresponsiveness. J Mol Med 1999;77(7):519–26.

26 Gandy KL, Domen J, Aguila H, Weissman IL. CD8+TCR+ and CD8+TCR- cells in whole bone marrow facilitate the engraftment of hematopoietic stem cells across allogeneic barriers. Immunity 1999;11(5):579–90.

27 Colson YL, Shinde Patil VR, Ildstad ST. Facilitating cells: novel promoters of stem cell alloengraftment and donor-specific transplantation tolerance in the absence of GVHD. Crit Rev Oncol Hematol 2007;61(1):26–43.

28 June CH, Blazar BR. Clinical application of expanded CD4(+)25(+) cells. Semin Immunol 2006;18(2):78–88.

29 Janeway CA, Jr, Bottomly K. Signals and signs for lymphocyte responses. Cell 1994;76(2):275–85.

30 Thompson CB. Distinct roles for the costimulatory ligands B7-1 and B7-2 in T helper cell differentiation? Cell 1995;81(7):979–82.

31 Bluestone JA. New perspectives of CD28-B7-mediated T cell costimulation. Immunity 1995;2(6):555–9.

32 Baxter AG, Hodgkin PD. Activation rules: the two-signal theories of immune activation. Nat Rev Immunol 2002;2(6):439–46.

33 Larsen CP, Elwood ET, Alexander DZ et al. Long-term acceptance of skin and cardiac allografts after blocking CD40 and CD28 pathways. Nature 1996;381(6581): 434–8.

34 Kirk AD, Harlan DM, Armstrong NN et al. CTLA4-Ig and anti-CD40 ligand prevent renal allograft rejection in primates. Proc Natl Acad Sci U S A 1997;94(16): 8789–94.

35 Kirk AD, Burkly LC, Batty DS et al. Treatment with humanized monoclonal antibody against CD154 prevents acute renal allograft rejection in nonhuman primates. Nat Med 1999;5(6):686–93.

36 Cobbold SP. T cell tolerance induced by therapeutic antibodies. Philos Trans R Soc Lond B Biol Sci 2005;360(1461):1695–705.

37 Waldmann H, Hale G. CAMPATH: from concept to clinic. Philos Trans R Soc Lond B Biol Sci 200 2;360(1461): 1707–11.

38 Larsen CP, Knechtle SJ, Adams A, Pearson T, Kirk AD. A new look at blockade of T-cell costimulation: a therapeutic strategy for long-term maintenance immunosuppression. Am J Transplant 2006;6(5, pt 1):876–83.

39 Aw MM. Transplant immunology. J Pediatr Surg 2003;38(9):1275–80.

40 Simpson D. T-cell depleting antibodies: new hope for induction of allograft tolerance in bone marrow transplantation? BioDrugs 2003;17(3):147–54.

41 Strober S, Lowsky RJ, Shizuru JA, Scandling JD, Millan MT. Approaches to transplantation tolerance in humans. Transplantation 2004;77(6):932–6.

42 Steinman RM, Hawiger D, Nussenzweig MC. Tolerogenic dendritic cells. Annu Rev Immunol 2003;21:685–711.

43 Redmond WL, Sherman LA. Peripheral tolerance of CD8 T lymphocytes. Immunity 2005;22(3):275–84.

44 Fitch FW, McKisic MD, Lancki DW, Gajewski TF. Differential regulation of murine T lymphocyte subsets. Annu Rev Immunol 1993;11:29–48.

45 Stockinger B, Bourgeois C, Kassiotis G. CD4+ memory T cells: functional differentiation and homeostasis. Immunol Rev 2006;211:39–48.

46 Waaga AM, Gasser M, Kist-van Holthe JE et al. Regulatory functions of self-restricted MHC class II allopeptide-specific Th2 clones in vivo. J Clin Invest 2001;107(7): 909–16.

47 Franzke A. The role of G-CSF in adaptive immunity. Cytokine Growth Factor Rev 2006;17(4):235–44.

48 Ringden O, Soderdahl G, Mattsson J et al. Transplantation of autologous and allogeneic bone marrow with liver from a cadaveric donor for primary liver cancer. Transplantation 2000;69(10):2043–8.

49 Matthes-Martin S, Peters C, Konigsrainer A et al. Successful stem cell transplantation following orthotopic liver transplantation from the same haploidentical family donor in a girl with hemophagocytic lymphohistiocytosis. Blood 2000;96(12):3997–9.

50 Gajewski JL, Ippoliti C, Ma Y, Champlin R. Discontinuation of immunosuppression for prevention of kidney graft rejection after receiving a bone marrow transplant from the same HLA identical sibling donor. Am J Hematol 2002;71(4):311–3.

51 Gardner CR. The pharmacology of immunosuppressant drugs in skin transplant rejection in mice and other rodents. Gen Pharmacol 1995;26(2):245–71.

52 Bickerstaff AA, Wang JJ, Pelletier RP, Orosz CG. The graft helps to define the character of the alloimmune response. Transpl Immunol 2002;9(2–4):137–41.

53 Owens ML, Maxwell JG, Goodnight J, Wolcott MW. Discontinuance of immunosuppression in renal transplant patients. Arch Surg 1975;110(12):1450–1.

54 Uehling DT, Hussey JL, Weinstein AB, Wank R, Bach FH. Cessation of immunosuppression after renal transplantation. Surgery 1976;79(3):278–82.

55 Zoller KM, Cho SI, Cohen JJ, Harrington JT. Cessation of immunosuppressive therapy after successful transplantation: a national survey. Kidney Int 1980;18(1): 110–4.

56 Strober S, Benike C, Krishnaswamy S, Engleman EG, Grumet FC. Clinical transplantation tolerance twelve years after prospective withdrawal of immunosuppressive drugs: studies of chimerism and anti-donor reactivity. Transplantation 2000;69(8):1549–54.

57 Roussey-Kesler G, Giral M, Moreau A et al. Clinical operational tolerance after kidney transplantation. Am J Transplant 2006;6(4):736–46.

58 Cai J, Lee J, Jankowska-Gan E *et al.* Minor H antigen HA-1-specific regulator and effector CD8+ T cells, and HA-1 microchimerism, in allograft tolerance. J Exp Med 2004;199(7):1017–23.

59 Lechler RI, Sykes M, Thomson AW, Turka LA. Organ transplantation—how much of the promise has been realized? Nat Med 2005;11(6):605–13.

60 Kirk AD, Hale DA, Mannon RB *et al.* Results from a human renal allograft tolerance trial evaluating the humanized CD52-specific monoclonal antibody alemtuzumab (CAMPATH-1H). Transplantation 2003;76(1):120–9.

61 Kirk AD, Mannon RB, Kleiner DE *et al.* Results from a human renal allograft tolerance trial evaluating T-cell depletion with alemtuzumab combined with deoxyspergualin. Transplantation 2005;80(8):1051–9.

62 Starzl TE, Murase N, Abu-Elmagd K *et al.* Tolerogenic immunosuppression for organ transplantation. Lancet 2003;361(9368):1502–10.

63 Starzl TE, Demetris AJ, Murase N *et al.* Cell migration, chimerism, and graft acceptance. Lancet 1992;339(8809):1579–82.

64 Starzl TE, Demetris AJ, Trucco M *et al.* Cell migration and chimerism after whole-organ transplantation: the basis of graft acceptance. Hepatology 1993;17(6):1127–52.

65 Slavin S, Fuks Z, Kaplan HS, Strober S. Transplantation of allogeneic bone marrow without graft-versus-host disease using total lymphoid irradiation. J Exp Med 1978;147(4):963–72.

66 Slavin S, Reitz B, Bieber CP, Kaplan HS, Strober S. Transplantation tolerance in adult rats using total lymphoid irradiation: permanent survival of skin, heart, and marrow allografts. J Exp Med 1978;147(3):700–7.

67 Slavin S, Strober S, Fuks Z, Kaplan HS. Induction of specific tissue transplantation tolerance using fractionated total lymphoid irradiation in adult mice: long-term survival of allogeneic bone marrow and skin grafts. J Exp Med 1977;146(1):34–48.

68 Lan F, Zeng D, Higuchi M, Higgins JP, Strober S. Host conditioning with total lymphoid irradiation and antithymocyte globulin prevents graft-versus-host disease: the role of CD1-reactive natural killer T cells. Biol Blood Marrow Transplant 2003;9(6):355–63.

69 Strober S, Modry DL, Hoppe RT *et al.* Induction of specific unresponsiveness to heart allografts in mongrel dogs treated with total lymphoid irradiation and antithymocyte globulin. J Immunol 1984;132(2):1013–8.

70 Strober S, Dhillon M, Schubert M *et al.* Acquired immune tolerance to cadaveric renal allografts. A study of three patients treated with total lymphoid irradiation. N Engl J Med 1989;321(1):28–33.

71 Ildstad ST, Sachs DH. Reconstitution with syngeneic plus allogeneic or xenogeneic bone marrow leads to

specific acceptance of allografts or xenografts. Nature 1984;307(5947):168–70.

72 Guzzetta PC, Sundt TM, Suzuki T *et al.* Induction of kidney transplantation tolerance across major histocompatibility complex barriers by bone marrow transplantation in miniature swine. Transplantation 1991;51(4):862–6.

73 Huang CA, Fuchimoto Y, Scheier-Dolberg R, Murphy MC, Neville DM, Jr, Sachs DH. Stable mixed chimerism and tolerance using a nonmyeloablative preparative regimen in a large-animal model. J Clin Invest 2000;105(2):173–81.

74 Kawai T, Cosimi AB, Colvin RB *et al.* Mixed allogeneic chimerism and renal allograft tolerance in cynomolgus monkeys. Transplantation 1995;59(2):256–62.

75 Kimikawa M, Kawai T, Sachs DH *et al.* Mixed chimerism and transplantation tolerance induced by a nonlethal preparative regimen in cynomolgus monkeys. Transplant Proc 1997;29(1–2):1218.

76 Spitzer TR, Delmonico F, Tolkoff-Rubin N *et al.* Combined histocompatibility leukocyte antigen-matched donor bone marrow and renal transplantation for multiple myeloma with end stage renal disease: the induction of allograft tolerance through mixed lymphohematopoietic chimerism. Transplantation 1999;68(4):480–4.

77 Cosimi AB, Sachs DH. Mixed chimerism and transplantation tolerance. Transplantation 2004;77(6):943–6.

78 Fudaba Y, Spitzer TR, Shaffer J *et al.* Myeloma responses and tolerance following combined kidney and nonmyeloablative marrow transplantation: in vivo and in vitro analyses. Am J Transplant 2006;6(9):2121–33.

79 Gandy KL. Tolerance induction for solid organ grafts with donor-derived hematopoietic reconstitution. Immunol Res 2000;22(2–3):147–64.

80 Sykes M, Sachs DH. Mixed chimerism. Philos Trans R Soc Lond B Biol Sci 2001;356(1409):707–26.

81 BitMansour A, Burns SM, Traver D *et al.* Myeloid progenitors protect against invasive aspergillosis and Pseudomonas aeruginosa infection following hematopoietic stem cell transplantation. Blood 2002;100(13):4660–7.

82 BitMansour A, Cao TM, Chao S, Shashidhar S, Brown JM. Single infusion of myeloid progenitors reduces death from Aspergillus fumigatus following chemotherapy-induced neutropenia. Blood 2005;105(9):3535–7.

83 Arber C, Shashidhar S, Wang S, Tseng B, Brown JM. Protection against lethal Aspergillus fumigatus infection in mice by allogeneic myeloid progenitors is not major histocompatibility complex restricted. J Infect Dis 2005;192(9):1666–71.

84 Manz MG, Miyamoto T, Akashi K, Weissman IL. Prospective isolation of human clonogenic common myeloid

progenitors. Proc Natl Acad Sci U S A 2002;99(18): 11872–7.

85 Calne R, Friend P, Moffatt S *et al.* Prope tolerance, perioperative campath 1H, and low-dose cyclosporin monotherapy in renal allograft recipients. Lancet 1998;351(9117):1701–2.

86 Monaco AP. Antilymphocyte serum, donor bone marrow and tolerance to allografts: the journey is the reward. Transplant Proc 1999;31(1–2):67–71.

87 Knechtle SJ, Burlingham WJ. Metastable tolerance in nonhuman primates and humans. Transplantation 2004;77(6):936–9.

88 Adams AB, Pearson TC, Larsen CP. Heterologous immunity: an overlooked barrier to tolerance. Immunol Rev 2003;196:147–60.

89 Melo LG, Pachori AS, Kong D *et al.* Molecular and cell-based therapies for protection, rescue, and repair of ischemic myocardium: reasons for cautious optimism. Circulation 2004;109(20):2386–93.

90 Dimmeler S, Zeiher AM, Schneider MD. Unchain my heart: the scientific foundations of cardiac repair. J Clin Invest 2005;115(3):572–83.

91 Taylor DA, Atkins BZ, Hungspreugs P *et al.* Regenerating functional myocardium: improved performance after skeletal myoblast transplantation. Nat Med 1998;4(8):929–33.

92 Orlic D, Kajstura J, Chimenti S *et al.* Bone marrow cells regenerate infarcted myocardium. Nature 2001;410(6829):701–5.

93 Balsam LB, Wagers AJ, Christensen JL *et al.* Haematopoieticstem cells adopt mature haematopoietic fates in ischaemic myocardium. Nature 2004;428(6983):668–73.

94 Stamm C, Liebold A, Steinhoff G, Strunk D. Stem cell therapy for ischemic heart disease: beginning or end of the road? Cell Transplant 2006;15(suppl 1):S47–56.

95 Gallo P, Peschle C, Condorelli G. Sources of cardiomyocytes for stem cell therapy: an update. Pediatr Res 2006;59(4, pt 2):79R–83R.

CHAPTER 21

Neutralization of Th2 cytokines in therapy of cardiovascular pathology

A. Mandel & A. E. Bolton

Introduction

The immune system is an extended family of inter-communicating cells that accept harmless and beneficial entities, while rejecting harmful ones. Cytokines play a central role in communication within the immune system. T-helper lymphocytes (Th cells) can differentiate, depending on the cytokine environment, from a common naive T-cell precursor into Th1 and Th2 subsets [1]. Typically, Th1 cells secrete proinflammatory cytokines including interferon-gamma (IFN-γ), tumor necrosis factor-alpha (TNF-α), and interleukin 1-beta (IL-1β), whereas Th2 cells produce a number of cytokines including IL-4, IL-5, IL-6, IL-9, and IL-13 but not IFN-γ [2–11], and are considered to be functionally opposed to Th1 cells [12].

Cytokines bind to specific cell receptors and initiate a cascade of immune-related functions that lead to induction, enhancement, or inhibition of gene transcription, and ultimately affect cell behavior [13]. Many cytokines interact with each other in complex ways that may be additive, synergistic, or antagonistic, or may involve the induction of one cytokine by another. Many cytokines are pleiotropic with multiple targets and have a range of physiological effects. A number of different cytokines can support the same physiological function, providing a degree of redundancy [2].

Cytokines generally act as local effectors and function within a highly confined environment. Local inflammatory responses are determined by the conditions within the immediate milieu. Therefore, responses could differ, for example, within unstable or stable atherosclerotic plaques [14]. However, a systemic inflammatory environment may have important effects, for example, on endothelial function [15]. A broad range of cardiac disease has been associated with inflammatory (Th1) cytokine signaling, including heart failure, cardiac reperfusion injury, myocarditis, cardiac allograft rejection, and sepsis-associated cardiac dysfunction [16]. Here, we provide evidence that Th2 cytokines may play a role in inflammatory responses, and that specific Th2 cytokine signaling is involved in cardiac and arterial pathology, particularly relating to endothelial function, atherogenesis and thrombosis.

The role of the immune system in cardiovascular pathology

Over the years, the accepted dogma has been that the immune system discriminates between "self" and "non-self," rejecting everything that is "non-self" and being unresponsive to "self." However, many observations are difficult to explain within the constraints of this concept. For example, why does the immune system not normally attack the "non-self" but beneficial commensal microflora (of the gastrointestinal, respiratory tract, vagina), or foreign antigens in food? Why are neo-antigens that appear at puberty not a target and attacked as "foreign?" To reconcile these issues, Matzinger has recently proposed that the immune system identifies and discriminates against "danger signals" rather than "non-self." Danger signals may be products derived from damaged or stressed tissues and cells [17], and are determined by the tissue in which the response occurs [18]. Under this model, antigen-presenting cells of the innate immune system (including macrophages and dendritic cells) are activated by these danger signals. Without this activation, no primary immune response can occur.

One route of activation of innate immune system cells is by interaction of pathogen-associated molecular patterns (PAMP) expressed on a number of bacteria with pattern recognition receptors including Toll-like receptors (TLR) present on antigen-presenting cells (APC) [19]. Studies directly implicate TLR/APC signaling in the progression of atherosclerotic plaques and provide a potentially important link between APC function and known cardiovascular risk factors, such as oxidized-LDL. Antigen presenting cells, particularly dendritic cells, which depend on signaling by pattern-recognition receptors via TLRs, are direct and important participants in atherogenesis and cardiovascular pathology [20]. Additionally, heat shock proteins, which could identify stressed cells, are also candidates for danger signals, as are endogenously produced PAMPs, perhaps released during cell necrosis [21]. In the context of cardiovascular disease, oxidative stress stimulates the release of proteins of the Hsp90 family from vascular smooth muscle cells [22], and levels of Hsp60 are elevated in patients with atherosclerosis [23], both observations being compatible with their role as danger signals in such conditions.

When activated, cells of the innate immune system up-regulate surface costimulatory molecules, providing the second signal that rescues antigen-stimulated T cells, enabling their differentiation and proliferation. One key co-stimulatory molecule, inducible co-stimulator (ICOS), plays a critical role in the pathway that regulates Th2 signaling [24]. ICOS blockade inhibits the ability of in vitro-generated Th2 cells to induce Th2-mediated inflammation [25], and Th2 effector function, but not Th2 differentiation, is inhibited by ICOS blockade [26]. ICOS-deficient mice have reduced amounts of Th2 immunoglobulin isotypes and produce little IL-4 after secondary stimulation [27]. Thus, a paradigm has developed in which ICOS provides a unique role in Th2 costimulation. Another integral component

of Th2 signaling is the signal transducer and activator of transcription-6 (STAT-6). STAT-6 is an essential component of IL-4-induced inflammation [28]. In mice, the disruption of the STAT-6 gene results in the failure of IL-4 signaling [29] and in a loss of Th2 responses [30].

Inflammatory and immune events play a central role in the development of atherosclerotic plaques. Cell populations detected at the shoulders of lesions include APC, T cells, B cells, and mast cells, influencing both the development and the stability of atheroma [14]. It has been suggested that APC, including macrophage, activation elicits T-cell activation, with subsequent cytokine secretion and antibody production [31]. Early in the development of plaque, these cells could become activated by different antigens, including modified lipoproteins, heat shock proteins, and PAMPs [32]. These findings suggest that it may be possible to target APCs as a strategy to regulate the inflammatory and immune response in cardiovascular pathology.

As mediators and modulators, Th2 cytokines regulate immunological responses, hematopoietic development and cell-to-cell communication at the level of both innate and adaptive immunity as well as host humoral responses to "danger" stimuli [2]. Generally, it was considered that anti-inflammatory (Th2) cytokines suppress the activity of proinflammatory (Th1) cytokines and reduce inflammation [33]. However, many Th2 cytokines modulate the synthesis or the action of Th1 cytokines in a complex network of interactions [34]. Thus, although IL-4 and IFN-gamma often have opposing effects, each suppressing the production of the other by T cells, recently it has been demonstrated that IL-4 can stimulate STAT6-dependent IFN-gamma production [35] and promote an antibody-mediated TNF-alpha/IL-1beta-dependent inflammation in vivo [36]. Not surprisingly, therefore, Th2 cytokines are implicated in a number of inflammatory diseases including cardiovascular pathology (Table 21.1).

The endothelium, immunology, and cardiovascular disease

The state of the endothelium is a key factor in the inflammatory mechanisms involved in the development of cardiovascular pathology. The endothelium

Table 21.1 Cardiovascular pathologies associated with Th2 cytokine activation.

Cytokines	Conditions	References
IL-4	Idiopathic dilated cardiomyopathy	[37]
	Atherosclerosis	[38–41]
	Abdominal aortic aneurysm (remodeling)	[42, 43]
	Myocarditis	[44–46]
	Cardiac allograft rejection	[47, 48]
IL-6	Atherosclerosis	[49–52]
	Myocarditis	[53]
	Acute myocardial infarction	[54]
	Unstable angina	[54]
	Congestive heart failure	[55]
	Idiopathic dilated cardiomyopathy	[56, 57]
	Arrhythmia	[58]
	Valvular heart diseases	[59]
	Cardiac reperfusion injury (coronary artery bypass surgery)	[60–62]
	Cardiac allograft rejection	[53, 63]
	Hypertension	[64]
	Type 2 diabetes and insulin resistance	[51, 52, 65]
IL-5	Myocarditis	[44–46, 66]
	Cardiac allograft rejection	[47, 48, 67]
IL-3	Myocarditis	[66]
	Arrhythmia	[58]
	Cardiac allograft rejection	[48, 67, 68]
IL-13	Myocarditis	[45, 46]
	Idiopathic dilated cardiomyopathy	[37]
	Atherosclerosis	[69]
	Type 2 diabetes	[70]
	Abdominal aortic aneurysm (remodeling)	[42, 43, 71]

is a major determinant of vascular tone and, therefore, of blood flow. Endothelial cells determine leucocyte and platelet adhesion, as well as smooth muscle cell proliferation [72]. When the endothelium becomes activated, the synthesis and release of vasodilators, such as nitric oxide (NO), prostacyclin, and endothelium-derived hyperpolarizing factor is reduced and the balance tips in favor of endothelium-derived vasoconstrictors, such as endothelin and thromboxane [73]. As a result of impaired endothelial function, there is a reduction in coronary blood flow, enhanced adhesion of inflammatory cells and smooth muscle cell proliferation contributing to an acceleration of inflammatory cytokine signaling. Recently, it has been suggested that Th2 cytokines, including IL-6 and IL-10, are involved in the modulation of arterial vascular tone [74].

Human endothelial cells potentially play multiple critical roles in innate and adaptive immunity. They are potent antigen presenting cells, and express CD40, CD58 (LFA-3), CD134 (OX40) ligand, CD200, and ICOS [75–79]. They are capable of expressing a range of pro- and anti-inflammatory cytokines, including members of Th2 functional groups of cytokines such as IL-5 and IL-6 [80, 81]. Moreover, the expression, by endothelial cells, of indoleamine 2,3-dioxygenase (IDO) [75], an important enzyme in the regulation of immune responses, and CD200 [78], a transmembrane glycoprotein that transmits an immunoregulatory signal through the CD200 receptor (CD200R) to attenuate inflammatory reactions and promote immune tolerance, suggest that ECs are direct and important participants in the induction and regulation of inflammatory and immune responses. Endothelial cells pervade virtually all tissues, and have been implicated in allograft rejection, protection against pathogens, and lymphocyte recruitment [82]. Recently, data suggest that ECs may enhance T-cell responses in vitro and are thought to stimulate immune responses in vivo [75, 83–85].

IL-4 in cardiovascular disease

Interleukin-4 (IL-4) is a pleiotropic Th2 cytokine that has been implicated in several major proinflammatory pathways, including the Janus kinase (JAK)-signal transducers and activation of transcription (STAT), as well as phosphoinositide-3 kinase (PI3K) and p38 MAPK pathways [86, 87]. IL-4 influences the recruitment of mononuclear cells by stimulating an increase in expression of macrophage chemoattractant protein-1 (MCP-1) by endothelial cells [38]. IL-4 also influences cell adhesion by causing an increase in expression of VCAM-1 and E-selectin by endothelial and vascular smooth muscle cells [39]. Moreover, IL-4 stimulates the production of 15-lipoxygenase [40], an

Table 21.2 IL-4 neutralization strategies in inflammatory diseases.

Treatment	Indication	Development status	Reference
Recombinant human IL-4 receptor (IL-4 antagonist)	Asthma	Phase II completed (S)	[89–91]
Epinastine hydrochloride (histamine H1 receptor antagonist)	Allergic conditions	Preclinical	[92]
IL-4DM DNA (DNA administration of murine IL-4 mutant Q116D/Y119D (IL-4 double mutant))	Asthma	Preclinical	[93]
AAV-mediated delivery of IL-4RA (IL-4 receptor antagonist)	Asthma	Preclinical	[94]

enzyme implicated in oxidizing LDL to its athero-genic form, and increases scavenger receptor expression by macrophages, which may increase their uptake of modified lipid and accelerate early atherosclerotic lesion development. Selective inhibition of the JAK/STAT, PI3K, and p38 MAPK signaling pathways abrogates overexpression of proinflammatory mediators such as IL-6, MCP-1, VCAM-1, and E-selectin in IL-4-stimulated human vascular endothelial cells [39], supporting the role of IL-4 in up-regulation of proinflammatory mediators in vascular endothelium. Hence, IL-4 appears to play a significant role in the inflammatory molecular signaling mechanisms involving vascular endothelial cell dysfunction and the development of atherosclerosis.

Myocarditis is a major cause of heart failure and sudden death among adolescents and young adults [88]. Recently, evidence has emerged of Th2-mediated signaling in the immunological pathogenesis of dilated cardiomyopathy and myocarditis in humans [45], and the role of Th2 signaling, associated with IL-4, IL-5, IL-10, and IL-13 production [46], is well established in animal models of myocarditis. Experimental autoimmune myocarditis (EAM) in murine models exhibits a Th2-like phenotype demonstrated both by the histological picture of the heart lesions and by the humoral response (predominance of IgG1). Moreover, it has been reported that IL-4 mediates the development of EAM in mice and is critical to the progression of severe forms of acute myocarditis [44].

Preclinically, anti-IL-4 treatment markedly reduced the severity of EAM and this was associated with a switch from a Th2-like to a Th1-like phenotype. These effects of anti-IL-4 treatment seem to be dependent on increased levels of IFN-γ and were associated with a decrease in IL-4, IL-5, and IL-13 [44]. However, although IL-4 neutral-ization strategies are under preclinical and clinical investigation for asthma and allergic conditions (Table 21.2), such studies do not yet appear to have been extended to focus on cardiovascular diseases.

IL-6 in cardiovascular disease

IL-6 is produced by a wide spectrum of cells including CD4+ Th2 cells, B cells, dendritic cells, endothelial cells, and macrophages. From an immunological point of view, APCs represent one of the major sources of IL-6 [2, 95, 96]. IL-6 promotes Th2 differentiation and simultaneously can inhibit Th1 polarization through two independent molecular mechanisms. IL-6 activates transcription mediated by nuclear factor of activated T cells (NFAT) leading to production of IL-4 by naive CD4+ T cells and their differentiation into effector Th2 cells. While the induction of Th2 differentiation by IL-6 is dependent upon endogenous IL-4, inhibition of Th1 differentiation by IL-6 appears to be IL-4- and NFAT-independent and involves up-regulation of supressor of cytokine signaling (SOCS)-1 expression interfering with IFN-γ signaling and the development of Th1 cells. Since IL-6 is abundantly produced by APCs, it is a likely source of early Th1/Th2 control during CD4+ T cell activation.

IL-6 is a major proinflammatory cytokine of the acute phase reaction; elevated levels in peripheral blood are associated with a worse prognosis in unstable angina and after acute myocardial infarction (MI). Each 1 pg/mL increase in IL-6 was associated with a 1.70-fold (range 1.23- to 2.45-fold) increase in relative risk of subsequent MI or sudden death [97]. Systemically, IL-6 induces CRP gene expression in the liver during the acute phase response [98–100]. Elevated plasma levels of CRP have been noted in a variety of cardiovascular conditions [101], and now C-reactive protein (CRP) is

Table 21.3 IL-6 neutralization strategies in inflammatory diseases.

Cytokines	Drug treatment	Indication	Development status	Reference
IL-6	Actemra (tocilizumab; MRA) (humanized anti-IL-6 receptor monoclonal antibody)	Rheumatoid arthritis	Filed (Japan), Phase III underway (US and Europe)	[103–108]
IL-6	Actemra (tocilizumab; MRA) (humanized anti-IL-6 receptor monoclonal antibody)	Multicentric Castleman's disease	Approved (Japan), Phase I underway (US)	[105, 109]
IL-6	Actemra (tocilizumab; MRA) (humanized anti-IL-6 receptor monoclonal antibody)	Multiple myeloma	Phase I underway (US), Phase II underway (France)	[105]
IL-6	Actemra (tocilizumab; MRA) (humanized anti-IL-6 receptor monoclonal antibody)	Systemic onset juvenile idiopathic arthritis	Filed (Japan), Phase II underway (UK)	[105, 110]
IL-6	Actemra (tocilizumab; MRA) (humanized anti-IL-6 receptor monoclonal antibody)	Crohn's disease	Phase II underway (Japan)	[105]
IL-6	Actemra (tocilizumab; MRA) (humanized anti-IL-6 receptor monoclonal antibody)	Systemic lupus erythematosus	Phase I underway (US)	[105, 111]
IL-6	CNTO 328 (chimeric anti-IL-6 monoclonal antibody)	Kidney cancer	Phase II underway (US)	[112, 113]
IL-6	Atiprimod (azaspirane; angiogenesis inhibitor and VEGF/IL-6 inhibitor)	Multiple myeloma	Phase I/IIa underway (US)	[114–120]

generally recognized as a marker of inflammation that predicts the incidence of myocardial infarction, stroke, peripheral arterial disease, and sudden cardiac death among healthy individuals with no history of cardiovascular disease, and recurrent events and death in patients with acute or stable coronary syndromes [101, 102]. CRP confers additional prognostic value at all levels of cholesterol, Framingham coronary risk score, severity of the metabolic syndrome, and blood pressure, and in those with and without subclinical atherosclerosis. CRP levels of less than 1, 1 to 3, and greater than 3 mg/L are associated with lower, moderate, and higher cardiovascular risks, respectively [102]. Therefore, elevated IL-6 levels are strongly associated with future cardiac events and mortality in a population with CVD.

Blocking strategies for IL-6 are being developed clinically for the treatment of a number of different disease states involving inflammation (Table 21.3). However, although, as described above, IL-6 is implicated in the development of cardiovascular disease pathology, and is a clearly de-fined cardiovascular risk factor, it is perhaps surprising that IL-6 blocking strategies do not yet appear to have been developed in the cardiovascular area.

IL-3, IL-5, and IL-13 in cardiovascular disease

IL-3 is a growth factor for a variety of hematopoietic cell precursors [2], and T lymphocytes, eosinophils, and mast cells are the major source of this cytokine. In myocarditis, IL-3 enhances eosinophilopoiesis and, in the presence of IL-5, which is typically produced in the heart, activates mature eosinophils [66]. Eosinophilia and eosinophil-mediated cardiac injury are involved in a number of myocardial diseases, including myocarditis. Eosinophil degranulation produces several toxic proteins that may play an important role in the pathogenesis of this cardiac disorder [117]. Extremely high concentrations of IL-5 in the pericardial effusion, rather than in the peripheral blood, is indicative of a role for IL-5 in the pathogenesis of human myocarditis [66].

IL-13 is homologous with IL-4 and shares many of its biological effects on "professional" phagocytic cells, epithelial cells, B cells, and endothelial cells, including stimulating VCAM-1 expression [118]. Both functional IL-4 and IL-13 receptors are heterodimers and share a common IL-4Rα peptide chain that activates the STAT6 signaling pathway. It would be expected, therefore, that these two cytokines would share many biological properties [2].

Conclusion

The pathology of cardiovascular diseases involves complex inflammatory and immune responses. Cytokine blocking strategies have been developed for a number of other inflammatory conditions, most notably rheumatoid arthritis, where TNF-alpha blocking using monoclonal antibodies or the TNF-alpha receptor fusion protein etanercept is an approved therapeutic approach. However, despite its initial promise [119], such a TNF-alpha blocking strategy failed to show a significant clinical benefit in chronic heart failure [120]. It is possible that the approach of blocking a single proinflammatory cytokine in such a complicated pathology as chronic heart failure, and, potentially other cardiovascular diseases, is over simplistic, particularly given the well-known redundancy in cytokine networks. Similar criticisms could be directed toward blocking strategies for Th2 cytokines such as IL-4 and IL-6 in cardiovascular diseases. A greater understanding of the role of the immune system in cardiovascular disease, including a more detailed knowledge of the immunological activities of the endothelium, should ultimately lead to the development of innovative treatments that will eventually alleviate or prevent the devastating human suffering inflicted by cardiovascular diseases.

References

1 Seder RA, Paul WE. Acquisition of lymphokine-producing phenotype by CD4+ T cells. Ann Rev Immunol 1994;12:635–73.

2 Borish LC, Steinke JW, II. Cytokines and chemokines. J Allergy Clin Immunol 2003;111(suppl 2):S460–75.

3 Lorentz A, Wilke M, Sellge G et al. IL-4-induced priming of human intestinal mast cells for enhanced survival and Th2 cytokine generation is reversible and associated with increased activity of ERK1/2 and c-Fos. J Immunol 2005;174(11):6751–6.

4 Yano S, Ghosh P, Kusaba H, Buchholz M, Longo DL. Effect of promoter methylation on the regulation of IFN-gamma gene during in vitro differentiation of human peripheral blood T cells into a Th2 population. J Immunol 2003;171(5):2510–6.

5 Gardner EM, Murasko DM. Age-related changes in type 1 and type 2 cytokine production in humans. Biogerontology 2002;3(5):271–90.

6 Hamelmann E, Gelfand EW. IL-5-induced airway eosinophilia—the key to asthma? Immunol 2001;179:182–91.

7 Miller AL. The etiologies, pathophysiology, and alternative/complementary treatment of asthma. Altern Med Rev 2001;6(1):20–47.

8 Saito S. Cytokine network at the feto-maternal interface. J Reprod Immunol 2000;47(2):87–103.

9 Romagnani S. T-cell subsets (Th1 versus Th2). Ann Allergy Asthma Immunol 2000;85(1):9–18; quiz 18, 21.

10 Trinchieri G, Peritt D, Gerosa F. Acute induction and priming for cytokine production in lymphocytes. Cytokine Growth Factor Rev 1996;7(2):123–32.

11 Wood PR, Seow HF. T cell cytokines and disease prevention. Vet Immunol Immunopathol 1996;54(1–4):33–44.

12 Mosmann TR, Sad S. The expanding universe of T-cell subsets: Th1, Th2 and more. Immunol Today 1996;17:138–46.

13 O'Garra A, Arai N. The molecular basis of T helper 1 and T helper 2 cell differentiation. Trends Cell Biol December 2000;10(12):542–50.

14 Businaro R, Digregorio M, Rigano R et al. Morphological analysis of cell subpopulations within carotid atherosclerotic plaques. Ital J Anat Embryol 2005;110(2, suppl 1):109–15.

15 Huang AL, Vita JA. Effects of systemic inflammation on endothelium-dependent vasodilation. Trends Cardiovasc Med 2006;16(1):15–20.

16 Prabhu SD. Cytokine-induced modulation of cardiac function. Circ Res 2004;95(12):1140–53.

17 Matzinger P. The danger model: a renewed sense of self. Science 2002;296:301–5.

18 Matzinger P. An innate sense of danger. Ann N Y Acad Sci 2002;961:341–2.

19 Akira S, Hemmi H. Recognition of pathogen-associated molecular patterns by TLR family. Immunol Lett 2003;85(2):85–95.

20 Weyand CM, Ma-Krupa W, Pryshchep O, Groschel S, Bernardino R, Goronzy JJ. Vascular dendritic cells in giant cell arteritis. Ann N Y Acad Sci 2005;1062:195–208.

21 Matzinger P. An innate sense of danger. Semin immunol 1998;10:399–415.

22 Liao D-F, Jin Z-G, Baas AS *et al.* Purification and identification of secreted oxidative stress-induced factors from vascular smooth muscle cells. J Biol Chem 2000;275:189–96.

23 Xu Q, Schett G, Perschinka H *et al.* Serum soluble heat shock protein 60 is elevated in subjects with atherosclerosis in a general population. Circulation 2000;192: 14–20.

24 Watanabe M, Watanabe S, Hara Y *et al.* ICOS-mediated costimulation on Th2 differentiation is achieved by the enhancement of IL-4 receptor-mediated signaling. J Immunol 2005;174(4):1989–96.

25 Coyle AJ, Lehar S, Lloyd C *et al.* The CD28-related molecule ICOS is required for effective T cell-dependent immune responses. Immunity 2000;13(1):95–105.

26 Tesciuba AG, Subudhi S, Rother RP *et al.* Inducible costimulator regulates Th2-mediated inflammation, but not Th2 differentiation, in a model of allergic airway disease. J Immunol 2001;167(4):1996–2003.

27 McAdam AJ, Greenwald RJ, Levin MA *et al.* ICOS is critical for CD40-mediated antibody class switching. Nature 2001;409(6816):102–5.

28 Das G, Augustine MM, Das J, Bottomly K, Ray P, Ray A. An important regulatory role for CD4+CD8 alpha alpha T cells in the intestinal epithelial layer in the prevention of inflammatory bowel disease. Proc Natl Acad Sci U S A 2003;100(9):5324–9.

29 Takeda K, Tanaka T, Shi W *et al.* Essential role of Stat6 in IL-4 signalling. Nature 1996;380(6575):627–30.

30 Shimoda K, van Deursen J, Sangster MY *et al.* Lack of IL-4-induced Th2 response and IgE class switching in mice with disrupted Stat6 gene. Nature 1996;380(6575): 630–3.

31 Ma-Krupa W, Jeon MS, Spoerl S, Tedder TF, Goronzy JJ, Weyand CM. Activation of arterial wall dendritic cells and breakdown of self-tolerance in giant cell arteritis. J Exp Med January 19, 2004;199(2):173–83.

32 Kalayoglu MV, Hoerneman B, LaVerda D, Morrison SG, Morrison RP, Byrne GI. Cellular oxidation of low-density lipoprotein by Chlamydia pneumoniae. J Infect Dis 1999;180(3):780–90.

33 Brune IB, Wilke W, Hensler T, Holzmann B, Siewert JR. Downregulation of T helper type 1 immune response and altered pro-inflammatory and anti-inflammatory T cell cytokine balance following conventional but not laparoscopic surgery. Am J Surg 1999;177(1): 55–60.

34 Souza VM, Jacysyn JF, Macedo MS. IL-4 and IL-10 are essential for immunosuppression induced by high molecular weight proteins from Ascaris suum. Cytokine 2004;28(2):92–100.

35 Morris SC, Orekhova T, Meadows MJ, Heidorn SM, Yang J, Finkelman FD. IL-4 induces in vivo produc-

tion of IFN-gamma by NK and NKT cells. J Immunol 2006;176(9):5299–305.

36 Nandakumar KS, Holmdahl R. Arthritis induced with cartilage-specific antibodies is IL-4-dependent. Eur J Immunol 2006;36(6):1608–18.

37 Ohtsuka T, Inoue K, Hara Y *et al.* Serum markers of angiogenesis and myocardial ultrasonic tissue characterization in patients with dilated cardiomyopathy. Eur J Heart Fail June 2005;7(4):689–95.

38 Walch L, Massade L, Dufilho M, Brunet A, Rendu F. Pro-atherogenic effect of interleukin-4 in endothelial cells: modulation of oxidative stress, nitric oxide and monocyte chemoattractant protein-1 expression. Atherosclerosis 2006;187(2):285–91.

39 Lee YW, Kuhn H, Kaiser S, Hennig B, Daugherty A, Toborek M. Interleukin 4 induces transcription of the 15-lipoxygenase I gene in human endothelial cells. J Lipid Res May 2001;42(5):783–91.

40 Lee YW, Hirani AA. Role of interleukin-4 in atherosclerosis. Arch Pharm Res 2006;29(1):1–15.

41 Lee YW, Kuhn H, Hennig B, Toborek M. IL-4 induces apoptosis of endothelial cells through the caspase-3-dependent pathway. FEBS Lett 2000;485(2–3):122–6.

42 Chan WL, Pejnovic N, Liew TV, Hamilton H. Predominance of Th2 response in human abdominal aortic aneurysm: mistaken identity for IL-4-producing NK and NKT cells? Cell Immunol February 2005;233(2):109–14.

43 Chen B, Tsui S, Boeglin WE, Douglas RS, Brash AR, Smith TJ. Interleukin-4 induces 15-lipoxygenase-1 expression in human orbital fibroblasts from patients with Graves disease. Evidence for anatomic site-selective actions of Th2 cytokines. J Biol Chem July 7, 2006;281(27):18296–306.

44 Afanasyeva M, Wang Y, Kaya Z *et al.* Experimental autoimmune myocarditis in A/J mice is an interleukin-4-dependent disease with a Th2 phenotype. Am J Pathol 2001;159(1):5–12.

45 Kuethe F, Braun RK, Foerster M *et al.* Immunopathogenesis of dilated cardiomyopathy. Evidence for the role of TH2-type CD4+T lymphocytes and association with myocardial HLA-DR expression. J Clin Immunol January 2006;26(1):33–9.

46 Cunningham MW. Cardiac myosin and the TH1/TH2 paradigm in autoimmune myocarditis. Am J Pathol 2001;159(1):5–12.

47 Poulin LF, Richard M, Le Moine A *et al.* Interleukin-9 promotes eosinophilic rejection of mouse heart allografts. Transplantation August 15, 2003;76(3):572–7.

48 Van Hoffen E, Van Wichen D, Stuij I *et al.* In situ expression of cytokines in human heart allografts. Am J Pathol December 1996;149(6):1991–2003.

49 Zambon A, Gervois P, Pauletto P, Fruchart JC, Staels B. Modulation of hepatic inflammatory risk markers of

cardiovascular diseases by PPAR-alpha activators: clinical and experimental evidence. Arterioscler Thromb Vasc Biol May 2006;26(5):977–86.

50 Lobbes MB, Lutgens E, Heeneman S et al. Is there more than C-reactive protein and fibrinogen? The prognostic value of soluble CD40 ligand, interleukin-6 and oxidized low-density lipoprotein with respect to coronary and cerebral vascular disease. Atherosclerosis July 2006;187(1):18–25.

51 Omoigui S. Cholesterol synthesis is the trigger and isoprenoid dependent interleukin-6 mediated inflammation is the common causative factor and therapeutic target for atherosclerotic vascular disease and age-related disorders including osteoporosis and type 2 diabetes. Med Hypotheses 2005;65(3): 559–69.

52 Tanko LB, Christiansen C. Adipose tissue, insulin resistance and low-grade inflammation: implications for atherogenesis and the cardiovascular harm of estrogen plus progestogen therapy. Climacteric July 2006;9(3): 169–80.

53 Kanda T, Takahashi T. Interleukin-6 and cardiovascular diseases. Jpn Heart J March 2004;45(2):183–93.

54 Carter AM. Inflammation, thrombosis and acute coronary syndromes. Diab Vasc Dis Res 2006;2(3):113–21.

55 Torre-Amione G. Immune activation in chronic heart failure. Am J Cardiol 2005;95(11A):3C–8C.

56 Hogye M, Mandi Y, Csanady M, Sepp R, Buzas K. Comparison of circulating levels of interleukin-6 and tumor necrosis factor-alpha in hypertrophic cardiomyopathy and in idiopathic dilated cardiomyopathy. Am J Cardiol July 15, 2004;94(2):249–51.

57 Buzas K, Megyeri K, Hogye M, Csanady M, Bogats G, Mandi Y. Comparative study of the roles of cytokines and apoptosis in dilated and hypertrophic cardiomyopathies. Eur Cytokine Netw January–March 2004;15(1):53–9.

58 Weisensee D, Bereiter-Hahn J, Schoeppe W, Low-Friedrich I. Effects of cytokines on the contractility of cultured cardiac myocytes. Int J Immunopharmacol July 1993;15(5):581–7.

59 Fox CS, Guo CY, Larson MG et al. Relations of inflammation and novel risk factors to valvular calcification. Am J Cardiol May 15, 2006;97(10):1502–5.

60 Nesher N, Frolkis I, Vardi M et al. Higher levels of serum cytokines and myocardial tissue markers during on-pump versus off-pump coronary artery bypass surgery. J Card Surg 2006;21(4):395–402.

61 Ustunsoy H, Sivrikoz MC, Tarakcioglu M, Bakir K, Guldur E, Celkan MA. The effects of pentoxifylline on the myocardial inflammation and ischemia-reperfusion injury during cardiopulmonary bypass. J Card Surg January–February 2006;21(1):57–61.

62 Franke A, Lante W, Fackeldey V et al. Pro-inflammatory cytokines after different kinds of cardio-thoracic surgical procedures: is what we see what we know? Eur J Cardiothorac Surg 2005;28(4):569–75.

63 Deng MC, Plenz G, Labarrere C et al. The role of IL6 cytokines in acute cardiac allograft rejection. Transpl Immunol May 2002;9(2–4):115–20.

64 Das UN. Hypertension as a low-grade systemic inflammatory condition that has its origins in the perinatal period. J Assoc Physicians India February 2006;54: 133–42.

65 Sjoholm A, Nystrom T. Inflammation and the etiology of type 2 diabetes. Diabetes Metab Res Rev January–February 2006;22(1):4–10.

66 Kazama R, Okura Y, Hoyano M et al. Therapeutic role of pericardiocentesis for acute necrotizing eosinophilic myocarditis with cardiac tamponade. Mayo Clin Proc 2003;78(7):901–7.

67 Smith CR, Mohanakumar T, Shimizu Y et al. Brief cyclosporine treatment prevents intrathymic (IT) tolerance induction and precipitates acute rejection in an IT rat cardiac allograft model. Transplantation January 27, 2000;69(2):294–9.

68 Zweifel M, Hirsiger H, Matozan K, Welle M, Schaffner T, Mohacsi P. Mast cells in ongoing acute rejection: increase in number and expression of a different phenotype in rat heart transplants. Transplantation 2002;73(11): 1707–16.

69 Foteinos G, Afzal AR, Mandal K, Jahangiri M, Xu Q. Anti-heat shock protein 60 autoantibodies induce atherosclerosis in apolipoprotein E-deficient mice via endothelial damage. Circulation 2005;112(8):1206–13.

70 Mentink-Kane MM, Wynn TA. Opposing roles for IL-13 and IL-13 receptor alpha 2 in health and disease. Immunol Rev December 2004;202:191–202.

71 Ma B, Liu W, Homer RJ et al. Role of CCR5 in the pathogenesis of IL-13-induced inflammation and remodeling. J Immunol April 15, 2006;176(8):4968–78.

72 Kofler S, Nickel T, Weis M. Role of cytokines in cardiovascular diseases: a focus on endothelial responses to inflammation. Clin Sci (Lond) March 2005;108(3): 205–13.

73 Mombouli JV, Vanhoutte PM. Endothelial dysfunction: from physiology to therapy. J Mol Cell Cardiol January 1999;31(1):61–74.

74 Iversen PO, Nicolaysen A, Kvernebo K, Benestad HB, Nicolaysen G. Human cytokines modulate arterial vascular tone via endothelial receptors. Pflugers Arch December 1999;439(1–2):93–100.

75 Beutelspacher SC, Tan PH, McClure MO, Larkin DF, Lechler RI, George AJ. Expression of indoleamine 2,3-dioxygenase (IDO) by endothelial cells: implications for

the control of alloresponses. Am J Transplant 2006;6(6): 1320–30.

76 Karmann K, Min W, Fanslow WC, Pober JS. Activation and homologous desensitization of human endothelial cells by CD40 ligand, tumor necrosis factor, and interleukin 1. J Exp Med 1996;184:173–82.

77 Kunitomi A, Hori T, Imura A, Uchiyama T. Vascular endothelial cells provide T cells with costimulatory signals via the OX40/gp34 system. J Leukoc Biol 2000;68:111–8.

78 Chen Z, Marsden PA, Gorczynski RM. Cloning and characterization of the human CD200 promoter region. Mol Immunol 2006;43(6):579–87.

79 Klingenberg R, Autschbach F, Gleissner C et al. Endothelial inducible costimulator ligand expression is increased during human cardiac allograft rejection and regulates endothelial cell-dependent allo-activation of CD8+ T cells in vitro. Eur J Immunol 2005;35(6): 1712–21.

80 Janssens S, Beyaert R. Role of Toll-like receptors in pathogen recognition. Clin Microbiol Rev 2003;16(4): 637–46.

81 Paterson HM, Murphy TJ, Purcell EJ et al. Injury primes the innate immune system for enhanced Toll-like receptor reactivity. J Immunol 2003;171(3):1473–83.

82 Pober JS, Cotran RS. The role of endothelial cells in inflammation. Transplantation 1990;50:537–44.

83 Pober JS, Orosz CG, Rose ML, Savage CO. Can graft endothelial cells initiate a host anti-graft immune response? Transplantation 1996;61(3):343–9.

84 Vora M, Yssel H, de Vries J, Karasek M. Antigen presentation by human dermal microvascular endothelial cells. Immunoregulatory effect of IFN-γ and IL-10. J Immunol 1994;152:5734–41.

85 Vichchatorn P, Wongkajornsilp A, Petvises S, Tangpradabkul S, Pakakasama S, Hongeng S. Dendritic cells pulsed with total tumor RNA for activation NK-like T cells. J Neurooncol November 2005;75(2):111–8.

86 Pernis A, Witthuhn B, Keegan AD et al. Interleukin 4 signals through two related pathways. Proc Natl Acad Sci U S A 1995;92(17):7971–5.

87 Kalayoglu MV, Hoerneman B, LaVerda D, Morrison SG, Morrison RP, Byrne GI. Cellular oxidation of low-density lipoprotein by Chlamydia pneumoniae. J Infect Dis 1999;180(3):780–90.

88 Drory Y, Turetz Y, Hiss Y et al. Sudden unexpected death in persons less than 40 years of age. Am J Cardiol 1991;68:1388–92.

89 Phase II Efficacy Study of Aerosolized Recombinant Human IL-4 Receptor in Asthma. Trial listed on FDA Clinicaltrials.gov website. Accessed June 2006. http:// www.clinicaltrials.gov/ct/show/NCT00001909?order=9.

90 Recombinant Human IL-4 Receptor Used in Treatment of Asthma. Trial listed on FDA Clinicaltrials.gov

website. Accessed June 2006. http://www.clinicaltrials .gov/ct/show/NCT00017693?order=4.

91 Borish LC, Nelson HS, Corren J et al., for IL-4R Asthma Study Group. Efficacy of soluble IL-4 receptor for the treatment of adults with asthma. J Allergy Clin Immunol June 2001;07(6):963–70.

92 Kanai K, Asano K, Watanabe S, Kyo Y, Suzaki H. Epinastine hydrochloride antagonism against interleukin-4-mediated T cell cytokine imbalance in vitro. Int Arch Allergy Immunol 2006;140(1):43–52.

93 Nishikubo K, Murata Y, Tamaki S et al. A single administration of interleukin-4 antagonistic mutant DNA inhibits allergic airway inflammation in a mouse model of asthma. Gene Ther December 10, 2003;26:2119–25.

94 Zavorotinskaya T, Tomkinson A, Murphy JE. Treatment of experimental asthma by long-term gene therapy directed against IL-4 and IL-13. Mol Ther February 7, 2003;2:155–62.

95 Rincon M, Anguita J, Nakamura T, Fikrig E, Flavell RA. Interleukin (IL)-6 directs the differentiation of IL-4-producing CD4+ T cells. J Exp Med 1997;185(3):461–9.

96 Diehl S, Rincon M. The two faces of IL-6 on Th1/Th2 differentiation. Mol Immunol 2002;39(9):531–6.

97 Fisman EZ, Benderly M, Esper RJ et al. Interleukin-6 and the Risk of future cardiovascular events in patients with angina pectoris and/or healed myocardial infarction. Am J Cardiol 2006;98(1):14–8.

98 Khreiss T, Jozsef L, Potempa LA, Filep JG. Opposing effects of C-reactive protein isoforms on shear-induced neutrophil-platelet adhesion and neutrophil aggregation in whole blood. Circulation 2004;110(17):2713–20.

99 Simon DI, Chen Z, Xu H et al. Platelet glycoprotein Ib is a counterreceptor for the leukocyte integrin Mac-1 (CD11b/CD18). J Exp Med 2000;192:193–204.

100 Santoso S, Sachs UJH, Kroll H et al. The junctional adhesion molecule 3 (JAM-3) on human platelets is a counterreceptor for the leukocyte integrin Mac-1. J Exp Med 2002;196:679–91.

101 Ridker PM, Morrow DA. C-reactive protein, inflammation, and coronary risk. Cardiol Clin 2003;21(3):315–25.

102 Bassuk SS, Rifai N, Ridker PM. High-sensitivity C-reactive protein: clinical importance. Curr Probl Cardiol 2004;8:439–93.

103 Nakahara H, Song J, Sugimoto M et al. Anti-interleukin-6 receptor antibody therapy reduces vascular endothelial growth factor production in rheumatoid arthritis. Arthritis Rheum June 2003;48(6):1521–9.

104 Press release dated April 28, 2006: "Actemra®," a humanized anti-human IL-6 receptor monoclonal antibody, filed for rheumatoid arthritis in japan. http:// www.chugai-pharm.co.jp/generalPortal/pages/detail Type Table.jsp;jsessionid=BWKJQI3OAGGMICSSUIH SFEQ?documentId=doc_6921&lang=en.

105 Chugai development pipeline as of April 25, 2006. Chugai website. Accessed June 2006. http://www.chugai-pharm.co.jp/pdf/pipeline/english/060425ePipeline.pdf.

106 A study to assess the safety and efficacy of tocilizumab in patients with active rheumatoid arthritis. Clinical trial listed on FDA ClinicalTrials.gov website. Accessed June 2006. http://www.clinicaltrials.gov/ct/show/NCT00109408?order=1.

107 Nishimoto N, Yoshizaki K, Miyasaka N et al. Treatment of rheumatoid arthritis with humanized anti-interleukin-6 receptor antibody: a multicenter, double-blind, placebo-controlled trial. Arthritis Rheum June 2004;50(6):1761–9.

108 Choy EH, Isenberg DA, Garrood T et al. Therapeutic benefit of blocking interleukin-6 activity with an anti-interleukin-6 receptor monoclonal antibody in rheumatoid arthritis: a randomized, double-blind, placebo-controlled, dose-escalation trial. Arthritis Rheum December 2002;46(12):3143–50.

109 Nishimoto N, Kanakura Y, Aozasa K et al. Humanized anti-interleukin-6 receptor antibody treatment of multicentric Castleman's disease. Blood October 15, 2005;106(8):2627–32.

110 Yokota S, Miyamae T, Imagawa T et al. Therapeutic efficacy of humanized recombinant anti-interleukin-6 receptor antibody in children with systemic-onset juvenile idiopathic arthritis. Arthritis Rheum March 2005;52(3):818–25.

111 Monoclonal Antibody Treatment for Systemic Lupus Erythematosus. Clinical trial listed on FDA ClinicalTrials.gov website. Accessed June 2006. http://www.clinicaltrials.gov/ct/show/NCT00046774?order=4.

112 CNTO 328 in Treating Patients With Unresectable or Metastatic Kidney Cancer. Clinical trial listed on FDA ClinicalTrials.gov website. Accessed June 2006. http://www.clinicaltrials.gov/ct/gui/show/NCT00311545; jsessionid=1AA9B3B8E120F916669213EE5817223D?order=36.

113 van Zaanen HC, Koopmans RP, Aarden LA et al. Endogenous interleukin 6 production in multiple myeloma patients treated with chimeric monoclonal anti-IL6 antibodies indicates the existence of a positive feed-back loop. Clin Invest September 15, 1996;98(6):1441–8.

114 Callisto Pharmaceuticals website. Accessed June 2006. http://www.calisto-pharma.com/.

115 Safety and Efficacy of Atiprimod for Patients With Refractory Multiple Myeloma. Trial listed on FDA clinicaltrials.org website. Accessed June 2006. http://www.clinicaltrials.gov/ct/show/NCT00086216?order=2.

116 Atiprimod in Treating Patients With Refractory or Relapsed Multiple Myeloma. Trial listed on FDA clinicaltrials.org website. Accessed June 2006. http://www.clinicaltrials.gov/ct/show/NCT00301977?order=1.

117 Olsen EG, Spry CJ. Relation between eosinophilia and endomyocardial disease. Prog Cardiovasc Dis January–February 1985;27(4):241–54.

118 Zurawski G, de Vries JE. Interleukin 13 elicits a subset of the activities of its close relative interleukin 4. Stem Cells 1994;12(2):169–74.

119 Deswal A, Bozkurt B, Seta Y et al. Safety and efficacy of a soluble P75 tumor necrosis factor receptor (Enbrel, etanercept) in patients with advanced heart failure. Circulation 1999;99:3224–6.

120 Mann DL, NcNurray JJV, Packer M et al. Targeted anticytokine therapy in patients with chronic heart failure. Results of the randomised etanercept worldwide evaluation (RENEWAL). Circulation 2004;109:1594–602.

CHAPTER 22

Anti-inflammatory immune therapy in heart disease

*David Chen, Christian Assad-Kottner, Francisco J. Cordova,
Carlos Orrego & Guillermo Torre-Amione*

Introduction

Our understanding of the pathogenesis of heart failure (HF) has evolved from a linear view of "pump
failure" to a more complex syndrome involving
overactivation of various compensatory systems of
hormones. This is supported by well-established
evidence that partial blockade of the rennin–
angiotensin system and β-adrenergic system leads
to improved survival.

There is an emerging area of focus in the role
of inflammatory mediators (i.e., proinflammatory
cytokines, activation of the complement cascade,
production of autoantibodies, and overexpression
of New York Heart Association (NYHA) class II major histocompatibility complex molecules as well
as adhesion molecules) that may perpetuate an inflammatory state in HF. Our expanding knowledge
of the various components of the immune system has led to newer treatment modalities. This
chapter will focus on the following topics: (1)
target-specific anticytokine therapy and (2) broad-
spectrum anti-inflammatory therapy in HF–IV
immunoglobulin, immune adsorption, plasmapheresis, statin therapy, and immune modulation
therapy.

Anticytokine therapy—why did it fail?

Tumor necrosis factor-α (TNF-α) is the most studied cytokine in chronic HF.

Normal myocardium does not contain TNF-α,
but as myocardial function starts deteriorating the
myocardium begins to express receptors Type I and
II of TNF-α. However, in the failing myocardium,
there is an increased expression of TNF-α and TNF
receptors are downregulated [1].

Proinflammatory cytokines, in particular
TNF-α, would appear to be an ideal target for
intervention. Indeed, in small preliminary studies,
pharmacologic blockade of the biologic effects of
TNF-α in humans was associated with improved
functional status as well as with improved myocardial function [2]. Following these positive
results, two large randomized clinical trials were
launched (the Randomized Etanercept North
American Strategy to Study Antagonism of Cytokines [RENAISSANCE] in the United States, and
the Research into Etanercept Cytokine Antagonism
in Ventricular Dysfunction [RECOVER] trial in
Europe and Australia) in which patients with
moderate-to-severe chronic HF were treated with
etanercept, a highly specific anti-TNF-α blocking
agent. However, the results were disappointing
[3]. These studies were terminated prematurely for
lack of clinical benefit. Furthermore, another study
with a different compound, infliximab, showed an
increased incidence of worsening HF.

Why did specific anti-TNF-α blocking agents fail
to show clinical improvement in these large studies?
There are at least two important explanations: (1)
TNF-α is a mediator of hypertrophy, and (2) the
immune system is redundant.

TNF-α and hypertrophy

There are a number of clinical settings in which
systolic function is preserved with high level of
cardiac TNF-α expression, including patients with

hypertrophic cardiomyopathy [4], aortic stenosis [5], and transplant myocardium [6]. Therefore, it appears that systolic dysfunction is not the direct result of cardiac TNF-α. However, persistent expression of TNF-α may result in hypertrophy and, at a later stage, dilated cardiomyopathy and death. In patients with established chronic HF, anti-TNF-α therapy may no longer have the ability to change outcomes because injury at that stage is not dependent on TNF-α expression only. Once persistent activation of TNF-α results in hypertrophy and dilation, therapy would only put patients at risk of potential side effects of the therapy with no potential clinical benefit.

Immune system redundancy

Etanercept, a highly selective TNF-α inhibitor, has no cross-reaction with any other known cytokine. It is logical to postulate after the demonstration of lack of benefit that the highly selective nature of this compound may also be among its disadvantages. The immune system is redundant, and other proinflammatory cytokines known to be elevated in chronic HF (e.g., interleukin (IL)-1, IL-6) can participate and/or substitute for the absence of TNF-α in etanercept-treated patients.

A new era of broad-spectrum anti-inflammatory treatments in HF

To tackle various components of the immune system, newer treatment modalities have emerged that widen the potential targets. There are four forms of broad-spectrum immunomodulatory strategies currently under investigation: (1) intravenous immunoglobulin (IVIG), (2) immunoadsorption, (3) plasmapheresis, and (4) immune-modulation therapy (IMT).

Immunoglobulin

Proposed mechanisms of IVIG in autoimmune diseases include Fc receptor blockade on macrophages, inactivation of circulating autoantibodies and complement proteins, and a decrease in proinflammatory cytokines [7]. A fair summary may be that γ-globulin represents a natural anti-inflammatory or anti-injury response of the host. Three small tri-

als were initiated to assess the efficacy of IVIG in acute HF. In the pediatric population with acute myocarditis, Drucker et al. [8] demonstrated an improvement in left ventricular (LV) function and a trend toward increased survival in the group of children treated with high-dose IVIG compared with historical controls. In the adult population, McNamara et al. [9] treated 10 patients with new-onset (within 6 mo) NYHA class III–IV HF with high-dose IVIG. At 1-year follow-up, all patients improved to NYHA class I or II with left ventricular ejection fraction (LVEF) improvement from 0.24 to 0.41 ($p = 0.003$). Bozkurt et al. [10] retrospectively studied the outcome of six women with peripartum cardiomyopathy treated with IVIG who presented within the first 6 months of delivery with NYHA class III–IV and LVEF <0.40, and compared with 11 historical control subjects. The IVIG group showed a significantly greater improvement in LVEF than the control group ($\Delta EF = 0.26$ versus 0.13, respectively; $p = 0.042$). With these promising results, two large randomized clinical trials were launched. The first study was the Intervention in Myocarditis and Acute Cardiomyopathy (IMAC) trial. In this study, 62 patients who presented with recent-onset cardiomyopathy (<6 mo) with an LVEF <0.40 and no evidence of coronary artery disease with or without evidence of inflammation were randomized to receive high-dose IVIG for two consecutive days. The primary endpoint of the study was the change in LVEF at 6 months. The surprising finding of the study was that the mean LVEF in the placebo-treated patients changed from 0.23 at baseline to 0.42 at 6 months. With this dramatic improvement in the placebo-treated patients, there was no further effect observed in the IVIG-treated patients [11]. However, a different trial, which included 40 ischemic and nonischemic patients with an LVEF <0.40 who were categorized as NYHA class II–IV and were treated for 6 months on a monthly basis, found that the LVEF increased from 0.26 to 0.31 in the treated patients, and that this change also occurred with improvements in functional class. More interestingly, it was found that there was an increase in three or more than three anti-inflammatory peptides, IL-10, and the soluble receptors for IL-1 and TNF [12]. Whether IVIG is useful in chronic HF is not known, but it will be the focus of further

Table 22.1 IVIG trials.

Author	EF (%)	N	Etiology of HF	Trial design	Outcome
Drucker et al.	NA	21	Actue myocarditis	Prospective	Significant LVEF improvement at 1 yr follow-up
McNamara et al.	<40	10	Idiopathic dilated cardiomyopathy (recent onset, <6 mo)	Retrospective	Significant LVEF increase (24–41%) and improvement in NYHA class
Bozkurt et al.	<40	6	Peripartum cardiomyopathy	Retrospective	Significant LVEF increase (26% vs. 13% in placebo group)
IMAC trial (McNamara et al.)	<40	62	NICMP (recent onset, <6 mo)	Prospective, randomized, placebo-controlled	No significant difference in LVEF, peak oxygen consumption, and 6-min walk distance between the IVIG and placebo groups
Gullestad et al.	<40	40	ICMP (n = 23) NICMP (n = 17) (chronic, >6 mo)	Randomized, double-blind, placebo controlled	Significant LVEF increase (26% to 31%) and improvement in NYHA class

ICMP, ischemic cardiomyopathy; NICMP, nonischemic cardiomyopathy.

investigation in patients with chronic HF. See Table 22.1 for the trials reviewed.

Immune adsorption

Recent concepts involving the pathophysiology of HF include disturbances in the cellular and humoral immune system. Studies have identified several antibodies against various cardiac proteins in patients with HF, for example, antibodies against mitochondrial proteins, contractile proteins, and $\beta1$ receptors [13].

Immunoadsorption, a technique used to remove specific antibodies from the circulation, has shown beneficial effects on patients with HF. The procedure is based on the utilization of ligands and adsorbers extracorporeally to remove serum immunoglobulins and immune complexes. In case that cardiac antibodies are, in part, a culprit for the cardiac dysfunction, it would be acceptable to assume that their removal would be expected to improve the patients' hemodynamics [14, 15]. Several trials have evaluated the efficacy of elimination of cardiac autoantibodies through immune adsorp-

tion in the stabilization or slowing of the progression of HF.

In a small, prospective case-control study, 34 patients (all listed for heart transplantation at the German Heart Institute who had high anti-$\beta1$-adrenoceptor antibodies) underwent immunoadsorption during five consecutive days. The study found that LVEF improved from 0.22 to 0.38, and that along with the change in LVEF, there were improvements in systolic and end-diastolic volumes. Furthermore, 3 months after completing therapy, there was no evidence of anti-$\beta1$-adrenoceptor antibodies. Although this was a small study, the magnitude of the change and the dramatic improvements in functional class merit further investigation. Whether the benefit was the result of removing $\beta1$ antibodies or some nonspecific suppression is not known [16].

Another study evaluated the effect of immune adsorption on hemodynamic patterns. Immunoadsorption was performed on nine patients with dilated cardiomyopathy (LVEF <25%) on five consecutive days. In these patients, a significant increase in cardiac output (from 3.7 ± 0.8 to 5.5 ± 1.8 L/min; $p < 0.01$) and a significant decrease in mean arterial pressure (from 76.0 ± 9.9 to 65 ± 11.2 mm Hg; $p < 0.05$) and mean pulmonary arterial pressure (from 27.6 ± 7.7 to 22.0 ± 6.5 mm Hg; $p < 0.05$) was noted [17].

Two further studies evaluated the effect of immune adsorption on clinical endpoints and LVEF. Felix et al. randomized 25 patients with dilated cardiomyopathy, LVEF <30% with evidence of β1 receptor autoantibody and, signs of myocardial inflammation on endomyocardial biopsy to immune adsorption versus conventional therapy. The treatment group underwent monthly immune adsorption followed by immunoglobulin substitution for 3 months. Immune adsorption led to a significant decrease in β1 receptor autoantibody levels. The increase in LVEF and improvement of NYHA class were significantly greater in the treatment group compared with the controls. Moreover, a significant decrease in inflammation on endomyocardial biopsy was noted in the treatment group compared with the control group [18, 19].

In a prospective case-control study, Muller et al. [20] evaluated 34 patients with nonischemic dilated cardiomyopathy with NYHA class II–IV HF, LVEF <29%, and evidence of elevated levels of β1 autoantibodies. The active treatment group of 17 patients underwent immune adsorption on five consecutive days. At 1 year, the treatment group experienced a significant increase in LVEF (0.223–0.379; $p = 0.0001$) and improvement in NYHA class compared

with no significant change in LVEF in the placebo group.

A recent study compared the results of patients undergoing repeated immunoadsorption at monthly intervals versus just one course of the therapy. Patients treated with only one immunoadsorption course experienced comparable improvement of LVEF after 6 months (from $26.5 \pm 2.2\%$ to $34.8 \pm 2.9\%$; $p < 0.01$ versus baseline) [13].

All of the trials mentioned have shown that patients with dilated cardiomyopathies have benefited from immunoadsorption therapy. Whether the benefit found in this group of patients are the result of the removal of antibodies or some nonspecific suppression is still unclear. A summary of these trials can be seen in Table 22.2.

Plasmapheresis

Plasma exchange or plasmapheresis is viewed as a broad-spectrum anti-inflammatory treatment strategy since it appears to target various aspects of inflammation.

During plasmapheresis, venous blood is removed and plasma is separated from the cells through either centrifugation or membrane filtration. The cells are then reinfused together with fresh frozen plasma, 5% albumin, or crystalloid solution. Plasmapheresis appears to exert its anti-inflammatory action by removing circulating autoantibodies, immune complexes, various

Table 22.2 Immune adsorption.

Author	EF (%)	N	Etiology of HF	Trial design	Outcome
Dorffel et al.	<25	18	NICMP	Prospective, observational	Improvement in hemodynamic parameters (↑cardiac ouput, ↓ pulmonary arterial pressure, ↓LV filling pressure, ↓systemic vascular resistance)
Staudt et al.	<30	25	NICMP	Prospective, randomized, controlled	Improvement in LVEF and NYHA class
Muller	<29	34	NICMP	Prospective, case—control	Improvement in LVEF, LV dimensions, and NYHA class
Staudt et al.	<35	22	NICMP	Prospective randomized	Improvement of LVEF in the single and multiple course regimen

NICMP, nonischemic cardiomyopathy.

immunoglobulins, complements, and other serum components such as cytokines, cryoglobulin, and fibrinogen.

The molecules most successfully removed by plasma exchange are those that are mainly present in the intravascular space and have a long half-life, such as IgG, IgM, and low-density lipoproteins. Molecules that are evenly distributed in the intravascular and extravascular space cannot be reliably and persistently removed by plasma exchange. Thus, the removal of complement factors and cytokines, proposed to be beneficial in certain disease states, has not been thoroughly validated [21].

Although IgG can be successfully removed by plasmapheresis, because 45% of total IgG is intravascular and 55% extravascular, this can lead to rapid reaccumulation of intravascular IgG, partially due to reequilibration with extravascular IgG. A reduction of intravascular IgG of up to 70–85% has been shown to be possible when combined with immunosuppression. The majority of IgM, on the other hand, is present intravascularly, and thus the removal of IgM by plasmapheresis is more efficacious and the result is more persistent [22].

The evidence of the use of plasmapheresis in HF is scarce. Case reports and case series have been presented in which plasmapheresis has been implemented successfully to treat HF in the setting of autoimmune diseases such as systemic lupus erythematosus [23], thrombotic thrombocytopenic purpura [24–26], antiphospholipid syndrome [27, 28], polymyositis [29], or a viral infection [30]. Plasmapheresis has also been used in the treatment of cardiac allograft dysfunction without evidence of cellular rejection. This type of rejection is presumed to be mediated by humoral immune response with deposition of immunoglobulins and complement factors in the vascular endothelium [31–33]. Thus, plasmapheresis has been postulated to be efficacious by the removal of immunoglobulins and immune complexes.

Berglin et al. [34] published a case series of five patients who presented with rejection resistant to conventional immunosuppressive treatment. Plasmapheresis resulted in improvement of HF symptoms in all patients. Furthermore, endomyocardial biopsies obtained after plasmapheresis revealed regression in vascular inflammation as evidenced by decreases in endothelial swelling, interstitial edema,

and lymphocytic infiltrates. All patients were alive 2–3.5 years after transplantation.

Grauhan et al. [35] compared six patients with vascular rejection treated with immunosuppressants and plasmapheresis to seven historical controls with vascular rejection treated with immunosuppressants only. All patients who received plasmapheresis survived. Only two of the seven patients who received immunosuppressive therapy survived.

In another observational case series, Olsen et al. [36] reported 13 patients with vascular rejection who underwent three sessions of plasmapheresis in addition to immunosuppressive therapy. One patient died during the rejection episode. The remaining 12 patients showed significantly improved LV function within 7 days of treatment. Long-term, event-free survival, however, was poor. Eight patients were alive 12–23 months after transplantation. Three patients suffered subsequent episodes of vascular rejection with hemodynamic compromise, of whom 1 patient died and 1 patient underwent re-transplantation and later died. Two additional patients died following medical noncompliance 8–18 months after transplantation.

In the pediatric population, Pahl et al. [37] described the use of plasmapheresis in seven episodes of vascular rejection in five pediatric cardiac transplant recipients. All patients survived with improved LV function. On long-term follow-up, three patients developed allograft vasculopathy, of whom one patient required re-transplantation.

In our institution, the Methodist DeBakey Heart Center, 10 heart transplant recipients have undergone plasmapheresis for graft failure without evidence of cellular rejection. Nine out of 10 patients experienced a significant increase in ejection fraction with plasmapheresis (mean, 26.3% increase in ejection fraction). On long-term follow-up, six patients are doing well without any major problems. Two patients died from infectious complications, 1 patient expired as a result of recurrent rejections, and 1 patient developed recurrent LV systolic dysfunction unresponsive to treatment. So far, the majority of data for plasmapheresis in HF is based on retrospective analyses in patients with cardiac allograft dysfunction. The majority of patients show initial improvement in clinical symptoms and LV function. On long-term follow-up, however, patients

Table 22.3 Plasmapheresis.

Author	N	Indication	Trial design	Outcome after plasmapheresis use
Berglin et al.	5	Resistance to conventional immunosuppressive treatment	Retrospective	Improvement of HF symptoms in all patients. Endomyocardial biopsies obtained after plasmapheresis revealed regression in vascular inflammation
Grauhan et al.	13	Resistance to conventional immunosuppressive treatment	Retrospective	Patients treated with plasmapheresis and immunosuppressants had 80% greater survival than immunosuppressants alone
Olsen et al.	13	Vascular rejection	Retrospective	Significant improved LV function within 7 days of treatment. Long-term event free survival was poor
Pahl et al.	5	Vascular rejection	Retrospective	All patients survived with improved LV function. Long-term event-free survival was poor

appear to suffer from recurrent vascular rejection and allograft vasculopathy.

Although there is ample evidence of activation of the humoral and cellular immune response during acute and chronic HF, to date there are no data on the efficacy of plasmapheresis in non-heart transplant recipients with LV dysfunction. Because of the evidence in support of broad-spectrum activation of the immune system in HF, coupled with the increasing clinical evidence of improvement in cardiac function with broad-spectrum anti-inflammatory strategies, we are currently conducting a nonrandomized clinical trial of plasmapheresis in patients with advanced cardiomyopathy, with LVEF less than 30% and NYHA functional class III–IV. Treatment protocol consists of five courses of plasmapheresis over a 3-hour period utilizing albumin reconstitution following each treatment and intravenous γ-globulin at 500 mg/kg after the fifth course of treatment. Baseline measurements of hemodynamics, echocardiography, plasma samples, and right ventricular endomyocardial biopsies are obtained.

Preliminary results of five completed patients showed a reduction in end-diastolic volume in three patients, and two patients with a significant increase in EF after the second course of treatment. No significant changes in blood pressure or heart rate were found during the study. In addition, there were no cases of fluid overload or the need of intravenous diuretics secondary to the use of albumin. There were no line infections and none of the patients studied were re-hospitalized for either infection or decompensated HF during follow-up.

These initial results suggest that plasmapheresis can be safely conducted in symptomatic patients with advanced HF and provide the basis for conducting clinical studies to further define its clinical utility. We are currently in the process of organizing a larger scale study. See Table 22.3 for a summary of trials reviewed.

Statin therapy

Previous studies have addressed the association between inflammatory mediators/receptors and the failing myocardium. For example, in the Studies on Left Ventricular Dysfunction (SOLVD) trial, a subset of patients who presented with TNF-α level below 6.5 pg/mL had better outcomes than patients who had higher concentrations [38]. Similarly, Vesnarinone Trial (VEST) confirmed this correlation by demonstrating that inflammatory cytokines, such as TNF-α and IL-6, as well as cytokine receptors were independent predictors of advanced HF [39].

Statin's cholesterol-lowering properties have been well established for several years, yet the utilization of statin therapy in ischemic and nonischemic cardiomyopathy patients remains controversial. Recently, there has been increasing evidence of anti-inflammatory and immunomodulation effects of statins in experimental animals as well as in humans. For example in our recent study, simvastatin treatment in heart transplant recipients significantly decreased myocardium TNF-α expression at the 24th week after transplant [40]. With

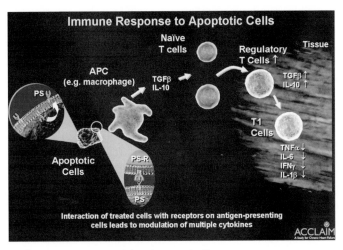

Figure 22.1 A schematic of immune response to Celacade-treated cells.

these positive results, several studies were launched to evaluate the role of this new pathway as a target of therapeutic intervention in ischemic and nonischemic HF.

We reviewed the most recent literature on this subject and the results have been promising. Six out of seven trials concluded that the group of patients utilizing HMG-CoA reductase blockade therapy showed improvement in one or more surrogate endpoints including LVEF, decrease in LV diameters and volumes, and reduction of inflammatory markers such as IL-6, TNF-αR1, and TNF-αR2. Only one trial failed to show positive results, Bleske *et al.* concluded that no difference in outcome was observed between the statins and the placebo-controlled group.

Current evidence of statins as a potential therapy in the treatment of HF appears to be a promising one, yet no conclusions should be taken until larger randomized clinical trials further address this issue. The GISSI-HF and CORONA trials are such examples of several ongoing trials.

Immune modulation therapy

IMT (Celacade, Vasogen Inc., Mississaugo, Ontario, Canada) involves the ex vivo treatment of a patient's blood with oxidative and thermal stressors (oxidizing agent, UV light, and elevated temperature), which leads to apoptosis of the treated cells. The treated sample is administered back to the patient

intramuscularly, at which point the apoptotic cells stimulate anti-inflammatory cytokines and suppress proinflammatory cytokines, thereby creating an anti-inflammatory effect [41–45] (Figure 22.1).

In our recent trial [44], 75 patients with NYHA class III–IV HF, LVEF <40%, and 6-minute walk distance < 300 m were randomized to either Celacade (38 patients) or placebo (37 patients). Celacade was given on two consecutive days followed by monthly treatments 2 weeks later for a total of eight treatments. There was an increase in 6-minute walk distance in both the treatment and control groups; however, no significant treatment effect could be shown. There was a trend toward improvement in NYHA class, with 42% of treated patients improving by at least one class, compared with 24% in the placebo arm. Surprisingly, fewer clinical events were noted in the Celacade group. There were a total of 25 events in the Celacade group versus 48 events in the placebo arm ($p = 0.035$). One patient died in the treated group, compared with seven in the placebo group (2.8% versus 19%; $p = 0.56$), resulting in a significant reduction in the risk of death with Celacade ($p = 0.022$). The Celacade group also had a trend toward fewer hospitalizations compared with the placebo group (24 versus 41; $p = 0.089$). This was a small efficacy and safety trial. These positive results lead to a large randomized, phase 3, controlled trial (Advanced Chronic HF Clinical Assessment of Immune Modulation Therapy [ACCLAIM]) aiming to assess the full clinical benefit of Celacade.

In this study, 2408 patients with NYHA class II–IV with LVEF ≤0.30, who had been hospitalized or receive IV drug therapy for HF within the previous 12 months, or NYHA class III or IV with LVEF ≤0.25, were randomized to receive either Celacade (1204 patients) or placebo (1204 patients). The IMT group received induction therapy at days 1, 2, and 14, and Celacade treatment was continued for a minimum of 22 weeks (8 treatments) or until the end of the study. The difference in time to death or first cardiovascular hospitalization (the primary endpoint) for the intent-to-treat study population was not statistically significant ($p = 0.22$); however, the risk reduction directionally favored the Celacade group (hazard ratio = 0.92). There was a significant improvement in quality of life (as measured by the Minnesota Living with Heart Failure Questionnaire) for the intent-to-treat study population ($n = 2408$ patients; $p = 0.04$). In patients with nonischemic HF, Celacade significantly reduced the risk of death or first cardiovascular hospitalization by 26% ($n = 919$ patients, 243 events; $p = 0.02$). In patients with NYHA class II HF at baseline, Celacade was also shown to significantly reduce the risk of death or first cardiovascular hospitalization by 39% ($n = 689$ patients, 216 events; $p = 0.0003$). A combined analysis of NYHA class III or IV patients with no prior history of heart attack and all NYHA class II patients demonstrated a 31% reduction in the risk of death or first cardiovascular hospitalization in the Celacade group compared to placebo ($n = 1305$ patients, 391 events; $p = 0.0003$). In addition, an exploratory analysis based on prespecified subgroups, which comprised 72% of the patient population and excluded only those patients in NYHA class III or IV with a prior history of heart attack and an ejection fraction equal to or below the median (EF ≤23%), showed that Celacade reduce the risk of death or first cardiovascular hospitalization by 21% ($n = 1746$ patients, 560 events; $p = 0.005$). Celacade was also shown to be safe and well tolerated, and there were no significant between-group differences for any serious adverse events.

These findings are consistent with the role that chronic inflammation plays in the development and progression of HF and are particularly impressive in the large subgroup of NYHA class III or IV patients who had not experienced a prior heart attack and in all NYHA class II patients. These results provide a strong basis for targeting Celacade's novel anti-inflammatory mechanism in this large and well-defined patient population. See Table 22.4 for a summary of these trials.

Conclusion

It has become increasingly clear that immune activation occurs in patients with HF, and for this reason the mediators responsible for inflammation and/or anti-inflammatory responses became new potential targets for therapeutic intervention.

Table 22.4 Immune modulation therapy.

Author	EF (%)	N	Etiology of HF	Trial design	Outcome
Torre et al.	<40	75	ICMP and NICMP	Prospective, randomized, placebo controlled	Significant reduction in mortality and clinical events and trend toward improved NYHA class
ACCLAIM	<30	2408	ICMP (68%) and NICMP (32%)	Prospective, randomized, placebo controlled	No significant difference in all-cause mortality. Reduction in mortality risk or CV hospitalization in nonischemic cardiomyopathy (CM) patients or ischemic CM patients with NYHA class II

ICMP, ischemic cardiomyopathy; NICMP, nonischemic cardiomyopathy.

Although previous trials have shown that specific-target therapy aimed to block TNF-α failed to demonstrate clinical efficacy, other broad-spectrum immune therapies were promising when applied to specific populations.

As we have discussed previously, IVIG, immunoadsorption, statin therapy, and plasmapheresis are all modalities currently being studied at an early stage of development for treatment of HF. Several trials showed promising yet inconclusive results for the treatment of HF. Recently, the largest trial utilizing Celacade immune modulation therapy (ACCLAIM™) demonstrated potential use in subgroups of nonischemic HF patients with NYHA class III or IV or ischemic HF patients with NYHA class II. These results show perhaps immune therapy is most effective at an early stage of the development of HF, and these findings will serve as a basis for future investigation. Further large randomized trials are needed to confirm the therapeutic role of anti-inflammatory immune therapy in HF.

References

1 Torre-Amione G, Kapadia S, Lee J, Bies RD, Lebovitz R, Mann DL. Expression and functional significance of tumor necrosis factor receptors in human myocardium. Circulation September 15, 1995;92(6):1487–93.

2 Bozkurt B, Torre-Amione G, Warren MS et al. Results of targeted anti-tumor necrosis factor therapy with etanercept (ENBREL) in patients with advanced heart failure. Circulation February 27, 2001;103(8):1044–7.

3 Mann DL. Inflammatory mediators and the failing heart: past, present, and the foreseeable future. Circ Res November 29, 2002;91(11):988–98.

4 Nagueh SF, Stetson SJ, Lakkis NM et al. Decreased expression of tumor necrosis factor-alpha and regression of hypertrophy after nonsurgical septal reduction therapy for patients with hypertrophic obstructive cardiomyopathy. Circulation April 10, 2001;103(14):1844–50.

5 Kapadia SR, Yakoob K, Nader S, Thomas JD, Mann DL, Griffin BP. Elevated circulating levels of serum tumor necrosis factor-alpha in patients with hemodynamically significant pressure and volume overload. J Am Coll Cardiol July 2000;36(1):208–12.

6 Sacher RA. Intravenous immunoglobulin consensus statement. J Allergy Clin Immunol October 2001; 108(suppl 4):S139–46.

7 Yu Z, Lennon VA. Mechanism of intravenous immune globulin therapy in antibody-mediated autoimmune diseases. N Engl J Med January 21, 1999;340(3):227–8.

8 Drucker NA, Colan SD, Lewis AB et al. Gamma-globulin treatment of acute myocarditis in the pediatric population. Circulation January 1994;89(1):252–7.

9 McNamara DM, Rosenblum WD, Janosko KM et al. Intravenous immune globulin in the therapy of myocarditis and acute cardiomyopathy. Circulation June 3, 1997;95(11):2476–8.

10 Bozkurt B, Villanueva FS, Holubkov R et al. Intravenous immune globulin in the therapy of peripartum cardiomyopathy. J Am Coll Cardiol July 1999;34(1):177–80.

11 McNamara DM, Holubkov R, Starling RC et al. Controlled trial of intravenous immune globulin in recent-onset dilated cardiomyopathy. Circulation May 8, 2001;103(18):2254–9.

12 Gullestad L, Aass H, Fjeld JG et al. Immunomodulating therapy with intravenous immunoglobulin in patients with chronic heart failure. Circulation January 16, 2001;103(2):220–5.

13 Staudt A, Hummel A, Ruppert J et al. Immunoadsorption in dilated cardiomyopathy: 6-month results from a randomized study. Am Heart J October 2006;152(4):712–6.

14 Torre-Amione G. Immune activation in chronic heart failure. Am J Cardiol June 5, 2005;95(11A):3C–8C.

15 Ramasubbu K, Oliveira G, Torre-Amione G. Novel therapies for heart failure: focus on anti-inflammatory strategies. Congest Heart Fail May 2006;12(3):153–9.

16 Muller J, Wallukat G, Dandel M et al. Immunoglobulin adsorption in patients with idiopathic dilated cardiomyopathy. Circulation February 1, 2000;101(4):385–91.

17 Dorffel WV, Felix SB, Wallukat G et al. Short-term hemodynamic effects of immunoadsorption in dilated cardiomyopathy. Circulation April 15, 1997;95(8):1994–7.

18 Felix SB, Staudt A, Dorffel WV et al. Hemodynamic effects of immunoadsorption and subsequent immunoglobulin substitution in dilated cardiomyopathy: three-month results from a randomized study. J Am Coll Cardiol May 2000;35(6):1590–8.

19 Staudt A, Schaper F, Stangl V et al. Immunohistological changes in dilated cardiomyopathy induced by immunoadsorption therapy and subsequent immunoglobulin substitution. Circulation June 5, 2001;103(22):2681–6.

20 Muller J, Wallukat G, Dandel M et al. Immunoglobulin adsorption in patients with idiopathic dilated cardiomyopathy. Circulation February 1, 2000;101(4):385–91.

21 McLeod BC. An approach to evidence-based therapeutic apheresis. J Clin Apheresis 2002;17(3):124–32.

22 Mahalati K, Dawson RB, Collins JO, Mayer RF. Predictable recovery from myasthenia gravis crisis with plasma exchange: thirty-six cases and review of current management. J Clin Apheresis 1999;14(1):1–8.

23 Habersetzer R, Samtleben W, Blumenstein M, Gurland HJ. Plasma exchange in systemic lupus erythematosus. Int J Artif Organs July 1983;6(suppl 1):39–41.

24 Webb JG, Butany J, Langer G, Scott G, Liu PP. Myocarditis and myocardial hemorrhage associated with thrombotic thrombocytopenic purpura. Arch Intern Med July 1990;150(7):1535–7.

25 Kelton JG. Thrombotic thrombocytopenic purpura and hemolytic uremic syndrome: will recent insight into pathogenesis translate into better treatment? Transfusion April 2002;42(4):388–92.

26 Byrnes JJ, Lian EC. Recent therapeutic advances in thrombotic thrombocytopenic purpura. Semin Thromb Hemost 1979;5(3):199–215.

27 Dornan RI. Acute postoperative biventricular failure associated with antiphospholipid antibody syndrome. Br J Anaesth May 2004;92(5):748–54.

28 Asherson RA, Cervera R, Piette JC et al. Catastrophic antiphospholipid syndrome. Clinical and laboratory features of 50 patients. Medicine (Baltimore) May 1998;77(3):195–207.

29 Yoshioka M, Okuno T, Mikawa H. Prognosis and treatment of polymyositis with particular reference to steroid resistant patients. Arch Dis Child March 1985;60(3):236–44.

30 Tabbutt S, Leonard M, Godinez RI et al. Severe influenza B myocarditis and myositis. Pediatr Crit Care Med July 2004;5(4):403–6.

31 Hammond EH, Yowell RL, Nunoda S et al. Vascular (humoral) rejection in heart transplantation: pathologic observations and clinical implications. J Heart Transplant November 1989;8(6):430–43.

32 Kemnitz J, Cohnert T, Schafers HJ et al. A classification of cardiac allograft rejection: a modification of the classification by Billingham. Am J Surg Pathol July 1987;11(7):503–15.

33 Hammond EH, Ensley RD, Yowell RL et al. Vascular rejection of human cardiac allografts and the role of humoral immunity in chronic allograft rejection. Transplant Proc April 1991;23(2, suppl 2):26–30.

34 Berglin E, Kjellstrom C, Mantovani V, Stelin G, Svalander C, Wiklund L. Plasmapheresis as a rescue therapy to resolve cardiac rejection with vasculitis and severe heart failure: a report of five cases. Transpl Int 1995;8(5):382–7.

35 Grauhan O, Knosalla C, Ewert R et al. Plasmapheresis and cyclophosphamide in the treatment of humoral rejection after heart transplantation. J Heart Lung Transplant March 2001;20(3):316–21.

36 Olsen SL, Wagoner LE, Hammond EH et al. Vascular rejection in heart transplantation: clinical correlation, treatment options, and future considerations. J Heart Lung Transplant March 1993;12(2):S135–42.

37 Pahl E, Crawford SE, Cohn RA et al. Reversal of severe late left ventricular failure after pediatric heart transplantation and possible role of plasmapheresis. Am J Cardiol March 15, 2000;85(6):735–9.

38 Seta Y, Shan K, Bozkurt B, Oral H, Mann DL. Basic mechanisms in heart failure: the cytokine hypothesis. J Card Fail September 1996;2(3):243–9.

39 Deswal A, Petersen NJ, Feldman AM, Young JB, White BG, Mann DL. Cytokines and cytokine receptors in advanced heart failure: an analysis of the cytokine database from the Vesnarinone trial (VEST). Circulation April 24, 2001;103(16):2055–9.

40 Wallace CK, Stetson SJ, Kucuker SA et al. Simvastatin decreases myocardial tumor necrosis factor alpha content in heart transplant recipients. J Heart Lung Transplant January 2005;24(1):46–51.

41 Fadok VA, Bratton DL, Konowal A, Freed PW, Westcott JY, Henson PM. Macrophages that have ingested apoptotic cells in vitro inhibit proinflammatory cytokine production through autocrine/paracrine mechanisms involving TGF-beta, PGE2, and PAF. J Clin Invest February 15, 1998;101(4):890–8.

42 Shivji GM, Suzuki H, Mandel AS, Bolton AE, Sauder DN. The effect of VAS972 on allergic contact hypersensitivity. J Cutan Med Surg July 2000;4(3):132–7.

43 Babaei S, Stewart DJ, Picard P, Monge JC. Effects of VasoCare therapy on the initiation and progression of atherosclerosis. Atherosclerosis May 2002;162(1):45–53.

44 Bolton AE. Biologic effects and basic science of a novel immune-modulation therapy. Am J Cardiol June 6, 2005;95(11A):24C–9C.

45 Torre-Amione G, Sestier F, Radovancevic B, Young J. Effects of a novel immune modulation therapy in patients with advanced chronic heart failure: results of a randomized, controlled, phase II trial. J Am Coll Cardiol September 15, 2004;44(6):1181–6.

CHAPTER 23

Cholesterol, interleukin-6 inflammation, and atherosclerosis—role of statins, bisphosphonates, and plant polyphenols in atherosclerosis and other diseases of aging

Sota Omoigui

Introduction

In 400 BC, Hippocrates recognized the relationship between health and food. He said, "Let food be your medicine and medicine be your food." In 1513, Spanish explorer Juan Ponce de Leon discovered Florida while searching for the Fountain of Youth, a mythical spring said to restore youth. Ponce de Leon died trying to find those waters. He should have been looking instead for the Flora of Youth and inhibitors of Interleukin-6 (IL-6)-mediated inflammation.

Aging is associated with increased frequency of several disorders including atherosclerosis, peripheral vascular disease, coronary artery disease, osteoporosis, type 2 diabetes, dementia and Alzheimer's disease, and some forms of arthritis and cancer. Aging is also characterized by a proinflammatory state that contributes to the onset of disability and age-related diseases. Proinflammatory cytokines play a central role in mediating cellular and physiological responses. Studies of the effects of aging on inflammatory response show IL-6, tumor necrosis factor-α (TNF)-α, and interleukin-1β (IL-1β) to be important [1]. This review will focus on inhibition of IL-6-mediated inflammation as key to the prevention and treatment of aging and age-related disorders.

Atherosclerosis

Cardiovascular disease (CVD) is the leading cause of death and disability in developed nations and is increasing rapidly in the developing world. By the year 2020, it is estimated that CVD will surpass infectious diseases as the world's leading cause of death and disability. Atherosclerotic vascular disease, which encompasses coronary heart disease, cerebrovascular disease, and peripheral arterial disease, is responsible for the majority of cases of CVD in both developing and developed countries [2]. Atherosclerosis, a progressive disease characterized by the accumulation of lipids and fibrous elements in the arteries, constitutes the single most important contributor to this growing burden of CVD. The link between lipid metabolism and atherosclerosis dominated the thinking until the 1980s [3]. Over the last 15 years, however, a prominent role for inflammation in the pathogenesis of atherosclerosis has been established [4]. Now atherosclerosis is considered as an inflammation-mediated disease driven by complex interactions between leukocytes, platelets, and cells of the vessel wall. Endothelial injury is the first and crucial step in the pathogenesis of atherosclerosis. A plethora of genetically determined and epigenetic factors, such as oxidized low-density lipoprotein

(Ox-LDL), free radicals (e.g., due to cigarette smoking), hypertension, diabetes mellitus (DM), elevated plasma homocysteine, infectious microorganisms, autoimmune reactions, and combinations thereof, have been identified as etiological principles. Endothelial injury triggers inflammation with increased adhesiveness and activation of leukocytes (mainly monocytes) and platelets, which is accompanied by the production of cytokines, chemokines, vasoactive molecules, and growth factors.

The hallmark of the early atherosclerotic lesion is the cholesterol ester-laden macrophage foam cell [5]. Progressive "free" cholesterol loading of lesional macrophages leads to a series of phospholipid-related adaptive responses. These adaptive responses eventually fail, leading to macrophage death. Macrophage death by necrosis leads to lesional necrosis, release of cellular proteases, inflammatory cytokines, and prothrombotic molecules, which could contribute to plaque instability, plaque rupture, and acute thrombotic vascular occlusion [6]. Indeed, necrotic areas of advanced atherosclerotic lesions are known to be associated with death of macrophages, and ruptured plaques from human lesions have been shown to be enriched in apoptotic macrophages. The presence of apoptotic and necrotic macrophages in atherosclerotic lesions has been well documented in many human and animal studies [7, 8].

Currently, the inflammatory mediators implicated in the pathogenesis of atherosclerosis include cytokines, chemokines, vasoactive molecules, and growth factors. The anti-inflammatory effects of statins are attributed to multifaceted mechanisms including inhibition of cell cycle progression, induction of apoptosis, reduction of cyclooxygenase-2 activity, and an enhancement of angiogenesis. At the center of these mechanisms stands the ability to inhibit G protein prenylation through a reduction of farnesylation and geranylgeranylation [9].

To advance the current theories and thinking [10], and clarify the relationship between these common illnesses, we submit our theory of the precise biochemical pathway, between cholesterol and inflammation, and between inflammation and aging and age-related disorders including atherosclerosis, peripheral vascular disease, coronary artery disease (CAD), osteoporosis, type 2 diabetes, dementia and Alzheimer's disease, and some forms of arthritis and cancer. By elaborating this biochemical pathway, we will delineate the precise mechanism of the pleiotropic effects of statins, bisphosphonate drugs, and polyphenolic compounds. The common mechanism of action and common pleiotropic effects of the statins, bisphosphonate drugs, and plant-derived and synthetic polyphenolic compounds in addition to our identification of the unique activity of the IL-6 cytokine among all the vast mediators of inflammation and the inflammatory response enabled us to reverse engineer this biochemical pathway. Each component of our theory is supported and validated by numerous research studies.

Acute phase response

The acute phase response occurs before antibody-mediated immunological defense. It occurs in response to an inflammatory response brought on by injury and trauma, neoplasm, or disordered immunological activity. A local reaction at the site of injury or infection leads to an activation of cytokines (specifically, IL-6, IL-1, TNF-α, and interferons) that triggers a systemic response consisting of leukocytosis; increases in glucocorticoid production; increases in erythrocyte sedimentation rates, fever, activation of complement, and clotting cascades; decreases in serum zinc and iron; and an increase in plasma levels of acute phase proteins, C-reactive protein (CRP), serum amyloid A, fibrinogen, and other proteins [11].

Levels of cytokines involved in the acute phase response—TNF-α, IL-1, IL-6, and fibrinogen— have been shown to be elevated in cases of unstable angina related to aneurysm [12–14] and have been positively correlated with the risk of primary and recurrent myocardial infarction and death [15–17]. The risk associated with these elevated levels remains constant even when the data is adjusted for other major risk factors: blood pressure, total and HDL cholesterol, body mass index (BMI), diabetes, alcohol use, family history, and exercise frequency [15]. Elevated levels of highly sensitive C-reactive protein (hs-CRP) have been related to increased risk of CVD, myocardial infarction, and CAD deaths among individuals with angina pectoris [18–20]. Assayed levels of hs-CRP can increase 100 times over normal levels within 24–48 hours after an acute inflammatory stimulus. However, in long-term prospective studies interindividual variations in hs-CRP levels may occur over long periods of time, in the absence of trauma or acute infection [21]. Elevated levels of hs-CRP have shown a doubling of risk both for ischemic stroke in hypertensive men and women [14, 22] and for peripheral artery disease [23].

Recent studies are now demonstrating that IL-6 and TNF-α are stronger predictors of CVD than CRP. In the Health, Aging and Body Composition study [24], done at the Wake Forest University School of Medicine, the researchers tracked the medical history of the 2225 participants for an average of 42 months after measuring their blood levels of CRP, IL-6, and TNF-α. People with the highest IL-6 levels were two to five times more likely to have a heart attack, stroke, or other cardiovascular episode than those with the lowest levels. High blood levels of TNF-α increased the risk of heart disease by 79% and of heart failure by 121%. High levels of CRP increased the risk of heart failure by 160% compared to those with low levels, but they did not significantly raise the risk of a first stroke or heart attack.

As expected, the incidence of CVD was high for people with the conventional risk factors: smoking, high blood pressure, high cholesterol, and the like. But for participants free of these risk factors, the inflammation-related molecules were better predictors of heart disease.

Cholesterol metabolism

Normal healthy adults synthesize cholesterol at a rate of approximately 1 g/day and consume approximately 0.3 g/day. A relatively constant level of cholesterol in the body (150–200 mg/dL) is maintained primarily by controlling the level of de novo synthesis. The level of cholesterol synthesis is regulated in part by the dietary intake of cholesterol. Cholesterol from both diet and synthesis is utilized in the formation of membranes and in the synthesis of the steroid hormones and bile acids. The greatest proportion of cholesterol is used in bile acid synthesis [25]. Cholesterol synthesis occurs in the cytoplasm and microsomes with initial synthesis of mevalonate from the two-carbon acetate group of acetyl-CoA (see Figure 23.1).

1 Synthesis begins when acetyl-CoA is derived from an oxidation reaction in the mitochondria and is transported to the cytoplasm.
2 Two moles of acetyl-CoA are condensed, forming acetoacetyl-CoA. Acetoacetyl-CoA and a third mole of acetyl-CoA are converted to 3-hydroxy-3-methylglutaryl-CoA (HMG-CoA) by the action of HMG-CoA synthase.
3 HMG-CoA is converted to mevalonate, in a rate-limiting step catalyzed by the enzyme HMG-CoA reductase (HMGR).

In human beings, cholesterol and isoprenoids are then synthesized via the mevalonate pathway (see Figure 23.2).
1 Mevalonate is activated by three successive phosphorylations, yielding 5-pyrophosphomevalonate.
2 After phosphorylation, an ATP-dependent decarboxylation yields isopentenyl pyrophosphate (IPP), an activated isoprenoid molecule. IPP is in equilibrium with its isomer, dimethylallyl pyrophosphate, DMAPP.
3 One molecule of IPP condenses with one molecule of DMAPP to generate geranyl pyrophosphate (GPP). This step is catalyzed by GPP synthase.
4 GPP further condenses with another IPP molecule to yield farnesyl pyrophosphate (FPP). This step is catalyzed by FPP synthase.
5 FPP condenses with another IPP molecule to yield geranylgeranyl pyrophosphate (GGPP). This step is catalyzed by GGPP synthase.
6 The head-to-tail condensation of two molecules of FPP yielding Squalene, is catalyzed by squalene synthase.
7 Squalene undergoes a two-step cyclization to yield lanosterol.
8 Lanosterol is converted to cholesterol, through a series of 19 additional reactions.

There is a complex regulatory system to coordinate the biosynthesis of cholesterol with the availability of dietary cholesterol. The cellular supply of cholesterol is maintained at a steady level by the following mechanisms:
1 Regulation of HMGR activity and levels.
2 Regulation of excess intracellular free cholesterol through the activity of acyl-CoA: cholesterol acyltransferase (ACAT).
3 Regulation of plasma cholesterol levels via LDL receptor-mediated uptake and HDL-mediated reverse transport.

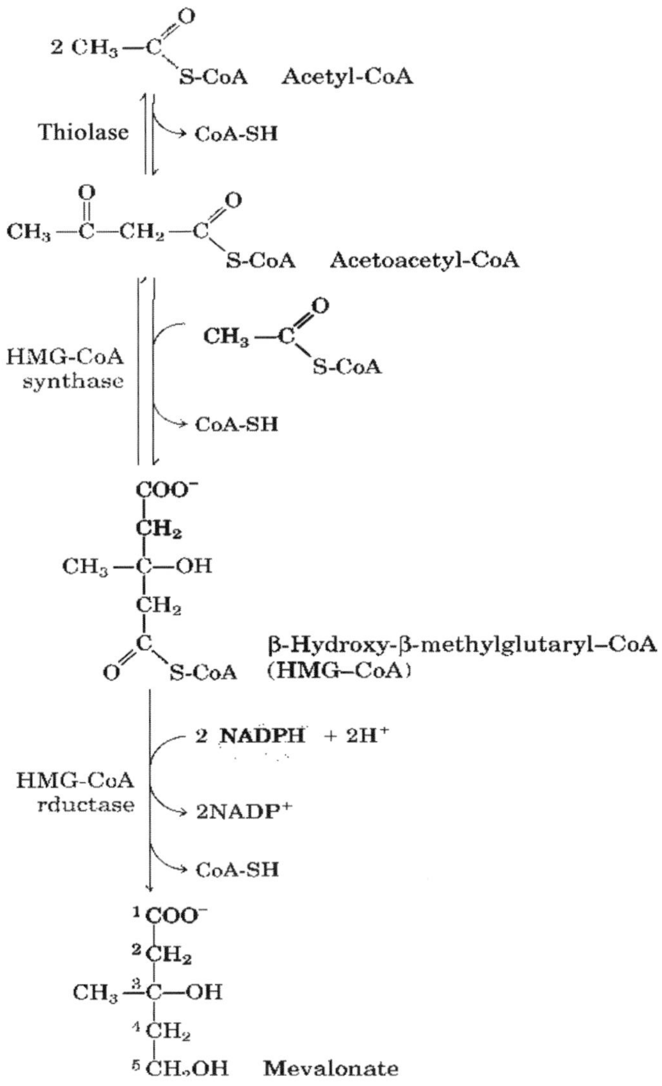

Figure 23.1 Mevalonate synthesis.

Interleukin-6

The IL-6 family of cytokines, signaling through the common receptor subunit (glycoprotein) subsequently activates signal transducers and activators of transcription (STAT3), mitogen-activated protein kinase (MAPK), and phosphatidylinositol 3-kinase [27]. The IL-6 family comprises IL-6, IL-11, leukemia inhibitory factor, oncostatin M, ciliary neurotrophic factor, and cardiotrophin-1. Among its many functions, IL-6 plays an active role in inflammation, immunology, bone metabolism, reproduction, arthritis, neoplasia, and aging. IL-6 expression is regulated by a variety of factors, including steroidal hormones, at both the transcriptional and posttranscriptional levels. Elevated levels of IL-6 are associated with the highest risks for subclinical CVD as well as for clinical CVD in older men and women [28]. Elevated levels of IL-6 are associated with a 34% increased likelihood of cognitive decline in older men and women [29]. IL-6-mediated inflammation contributes to bone resorption and osteoporosis by stimulating osteoclastogenesis and osteoclast activity [30–32]. IL-6

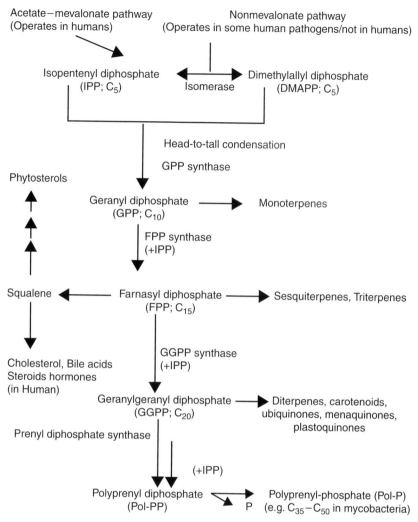

Figure 23.2 Cholesterol and isoprenoid synthesis [26].

production is considerably enhanced and associated with bone destruction in *Staphylococcus aureus* and mycobacterial arthritis, osteitis or osteomyelitis [33–35]. During times of stress or depression, IL-6 levels are increased. In a study of older adults undergoing a chronic stressor (men and women who were caregiving for a spouse with dementia), caregivers' average rate of increase in IL-6 was about four times as large as that of noncaregivers [36, 37].

IL-6 transmits its biological signal through two proteins on the cell. One of them is IL-6 receptor (IL-6R), an IL-6-specific binding molecule with a molecular weight of about 80 kDa. The other is a membrane-bound protein gp130 having a molecular weight of about 130 kDa, which is involved in non-ligand-binding signal transduction. IL-6R exists not only in the membrane-bound form with transmembrane domain expressed on the cell surface but also as a soluble IL-6R consisting mainly of the extracellular region. IL-6 and IL-6R form the IL-6/IL-6R complex, which after binding to gp130 transmits its biological signal to the cell. The important participants in the IL-6 signaling pathway include the Janus kinases (JAKs) JAK1, JAK2, and Tyk2, the signal transducers and activators of transcription STAT1 and STAT3, the tyrosine phosphatase SHP2 [SH2 (Src homology 2) domain-containing tyrosine phosphatase], and transcription factor NF-κB.

Protein kinases

Protein kinases are a class of allosteric enzymes that possess a catalytic subunit which transfers a phosphate from ATP to one or more amino acid residues (as serine, threonine, or tyrosine) in a protein's side chain resulting in a conformational change affecting protein function, and these play a role in regulating intracellular processes. JAKs (abbreviation for janus-activated kinase) is the name given to a family of nonreceptor protein tyrosine kinases, comprising JAK1, JAK2, Tyk2 (nonreceptor protein tyrosine kinase-2), which are widely expressed and JAK3 which is mainly found in cells of haematopoietic origin. STATS comprise a family of seven transcription factors that are activated by a variety of cytokines, hormones, and growth factors [1]. Engagement of cell surface IL-6 receptors activates the JAK family of tyrosine kinases, which in turn phosphorylate the cytoplasmic part of gp130, thereby creating docking sites for STAT factors STAT1 and STAT3 [2, 3]. Activated STATs dimerize upon activation by JAKs and translocate to the nucleus where they bind specific DNA response elements and regulate the expression of certain genes. Following gp130 dimerization, IL-6 activates multiple signaling pathways (Ras-dependent MAP kinase cascade, STAT1–STAT3 heterodimer pathway, and STAT3 homodimer pathway) [4–6].

Tyrosine kinase

Tyrosine-specific protein kinases (tyrosine kinases) represent a family of enzymes, which catalyze the transfer of the terminal phosphate of adenosine triphosphate to tyrosine residues in protein substrates. Tyrosine kinases consist of three general subclasses: (1) membrane receptor tyrosine kinases, including the insulin receptor and receptors for epidermal growth factor and platelet-derived growth factor; (2) cytosolic nonreceptor protein tyrosine kinases which include members of the Src, Tec, JAK, Fes, Abl, FAK, Csk, and Syk families; and (3) membrane-associated nonreceptor tyrosine kinases

which are associated with viral genes (oncogenes), capable of cell transformation and related closely to pp60^{v-src} [14]. Tyrosine-kinase receptors exist as single polypeptides in the plasma membrane. The extracellular portion of the protein, with the signal-molecule binding site, is connected by a single transmembrane a helix to the protein's cytoplasmic portion. This part of the protein is responsible for the receptor's tyrosine-kinase activity and also has a series of tyrosine amino acids. When signals molecules (such as a growth factor) attach to their binding sites, two polypeptides aggregate, forming a dimer. Using phosphate groups from ATP, the tyrosine-kinase region of each polypeptide phosphorylates the tyrosines on the other polypeptide. Thus, the dimer is both an enzyme and its own substrate. Now fully activated, the receptor protein can bind specific intracellular proteins, which attach to specific phosphorylated tyrosines and are themselves activated. Each can then initiate a signal-transduction pathway leading to a specific cellular response. Tyrosine-kinase receptors often activate several different signal-transduction pathways at once, helping regulate such complicated functions as cell reproduction (cell divisions). Inappropriate activation of these receptors can lead to uncontrolled cell growth—cancer. Tyrosine kinases are key elements in cellular signal transduction pathways. Small GTPases of the Ras protein superfamily stimulate the tyrosine phosphorylation and activation of the JAK family of intracellular kinases. This in turn activates the STAT family of transcription factors and results in the induction of IL-6 and IL-6R gene.

Serine/threonine kinases

Serine/threonine kinases include phosphorylase kinase (GPK), pyruvate dehydrogenase kinase, cAMP-dependent protein kinases (PKA), cGMP-dependent protein kinases (PKG), protein kinase C (PKC), Ca^{2+}/calmodulin-dependent protein kinases, G-protein-coupled receptor kinases (GRKs), mitogen-activated protein kinases (MAP kinase), several oncogenes (including mil, raf, and mos), heme-regulated protein kinase, plant-specific serine/threonine kinases, and receptor serine/threonine kinases (receptors for transforming growth factor TGF-β superfamily).

Dimeric transcription factors

Activator protein-1 (AP-1) is a collective term referring to dimeric transcription factors composed of Jun, Fos, or ATF (activating transcription factor) subunits that bind to the AP-1 binding site on the several proinflammatory genes including the IL-6 promoter [38]. AP-1 activity plays an important role in the inflammatory response by modulating gene expression of several inflammatory mediators including IL-6 transcription. Phosphorylation of c-Jun is a prerequisite of AP-1 dimerization and activation. AP-1 activity is controlled by signaling through the JNK family of MAP kinases. It has been demonstrated that during reperfusion, oxidative stress leads to activation and translocation of JNK to the nucleus, where phosphorylation of transcription factors such as c-Jun occurs.

Nuclear factor-κB

Nuclear factor-κB (NF-κB) is a widely expressed, inducible transcription factor of particular importance to cells of the immune system. It was originally identified as an enhancer binding protein for the Ig κ-light chain gene in B cells [39]. NF-κB regulates the expression of many genes involved in mammalian immune and inflammatory responses, including cytokines, cell adhesion molecules, complement factors, and a variety of immunoreceptors. The NF-κB transcription factor is a heterodimeric protein that comprises the p50 and p65 (Rel A) subunits. These subunits are proteins of the Rel family of transcriptional activators. Members of the Rel family share a conserved 300-amino acid Rel homology domain responsible for DNA binding, dimerization, and nuclear localization. While transcriptionally active homodimers of both p50 and p65 can form, the p50/65 heterodimer is preferentially formed in most cell types [40].

In the absence of stimulatory signals, the NF-κB heterodimer is retained in the cytoplasm by its physical association with an inhibitory phosphoprotein, IκB. Multiple forms of IκB have been identified [41]. Two of these forms, IκBα and IκBß, have been shown to modulate the function of the NF-κB heterodimer, and these two IκBs are phosphorylated in response to differ-ent extracellular stimuli [42]. Recent studies indicate that the catalytic subunit of protein kinase A (PKA$_C$) is associated with the NF-κB/IκBα complex [43]. In this p50/p65/IκBα/PKA$_C$ tetrameric configuration, IκBα renders PKA$_C$ inactive and masks the nuclear localization signal on NF-κB. Proinflammatory stimuli can activate a number of protein kinases, which have the capacity to modulate nuclear factor-κB (NF-κB) or AP-1 activity. A variety of extracellular stimulatory signals, such as cytokines, viruses, and oxidative stressors [44] activate kinases that phosphorylate IκB. The cytokine-activated IκB kinase termed IKK is the key regulatory kinase for IκBα [42]. IκB kinase (IKK) complex is composed of subunits, IKK-α, IKK-β, and IKK-γ, which are serine/threonine protein kinases whose function is needed for NF-κB activation by proinflammatory stimuli [45]. Phosphorylation at serines 32 and 36 targets IκBα for ubiquitination and subsequent rapid proteolysis via a proteasome-mediated pathway [46–49] resulting in the release of NF-κB/PKA$_C$. The now active PKA$_C$ subunit dissociates and phosphorylates the p65 subunit of NF-κB. Phosphorylated NF-κB then translocates to the cell nucleus, where it binds to target sequences in the chromatin and activates specific gene subsets, particularly those important to immune and inflammatory function [50–52]. PPAR-α (peroxisome proliferator-activated receptor-α) negatively interferes with inflammatory gene expression by upregulation of the cytoplasmic inhibitor molecule IκB-α, thus establishing an autoregulatory loop. This induction takes place in the absence of peroxisome proliferator-response elements, but requires the presence of NF-κB and Sp1 elements in the IκB-α promoter sequence as well as DRIP250 cofactors [53].

Nuclear factor-κB (NF-κB) is a required transcription factor for angiotensin II (Ang II)-inducible IL-6 expression. IL-6 is expressed by Ang II-stimulated vascular smooth muscle cells (VSMCs). In one study, Ang II treatment induced IL-6 transcription by inducing cytoplasmic-to-nuclear translocation of the NF-κB subunits Rel A and NF-κB1 with parallel changes in DNA-binding activity in a biphasic manner, which produced an early peak at 15 minutes followed by a nadir 1–6 hours later and a later peak at 24 hours [54].

Peroxisome proliferator-activated receptors

Peroxisome proliferator-activated receptors (PPARs) are ligand-activated transcription factors, which form a subfamily of the nuclear receptor gene family. The PPAR subfamily consists of three isotypes, α (NR1C1), γ (NR1C3), and β/δ (NRC1C2) with a differential tissue distribution. PPARs are activated by ligands, such as naturally occurring fatty acids, which are activators of all three PPAR isotypes. In addition to fatty acids, several synthetic compounds, such as fibrates and thiazolidinediones, bind and activate PPARα and PPARγ, respectively. PPARα is expressed primarily in tissues with a high level of fatty acid catabolism such as liver, brown fat, kidney, heart, and skeletal muscle. PPARβ is ubiquitously expressed, and PPARγ has a restricted pattern of expression, mainly in white and brown adipose tissues, whereas other tissues such as skeletal muscle and heart contain limited amounts. Furthermore, PPARα and PPARγ isotypes are expressed in vascular cells including endothelial and smooth muscle cells and macrophages/foam cells. In order to be transcriptionally active, PPARs need to heterodimerize with the retinoid-X-receptor (RXR). Upon activation, PPAR-RXR heterodimers bind to DNA-specific sequences called peroxisome proliferator-response elements and stimulate transcription of target genes. PPARs play a critical role in lipid and glucose homeostasis, but lately they have been implicated as regulators of inflammatory responses. The first evidence of the involvement of PPARs in the control of inflammation came from the PPARα null mice, which showed a prolonged inflammatory response. PPARα activation results in the repression of NF-κB signaling and inflammatory cytokine production in different cell types. A role for PPARγ in inflammation has also been reported in monocyte/macrophages, where ligands of this receptor inhibited the activation of macrophages and the production of inflammatory cytokines (TNFα, IL-6, and 1β) [55]. PPAR activators have effects on both metabolic risk factors and on vascular inflammation related to atherosclerosis. PPAR have profound effects on the metabolism of lipoproteins and fatty acids. PPARα binds hypolipidemic fibrates, whereas PPARγ has a high affinity for antidiabetic glitazones. Both PPARα and PPARγ are activated by fatty acids and their derivatives. Activation of PPARα increases the catabolism of fatty acids at several levels. In the liver, it increases uptake of fatty acids and activates their β-oxidation. The effects that PPARα exerts on triglyceride-rich lipoproteins is due to their stimulation of lipoprotein lipase and repression of apolipoprotein CIII expression, while the effects on high-density lipoproteins depend upon the regulation of apolipoproteins AI and AII. PPARγ has profound effects on the differentiation and function of adipose tissue, where it is highly expressed. PPAR are also expressed in atherosclerotic lesions and are present in vascular endothelial cells, smooth muscle cells, monocytes, and monocyte-derived macrophages. Via negative regulation of nuclear factor-κB and AP-1 signaling pathways, PPARα inhibits expression of inflammatory genes, such as IL-6, cyclooxygenase-2, and endothelin-1. Furthermore, PPARα inhibits expression of monocyte-recruiting proteins such as vascular cell adhesion molecule (VCAM)-1 and induces apoptosis in monocyte-derived macrophages. PPARγ activation in macrophages and foam cells inhibits the expression of activated genes such as inducible nitric oxide synthase, matrix metalloproteinase-9, and scavenger receptor A. PPARγ may also affect the recruitment of monocytes in atherosclerotic lesions as it is involved in the expression of VCAM-1 and intracellular adhesion molecule-1 in vascular endothelial cells [56].

Activation of IL-6 inflammation by isoprenoids

Cytokine receptors act through a complex signaling network involving GTPase proteins such as Ras, Rho, Rac, and Rab (particularly Rho), JAKs, and the signal transducers and activators of transcription (STATs) to regulate diverse biological processes controlling immune function, growth, development, and homeostasis [57].

Isoprenoids are necessary for posttranslational lipid modification (prenylation) and, hence, the function of Ras and other small guanosine triphosphatases (GTPases) [58].

GTPase proteins such as Ras, Rho, Rac, and Rab (particularly Rho) are intracellular signaling proteins that, when activated, are involved in receptor-coupled transduction of signals from extracellular stimuli to cytoplasm and the nucleus. Small GTPase proteins constitute a Ras superfamily, which comprises at least five major branches. Members of the Ras branch include the Ras, Rap, Ral, and R-Ras family proteins [59, 60]. The Ras family regulates gene expression. The Rho branch constitutes a second major branch, with RhoA, Rac1, and Cdc42 the most studied members. The Rho family regulates cytoskeletal reorganization and gene expression. The Rab branch is the largest, and, together with members of the Arf/Sar branch, serve as regulators of intracellular vesicular transport. Ran is the sole member of its branch and is a crucial regulator of nucleocytoplasmic transport of proteins and RNA. The Ras superfamily proteins alternate between an inactivated GDP-bound form and activated GTP-bound form, allowing them to act as molecular switches for growth and differentiation signals. Prenylation is a process involving the binding of hydrophobic isoprenoid groups consisting of farnesyl or geranylgeranyl residues to the C-terminal region of Ras protein superfamily. FPP and GGPP are metabolic products of mevalonate that are able to supply prenyl groups. The prenylation is conducted by prenyl transferases. The hydrophobic prenyl groups are necessary to anchor the Ras superfamily proteins to intracellular membranes so that they can be translocated to the plasma membrane [61]. The final cell-membrane fixation is necessary for Ras proteins to participate in their specific interactions [62, 63]. The activity of the small GTPase, Rac1, plays a role in various cellular processes including cytoskeletal rearrangement, gene transcription, and malignant transformation. Small GTPases of the Ras protein superfamily stimulate the tyrosine phosphorylation and activation of the JAK family of intracellular kinases. This in turn activates the STAT family of transcription factors and results in the induction of IL-6 and IL-6R gene. Persistent Rac1 activity leads to the autocrine production and signal transduction of IL-6 [36]. IL-6 itself may produce a delayed phosphorylation and activation of STAT3, and the JAK/STAT3 pathway is an indirect target of Ras and Rho GTPases [64]. Blocking the IL-6 signaling pathway inhibits Rac1-mediated STAT3-dependent gene expression. In one study [65], constitutively active Rac1 (Rac

V12) is shown to stimulate the activation of STAT3. The activity of Rac1 leads to STAT3 translocation to the nucleus coincident with STAT3-dependent gene expression [66]. Rac1 expression results in the induction of the IL-6 and IL-6R genes and neutralizing antibodies directed against the IL-6R block Rac1-induced STAT3 activation. Inhibition of nuclear factor-κB activation or disruption of IL-6-mediated signaling through the expression of IκB-α S32AS36A and suppressor of cytokine signaling 3, respectively, blocks Rac1-induced STAT3 activation. The study also investigated whether the other Rho family members mediate STAT3 activation in an IL-6-dependent pathway. The expression of constitutively active RhoG, Cdc42, and RhoA caused the translocation from the cytoplasm to the nucleus of cotransfected STAT3-GFP. This GTPase-induced STAT3 translocation was blocked to varying degrees by neutralizing IL-6R antibodies, supporting a role for autocrine IL-6 in Rho family-induced STAT3 activation. These findings elucidate a mechanism dependent on the induction of an autocrine IL-6 activation loop through which Rac1 and the Rho family mediate STAT3 activation establishing a link between GTPase activity and Janus kinase/STAT signaling. Interestingly, STAT3 is persistently activated in many human cancers and transformed cell lines. In cell culture, active STAT3 is either required for transformation, enhances transformation, or blocks apoptosis.

In one study [67], leukemic cells from 50 patients with acute myeloid leukemia (AML) were analyzed for the presence of activating point mutations of the N-RAS gene using polymerase chain reaction (PCR) and differential oligonucleotide hybridization. Clonal activation of N-RAS, noted in the large majority of leukemic cells of the six of these patients, was correlated significantly ($p = 0.0003$) with the ability of these cells to express IL-6, previously shown to be expressed at high levels in approximately 30% of primary AML cells.

In summary, isoprenoids FPP and GGPP are necessary for posttranslational lipid modification (prenylation) and, hence, the function of Ras and other small GTPase proteins such as Ras, Rho, Rac, and Rab [51]. Persistently active Rho family and Rac1 results in the activation of JAKs and subsequent tyrosine phosphorylation and activation of STAT3 [68]. Tyrosine-phosphorylated

STAT3 forms dimers that translocate to the nucleus to bind DNA target sites in responsive genes [58]. IL-6 and IL-6R gene induction occurs as a result of activated STAT proteins and IL-6 mediates the long-term activation of STAT3 through an autocrine loop.

Inhibition of cholesterol pathway by statins

The main effect of statins is the decrease of serum level of low-density lipoprotein (LDL) cholesterol, due to the inhibition of intracellular cholesterol biosynthesis. A minor effect is the decrease of serum triglycerides. Statins inhibit HMG-CoA reductase and decrease the production of mevalonate, GPP, and FPP, and subsequent products on the way to construction of the cholesterol molecule. Thus, statins could inhibit inflammation by inhibition of the cholesterol pathway and intracellularly interfering with Ras superfamily protein function [69]. Ikeda *et al.* [70] recently showed that statins decrease matrix metalloproteinase-1 expression through inhibition of Rho. Statin therapy has been demonstrated to provide significant reductions in nonhigh-density lipoprotein cholesterol and to decrease cardiovascular morbidity and mortality.

Inhibition of cholesterol pathway by bisphosphonates

Recent findings suggest that alendronate and other N-containing bisphosphonates inhibit the isoprenoid biosynthesis pathway and interfere with protein prenylation, as a result of reduced geranylgeranyl diphosphate levels. One study [71] utilizing high-performance liquid chromatography (HPLC) analysis of products from a liver cytosolic extract, identified farnesyl disphosphate (FPP) synthase as the mevalonate pathway enzyme inhibited by bisphosphonates. Recombinant human farnesyl diphosphate synthase was inhibited by alendronate with an IC50 of 460 nM (following 15 minutes preincubation). Alendronate did not inhibit isopentenyl diphosphate isomerase or GGPP synthase. Recombinant farnesyl diphosphate synthase was also inhibited by pamidronate (IC50 = 500 nM) and risedronate (IC50 = 3.9 nM), negligi-

bly by etidronate (IC50 = 80 μM), and not at all by the non-nitrogen-containing bisphosphonate clodronate. In another study, a wide range of bisphosphonates were found to have a significant correlation between potency for inhibition of recombinant human FPP synthase in vitro and antiresorptive potency in vivo, suggesting that this enzyme is the major pharmacologic target of these drugs. The most potent antiresorptive bisphosphonates such as zoledronic acid and risedronate are very potent inhibitors of FPP synthase, with IC50 values as low as 3 nM and 10 nM, respectively. Inhibition of FPP synthase prevents the formation of FPP and its derivative GGPP. These isoprenoid lipids are necessary for the posttranslational lipid modification (prenylation) of small GTPase proteins such as Ras, Rho, Rac, and Rab. The effects of nitrogen-containing bisphosphonates on osteoclasts can be overcome by addition of components of the mevalonate pathway, which bypass the inhibition of FPP synthase and restore protein prenylation. In particular, geranylgeraniol (a cell-permeable form of GGPP) prevents inhibition of resorption by nitrogen-containing bisphosphonates in vitro [72].

Plant products—fungi, polyphenolic compounds, and fatty acids

Statins identical to the cholesterol lowering pharmaceutical lovastatin and its derivatives of simvastatin, pravastatin, and mevastatin can be produced by a variety of filamentous fungi, including *Monascus, Aspergillus, Penicillium, Pleurotus, Pythium, Hypomyces, Paelicilomyces, Eupenicillium,* and *Doratomyces* [73]. As a food product, rice fermented with a red Monascus fungus (red rice) has been known to contain low amounts of statins and used for hundreds of years in China. Red rice is used in wine making, as a food-coloring agent and as a drug in traditional Chinese medicine.

Several hundred molecules having a polyphenol (polyhydroxyphenol) structure (i.e., several hydroxyl groups on aromatic rings) have been identified in edible plants. These molecules are secondary metabolites of plants and are generally involved in defense against ultraviolet radiation or aggression by pathogens. Polyphenols are widespread constituents of fruits, vegetables, cereals, dry legumes, chocolate, and beverages, such as tea, coffee, or wine. These compounds may be classified into different groups as a function of the number of phenol rings that they contain and of the structural elements that bind these rings to one another. Classes of polyphenols include the phenolic acids, flavonoids, stilbenes, and lignans. There are two classes of phenolic acids: derivatives of benzoic acid and derivatives of cinnamic acid.

Hydroxybenzoic acids are components of complex structures such as hydrolyzable tannins (gallotannins in mangoes and ellagitannins in red fruit such as strawberries, raspberries, and blackberries). Hydroxycinnamic acids are more common than are the hydroxybenzoic acids and consist chiefly of *p*-coumaric, caffeic, ferulic, and sinapic acids. Caffeic and quinic acid combine to form chlorogenic acid, which is found in many types of fruit and in high concentrations in coffee.

Flavonoids are the largest single class as far as total numbers of known compounds. About two-thirds of the polyphenols we obtain in our diets are flavonoids. Flavonoids share a common structure consisting of two aromatic rings that are bound together by three carbon atoms that form an oxygenated heterocycle and may be divided into six major subclasses: anthocyanidins (e.g., cyanidin, pelargonidin); flavanols (e.g., epicatechin, gallocatechin); flavones (e.g., apigenin, luteolin); flavonols (e.g., kaempferol, myricetin, quercetin); flavanones (e.g., hesperidin, naringenin); isoflavones (e.g., genistein, daidzein, biochanin); and proanthocyanidins [74].

Proanthocyanidins (condensed tannins) are a class of polyphenolic compounds found in several plant species. They include procyanidins, which are chains of catechin, epicatechin, and their gallic acid esters and the prodelphinidins, which consist of gallocatechin, epigallocatechin, and their gallic acid esters as the monomeric units.

Isoflavones are flavonoids with structural similarities to estrogens. Although they are not steroids, they have hydroxyl groups in positions 7 and 4 in a configuration analogous to that of the hydroxyls in the estradiol molecule. This confers pseudohormonal properties on them, including the ability to bind to estrogen receptors, and they are consequently classified as phytoestrogens. Phytoestrogenic isoflavones including genistein, daidzein,

glycitein, biochanin A, formononetin, and their respective naturally occurring glycosides and glycoside conjugates are found in plants such as legumes, clover, and the root of the kudzu vine (pueraria root). Common legume sources of these isoflavone compounds include soybeans, chick peas, ground nuts, lentils, and various other types of beans and peas. Clover sources of these isoflavone compounds include red clover and subterranean clover.

Fatty acids consist of chains of carbon atoms linked together by chemical bonds. Fatty acids come in different lengths: short chain fatty acids have fewer than 6 carbons, while long chain fatty acids have 12 or more carbons. On one terminal of the carbon chain is a methyl group and on the other terminal is a carboxyl group. The chemical bonds between the carbon atoms determine whether a fatty acid is saturated or unsaturated. Saturated fatty acids contain single bonds only. Examples of foods high in saturated fats include lard, butter, whole milk, cream, eggs, red meat, chocolate, and solid shortenings. An excess intake of saturated fat can raise blood cholesterol and increase the risk of developing coronary heart disease. Monounsaturated fatty acids contain one double bond. Examples of foods high in monounsaturated fat include avocados, nuts, and olive, peanut, and canola oils. Polyunsaturated fatty acids contain more than one double bond. Examples of foods high in polyunsaturated fats include vegetable oils, corn, sunflower, and soy. Essential fatty acids are polyunsaturated fatty acids that the human body needs for metabolic functioning but cannot produce, and therefore has to be acquired from food. Omega-3 fatty acids are a class of essential polyunsaturated fatty acids with the double bond in the third carbon position from the methyl terminal (hence the use of "3" in their description). Foods high in omega-3 fatty acids include cold-water fatty fish such as salmon, herring, mackerel, anchovies, and sardines, and vegetable sources such as the oil from the seeds of chia, perilla, flax, purslane, hemp, and canola. Other foods that contain omega-3 fatty acids include whole grains, beans, green leafy vegetables such as spinach and seafood such as shrimp, clams, light chunk tuna, catfish, and cod. Omega-6 fatty acids are a class of essential polyunsaturated fatty acids with the initial double bond in the sixth carbon position from the methyl group. Examples of foods rich in omega-6 fatty acids include corn, safflower, sunflower, soybean, and cottonseed oil.

Omega-3 and omega-6 fatty acids are also referred to as n-3 and n-6 fatty acids, respectively.

Atherosclerosis and IL-6

Macrophage uptake of Ox-LDL is a hallmark of the early atherosclerotic lesion and may be mediated by IL-6. Incubation of IL-6 with MPM or IL-6 administration in mice increased macrophage Ox-LDL degradation and CD36 mRNA expression. Ang II plays an important role in atherogenesis. Ang II increases macrophage cholesterol accumulation and foam cell formation, increases contraction of blood vessels, and induces hypertrophy and hyperplasia of VSMC. Ang II significantly increases the expression of IL-6 mRNA and protein in vascular smooth muscle, in a dose-dependent manner. The induction of IL-6 expression by Ang II is dependent on intracellular Ca^{2+}, tyrosine phosphorylation, and MAPK [75]. Ang II administration to apolipoprotein E-deficient atherosclerotic mice increases Ox-LDL degradation, CD36 mRNA expression, and CD36 protein expression by their peritoneal macrophages (MPMs). Ang II treatment of IL-6-deficient mice did not affect their MPM Ox-LDL uptake and CD36 protein levels. Furthermore, injection of IL-6R antibodies in mice during Ang II treatment reduced macrophage Ox-LDL uptake and CD36 expression [76].

Enzymatic, nonoxidative modification transforms low-density lipoprotein (LDL) to an atherogenic molecule (E-LDL) that activates complement and macrophages and is present in early atherosclerotic lesions. E-LDL accumulates in human VSMC, where it stimulates the expression of gp130, the signal-transducing chain of the IL-6R family, and the secretion of IL-6 [77]. IL-6/sIL-6R provokes marked upregulation of gp130 mRNA and surface protein expression in VSMC. This is accompanied by secretion of IL-6 by the cells, so that an autocrine stimulation loop is created. In the wake of this self-sustaining system, there is a selective induction and secretion of monocyte chemotactic protein-1 (MCP-1), upregulation of ICAM-1, and marked vascular smooth mus-

cle proliferation [78]. IL-6 induces proliferation of VSMCs and the release of monocyte chemoattractant protein-1 (MCP-1) [79]. One study investigated IL-6 mRNA expression in atherosclerotic arteries from patients undergoing surgical vascularization, utilizing reverse transcription polymerase chain reaction (RT-PCR) and in situ hybridization analyses. In RT-PCR analysis, the atherosclerotic arteries showed 10- to 40-fold levels of IL-6 mRNA expression over the nonatherosclerotic artery. In in situ hybridization analysis, IL-6 gene transcripts were observed in the thickened intimal layer of atherosclerotic lesions. These results strongly suggest the involvement of IL-6 in the development of human atherosclerosis [80]. Thrombin is a potent mitogen for VSMCs and plays an important role in the progression of atherosclerosis. Thrombin induces IL-6 mRNA and protein expression in a dose-dependent manner. Pharmacological inhibition of extracellular signal-regulated protein kinase (ERK), p38 MAPK, or epidermal growth factor receptor (EGF-R) suppresses thrombin-induced IL-6 expression [81]. IL-6 increases the number of platelets in the circulation [82] and activates platelets through arachidonic acid metabolism in vitro [83]. IL-6 is reported to increase plasma fibrinogen and decrease free protein S concentration. These IL-6-induced modifications of platelet and the coagulant phase of the clotting mechanism may lead to pathological thrombosis and instability of plaque [84]. IL-6 stimulation of VSMCs occurs via the JAK/STAT signaling pathway. In one study, Rat VSMC were stimulated with IL-6 in the presence or absence of a JAK 2 inhibitor, and the activation of STAT 3 (by Western), MCP-1 (by ELISA), and DNA synthesis (by (3)H-thymidine incorporation) was determined. IL-6 rapidly induced phosphorylation of STAT 3 in a dose- and time-dependent manner with a peak expression at 30 minutes. IL-6 also stimulated MCP-1 protein production and DNA synthesis dose dependently. A total of 50 μM of AG490, a specific JAK2 inhibitor, partially inhibited STAT 3 activation and MCP-1 production, with near complete inhibition of DNA synthesis [85]. Levels of IL-6 are significantly higher in patients with dyslipidemia IIa and IIb biochemically confirmed, and IL-6 levels are significantly correlated to intima-media complex thickness [86].

Statins and IL-6

The ability of HMG-CoA reductase inhibitors to lower CRP levels has recently brought into question the mechanisms of action of the statin drugs. Because these medications lower incidences of acute cardiovascular events as well as decreasing morbidity and mortality well before the effects of lowered LDL cholesterol can be expected to occur, questions have been asked about whether they may work independently of LDL-lowering mechanisms. One study examined the effects of atorvastatin on soluble adhesion molecules, IL-6, and brachial artery endothelial-dependent flow mediated dilatation (FMD) in patients with familial (FH) and non-familial hypercholesterolemia (NFH) [87]. A total of 74 patients (27 FH and 47 NFH) were recruited. Fasting lipid profiles, soluble intercellular adhesion molecule-1 (sICAM-1), soluble vascular–cellular adhesion molecule-1 (sVCAM-1), E-selectin, IL-6, and FMD were measured at baseline, 2 weeks, 3 and 9 months postatorvastatin treatment (FH—80 mg/day, NFH—10 mg/day). In both groups, compared to baseline, sICAM-1 levels were significantly reduced at 2 weeks, further reduced at 3 months and maintained at 9 months ($p < 0.0001$). The IL-6 levels were significantly reduced at 3 months and 9 months compared to baseline for FH ($p < 0.005$) and NFH ($p < 0.0001$). In both groups, the FMD at 2 weeks was higher than baseline ($p < 0.005$), with progressive improvement up to 9 months. FMD was negatively correlated with sICAM-1 and IL-6.

Bisphosphonates and IL-6

Because of various modes of action observed in studies, bisphosphonates have been classified into two groups. Bisphosphonates (such as clodronate and etidronate) that closely resemble pyrophosphate—a normal byproduct of human metabolism—are incorporated into adenosine triphosphate (ATP) analogues, which create compounds that are believed to build up and lead to osteoclast death [88]. The newest generation of bisphosphonates, which contain nitrogen (such as pamidronate, alendronate, risedronate, and ibandronate), are believed to inhibit protein prenylation (posttranslational modification) within the mevalonate pathway. The mevalonate pathway is responsible for the biosynthesis of cholesterol, other sterols, and isoprenoid lipids. Isoprenoid lipids are key in the prenylation of intracellular signaling proteins (GTPases) that, when activated, regulate a number of processes, including osteoclast activity. It is believed that by impeding the function of these regulatory proteins, bisphosphonates block osteoclast functioning and cause apoptosis [89].

In patients with Paget's disease of bone, bisphosphonate therapy is associated with a significant reduction of IL-6 soluble receptor (sIL-6R) serum levels [90]. Bisphosphonates inhibit the production of proinflammatory cytokine IL-6 in tumoral cell lines of human osteoblastic phenotype (MG63 and SaOs cells) and in peripheral blood mononuclear cells (PBMC) [91]. Bisphosphonates also inhibit IL-1 and TNF-α stimulated IL-6 release in cultures of human osteoblastic osteosarcoma cells [92]. Osteoblasts exposed to small amounts of bisphosphonate elaborate a soluble inhibitor, which interferes with osteoclast formation and development [93]. Bisphosphonates prevent apoptosis of murine osteocytic MLO-Y4 cells, whether it is induced by etoposide, TNF-α, or glucocorticoid dexamethasone [94]. Pamidronate and other bisphosphonates inhibit the production by osteoblasts of the inflammatory cytokine IL-6, a growth factor essential to myeloma cells [95].

Plant polyphenols, fatty acids, and IL-6

The beneficial skeletal effects of genistein, at dietarily achievable levels, are mediated, by IL-6. IL-6 production was decreased 40% in osteoblastic cells treated with genistein from either Day 8–16 or Day 12–16 at dietarily achievable concentrations (10(−10) to 10(−8) M) ($p < 0.05$) [96]. In one study, Sophoricoside (SOP), an isoflavone glycosid isolated from immature fruits of Sophora japonica (Leguminosae family) inhibited the IL-6 bioactivity with an IC50 value of 6.1 μM [97]. In another study, treatment with soybean isoflavones (10(−5) M), in the presence of TNF-α (10(−10) M), for 48 hours inhibited production of IL-6 and PGE(2). The authors suggested that the antiresorptive action of soy phytoestrogen may be mediated by decreases in these local factors [98]. One study investigated the mechanisms of drug resistance associated with the human prostate carcinoma PC-3 cell line. Endogenous and exogenous IL-6 and exogenous OM upregulated cell growth and enhanced resistance of PC-3 tumor cells to both etoposide and cisplatin. Both IL-6- and OM-mediated effects were inhibited by the treatment of PC-3 with an antisense oligodeoxynucleotide against gp130, the protein kinase inhibitor genistein (GNS), or the monoterpene perillic acid (PA), a posttranslational inhibitor of p21ras isoprenylation [99]. In another study, the effect of inhibition of tyrosine kinase activity on thymidine uptake into cultured human pituitary adenoma cells was studied using two inhibitors, genestein and methyl-2,3-dihydroxycinnamate (MDHC). Of 33 pituitary adenomas, 7 incorporated sufficient [3H]thymidine to be investigated in the experiments. Genestein and MDHC both potently inhibited thymidine uptake into these tumors, with a mean inhibition by 74 μmol/L genestein of $61.96 \pm 18.96\%$ ($\pm$ SD inhibition of basal), by 740 μmol/L genestein of $92.65 \pm 8.59\%$, and by 100 μmol/L MDHC of $93.84 \pm 3.85\%$. Epidermal growth factor stimulated thymidine uptake in two of the three clinically nonfunctioning adenomas studied, and this stimulation was inhibited by genestein. The authors concluded that tyrosine kinase activity is crucial for the integrity and growth of pituitary adenomas in culture and that growth factors released by pituitary adenomas potentially may maintain and promote tumor growth by stimulating tyrosine kinase activity [100].

Bacterial LPS induce a 12- to 16-fold increase in IL-1β, IL-6, and TNF-α mRNA levels. In one study, this increase was completely or more than 80% blocked by the protein tyrosine kinase-specific inhibitors herbimycin A and genistein at the concentrations of 1.7 and 37 μM, respectively. LPS-induced IL-6 protein synthesis and IL-6 bioactivity were also reduced to baseline levels by the PTK inhibitors herbimycin A and genistein. Both PTK inhibitors also reduced the LPS activation of nuclear factor-κB (NF-κB), which is a transcription factor involved in the expression of cytokine genes such as IL-6 and TNF-α [101].

Epidemiological evidence suggests that tea consumption may have a strong effect on CVD, but there has been no prior description of the molecular mechanisms involved. Epigallocatechin-3-gallate (EGCG) is a prominent catechin present in green tea. Several experimental studies have re-ported beneficial effects of EGCG in inflammation and cancer [102–104]. NF-κB is a transcription factor centrally involved in the signal transduction of the inflammatory process. The common pathway for activation of NF-κB involves phosphorylation of its inhibitor protein IκBα by IKK. Activation of IKK complex is an essential step for NF-κB activation because the kinase phosphorylates IκB-α and allow its degradation. Several studies have demonstrated that EGCG is an effective inhibitor of IKK activity. EGCG inhibits TNF-α-mediated IKK activation in human epithelial cells. Yang and colleagues showed that EGCG in concentrations of 50–200 μM inhibited IKK activity in an intestinal epithelial cell line [105]. In the Myocardial ischemia reperfusion study, EGCG reduced reperfusion-induced activation of IKK, degradation of IκBα, and activation of NF-κB [106]. EGCG has been demonstrated to dramatically inhibit chemokine-induced neutrophil chemotaxis in vitro [107]. Tea polyphenols have also been noted to induce apoptosis and cell cycle arrest in a wide array of cell lines [108–110]. EGCG affects several signaling mechanisms in inflammation. Menegazzi and colleagues showed that interferon-γ-induced STAT-1 activation in carcinoma-derived cell lines of nongut origin was blocked by EGCG [111]. In another study, Watson and colleagues demonstrated that EGCG significantly reduced INF-γ-induced STAT1 activation in T84 epithelial and THP-1 monocytes/macrophages [112].

Polyunsaturated omega-3 fatty acids reduce the secretion of proinflammatory cytokines and downregulate the inflammatory process. A total of 18-week n-3 PUFA diet supplementation exerts a significant inhibitory effect on basal and lipopolysaccharide (LPS)-stimulated IL-6 monocyte production (50 and 46%, respectively, $p < 0.05$) [113].

Atherosclerosis and statins

Changes in intima-media thickness (IMT) and arterial lumen diameter—as measured by B-mode high-resolution ultrasonography and quantitative coronary angiography, respectively—are currently the only surrogate markers for progression of atherosclerotic disease. There has been increasing use of this imaging technique in observational studies and interventional studies of lipid-lowering agents over the last decade. These observational studies clearly demonstrated an association between carotid IMT and atherosclerotic disease. Of the interventional studies, the recent Arterial Biology for the Investigation of the Treatment Effects of Reducing Cholesterol (ARBITER) trial found that use of atorvastatin 80 mg daily for aggressive lowering of plasma low-density lipoprotein cholesterol (LDL-C) concentrations to below current target levels was associated with significant IMT regression compared with results obtained with less aggressive plasma LDL-C lowering [114, 115].

Atherosclerosis and bisphosphonates

In one study, the effect of etidronate treatment on carotid arterial intima-media thickness was prospectively examined in 57 subjects with type 2 diabetes associated with osteopenia. After 1 year of therapy with cyclical etidronate (200 mg/day for 2 weeks every 3 months), intima-media thickness showed a decrease (mean $\pm$ SE, -0.038 ± 0.011 mm), which was significantly different from a change in 57 control subjects (0.023 ± 0.015 mm; $p < 0.005$). Cardiovascular parameters were not changed after etidronate treatment. The authors concluded that etidronate in clinical dosage may have an antiatherogenic action, at least in type 2 diabetes [116]. In another study, administration of ethane-1-hydroxy-1,1-diphosphonate (EHDP) to swine with preestablished atherosclerosis resulted in lower lesion calcium concentration, smaller lesions, and a decrease in the area of lesions involved in necrosis [117].

Atherosclerosis, plant polyphenols, and fatty acids

Cupric-ion-oxidized LDL (CuLDL) or endothelial cell-oxidized LDL (ELDL) induces the activation by Tyr-phosphorylation of JAK2, one of the Janus kinase involved upstream of STATs in the JAK/STAT pathway of cytokine transduction. Oxidized LDL (Ox-LDL) also initiates STAT1 and STAT3 Tyr-phosphorylation and translocation to the nucleus, with a more marked effect for the extensively modified Cu-LDL. In one study, Genistein, a nonspecific Tyr-kinase inhibitor, and AG490, a specific in-

hibitor of JAKs, markedly prevented the Cu-LDL-induced enhancement of STAT1 and STAT3 Tyr-phosphorylation and DNA-binding activity, suggesting that JAKs are the main kinases involved in STATs' activation by oxidized LDL [118]. The effect of genistein on aortic atherosclerosis was studied in New Zealand White rabbits. After provocation of atherosclerosis with hyperlipidemic diet, the rabbits were divided as hyperlipidemic diet group (HD), normal diet group (ND), and hyperlipidemic plus genistein diet group (HD + genistein) for 4 and a half months. The average cross-sectional area of atherosclerotic lesion was 0.269 mm^2 after provocation. The lesion was progressed by continuous hyperlipidemic diet (10.06 mm^2) but was increased mildly by genistein (0.997 mm^2), and decreased by normal diet [119]. Ang II plays an important role in atherogenesis. One study investigated the effect of Ang II on the production of IL-6 in rat VSMCs. Ang II significantly increased the expression of IL-6 mRNA and protein in a dose-dependent manner (10(−10) to 10(−6) mol/L). The expression of IL-6 mRNA induced by Ang II was completely blocked by an Ang II type 1 receptor antagonist, CV11974. Inhibition of tyrosine kinase with genistein and inhibition of MAPK with PD98059 completely abolished the effect of Ang II [120]. The potent endothelium-derived vasoactive factor endothelin-1 (ET-1) has been implicated in the pathophysiology of atherosclerosis and its complications. ET-1 stimulates the formation of proinflammatory cytokines including IL-6 and tumor necrosis factor-α (TNF-α) [121]. In one study, ET-1 transiently increased IL-6 mRNA compatible with regulation of IL-6 release at the pretranslational level. Electrophoretic mobility shift assays demonstrated time- and concentration-dependent activation of the proinflammatory transcription factor nuclear factor-κB (NF-κB) in ET-1-stimulated human vascular SMC. A decoy oligodeoxynucleotide bearing the NF-κB binding site inhibited ET-1-stimulated IL-6 release to a great extent suggesting that this transcription factor plays a key role for cytokine production elicited by ET-1 [122]. In one study, researchers investigated the suppressive effect of cocoa powder (cacao polyphenol content: 7.8%) on atherosclerosis in a spontaneous familial hypercholesterolemic model, Kurosawa and Kusanagi-hypercholesterolemic (KHC) rabbits. Six-month dietary administration of cocoa powder had no effects on body weight, hematology, or blood chemistry parameters or a lipid profile in KHC rabbits. Thiobarbituric acid reactive substances (TBARS), the marker of lipid peroxidation, in plasma were decreased in the cocoa-powder-treated group from the second month of administration during the study period compared to that in the control group. The area of atherosclerotic lesions in the aorta was significantly smaller in the cocoa powder group (30.87%) than in the control (52.39%). Tissue cholesterol content also tended to decrease. Distensibility of the aortic wall was improved significantly in the cocoa-powder-treated group due to decreases in fatty streaks and intimal thickening compared to that in the control group. These results suggest that cocoa powder has suppressive effect on development of atherosclerotic lesions [123]. One study determined the effects of green tea polyphenols on the proliferation and p44/42 MAPK activity in rat VSMCs simulated by native LDL. Rat aortic VSMCs were cultured and treated with LDL (100 μg/mL) in the absence or presence of green tea polyphenols, and the cell proliferation was subsequently quantified by nonradioactive MTS/PES assay and the cell cycle analyzed by flow cytometry. The p44/42 MAPK activity was evaluated by immunoblotting using anti-p44/42 phospho-MAPK antibody. Compared with the cells without polyphenol treatment, the proliferation of the VSMCs induced by LDL was dose-dependently inhibited by green tea polyphenols ($p < 0.05$), with more numerous cells in G(0)G(1) phase ($p < 0.05$) as shown by flow cytometry analysis. LDL significantly enhanced the p44/42 MAPK activity, an effect obviously inhibited by green tea polyphenols (at 100 μg/mL). These results suggest that green tea polyphenols can inhibit high levels of LDL-induced proliferation of phosphorylated p44/42 MAPK expression in rat VSMCs [124]. In another study, hamsters (nine in each group) were given a cholesterol/saturated fat for 10 weeks to induce foam cell formation. Water or 6.75% ethanol was given to the control groups. Beverages tested included red wine, dealcoholized red wine, and red grape juice, all diluted in half. Ethanol and all beverages caused a significant reduction in atherosclerosis. The combination of ethanol in red wine had the largest effect in decreasing atherosclerosis. When compared with dealcoholized wine and normalized to polyphenol dose, red wine's beneficial effects can be attributed entirely to the polyphenols. Grape juice had a significant benefit at a much lower dose of polyphenols than the wines. Grape juice was calculated to be much more effective than red wine or dealcoholized red wine at the same polyphenol dose in inhibiting atherosclerosis and improving lipids and antioxidant parameters. The authors suggest that polyphenolic beverages from grapes are beneficial in inhibiting atherosclerosis by several mechanisms [125]. The low incidence of CVD associated epidemiologically with high consumption of food rich in n-3 fatty acids suggests the possibility that part of the beneficial cardiovascular effects of these natural substances may be due to a reduction of atherosclerosis [126]. Dietary intervention trials using coronary heart disease (CHD) mortality and morbidity as endpoints have demonstrated that restriction of dietary total and saturated fat or replacement of the latter with polyunsaturated fatty acids (PUFAs), in particular n-3 PUFAs, is of great benefit with respect to CHD risk [127]. A range of prospective studies have proven high efficacy of omega-3-polyunsaturated fatty acids in secondary prophylaxis of atherosclerosis and its complications [128, 129].

Type 2 diabetes and IL-6

Circulating levels of IL-6 are raised in insulin resistant states such as obesity, impaired glucose tolerance (IGT), and type 2 DM. Growing evidence suggests that IL-6 is not only produced by fat cells but is also capable of inducing insulin resistance in these cells. The expected result of this in vivo would be to increase adipose mass and subsequently BMI. The IL-6–174G > C common functional gene variant has consistently been associated with increased plasma IL-6, insulin resistance, and increased cardiovascular risk [130]. In The Women's Health Study (an ongoing US primary prevention, randomized clinical trial initiated in 1992), the authors determined whether elevated levels of the inflammatory markers IL-6 and CRP are associated with development of type 2 DM in healthy middle-aged women. From a nationwide cohort of 27,628 women free of diagnosed DM, CVD, and cancer at baseline, 188 women who developed diagnosed DM over a 4-year follow-up period were defined as cases and matched by age and fasting status with 362 disease-free controls. Study results showed that baseline levels of IL-6 ($p < 0.001$) and CRP ($p < 0.001$) were significantly higher among cases than among controls. The relative risks of future DM for women in the highest versus lowest quartile of these inflammatory markers were 7.5 for IL-6 (95% CI, 3.7–15.4) and 15.7 for CRP (95% CI, 6.5–37.9). Positive associations persisted after adjustment for BMI, family history of diabetes, smoking, exercise, use of alcohol, and hormone replacement therapy. The authors concluded that elevated levels of CRP and IL-6 predict the development of type 2 DM, and the data support a possible role for inflammation in diabetogenesis.

Type 2 diabetes and bisphosphonates

Advanced glycation end products (AGE), senescent macroprotein derivatives form at an accelerated rate in diabetes and induce angiogenesis through overgeneration of autocrine vascular endothelial growth factor (VEGF). In one study, incadronate disodium, a nitrogen-containing bisphosphonate, was found to completely inhibit AGE-induced increase in DNA synthesis as well as tube formation of human microvascular endothelial cells (EC). Furthermore, incadronate disodium significantly prevented transcriptional activation of nuclear factor-κB and AP-1 and the subsequent upregulation of VEGF mRNA levels in AGE-exposed EC. FPP, but not GGPP, was found to completely reverse the anti-angiogenic effects of incadronate disodium on EC. These results suggest that incadronate disodium could block the AGE-signaling pathway in microvascular EC through inhibition of protein farnesylation [131, 132]. In another study, the bisphosphonate, pamidronate, given as a single dose led to a reduction in bone turnover, symptoms, and disease activity in diabetic patients with active Charcot neuroarthropathy [133].

Type 2 diabetes and statins

In West of Scotland Coronary Prevention Study (WOSCOPS) [134], development of type 2 DM was found to decrease by 30% in pravastatin-treated patients. One study investigated the effects of an HMG-CoA reductase inhibitor, atorvastatin, on insulin sensitization in performed in chow fed Zucker lean and fatty rats treated with atorvastatin 50 mg/kg/day (ATORVA_50) and results were compared to Zucker lean and fatty rats treated with drug vehicle only (CONT). Treatment with atorvastatin resulted in a dose-dependent improvement in whole body insulin sensitivity in both lean and fatty rats, with an approximately twofold increase in glucose infusion rate and glucose disposal (Rd) in ATORVA_50 versus CONT ($p < 0.01$) [135]. Another study investigated the effects of atorvastatin on the glucose metabolism and insulin resistance of KK/Ay mice, an animal model of type 2 diabetes, were investigated. Atorvastatin significantly decreased the non-HDL-cholesterol level in the oral glucose tolerance test, inhibited increase in the 30-minutes glucose level, decreased plasma insulin levels before and 30 and 60 minutes after glucose loading, and decreased the insulin resistance index, compared with corresponding values in controls, indicating that atorvastatin appeared to improve glucose metabolism by improving insulin resistance [136].

Type 2 diabetes, plant polyphenols, and fatty acids

Nutritional intervention studies performed in animals and humans suggest that the ingestion of soy protein associated with isoflavones and flaxseed rich in lignans improves glucose control and insulin resistance. In animal models of obesity and diabetes, soy protein has been shown to reduce serum insulin and insulin resistance. In studies of human subjects with or without diabetes, soy protein also appears to moderate hyperglycemia and reduce body weight, hyperlipidemia, and hyperinsulinemia, supporting its beneficial effects on obesity and diabetes [137]. Recent studies have provided evidence that soy consumption alleviates some of the symptoms associated with type 2 diabetes such as insulin resistance and glycemic control [138, 139]. Isoflavones may improve lipid and glucose metabolism by acting as an antidiabetic PPAR agonist [140] The β subunit of the signalsome—IKKβ, a crucial catalyst of NF-κB activation—is an obligate mediator of the disruption of insulin signaling induced by excessive exposure of tissues to free fatty acids and by hypertrophy of adipocytes. IKKβ plays a crucial role, not only in the induction of insulin resistance, but also atherogenesis, a host of inflammatory disorders, and the survival and spread of cancer. The polyphenols resveratrol and silibinin inhibit or suppress the activation of IKKβ [141]. Epidemiologic studies have reported a lower prevalence of impaired glucose tolerance and type 2 diabetes in populations consuming large amounts of the n-3 long-chain polyunsaturated fatty acids (n-3 LC-PUFAs) found mainly in fish. In one study, the hypoglycemic and hypolipidemic effect of docosahexaenoic acid (DHA; C22: 6omega-3) ethyl ester was examined in KK-Ay mice and neonatal streptozotocin-induced diabetic (NSZ) which are respectively obese and lean animal models of noninsulin-dependent diabetes mellitus (NIDDM), and in ddY normal mice. Single administration of DHA (500 mg/kg body weight) to KK-Ay mice significantly reduced ($p < 0.05$) the blood glucose levels (BG) ($p < 0.05$) and plasma free fatty acid levels (FFA) ($p < 0.05$) at 10 hours after oral administration when compared with control group. DHA (500 mg/kg body weight)-treated NSZ and normal mice, however, showed no change in these parameters. In addition, repeated administration of DHA (100 mg/kg) to KK-Ay mice significantly suppressed the increment of BG ($p < 0.05$) and plasma triglyceride levels (TG) ($p < 0.01$), and significantly decreased FFA ($p < 0.05$) at 30 days compared with control group. DHA also significantly decreased the blood glucose at 60 and 120 minutes on insulin tolerance test (ITT) [142].

Osteoporosis and IL-6

Osteoporosis is a condition that is common with aging and especially in postmenopausal women. The etiology has often been ascribed to abnormalities in calcium metabolism. However, many patients with osteopenia/osteoporosis have in common pain and inflammation and many inflammatory pain syndromes have osteopenia/osteoporosis as an accompanying feature [143]. Inflammatory joint disease, particularly rheumatoid arthritis [144], is associated with bone resorption and increased synovial fluid levels of IL-6 [145]. Another example is the osteoporosis that is often present in Complex Regional Pain Syndrome/Reflex sympathetic dystro-

phy (CRPS-I/RSD) [146]. IL-6-mediated inflammation has been shown to contribute to the process of bone remodeling. This is done by stimulating osteoclastogenesis and osteoclast activity [147]. Elevated levels of IL-6 have been observed in conditions of rapid skeletal turnover and hypercalcemia as in Paget's disease and multiple myeloma [148]. In multiple myeloma, radiologic examinations reveals osteolytic lesion and the most common finding is diffuse osteopenia [149]. Adhesion of multiple myeloma cells to stromal cells triggers IL-6 secretion by the stromal cells [150]. This results in increased osteoclastic activity that in turn results in osteoporosis, painful osteolytic lesions, and hypercalcemia characteristic of multiple myeloma [150]. In their youth, women are protected from osteoporosis because of the presence of sufficient levels of estrogen. Estrogen blocks the osteoblast's synthesis of IL-6. Estrogen may also antagonize the IL-6 receptors. Decline in estrogen production is often associated with osteopenia/osteoporosis in postmenopausal women. Estrogen's ability to repress IL-6 expression was first recognized in human endometrial stromal cells [151]. Additional clues came from the observations that menopause or ovariectomy resulted in increased IL-6 serum levels [152], increased IL-6 mRNA levels in bone cells [153], and increased IL-6 secretion by mononuclear cells [154–156]. Further evidence for estrogen's ability to repress IL-6 expression is derived from studies, which demonstrated that estradiol inhibits bone marrow stromal cell and osteoblastic cell IL-6 protein and mRNA production in vitro [157] and that estradiol was as effective as neutralizing antibody to IL-6 in suppressing osteoclast development in murine bone cell cultures [157] or in ovariectomized mice [158].

Osteoporosis and bisphosphonates

Bisphosphonates are inorganic chemical compounds that bind to hydroxyapatite in bone and prevent osteoclastic absorption of bone. Nitrogen-containing bisphosphonates (N-BPs) are potent inhibitors of bone resorption widely used in the treatment of osteoporosis and other bone degrading disorders including Paget's disease of bone, hypercalcemia associated with malignancy, metastatic bone diseases, such as breast cancer, multiple myeloma, and arthritis [143, 159]. At the tissue level, N-BPs reduce bone turnover and increase bone mass and mineralization. This is measured clinically as an increase in bone mineral density and bone strength and a decrease in fracture risk. N-BPs localize preferentially at sites of bone resorption, where mineral is exposed, are taken up by ostoclasts and inhibit osteoclastic activity. At the molecular level, N-BPs inhibit an enzyme in the cholesterol synthesis pathway, farnesyl diphosphate synthase. As a result, there is a reduction in the lipid geranylgeranyl diphosphate, which prenylates GTPases required for cytoskeletal organization and vesicular traffic in the osteoclast, leading to osteoclast inactivation [160, 161].

Osteoporosis and statins

3-Hydroxy-3-methylglutaryl coenzyme A reductase inhibitors (statins) have been shown to stimulate bone formation in laboratory studies, both in vitro and in vivo. Statin use in most, but not all, observational studies is associated with a reduced risk of fracture, particularly hip fracture, even after adjustment for the confounding effects of age, weight, and other medication use. This beneficial effect has not been observed in clinical trials designed to assess cardiovascular endpoints [162]. Men using statin drugs are more likely to have a greater BMD of the spine ($p < 0.005$), and men who receive statin drugs for more than 2 years are approximately half as likely to develop osteoporosis. A similar effect is observed in women taking statins for any length of time [163]. Statin use in women is associated with a 3% greater adjusted BMD at the femoral neck, and BMD tends to be greater at the spine and whole body [164]. Nitrogen-containing bisphosphonate drugs inhibit the mevalonate pathway, preventing the production of isoprenoids, which consequently results in the inhibition of osteoclast formation and osteoclast function. Statins decrease the hepatic biosynthesis of cholesterol by blocking the mevalonate pathway, and can affect bone metabolism in vivo through effects on osteoclastic bone resorption. The ability of statin compounds to inhibit bone resorption is directly related to HMG-CoA reductase activity [165].

Osteoporosis, plant polyphenols, and fatty acids

Dietary supplementation with soybean isoflavone can prevent postmenopausal bone loss. In one study, postmenopausal women ($n = 19$), mean age 70.6 ± 6.3 years and mean time since menopause 19.1 ± 5.5 years, were given isoflavone supplements for 6 months. There was a 37% decrease in urinary concentrations of type 1 collagen α1-chain helical peptide (HP), a marker of bone resorption, during the isoflavone supplementation compared with baseline ($p < 0.05$) and a significant difference in mean (SE) HP excretion levels when isoflavone was compared with placebo (43.4 ± 5.2 versus 56.3 ± 7.2 μg/mmol creatinine [cr], $p < 0.05$). With isoflavone supplementation, mean spine BMD at L2 and L3 was significantly greater when treatment was compared with control, with a difference between means of 0.03 ± 0.04 g and 0.03 ± 0.04 g ($p < 0.05$), respectively. There were nonsignificant increases from baseline for total spine BMC (3.5%), total spine BMD (1%), total hip BMC (3.6%), and total hip BMD (1.3%) with the isoflavone treatment [166]. Data from a randomized, double-blind, placebo-controlled, yearlong clinical trial has also suggested that supplementation with the dietary phytoestrogen genistein (54 mg/day) may be as effective as hormone replacement therapy in attenuating menopause-related bone loss [167].

Beneficial effects of omega-3 fatty acids on bone mineral density have been reported in rats and humans. In one study, sham and ovariectomized (OVX) mice were fed diets containing either 5% corn oil (CO), rich in omega-6 fatty acids or 5% fish oil (FO), rich in omega-3 fatty acids. Bone mineral density was analyzed by DXA. The serum lipid profile was analyzed by gas chromatography. Receptor activator of NF-κB ligand (RANKL) expression and cytokine production in activated T-cells were analyzed by flow cytometry and ELISA, respectively. Significantly increased bone mineral density loss (20% in distal left femur and 22.6% in lumbar vertebrae) was observed in OVX mice fed CO, whereas FO-fed mice showed only 10% and no change, respectively. Bone mineral density loss was correlated with increased RANKL expression in activated CD4+ T-cells from CO-fed OVX mice, but there was no change in FO-fed mice. Selected n-3 fatty acids (docosahexaenoic acid [DHA] and eicosapentaenoic acid [EPA]) added in vitro caused a significant decrease in TRACP activity and TRACP+ multinuclear cell formation from BM cells compared with selected n-6 fatty acids (linoleic acid [LA] and arachidonic acid [AA]). DHA and EPA also inhibited BM macrophage NF-κB activation induced by RANKL in vitro. TNF-α, interleukin (IL)-2, and interferon (IFN)-γ concentrations from both sham and OVX FO-fed mice were decreased in the culture medium of splenocytes, and IL-6 was decreased in sham-operated FO-fed mice [168].

Aging, age-related disorders, and IL-6

Evidence has linked IL-10 and IL-6 cytokine polymorphisms to longevity. Individuals who are genetically predisposed to produce high levels of IL-6 have a reduced capacity to reach the extreme limits of human life, whereas the high IL-10-producer genotype is increased among centenarians [169].

Telomere length is linked to age-associated diseases, with shorter telomeres in blood associated with an increased probability of mortality from infection or heart disease. In patients with multiple myeloma (MM), telomere length (TL) of MM cells is significantly shorter than that of the patients' own leukocytes. In one study, TL negatively correlated with age and with IL-6 and β2-microglobulin levels [170]. Overproduction of IL-6, a proinflammatory cytokine, is associated with a spectrum of age-related conditions including CVD, osteoporosis, arthritis, type 2 diabetes, certain cancers, periodontal disease, frailty, and functional decline. To describe the pattern of change in IL-6 over 6 years among older adults undergoing a chronic stressor, this longitudinal community study assessed the relationship between chronic stress and IL-6 production in 119 men and women who were caregiving for a spouse with dementia and 106 noncaregivers, with a mean age at study entry of 70.58 (SD = 8.03) for the full sample. On entry into this portion of the longitudinal study, 28 of the caregivers' spouses had already died, and an additional 50 of the 119 spouses died during the 6 years of this study. Levels of IL-6

and health behaviors associated with IL-6 were measured across 6 years. Caregivers' average rate of increase in IL-6 was about four times as large as that of noncaregivers. Moreover, the mean annual changes in IL-6 among former caregivers did not differ from that of current caregivers even several years after the death of the impaired spouse. There were no systematic group differences in chronic health problems, medications, or health-relevant behaviors that might have accounted for caregivers' steeper IL-6 slope. These data provide evidence of a key mechanism through which chronic stressors may accelerate risk of a host of age-related diseases by prematurely aging the immune response [171]. Aortic VSMCs isolated from spontaneously hypertensive rats (SHR) grow nearly twice as fast in vitro as cells isolated from several normotensive control strains of rats. DNA synthesis in SHR cells from both young and adult animals in response to epidermal growth factor is selectively enhanced compared with normotensive controls, suggesting that epidermal growth factor may be at least partly responsible for the enhanced growth rate. One study determined whether the enhanced DNA synthesis in response to epidermal growth factor in SHR cells is mediated via an enhanced epidermal growth factor receptor tyrosine kinase. The researchers measured thymidine incorporation in epidermal growth factor-stimulated VSMCs in the presence of the highly specific tyrosine kinase inhibitor genistein. The 50% inhibitory dose (IC50) of genistein was higher for the SHR VSMCs than for the normotensive Wistar rat (NBR; National Institutes of Health Black rat). The researchers suggest that the increased DNA synthesis in response to epidermal growth factor in SHR cells is a result of higher receptor tyrosine kinase activity initiating further intracellular signals [172]. IL-6 is also a causative factor in other manifestations of aging.

Wrinkles on the skin are a manifestation of aging. Excess sunlight, smoking, and exposure to wind, heat, and harsh chemicals cause the outer layers of the skin to thicken and cause skin to wrinkle, sag, and become leathery. Ultraviolet (UV) radiation from the sun is widely considered as a major cause of human skin photoaging and skin cancer. IL-6 is produced by keratinocytes in vivo and in vitro and the release is enhanced by UV light. A study was performed to investigate the effect of a single

UV dose eliciting moderate to severe sunburn reaction on the production of IL-6 in vivo. Plasma of UV-treated human subjects was evaluated for IL-6 activity by testing its capacity to induce the proliferation of an IL-6-dependent hybridoma cell line (B9). In contrast to plasma samples obtained before UV exposure, post-UV-specimens contained significant levels of IL-6 peaking at 12 hours after UV irradiation. Plasma IL-6 activity was neutralized by an antiserum directed against recombinant human IL-6 [173]. UV radiation-induced proinflammatory cytokines mediated by NF-κB reportedly play important roles in sunburn, skin damage, premature aging, and increase the risk of developing melanomas and other types of skin cancer. In one study, immunohistochemical and Western blot analysis and ELISA indicated that both nuclear p65 and secreted IL-6 were significantly ($p < 0.05$) induced by UVB (20, 30 mJ/cm^2) and UVA irradiation (10, 20 J/cm^2). NF-κB nuclear translocation and IL-6 secretion induced by UVB and UVA were dramatically inhibited by treatment of EGCG [174]. Higher levels of the systemic inflammatory markers CRP and IL-6 are independently associated with progression of age-related macular degeneration (AMD). One study tested the hypothesis that baseline CVD biomarkers are associated with subsequent increased risk for progression of AMD. This prospective cohort study involved 251 participants aged 60 years and older who had some sign of nonexudative AMD and visual acuity of 20/200 or better in at least one eye at baseline. The AMD status was assessed by standardized grading of fundus photographs, and stored fasting blood specimens obtained at baseline were analyzed for levels of the various biomarkers. The average follow-up time was 4.6 years. Comparing the highest quartile with the lowest quartile, CRP was associated with progression of AMD, with a multivariate adjusted relative risk (RR) of 2.10 (95% CI, 1.06–4.18; p for trend, 0.046) controlling for BMI, smoking, and other cardiovascular variables and a multivariate adjusted RR of 2.02 (95% CI, 1.00–4.04; p for trend, 0.06) controlling additionally for antioxidant nutrients. IL-6 was also related to progression of AMD, with a multivariate adjusted RR of 1.81 (95% CI, 0.97–3.36; p for trend, 0.03). Comparing the highest quartile with the lowest quartile, the effect estimates for VCAM-1 (multivariate adjusted

RR, 1.94) and apolipoprotein B (adjusted RR, 1.39) were in the positive direction but were not statistically significant (p for trend, 0.08 and 0.24, respectively). The CRP and IL-6 levels were both significantly related to higher BMI and current smoking [175].

Aging, age-related disorders, IL-6, and gene therapy/modulation

Genetic polymorphisms involving a change of a single base, from guanine to cytosine, at position—174 in the 5′ flanking region of the IL-6 gene is of great importance because the G allele is associated with higher IL-6 production than the C allele. In vivo studies have found basal IL-6 levels to be twice as high in volunteers with the GG allele than in those with the CC allele. The polymorphism in the 5′ flanking region (an area important in the regulation of gene expression) alters the transcriptional response to stimuli such as LPS and IL-1 [176]. An increased frequency of an Xba I Restriction Fragment Length Polymorphism (RFLP) likely to be due to 3′ flanking region insertions, has been described in some patients with SLE and elevated IL-6 levels [177]. By using PCR-RFLP and sensitive polyacrylamide gel electrophoresis, an association between genotype for the 3′ flanking region polymorphism and peak bone mineral density in women has been demonstrated [178]. Manipulating the genetic mechanisms controlling the IL-6 levels and increasing the frequency of GG alleles in the population would prevent aging and age-related diseases and be the key to eternal youth and immortality. Gene therapy will aim to provide for targeted gene transfer, controlled expression of the gene transferred, and enhanced activity of the transferred gene product. An alternate means of gene therapy is gene modulation. In gene modulation, expression of an already expressed gene is increased by introducing exogenous normal genetic sequences and decreased by introducing antisense genes or gene fragments, or by introducing vectors that can produce ribozymes that can cleave specific mRNAs. Gene modulation can also be achieved by the introduction of exogenous normal genetic sequences that code for proteins that modulate the extent of gene expression, or affect the processing, assembly, or secretion of gene products.

Conclusion

In conclusion, we have described the biochemical pathway from cholesterol to IL-6-mediated inflammation. IL-6-mediated inflammation is the gatekeeper and common causative factor for aging and age-related disorders including atherosclerosis, peripheral vascular disease, CAD, osteoporosis, type 2 diabetes, dementia and Alzheimer's disease, and some forms of arthritis and cancer. We have clarified the relationship between some of these common illnesses and we determine that pleiotropic effects of bisphosphonates, statins, and polyphenolic compounds are mediated by inhibition of IL-6-mediated inflammation.

Isoprenoids, which are intermediates, generated in the cholesterol biosynthesis pathway, play a role as significant as the end product cholesterol, in activation of IL-6-mediated inflammation. Isoprenoids are generated by endogenous cellular cholesterol synthesis in the body as well as by cholesterol synthesis in activated monocytes during the inflammatory response. However, isoprenoids are but one component of the signaling pathway for IL-6-mediated inflammation.

Inhibition of the signal transduction pathway for IL-6-mediated inflammation is key to the prevention and treatment of aging and age-related disorders including atherosclerosis, peripheral vascular disease, CAD, osteoporosis, type 2 diabetes, dementia, Alzheimer's disease, and some forms of arthritis and cancer. Inhibition of IL-6-mediated inflammation may be achieved indirectly through regulation of endogenous cholesterol synthesis and isoprenoid depletion or by direct inhibition of the IL-6 signal transduction pathway.

Statins, bisphosphonates, and polyphenolic compounds have similar mechanisms of action and act on similar diseases in the following ways:

1 Statins and bisphosphonates inhibit the mevalonate to cholesterol conversion pathway and cause isoprenoid depletion; with inhibition of IL-6 inflammation. Statins inhibit the enzyme HMG-CoA reductase and bisphosphonates inhibit the enzyme FPP synthase. Polyphenolic compounds inhibit multiple pathways of signal transduction for IL-6-mediated inflammation including inhibition of tyrosine kinase activity, inhibition of activa-tion of NF-κB, and inhibition of activation of IKK complex.

2 Statins, bisphosphonates, and polyphenolic compounds inhibit the JAK/STAT3 signaling pathway for IL-6-mediated inflammation.

3 Statins, bisphosphonates, and polyphenolic compounds have common pleiotropic effects and decrease the progression of atherosclerotic vascular disease and inhibit bone resorption.

4 Combination treatment with agents that inhibit different aspects of the signal transduction pathways for IL-6-mediated inflammation, including statins, bisphosphonates, and polyphenolic compounds, will be transformational and have better efficacy with fewer side-effects in the prevention and treatment of aging and age-related disorders including atherosclerosis, peripheral vascular disease, CAD, osteoporosis, type 2 diabetes, dementia, and some forms of arthritis and tumors. Evidence of safety and efficacy of combination treatment with inhibitors of IL-6-mediated inflammation should be sought from new clinical trials.

Statins and bisphosphonates are just indirect inhibitors of IL-6 inflammation, yet both class of drugs have enabled a significant decrease in mortality and morbidity from these common illnesses.

Epidemiological evidence suggests that increased consumption of plant-derived polyphenolic compounds is associated with decrease in mortality and morbidity from these common illnesses. Newer therapies will include delivering by gene therapy or gene modulation variations and/or modifications of the IL-6 gene associated with decreased or absent IL-6 production. Newer drugs will include IL-6 inhibitor/antibody, IL-6 receptor inhibitor/antibody, IL-6 antisense oligonucleotide (ASON), gp130 protein inhibitor/antibody, tyrosine kinases inhibitors/antibodies, serine/threonine kinases inhibitors/antibodies, mitogen-activated protein (MAP) kinase inhibitors/antibodies, phosphatidylinositol 3-kinase inhibitors/antibodies, nuclear factor κB (NF-κB) inhibitors/antibodies, IKK inhibitors/antibodies, AP-1 inhibitors/antibodies, STAT transcription factors inhibitors/antibodies, altered IL-6, partial peptides of IL-6 or IL-6R, or SOCS (suppressors of cytokine signaling) protein, PPARγ and/or PPARβ/δ activators/ligands or a functional fragment thereof.

The public health significance of such new drugs and gene therapy will be transformational.

References

1 Huang H, Patel DD, Manton KG. The immune system in aging: roles of cytokines, T cells and NK cells. Front Biosci January 1, 2005;10:192–215.

2 Hackam DG, Anand SS. Emerging risk factors for atherosclerotic vascular disease: a critical review of the evidence. JAMA August 20, 2003;290(7):932–40.

3 Ross R. Atherosclerosis an inflammatory disease. N Engl J Med 1999;340:115–26.

4 Libby P, Ridker PM, Maser A. Inflammation and atherosclerosis. Circulation 2002;105:1135–43.

5 Ross R. Cell biology of atherosclerosis. Annu Rev Physiol 1995;57:791–804.

6 Tabas I. Free cholesterol-induced cytotoxicity. A possible contributing factor to macrophage foam cell necrosis in advanced atherosclerotic lesions. Trends Cardiovasc Med 1997;7:256–63.

7 Kockx MM. Apoptosis in the atherosclerotic plaque: quantitative and qualitative aspects. Arterioscler Thromb Vasc Biol 1998;18:1519–22.

8 Mitchinson MJ, Hardwick SJ, Bennett MR. Cell death in atherosclerotic plaques. Curr Opin Lipidol 1996;7:324–9.

9 Davignon J, Mabile L. Mechanisms of action of statins and their pleiotropic effects. [Article in French] Ann Endocrinol (Paris) February 2001;62(1, pt 2):101–12.

10 McFarlane SI, Muniyappa R, Shin JJ, Bahtiyar G, Sowers JR. Osteoporosis and cardiovascular disease: brittle bones and boned arteries, is there a link? Endocrine February 2004;23(1):1–10.

11 Heinrich PC, Castell JV, Andus T. Interleukin-6 and the acute phase response. Biochem J 1990;265:621–36.

12 Biasucci LM, Vitelli A, Liuzzo G et al. Elevated levels of interleukin-6 in unstable angina. Circulation 1996;94:874–7.

13 Biasucci LM, Liuzzo G, Fantuzzi G et al. Increasing levels of interleukin (IL)-1Ra and IL-6 during the first 2 days of hospitalization in unstable angina are associated with increasing risk of in-hospital coronary events. Circulation 1999;99:2079–84.

14 Szekanecz Z, Shah MR, Pearce WH, Koch AE. Human atherosclerotic abdominal aortic aneurysms produce interleukin (IL)-6 and interferon-gamma but not IL-2 and IL-4: the possible role for IL-6 and interferon-gamma in vascular inflammation. Agents Actions 1994;42:159–62.

15 Ridker PM, Rifai N, Pfeifer M et al. Elevation of tumor necrosis factor-alpha and increased risk of recurrent coronary events after myocardial infarction. Circulation 2000;101:2149–53.

16 Ridker PM, Rifai N, Stampfer MJ, Hennekens CH. Plasma concentration of interleukin-6 and the risk of future myocardial infarction among apparently healthy men. Circulation 2000;101:1767–72.

17 Ma J, Hennekens CH, Ridker PM, Stampfer MJ. A prospective study of fibrinogen and risk of myocardial infarction in the physicians' health study. J Am Coll Cardiol 1999;33:1347–52.

18 Berk BC, Weintraub WS, Alexander RW. Elevation of C-reactive protein in "active" coronary artery disease. Am J Cardiol 1990;65:168–72.

19 Ford ES, Giles WH. Serum C-reactive protein and fibrinogen concentrations and self-reported angina pectoris and myocardial infarction: findings from national health and nutrition examination survey III. J Clin Epidemiol 2000;53:95–102.

20 Morrow DA, Ridker PM. C-reactive protein, inflammation, and coronary risk. Med Clin North Am 2000; 84:149–61.

21 Ridker PM, Rifai N, Pfeifer MA et al. Long-term effects of pravastatin on plasma concentration of C-reactive protein. The cholesterol and recurrent events (CARE) investigators. Circulation 1999;100:230–5.

22 Schaumberg DA, Ridker PM, Glynn RJ et al. High levels of plasma C-reactive protein and future risk of age-related cataract. Ann Epidemiol 1999;9:166–71.

23 Ridker PM, Cushman M, Stampfer MJ et al. Plasma concentration of C-reactive protein and risk of developing peripheral vascular disease. Circulation 1998;97:425–8.

24 Cesari M, Penninx BW, Newman AB et al. Inflammatory markers and onset of cardiovascular events: results from the health ABC study. Circulation November 11, 2003;108(19):2317–22.

25 King MW. *Cholesterol and Bile Metabolism*, Medical Biochemistry Course Guide, Indiana University School of Medicine, 2004.

26 Dubey VS. Mevalonate-independent pathway of isoprenoids synthesis: a potential target in some human pathogens. Curr Sci September 25, 2002;83(6):685–7.

27 Zhao L, Hart S, Cheng J et al. Mammary gland remodeling depends on gp130 signaling through Stat3 and MAPK. J Biol Chem October 15, 2004;279(42):44093–100.

28 Cesari M, Penninx BW, Newman AB et al. Inflammatory markers and cardiovascular disease (The Health, Aging and Body Composition [Health ABC] Study). Am J Cardiol September 1, 2003;92(5):522–8.

29 Yaffe K, Lindquist K, Penninx BW et al. Inflammatory markers and cognition in well-functioning African-American and white elders. Neurology July 8, 2003;61(1):76–80.

30 Kurihara N, Bertolini D, Suda T, Akiyama Y, Roodman GD. IL-6 stimulates osteoclast-like multinucleated cell

formation in long term human marrow cultures by inducing IL-1 release. J Immunol 1990;144:4226–30.

31 Tamura T, Udagawa N, Takahashi N *et al.* Soluble interleukin-6 receptor triggers osteoclast formation by interleukin-6. Proc Natl Acad Sci USA 1993;90:11924–8.

32 Manolagas SC, Jilka RL. Bone marrow, cytokines, and bone remodeling. Emerging insights into the pathophysiology of osteoporosis. N Engl J Med February 2, 1995;332(5):305–11.

33 Yoshii T, Magara S, Miyai D *et al.* Local levels of interleukin-1beta, −4, −6 and tumor necrosis factor alpha in an experimental model of murine osteomyelitis due to staphylococcus aureus. Cytokine July 21, 2002;19(2):59–65.

34 Meghji S, Crean SJ, Hill PA *et al.* Surface-associated protein from *Staphylococcus aureus* stimulates osteoclastogenesis: possible role in *S. aureus*-induced bone pathology. Br J Rheumatol October 1998;37(10):1095–101.

35 Hotokezaka H, Kitamura A, Matsumoto S, Hanazawa S, Amano S, Yamada T. Internalization of Mycobacterium bovis Bacillus Calmette-Guerin into osteoblast-like MC3T3-E1 cells and bone resorptive responses of the cells against the infection. Scand J Immunol May 1998;47(5):453–8.

36 Kiecolt-Glaser JK, Preacher KJ, MacCallum RC, Atkinson C, Malarkey WB, Glaser R. Chronic stress and age-related increases in the proinflammatory cytokine IL-6. Proc Natl Acad Sci U S A July 22, 2003;100(15):9090–5.

37 Lutgendorf SK, Garand L, Buckwalter KC, Reimer TT, Hong SY, Lubaroff DM. Life stress, mood disturbance, and elevated interleukin-6 in healthy older women. J Gerontol A Biol Sci Med Sci September 1999;54(9):M434–9.

38 Karin M. The regulation of AP-1 activity by mitogen-activated protein kinases. J Biol Chem 1995;270:16483–6.

39 Sen R, Baltimore D. Multiple nuclear factors interact with the immunoglobulin enhancer sequences. Cell 1986;46:706–16.

40 Fujita T, Nolan GP, Ghosh S, Baltimore D. Independent modes of transcriptional activation by the p50 and p65 subunits of NF-κβ. Genes Dev 1992;6:775–87.

41 Zhong H, SuYang H, Erdjument-Bromage H, Tempst P, Ghosh S. The transcriptional activity of NF-κβ is regulated by the I-κβ-associated PKAc subunit through a cyclic AMP-independent mechanism. Cell 1997;89:413–24.

42 Verma I, Stevenson JK, Schwarz EM, Van Antwerp D, Miyamoto S. Rel/NFκβ/Iκβ family: intimate tales of association and dissociation. Genes Dev 1995;9:2723–35.

43 Chen Z, Parent L, Maniatis T. Site-specific phosphorylation of Iκβα by a novel ubiquitination-dependent pathway. Cell 1996;84:853–62.

44 Baeuerle PA, Henkel T. Function and activation of NF-κB 1995 Rel/NF T 1996 Site-specific phosphorylation of in vitro cell mediated immune assay predicts in vivo response. J Rheumatol 1994;18:1130–3.

45 Rothwarf DM, Zandi E, Natoli G, Karin M. IKK-gamma is an essential regulatory subunit of the IkappaB kinase complex. Nature September 17, 1998;395(6699):297–300.

46 Alkalay I, Yaron A, Hatzubai A, Orian A, Ciechanover A, Ben-Neriah Y. Stimulation-dependent Iκβα phosphorylation marks the NFκβ inhibitor for degradation via the ubiquitin-proteasome pathway. Proc Natl Acad Sci U S A 1995;92:10599–603.

47 Palombella VJ, Rando OJ, Goldberg AL, Maniatis T. The ubiquitin-proteasome pathway is required for processing the NF-κβ 1 precursor protein and the activation of NF-κβ. Cell 1994;78:773–85.

48 Baldwin AS. The NFκβB and IκβB proteins: new discoveries and insights. Annu Rev Immunol 1996;14:649–81.

49 Adcock IM, Lane SJ, Brown CR, Lee TH, Barnes PJ. Abnormal glucocorticoid receptor-activator protein 1 interaction in steroid-resistant asthma. J Exp Med 1995;182:1951–8.

50 McKay LI, Cidlowski JA. Cross-talk between nuclear factor-B and the steroid hormone receptors: mechanisms of mutual antagonism. Mol Endocrinol 1998;12(1):45–56.

51 Zhong H, SuYang H, Erdjument-Bromage H, Tempst P, Ghosh S. The transcriptional activity of NF-κβ is regulated by the I-κβ-associated PKAc subunit through a cyclic AMP-independent mechanism. Cell 1997;89:413–24.

52 Karin M, Ben-Neriah Y. Phosphorylation meets ubiquitination: the control of NF-κB activity. Annu Rev Immunol 2000;18:621–63.

53 Vanden Berghe W, Vermeulen L, Delerive P, De Bosscher K, Staels B, Haegeman G. A paradigm for gene regulation: inflammation, NF-κB and PPAR. Adv Exp Med Biol 2003;544:181–96.

54 Han Y, Runge MS, Brasier AR. Angiotensin II induces interleukin-6 transcription in vascular smooth muscle cells through pleiotropic activation of nuclear factor-kappa B transcription factors. Circ Res April 2, 1999;84(6):695–703.

55 Cabrero A, Laguna JC, Vazquez M. Peroxisome proliferator-activated receptors and the control of inflammation. Curr Drug Targets Inflamm Allergy September 2002;1(3):243–8.

56 Neve BP, Fruchart JC, Staels B. Role of the peroxisome proliferator-activated receptors (PPAR) in atherosclerosis. Biochem Pharmacol October 15, 2000;60(8):1245–50.

57 Leung KC. Regulation of cytokine receptor signaling by nuclear hormone receptors: a new paradigm for receptor interaction. DNA Cell Biol August 2004;23(8):463–74.

58 Das UN. Statins and the prevention of dementia. CMAJ October 2, 2001;165(7):908–9.

59 Takai Y, Sasaki T, Matozaki T. Small GTP-binding proteins. Physiol Rev January 2001;81(1):153–208.

60 Wennerberg K, Rossman KL, Der CJ. The Ras superfamily at a glance. J Cell Sci March 1, 2005;118(pt 5): 843–6.

61 Magee T, Marshall C. New insights into the interaction of Ras with the plasma membrane. Cell 1999;98:9–12.

62 Dechend R, Müller D, Park JK, Fiebeler A, Haller H, Luft FC. Statins and angiotensin II-induced vascular injury. Nephrol Dial Transplant 2002;17:349–53.

63 Beaupre DM, Kurzrock R. RAS and leukemia: from basic mechanisms to gene-directed therapy. J Clin Oncol March 1999;17(3):1071–9.

64 Sano M, Fukuda K, Kodama H *et al.* Autocrine/Paracrine secretion of IL-6 family cytokines causes angiotensin II-induced delayed STAT3 activation. Biochem Biophys Res Commun March 24, 2000;269(3):798–802.

65 Faruqi TR, Gomez D, Bustelo XR, Bar-Sagi D, Reich NC. Rac1 mediates STAT3 activation by autocrine IL-6. Proc Natl Acad Sci U S A July 31, 2001;98(16):9014–9.

66 Aznar S, Valeron PF, del Rincon SV, Perez LF, Perona R, Lacal JC. Simultaneous tyrosine and serine phosphorylation of STAT3 transcription factor is involved in Rho A GTPase oncogenic transformation. Mol Biol Cell October 2001;12(10):3282–94.

67 Lubbert M, Oster W, Knopf HP, McCormick F, Mertelsmann R, Herrmann F. N-RAS gene activation in acute myeloid leukemia: association with expression of interleukin-6. Leukemia December 1993;7(12):1948–54.

68 Pelletier S, Duhamel F, Coulombe P, Popoff MR, Meloche S. Rho family GTPases are required for activation of Jak/STAT signaling by G protein-coupled receptors. Mol Cell Biol February 2003;23(4):1316–33.

69 Khwaja A, O'Connolly J, Hendry BM. Prenylation inhibitors in renal disease. Lancet 2000;355:741–4.

70 Ikeda U, Shimpo M, Ohki RK *et al.* Fluvastatin inhibits matrix metalloproteinase-1 expression in human vascular endothelial cells. Hypertension 2000;36:325–9.

71 Bergstrom JD, Bostedor RG, Masarachia PJ, Reszka AA, Rodan G. Alendronate is a specific, nanomolar inhibitor of farnesyl diphosphate synthase. Arch Biochem Biophys January 1, 2000;373(1):231–41.

72 Rogers MJ. New insights into the molecular mechanisms of action of bisphosphonates. Curr Pharm Des 2003;9(32):2643–58.

73 Manzoni M, Rollini M. Biosynthesis and biotechnological production of statins by filamentous fungi and ap-

plication of these cholesterol-lowering drugs. Appl Microbiol Biotechnol April 2002;58(5):555–64.

74 Manach C, Scalbert A, Morand C, Remesy C, Jimenez L. Polyphenols: food sources and bioavailability. Am J Clin Nutr May 2004;79(5):727–47.

75 Funakoshi Y, Ichiki T, Ito K, Takeshita A. Induction of interleukin-6 expression by angiotensin II in rat vascular smooth muscle cells. Hypertension July 1999;34(1):118–25.

76 Keidar S, Heinrich R, Kaplan M, Hayek T, Aviram M. Angiotensin II administration to atherosclerotic mice increases macrophage uptake of oxidized LDL: a possible role for interleukin-6. Arterioscler Thromb Vasc Biol September 2001;21(9):1464–9.

77 Klouche M, Rose-John S, Schmiedt W, Bhakdi S. Enzymatically degraded, nonoxidized LDL induces human vascular smooth muscle cell activation, foam cell transformation, and proliferation. Circulation April 18, 2000;101(15):1799–805.

78 Klouche M, Bhakdi S, Hemmes M, Rose-John S. Novel path to activation of vascular smooth muscle cells: upregulation of gp130 creates an autocrine activation loop by IL-6 and its soluble receptor. J Immunol October 15, 1999;163(8):4583–9.

79 Nabata T, Morimoto S, Koh E, Shiraishi T, Ogihara T. Interleukin-6 stimulates c-myc expression and proliferation of cultured vascular smooth muscle cells. Biochem Int 1990;20(3):445–53.

80 Seino Y, Ikeda U, Ikeda M *et al.* Interleukin 6 gene transcripts are expressed in human atherosclerotic lesions. Cytokine January 1994;6(1):87–91.

81 Tokunou T, Ichiki T, Takeda K *et al.* Thrombin induces interleukin-6 expression through the cAMP response element in vascular smooth muscle cells. Arterioscler Thromb Vasc Biol November 2001;21(11): 1759–63.

82 Williams N, Bertoncello I, Jackson H, Arnold J, Kavnoudias H. The role of interleukin 6 in megakaryocyte formation, megakaryocyte development and platelet production. Ciba Found Symp 1992;167:160–70;discussion 170–3.

83 Oleksowicz L, Mrowiec Z, Zuckerman D, Isaacs R, Dutcher J, Puszkin E. Platelet activation induced by interleukin-6: evidence for a mechanism involving arachidonic acid metabolism. Thromb Haemost 1994; 72:302–8.

84 Burstein SA. Effects of interleukin 6 on megakaryocytes and on canine platelet function. Stem Cells 1994;12:386–93.

85 Watanabe S, Mu W, Kahn A *et al.* Role of JAK/STAT pathway in IL-6-induced activation of vascular smooth muscle cells. Am J Nephrol July–August 2004;24(4):387–92.

86 Okopien B, Hyper M, Kowalski J *et al.* A new immunological marker of atherosclerotic injury of arterial wall. Res Commun Mol Pathol Pharmacol March–April 2001;109(3–4):241–8.

87 Nawawi H, Osman NS, Annuar R, Khalid BA, Yusoff K. Soluble intercellular adhesion molecule-1 and interleukin-6 levels reflect endothelial dysfunction in patients with primary hypercholesterolaemia treated with atorvastatin. Atherosclerosis August 2003;169(2):283–91.

88 Martin TJ, Grill V. Experimental and clinical pharmacology: bisphosphonates-mechanisms of action. Aust Prescriber 2000;23(6):130–2.

89 Wuster C, Heilmann P. Bisphosphonate therapy in osteoporosis. Inhibition of trabecular perforation by aminobisphosphonate. Fortschr Med October 20, 1997;115(29):37–42.

90 Rendina D, Postiglione L, Vuotto P *et al.* Clodronate treatment reduces serum levels of interleukin-6 soluble receptor in Paget's disease of bone. Clin Exp Rheumatol May–June 2002;20(3):359–64.

91 Olmos JM, De Vega T, Perera L, Riancho JA, Amado JA, Gonzalez-Macias J. Etidronate inhibits the production of IL-6 by osteoblast-like cells. Methods Find Exp Clin Pharmacol October 1999;21(8):519–22.

92 Giuliani N, Pedrazzoni M, Passeri G, Girasole G. Bisphosphonates inhibit IL-6 production by human osteoblast-like cells. Scand J Rheumatol 1998;27(1):38–41.

93 Vitte C, Fleisch H, Guenther HL. Bisphosphonates induce osteoblasts to secrete an inhibitor of osteoclast-mediated resorption. Endocrinology June 1996;137(6):2324–33.

94 Plotkin LI, Weinstein RS, Parfitt AM, Roberson PK, Manolagas SC, Bellido T. Prevention of osteocyte and osteoblast apoptosis by bisphosphonates and calcitonin. J Clin Invest November 1999;104(10):1363–74.

95 Abildgaard N, Rungby J, Glerup H *et al.* Long-term oral pamidronate treatment inhibits osteoclastic bone resorption and bone turnover without affecting osteoblastic function in multiple myeloma. Eur J Haematol August 1998;61(2):128–34.

96 Chen X, Garner SC, Quarles LD, Anderson JJ. Effects of genistein on expression of bone markers during MC3T3-E1 osteoblastic cell differentiation. J Nutr Biochem June 2003;14(6):342–9.

97 Kim BH, Chung EY, Ryu JC, Jung SH, Min KR, Kim Y. Anti-inflammatory mode of isoflavone glycoside sophoricoside by inhibition of interleukin-6 and cyclooxygenase-2 in inflammatory response. Arch Pharm Res April 2003;26(4):306–11.

98 Suh KS, Koh G, Park CY *et al.* Soybean isoflavones inhibit tumor necrosis factor-alpha-induced apoptosis and the production of interleukin-6 and prostaglandin E2 in osteoblastic cells. Phytochemistry May 2003;63(2):209–15.

99 Borsellino N, Bonavida B, Ciliberto G, Toniatti C, Travali S, D'Alessandro N. Blocking signaling through the Gp130 receptor chain by interleukin-6 and oncostatin M inhibits PC-3 cell growth and sensitizes the tumor cells to etoposide and cisplatin-mediated cytotoxicity. Cancer January 1, 1999;85(1):134–44.

100 Jones TH, Justice SK, Price A. Suppression of tyrosine kinase activity inhibits [3H]thymidine uptake in cultured human pituitary tumor cells. J Clin Endocrinol Metab July 1997;82(7):2143–7.

101 Geng Y, Zhang B, Lotz M. Protein tyrosine kinase activation is required for lipopolysaccharide induction of cytokines in human blood monocytes. J Immunol December 15, 1993;151(12):6692–700.

102 Lin JK, Liang YC, Lin-Shiau SY. Cancer chemoprevention by tea polyphenols through mitotic signal transduction blockade. Biochem Pharmacol 1999;58:911–5.

103 Pan MH, Lin-Shiau SY, Ho CT, Lin JH, Lin JK. Suppression of lipopolysaccharide-induced nuclear factor-kappaB activity by theaflavin-3,3-digallate from black tea and other polyphenols through down-regulation of IkappaB kinase activity in macrophages. Biochem Pharmacol 2000;59:357–67.

104 Wang ZY, Huang MT, Lou YR *et al.* Inhibitory effects of black tea, green tea, decaffeinated black tea, and decaffeinated green tea on ultraviolet B light-induced skin carcinogenesis in 7,12-dimethylbenz[a]anthracene-initiated SKH-1 mice. Cancer Res 1994;54:3428–35.

105 Yang F, Oz HS, Barve S, de Villiers WJ, McClain CJ, Varilek GW. The green tea polyphenol (–)-epigallocatechin-3-gallate blocks nuclear factor-kappa B activation by inhibiting I kappa B kinase activity in the intestinal epithelial cell line IEC-6. Mol Pharmacol September 2001;60(3):528–33.

106 Aneja R, Hake P, Denenberg AG, Wong H, Zingarelli B. Epigallocatechin, a green tea polyphenol, attenuates myocardial ischemia reperfusion injury in rats. Mol Med January–June 2004;10:1–6.

107 Dona M, Dell'Aica I, Calabrese F *et al.* Neutrophil restraint by green tea: inhibition of inflammation, associated angiogenesis, and pulmonary fibrosis. J Immunol 2003;170:4335–41.

108 Levites Y, Amit T, Youdim MB, Mandel S. Involvement of protein kinase C activation and cell survival/cell cycle genes in green tea polyphenol (–)-epigallocatechin 3-gallate neuroprotective action. J Biol Chem 2002;277:30574–80.

109 Levites Y, Youdim MB, Maor G, Mandel S. Attenuation of 6-hydroxydopamine (6-OHDA)-induced nuclear factor-kappaB (NF-κB) activation and cell death

by tea extracts in neuronal cultures. Biochem Pharmacol 2002;63:21–9.

110 Ahmad N, Feyes DK, Nieminen AL, Agarwal R, Mukhtar H. Green tea constituent epigallocatechin-3-gallate and induction of apoptosis and cell cycle arrest in human carcinoma cells. J Natl Cancer Inst 1997;89:1881–6.

111 Tedeschi E, Suzuki H, Menegazzi M. Antiinflammatory action of EGCG, the main component of green tea, through STAT-1 inhibition. Ann N Y Acad Sci November 2002;973:435–7.

112 Watson JL, Ansari S, Cameron H, Wang A, Akhtar M, McKay DM. Green tea polyphenol (–)-epigallocatechin gallate blocks epithelial barrier dysfunction provoked by IFN-gamma but not by IL-4. Am J Physiol Gastrointest Liver Physiol November 2004;287(5):G954–61.

113 Abbate R, Gori AM, Martini F *et al.* n-3 PUFA supplementation, monocyte PCA expression and interleukin-6 production. Prostaglandins Leukot Essent Fatty Acids June 1996;54(6):439–44.

114 Taylor AJ, Kent SM, Flaherty PJ, Coyle LC, Markwood TT, Vernalis MN. ARBITER: arterial biology for the investigation of the treatment effects of reducing cholesterol: a randomized trial comparing the effects of atorvastatin and pravastatin on carotid intima medial thickness. Circulation October 15, 2002;106(16):2055–60.

115 Kastelein JJ, de Groot E, Sankatsing R. Atherosclerosis measured by B-mode ultrasonography: effect of statin therapy on disease progression. Am J Med March 22, 2004;116(suppl 6A):31S–6S.

116 Koshiyama H, Nakamura Y, Tanaka S, Minamikawa J. Decrease in carotid intima-media thickness after 1-year therapy with etidronate for osteopenia associated with type 2 diabetes. J Clin Endocrinol Metab 2000; 85(8):2793–6.

117 Daoud AS, Frank AS, Jarmolych J, Fritz KE. The effect of ethane-1-hydroxy-1,1-diphosphonate (EHDP) on necrosis of atherosclerotic lesions. Atherosclerosis September 1987;67(1):41–8.

118 Maziere C, Conte MA, Maziere JC. Activation of JAK2 by the oxidative stress generated with oxidized low-density lipoprotein. Free Radic Biol Med December 1, 2001;31(11):1334–40.

119 Lee CS, Kwon SJ, Na SY, Lim SP, Lee JH. J Korean Med Sci October 2004;19(5):656–61.

120 Funakoshi Y, Ichiki T, Ito K, Takeshita A. Induction of interleukin-6 expression by angiotensin II in rat vascular smooth muscle cells. Hypertension July 1999;34(1):118–25.

121 Ruetten H, Thiemermann C. Endothelin-1 stimulates the biosynthesis of tumour necrosis factor in macrophages: ET-receptors, signal transduction and inhibition by dexamethasone. J Physiol Pharmacol December 1997;48(4):675–88.

122 Browatzki M, Schmidt J, Kubler W, Kranzhofer R. Endothelin-1 induces interleukin-6 release via activation of the transcription factor NF-kappaB in human vascular smooth muscle cells. Basic Res Cardiol April 2000;95(2):98–105.

123 Kurosawa T, Itoh F, Nozaki A *et al.* Suppressive effect of cocoa powder on atherosclerosis in Kurosawa and Kusanagi-hypercholesterolemic rabbits. J Atheroscler Thromb 2005;12(1):20–8.

124 Ouyang P, Peng WL, Lai WY, Xu AL. Green tea polyphenols inhibit low-density lipoprotein-induced proliferation of rat vascular smooth muscle cells. [Article in Chinese]. Di Yi Jun Yi Da Xue Xue Bao September 2004;24(9):975–9.

125 Vinson JA, Teufel K, Wu N. Red wine, dealcoholized red wine, and especially grape juice, inhibit atherosclerosis in a hamster model. Atherosclerosis May 2001;156(1):67–72.

126 De Caterina R, Zampolli A. n-3 Fatty acids: antiatherosclerotic effects. Lipids 2001;36(suppl):S69–78.

127 Brousseau ME, Schaefer EJ. Diet and coronary heart disease: clinical trials. Curr Atheroscler Rep November 2000;2(6):487–93.

128 Vermel' AE. Clinical application of omega-3-fatty acids (cod-liver oil). Klin Med (Mosk) 2005;83(10): 51–7.

129 Hino A, Adachi H, Toyomasu K *et al.* Very long chain N-3 fatty acids intake and carotid atherosclerosis: an epidemiological study evaluated by ultrasonography. Atherosclerosis September 2004;176(1):145–9.

130 Stephens JW, Hurel SJ, Cooper JA, Acharya J, Miller GJ, Humphries SE. A common functional variant in the interleukin-6 gene is associated with increased body mass index in subjects with type 2 diabetes mellitus. Mol Genet Metab June 2004;82(2):180–6.

131 Okamoto T, Yamagishi S, Inagaki Y *et al.* Incadronate disodium inhibits advanced glycation end products-induced angiogenesis in vitro. Biochem Biophys Res Commun September 20, 2002;297(2):419–24.

132 Yamagishi S, Abe R, Inagaki Y *et al.* Minodronate, a newly developed nitrogen-containing bisphosphonate, suppresses melanoma growth and improves survival in nude mice by blocking vascular endothelial growth factor signaling. Am J Pathol December 2004;165(6):1865–74.

133 Jude EB, Selby PL, Burgess J *et al.* Bisphosphonates in the treatment of Charcot neuroarthropathy: a double-blind randomised controlled trial. Diabetologia November 2001;44(11):2032–7.

134 The West of Scotland Coronary Prevention Study Group. A coronary primary prevention study of Scottish men aged 45–64 years: trial design. J Clin Epidemiol August 1992;45(8):849–60.

135 Wong V, Stavar L, Szeto L *et al.* Atorvastatin induces insulin sensitization in Zucker lean and fatty rats. Atherosclerosis July 2, 2005;184(2):348–55.

136 Suzuki M, Kakuta H, Takahashi A *et al.* Effects of atorvastatin on glucose metabolism and insulin resistance in KK/Ay mice. J Atheroscler Thromb 2005;12(2): 77–84.

137 Bhathena SJ, Velasquez MT. Beneficial role of dietary phytoestrogens in obesity and diabetes. Am J Clin Nutr December 2002;76(6):1191–201.

138 Jayagopal V, Albertazzi P, Kilpatrick ES. Beneficial effects of soy phytoestrogen intake in postmenopausal women with type 2 diabetes. Diabetes Care 2002;25:1709–14.

139 Bhathena SJ, Velasquez MT. Beneficial role of dietary phytoestrogens in obesity and diabetes. Am J Clin Nutr 2002;76:1191–201.

140 Mezei O, Banz WJ, Steger RW, Peluso MR, Winters TA, Shay N. Soy Isoflavones exert antidiabetic and hypolipidemic effects through the PPAR pathways in obese Zucker rats and murine RAW 264.7 Cells. J Nutr May 2003;133:1238–43.

141 McCarty MF. Potential utility of natural polyphenols for reversing fat-induced insulin resistance. Med Hypotheses 2005;64(3):628–35.

142 Shimura T, Miura T, Usami M *et al.* Docosahexanoic acid (DHA) improved glucose and lipid metabolism in KK-Ay mice with genetic non-insulin-dependent diabetes mellitus (NIDDM). Biol Pharm Bull May 1997;20(5):507–10.

143 Omoigui S. *The Biochemical Origin of Pain: How a New Law and New Drugs Have Led to a Medical Breakthrough in the Treatment of Persistent Pain.* State-of-the-Art Technologies Publishers, Hawthorne, CA, 2004.

144 Kotake S, Sato K, Kim KJ *et al.* Interleukin-6 and soluble interleukin-6 receptors in the synovial fluids form rheumatoid arthritis patients are responsible for osteoclast-like cell formation. J Bone Miner Res 1996;11:88–95.

145 Houssiau F, Devoglaer JP, Van Damme J, Nagant de Deuxchaisnes C, Van Snick J. Interleukin 6 in synovial fluid and serum of patients with rheumatoid arthritis and other inflammatory arthritides. Arthritis Rheum 1988;31:784–8.

146 Veldman PH, Reynen HM, Arntz IE, Goris RJ. Signs and symptoms of reflex sympathetic dystrophy: prospective study of 829 patients. Lancet October 23, 1993;342(8878):1012–6.

147 Manolagas SC, Jilka RL. Bone marrow, cytokines, and bone remodeling. Emerging insights into the pathophysiology of osteoporosis. N Engl J Med February 2, 1995;332(5):305–11.

148 Roodman GD. Osteoclast function in Paget's disease and multiple myeloma. Bone 1995;17:57S–61S.

149 Ravaud P, Thepot C, Auleley GR, Amor B. Imaging of multiple myeloma. Ann Med Interne (Paris) 1996;147:370–5.

150 Teoh G, Anderson KC. Interaction of tumor and host cells with adhesion and extracellular matrix molecules in the development of multiple myeloma. Hematol Oncol Clin North Am 1997;11:27–42.

151 Tabibzadeh SS, Santhanam U, Sehgal PB, May LT. Cytokine-induced production of IFN-ß2/IL-6 by freshly explanted human endometrial stromal cells. Modulation by estradiol-17β. J Immunol 1989;142: 3134–9.

152 Kania DM, Binkley N, Checovich M, Havighurst T, Schilling M, Ershler WB. Elevated plasma levels of interleukin-6 in postmenopausal women do not correlate with bone density. J Am Geriatr Soc 1995;43:236–9.

153 Ralston SH. Analysis of gene expression in human bone biopsies by polymerase chain reaction: evidence for enhanced *Cytokine* expression in post-menopausal osteoporosis. J Bone Miner Res 1994;9:883–90.

154 Daynes RA, Araneo BA, Ershler WB, Maloney C, Li GZ, Ryu SY. Altered regulation of IL-6 production with normal aging. Possible linkage to the age-associated decline in dehydroepiandrosterone and its sulfated derivative. J Immunol 1993;150:5219–30.

155 Pacifici R, Brown C, Puscheck E *et al.* Effect of surgical menopause and estrogen replacement on *Cytokine* release from human blood mononuclear cells. Proc Natl Acad Sci U S A 1991;88:5134–8.

156 Pioli G, Basini G, Pedtazzoni M *et al.* Spontaneous release of interleukin-1 and interleukin-6 by peripheral blood mononuclear cells after oophorectomy. Clin Sci 1992;83:503–7.

157 Girasole G, Jilka RL, Passeri F *et al.* 17β-Estradiol inhibits interleukin-6 production by bone marrow-derived stromal cells and osteoblasts in vitro: a potential mechanism for the antiosteoporotic effect of estrogens. J Clin Invest 1992;89:883–91.

158 Jilka RL, Hangoc C, Girasole G *et al.* Increased osteoclast development after estrogen loss: mediation by interleukin-6. Science 1992;257:88–91.

159 Nakatsuka K. Development of bisphosphonates. Nippon Rinsho February 2003;61(2):219–25.

160 Rodan GA, Reszka AA. Bisphosphonate mechanism of action. Curr Mol Med September 2002;2(6):571–7.

161 Reszka AA, Rodan GA. Bisphosphonate mechanism of action. Curr Rheumatol Rep February 2003;5(1):65–74.

162 Bauer DC. HMG CoA reductase inhibitors and the skeleton: a comprehensive review. Osteoporos Int June 2003;14(4):273–82.

163 Funkhouser HL, Adera T, Adler RA. Effect of HMG-CoA reductase inhibitors (statins) on bone mineral density. J Clin Densitom 2002 Summer;5(2):151–8.

164 Pasco JA, Kotowicz MA, Henry MJ, Sanders KM, Nicholson GC. Geelong osteoporosis study. Statin use, bone mineral density, and fracture risk: Geelong osteoporosis study. Arch Intern Med March 11, 2002;162(5):537–40.

165 Staal A, Frith JC, French MH *et al.* The ability of statins to inhibit bone resorption is directly related to their inhibitory effect on HMG-CoA reductase activity. J Bone Miner Res January 2003;18(1):88–96.

166 Harkness LS, Fiedler K, Sehgal AR, Oravec D, Lerner E. Decreased bone resorption with soy isoflavone supplementation in postmenopausal women. J Womens Health (Larchmt) November 2004;13(9):1000–7.

167 Cotter A, Cashman KD. Genistein appears to prevent early postmenopausal bone loss as effectively as hormone replacement therapy. Nutr Rev October 2003;61(10):346–51.

168 Sun D, Krishnan A, Zaman K, Lawrence R, Bhattacharya A, Fernandes G. Dietary n-3 fatty acids decrease osteoclastogenesis and loss of bone mass in ovariectomized mice. J Bone Miner Res July 2003;18(7):1206–16.

169 Caruso C, Lio D, Cavallone L, Franceschi C. Aging, longevity, inflammation, and cancer. Ann N Y Acad Sci December 2004;1028:1–13.

170 Wu KD, Orme LM, Shaughnessy J, Jr, Jacobson J, Barlogie B, Moore MA. Telomerase and telomere length in multiple myeloma: correlations with disease heterogeneity, cytogenetic status, and overall survival. Blood June 15, 2003;101(12):4982–9.

171 Kiecolt-Glaser JK, Preacher KJ, MacCallum RC, Atkinson C, Malarkey WB, Glaser R. Chronic stress and age-related increases in the proinflammatory cytokine IL-6. Proc Natl Acad Sci U S A July 22, 2003;100(15):9090–5.

172 Clegg KB, Sambhi MP. Inhibition of epidermal growth factor-mediated DNA synthesis by a specific tyrosine kinase inhibitor in vascular smooth muscle cells of the spontaneously hypertensive rat. J Hypertens Suppl December 1989;7(6):S144–5.

173 Urbanski A, Schwarz T, Neuner P *et al.* Ultraviolet light induces increased circulating interleukin-6 in humans. J Invest Dermatol June 1990;94(6):808–11.

174 Xia J, Song X, Bi Z, Chu W, Wan Y. UV-induced NF-kappaB activation and expression of IL-6 is attenuated by (−)-epigallocatechin-3-gallate in cultured human keratinocytes in vitro. Int J Mol Med November 2005;16(5):943–50.

175 Seddon JM, George S, Rosner B, Rifai N. Progression of age-related macular degeneration: prospective assessment of C-reactive protein, interleukin 6, and other cardiovascular biomarkers. Arch Ophthalmol June 2005;123(6):774–82.

176 Fishman D, Faulds G, Jeffery R *et al.* The effect of novel polymorphisms in the interleukin-6 (IL-6) gene on IL-6 transcription and plasma IL-6 levels, and an association with systemic-onset juvenile chronic arthritis. J Clin Invest 1998;102:1369–76.

177 Linker-Israeli M, Wallace DJ, Prehn JL, Nand R, Li L, Klinenberg JR. A greater variability in the 3′ flanking region of the IL-6 gene in patients with systemic lupus erythematosus (SLE). Autoimmunity 1996;23:199–209.

178 Murray R, McGuigan F, Grant S, Reid D, Ralston S. Polymorphisms of the interleukin-6 gene are associated with bone mineral density. Bone 1997;21:89–92.

CHAPTER 24

Autoimmune myocarditis: treatment with anti-T-cell antibodies

Zofia T. Bilińska & Witold Rużyłło

Introduction

Autoimmunity is an immune response to self-tissues [1]. Autoimmune myocarditis may be induced by any cardiac injury that releases myocellular proteins. Autoimmune myocarditis may be postinfectious or noninfectious. Patients who survive acute phase of infection, most frequently viral myocarditis, can develop dilated cardiomyopathy possibly due to chronic, autoimmune-mediated injury. Noninfectious form of myocarditis is often associated with systemic diseases or idiopathic diseases. In autoimmune myocarditis, myocardial lesions usually consist of lymphocytic myocarditis. Immunohistochemical studies provide evidence that lymphocytes positive for T-cell antigens are predominant in the inflammatory infiltrate [2–4]. A rare and frequently fatal form of autoimmune myocarditis is giant cell myocarditis [5, 6]. In giant cell myocarditis, giant cells that are usually positive for macrophage antigens have to be identified. In both types of myocarditis, fulminant course of the disease can occur with circulatory collapse, severe arrhythmia, or both. Histopathological equivalent of fulminant course of the disease is massive inflammatory infiltrate along with severe myocardial necrosis. Anti-T-cell antibodies are an attractive option for treatment of fulminant myocarditis, since they could rapidly induce potent lymphopenia and immunosuppression, thus halting the progression of T-cell-mediated myocardial injury [7]. In humans, murine, antihuman mature T-cell monoclonal antibody (OKT3) [5–14], and rabbit polyclonal antithymocyte globulin (rATG) [15] have been used in this setting. This chapter will review available evidence on mechanism of action and the use of anti-T-cell antibodies in the treatment of experimental and human myocarditis.

Anti-T-cell antibodies: mechanism of action

T-cell-specific antibodies have been used in solid organ transplant recipients as well as in the treatment of graft versus host disease after allogeneic stem cell transplantation [16]. Immunotherapies using monoclonal antibodies against T-cell molecules are also efficacious in human autoimmune diseases, for instance, rheumatoid arthritis and multiple sclerosis. Muromonab, or OKT3, is first generation, an IgG2a monoclonal antibody against human CD3 molecule raised in mouse [17]. Following intravenous administration, anti-CD3 antibodies first bind to circulating T cells and subsequently to the target cells present in the peripheral lymphoid organs, such as lymph nodes and spleen [18]. T cells with bound anti-T-cell antibodies on their surface disappear from circulation rapidly (30–60 min). The number of circulating T cells gradually increase after the cessation of treatment reaching pretreatment values within 1–6 weeks.

Several mechanisms of action of anti-T-cell antibodies have been suggested. Induction of lymphocytopenia may result from complement-dependent cytolysis, antibody-dependent cell-mediated cytolysis by Fc receptor bearing cells, and opsonization with subsequent phagocytosis by macrophages [16–18]. Another mechanism that could be relevant to T-cell depletion is activation-induced cell death. Anti-CD3/TCR antibodies were reported to trigger apoptosis in activated mature T lymphocytes [18, 19]. Wong *et al.* in turn found that T cells may lyse other T cells in the presence of OKT3 [20]. Margination of T cells caused by adhesion of lymphocytes to vascular endothelial cells and redistribution of T cells to nonlymphoid organs, such as the lung, could also account for the rapid disappearance of T cells from peripheral blood.

Anti-T-cell antibodies are also responsible for direct functional effects on T cells [16]. They block the T-cell receptor that is closely related to CD3 molecule through interference with the antigen recognition sequence and make T cells incapable of interacting with foreign antigen. This results in the removal of the T-cell receptor complex from the T-cell surface by a process termed *internalization*. Internalization of the T-cell receptor prevents subsequent recognition of any specific antigen. Anti-CD3 antibody also induces a downregulation of the function of nondepleted T cells, as defined by lack of IL-2 production and a great reduction in the production of multiple cytokines [16]. Of note, anti-CD3 antibody neither alters granulocyte function nor significantly affects production of antibodies by B lymphocytes. To summarize, both depletion of T cells from circulation and the influence on T-cell function lead to profound and long-lasting immunosuppression after treatment cessation.

The use of OKT3 antibody has been associated with significant first-dose side effects and possibly with lymphoma [16–18]. First doses of OKT3 antibody have been associated with many life-threatening complications due to systemic cytokine release syndrome. Usually, only first administration of anti-CD3 monoclonal antibody induces these side effects because internalized T-cell receptor after the initial dose is not susceptible subsequently to stimulation by the monoclonal antibody.

Another concern associated with the use of OKT3 antibody is the increased risk of occurrence of lymphoproliferative disorders found in patients after solid organ transplantation. This well-known complication of immunosuppression may be related to Epstein-Barr virus infection.

Polyclonal antithymocyte globulin (ATG) is raised in sheep, horses, or rabbits immunized with human lymphoid cells such as peripheral blood lymphocytes, thymocytes; separation of the resulting immune sera is necessary to obtain the γ-globulin fraction [16, 18]. Preparations of ATG vary in their potency and selectivity for T cells, and their antigenic specificity is not well defined and controlled. ATG induces only minor first-infusion reactions. Reasons for the difference between OKT3 and ATG in this respect are not clear. They may be related to the dosage but also to the relative proportions of activating (anti-CD2, -CD3) and blocking (anti-CD4, -CD11a, -CD18, anti- HLA DR) antibodies in ATG [18].

It is possible that newer generation, chimeric or humanized (with grafted CD molecule) anti-T-cell antibodies will be considered in the treatment of human myocarditis in the near future.

The use of anti-T-cell antibodies in experimental myocarditis

In experimental studies, immunotherapy directed against T cells has been shown to be effective for the prevention of acute Coxsackie virus myocarditis in mice. Antibodies against pan T cells were more effective than those to T-cell subsets; this form of therapy was effective even in the presence of virus in the host [21]. The therapy does not suppress formation of neutralizing antibodies in the host, and therefore protects the host from virus entrance. The worsening of myocarditis observed with immunosuppressive agents such as cyclosporine and prednisone is probably due to their inhibition of neutralizing antibody production by lymphocytes B and a resultant increase in viral replication [22].

Experimental autoimmune myocarditis is a T-cell-mediated disease produced most frequently by immunization of rats or mice with cardiac myosin [23]. Antibodies against αβT-cell receptors, blocking directly the process of antigen recognition, have shown to be effective in preventing the induction of giant cell myocarditis in rats [24]. Similarly, a combination of monoclonal antibodies against leukocyte function-associated molecule-1 and intercellular adhesion molecule-1, blocking costimulatory signals provided by the interaction between T-cell surface receptor and adhesion molecule, prevents the induction of experimental autoimmune myocarditis in the same model [25].

CD2 molecule has been shown to function both as an adhesion and signal molecule in T-cell recognition. This molecule is also present on undifferentiated T cells in the thymus and on NK cells. Anti-CD2 monoclonal antibodies were reported to be effective in preventing the induction of experimental autoimmune myocarditis induced by immunizing Lewis rats with cardiac myosin [25].

Yuan et al. in turn studied the influence of selective anti-L3T4 monoclonal antibody, which is equivalent to anti-CD4 antibody in humans, in prevention of myosin-induced autoimmune myocarditis in mice [26]. Authors attained the immune tolerance to cardiac myosin and accordingly prevention of myocardial injury. Similar results with anti-CD4 monoclonal antibodies have been shown in the model of autoimmune myocarditis in rats by Qing-Qing et al. [27].

Another approach was to study the use of monoclonal antibodies directed against activated T cells. Activated T cells bear detectable amounts of IL-2R. AMT13, a rat monoclonal antibody against mouse IL-2R, did not exert a beneficial effect on acute Coxsackie virus B3 myocarditis in mice [28].

Thus, antibodies that could selectively and temporarily inactivate or eliminate CD2+, CD3+, CD4+ cells, but not activated T cells are effective in prevention of experimental myocarditis.

The use of anti-T-cell antibodies in human myocarditis

The use of immunosuppressive and immunomodulatory therapies for autoimmune myocarditis is still hotly debated issue. It is recommended to use immunosuppression in the treatment of giant cell myocarditis and in those patients with lymphocytic myocarditis in whom the presence of viral genome in endomyocardial biopsy has been excluded [4–6]. In the literature there is very few data on the use of anti-T-cell antibodies in the treatment of human myocarditis. Since its first use by Gilbert et al. in 1988 [7], 10 papers have included information on the use of OKT3 antibody [5–14] and 1 on the use of rabbit ATG in patients with myocarditis [15]. All patients but one presented with fulminant

or rapidly progressive heart failure (Table 24.1). The one patient had sustained ventricular tachycardia refractory to treatment. The age of patients ranged from 15 months to 67 years. Of interest, viral-like syndrome preceded onset of symptoms in 11 patients (68.8%), and time from onset of symptoms to diagnosis ranged from 2 days to 8 years and was shorter than 1 month in 8 patients (50%). As far as histopathological diagnosis is concerned, lymphocytic myocarditis was present in 8 patients, nonspecific in 2 patients, and giant cell myocarditis in 6 patients. The dose and regimen of the use of OKT3 antibody was variable (see Table 24.1). The outcome in this patient population was favorable in majority of patients. Full or partial recovery was reported in 13 patients (82.5%), 1 died of heart failure 13 days after initiation of combined immunosuppression, 1 had heart transplantation a few months later, and 1 died of stroke 30 months after the diagnosis. Of importance, OKT3 antibody was used with other immunosuppressives, like corticosteroids, cyclophosphamide, cyclosporine, azathioprine, but also with intravenous immunoglobulin in 6 patients (37.5%). Furthermore, use of this combined aggressive immunosuppressive therapy could not be possible in this patient population, if 10 of those patients (62.5%) had not received any mechanical support. Five of the patients received temporarily ventricular assist devices, 2 intraaortic balloon pump, 2 received extracorporeal membrane oxygenation, and 1 both extracorporeal membrane oxygenation and left ventricular assist device. Therefore, the real influence of anti-T-cell antibodies on the survival of patients with fulminant myocarditis is uncertain. McCarthy et al. reported on patients with fulminant myocarditis who were treated with inotropes and mechanical support only without use of any immunosuppressives and had excellent long-term survival [29].

The Myocarditis Treatment Trial did not show benefit in patients treated with immunosuppression in comparison to patients treated with conventional therapy only [30]. However, in the trial there were few patients with fulminant course of the disease, T-cell cytolytic therapy has not been considered, and patients with giant cell myocarditis were not included in the study.

The only one study on the use of OKT3 antibody in human myocarditis is the multicenter Giant Cell

Table 24.1 Anti-T-cell antibodies used in human myocarditis.

Intervention	Symptoms, pretreatment LVEF, if available	Sex and age	Viral-like syndrome preceding onset of symptoms	Time from onset of symptoms to diagnosis	Associated disease	Pathology	Dose and duration	Additional immunosuppressive and/or immunomodulatory therapies	Mechanical support	Outcome/ posttreatment LVEF (%)/duration of follow-up	Reference
OKT3, muromonab	CHF, NYHA IV, dobutamine-dependent	F, 31 yr	Yes	Not available	Mixed connective tissue disease	Lymphocytic myocarditis	Dose not available, 7 days	Cyclophosphamide, prednisone	No	Normal LV function after treatment	[7]
	CHF, heart block, VT, LVEF 24%	F, 42 yr	No	8 yr	Chronic ulcerative colitis	Giant cell myocarditis	5 mg q.d. for 10 days	Cyclosporine, corticosteroids	No	HTX a few months later/Not available/8 yr	[5, 11]
	CHF, LVEF 5%	M, 33 yr	Yes	2 days	No	Lymphocytic myocarditis	5 mg q.d. for 8 days	No	BVAD	Quick recovery/LVEF 60–65%/8 mo	[8]
	CHF, LBBB, LVEF 35%	F, 67 yr	No	18 days	No	Giant cell myocarditis	10 mg q.d. for 1 day, 5 mg q.d. for 12 days	Corticosteroids,	IABP	Died of heart failure 13 days after initiation of immunosuppression	[6, 11]
	CHF, LVEF 20% CHF, LVEF 5%	M, 16 yr M, 33 yr	Yes	20 days, 4 days	No	Nonspecific myocarditis	Data not available	Corticosteroids +IVIG Corticosteroids	LVAD BVAD	Quick recovery LVEF 45% LVEF 50% >6 mo and <3 y	[9]
	CHF, LVEF 10%	F, 34 yr	Yes	12 days	No	Giant cell myocarditis	5 mg q.d. for 10 days, followed by 2.5 mg q.d. for 10 days	Cyclosporine, prednisone, azathioprine	No	LVEF 37%/4.5 yr	[10, 11]
	AMI, CHF LVEF 25%	M, 47 yr	No	6 mo	No	Giant cell myocarditis	5 mg q.d. for 7 days, 2.5 mg q.d. for 7 days	Corticosteroids, azathioprine, cyclosporine	No	Quick recovery, LVEF 55% by day 13, 1 yr on immunosuppression	[11]

Clinical presentation	Patient		Duration	Associated condition	Diagnosis	RATG dose	Immunosuppression	Mechanical support	Outcome	Ref
CHF, severe ventricular arrhythmia LVEF ranging from 5 to 20%	5 patients 3 M/2 F: aged 15 mo -16 yr	Yes	Not available	Not available	Lymphocytic myocarditis	0.1 mg/kg q.d. for 10–14 days	IVIG in all patients, corticosteroids, cyclosporine+ azthioprine (3 patients), cyclosporine (1 patient)	IABP, LVAD, ECMO, LVAD+ ECMO	LVEF 50–74% by 2 wk, no progression to DCM during 3–56 mo	[12]
Inferior MI, LVEF <10%	M, 40 yr	Yes 2 days		No	Giant cell myocarditis	Not available	Corticosteroids, cyclophosphamide	BVAD	Quick recovery, LVEF– 50% by day 17, 9 mo	[13]
Intractable VT LVEF 30%	F, 33 yr	No 5 wk		Helicobacter pylori associated gastric inflammation	Lymphocytic myocarditis	5 mg q.d. for 5 days	Corticosteroids	No	Short-term recovery LVEF 30%, recurrent VT treated with catheter ablation, died of stroke 30 mo after initial episode, postcholecystectomy	[14]
RATG	Acute MI, cardiogenic shock	M, 64 yr	No 2 days	Not available	Giant cell myocarditis	75 mg q.d. for 3 days	Cyclosporine, prednisolone in the acute event, replaced by mycophenolate mofetil+prednisone	Femoral venoarterial ECMO	Quick recovery, LVEF 55%, 1 yr	[15]

BVAD, biventricular assist device; CHF, congestive heart failure; ECMO, extracorporeal membrane oxygenation; F, female; HTX, heart transplantation; IABP, intraaortic balloon pump; IVIG, intravenous immunoglobulin; LBBB, left bundle branch block; LV, left ventricular; LVAD, left ventricular assist device; LVEF, left ventricular ejection fraction; M, male; MI, myocardial infarction; NYHA, New York Heart Association functional class; OKT3, murine monoclonal antibody against human CD3; q.d., once daily; rATG, rabbit antithymocyte globulin; VT, ventricular tachycardia.

Myocarditis Treatment Trial [31]. This study is a randomized, open-label trial of muromonab-CD3, cyclosporine, and steroids versus cyclosporine and steroids for giant cell myocarditis diagnosed by endomyocardial biopsy. The primary endpoint is to compare the rate of death, transplantation, and ventricular assist device placement at 1 year. The results of the study have not been published so far.

Administration of corticosteroids prior to the use of OKT3 antibody is considered a standard procedure that has improved tolerance to the drug [16].

In summary, there is growing body of evidence that selective anti-T-cell antibodies exert a beneficial effect in experimental and clinical myocarditis. However, there are no large series or controlled trials adequately testing anti-T-cell therapy in humans. Therefore, the routine use of this biological therapy for autoimmune myocarditis is not justified.

References

1 Huber S. Cellular autoimmunity in myocarditis. In: Cooper LT, Jr, ed. *Myocarditis: From Bench to Bedside.* Humana Press, Totowa, NJ, 2003:55–76.

2 Davies MJ, Ward DE. How can myocarditis be diagnosed and should it be treated? Br Heart J 1992;68:346–7.

3 Kuhl U, Noutsias M, Schultheiss H-P. Immunohistochemistry in dilated cardiomyopathy. Eur Heart J 1995;16(suppl O):100–6.

4 Schultheiss H-P, Kuhl U. Myocarditis and inflammatory cardiomyopathy. In: Crawford MH, DiMarco JP, Paulus WJ, eds. *Cardiology*, 2nd edn. Mosby, Edinburgh, 2004:937–49.

5 Davidoff R, Palacios I, Southern J, Fallon JT, Newell J, Dec GW. Giant cell versus lymphocytic myocarditis: a comparison of their clinical features and long-term outcomes. Circulation 1991;83:953–61.

6 Cooper LT, Jr, Berry GJ, Shabetai R, for the Multicenter Giant Cell Myocarditis Study Group Investigators. Idiopathic giant-cell myocarditis—natural history and treatment. N Engl J Med 1997;336:1860–6.

7 Gilbert EM, O'Connell JB, Hammond ME, Renlund DG, Watson FS, Bristow MR. Treatment of myocarditis with OKT3 monoclonal antibody. Lancet 1988;1:759.

8 Jett GK, Miller A, Savino D, Gonwa T. Reversal of acute fulminant lymphocytic myocarditis with combined technology of OKT3 monoclonal antibody and mechanical circulatory support. J Heart Lung Transplant 1992;11(4, pt 1):733–8.

9 Marelli D, Laks H, Amsel B *et al.* Temporary mechanical support with the BVS 5000 assist device during treatment of acute myocarditis. J Card Surg 1997;12:55–9.

10 Levy NT, Olson LJ, Weyand C *et al.* Histologic and cytokine response to immunosuppression in giant-cell myocarditis. Ann Intern Med 1998;128:648–50.

11 Menghini VV, Savcenko V, Olson LJ *et al.* Combined immunosuppression for the treatment of idiopathic giant cell myocarditis. Mayo Clin Proc 1999;74:1221–6.

12 Ahdoot J, Galindo AJ, Alejos JC *et al.* Use of OKT3 for acute myocarditis in infants and children. J Heart Lung Transplant 2000;19:1118–21.

13 Pinderski LJ, Fonarow GC, Hamilton M *et al.* Giant cell myocarditis in a young man responsive to T-lymphocyte cytolytic therapy. J Heart Lung Transplant 2002;21:818–21.

14 Bilinska ZT, Grzybowski J, Szajewski T *et al.* Active lymphocytic myocarditis treated with murine OKT3 monoclonal antibody. Tex Heart Inst J 2002;29:113–7.

15 Ankersmit HJ, Ulrich R, Moser B *et al.* Recovery from giant cell myocarditis with ECMO support and utilization of polyclonal antithymocyte globulin: a case report. Thorac Cardiovasc Surg 2006;54:278–80.

16 Allegre M-L, Bluestone JA. T cell antigen and costimulatory receptors as therapeutic targets. In: Austen KF, Frank MH, Atkinson JP, Cantor H, eds. *Samster's Immunologic Diseases.* Lippincot Williams and Wilkins, Philadelphia, 2001:1155–74.

17 Cosimi AB. Clinical development of Orthoclone OKT3. Transplant Proc 1987;19(suppl 1):7–16.

18 Bonnefoy-Berard N, Revillard J-P. Mechanisms of immunosuppression induced by antithymocyte globulins and OKT3. J Heart Lung Transplant 1996;15:435–42.

19 Janssen O, Wesselborg S, Kabelitz D. Immunosuppression by OKT3: induction of programmed cell death (apoptosis) as a possible mechanism of action. Transplantation 1992;53:233–4.

20 Wong JT, Eylath AA, Ghobrial I, Colvin RB. The mechanism of anti-CD3 monoclonal antibodies. Mediation of cytolysis by inter-T cell bridging. Transplantation 1990;50:683–9.

21 Kishimoto C, Abelmann WH. Monoclonal antibody therapy for prevention of acute Coxsackievirus B3 myocarditis in mice. Circulation 1989;79:1300–8.

22 Matsumori A, Tomiaka N, Kawai C. Viral myocarditis: immunopathogenesis and the effect of immunosuppressive treatment in a murine model. Jpn Circ J 1989;53:58–60.

23 Smith SC, Allen PM. Myosin-induced acute myocarditis is a T cell mediated disease. J Immunol 1991;147:2141–7.

24 Hanawa H, Kodama M, Inomata T *et al.* Anti-alpha beta T cell receptor antibody prevents the progression of experimental autoimmune myocarditis. Clin Exp Immunol 1994;96:470–5.

25 Inomata T, Watanabe T, Haga M *et al.* Anti-CD2 monoclonal antibodies prevent the induction of experimental autoimmune myocarditis. Jpn Heart J 2000;41:507–17.

26 Yuan H-T, Liao Y-H, Wang Z *et al.* Prevention of myosin-induces autoimmune myocarditis in mice by anti-L3T4 monoclonal antibody. Can J Physiol Pharmacol 2003;81:84–8.

27 Qing-Qing W, Yu-Lin W, Hai-Tao Y, Feng-Qin L, You-Peng J, Bo H. Immune tolerance to cardiac myosin induced by anti-CD4 monoclonal antibody in autoimmune myocarditis rats. J Clin Immunol 2006;26:213–21.

28 Kishimoto C, Hiraoka Y, Takada H, Kurokawa M, Ochiai H. Failure of treatment with interleukin-2 receptor-specific monoclonal antibody in acute coxsackievirus B3 myocarditis in mice. Heart Vessels 1997;12:221–8.

29 McCarthy RE, Boehmer JP, Hruban RH *et al.* Long-term outcome of fulminant myocarditis as compared with acute (nonfulminant) myocarditis. N Engl J Med 2000;342:690–5.

30 Mason JW, O'Connell JB, Herskowitz A *et al.* A clinical trial of immunosuppressive therapy in myocarditis. N Engl J Med, 1995;333:269–75.

31 Cooper LT, Okura Y. Idiopathic giant cell myocarditis. Curr Treat Options Cardiovasc Med 2001;3:463–7.

CHAPTER 25

Immunosuppressive therapy to counter cardiac allograft vasculopathy

Carl V. Leier

Overview

Immunologic mechanisms play a major role in the development of cardiac allograft vasculopathy (CAV) throughout the clinical course following transplantation. It is the principal culprit in hyperacute rejection, typically occurring in close proximity to the transplant, and serves as a major contributor to less acute forms of graft vasculopathy. Advances in immunosuppressive therapy (e.g., mycophenolate mofetil, sirolimus) have improved posttransplant outcomes, in large part related to a reduction in the development of CAV. Preliminary reports indicate that some reversal of posttransplant vasculopathy may be achievable, but this challenge has not yet been studied in major trials.

Cardiac allograft vasculopathy: general concepts

The entire clinical course following cardiac transplantation is threatened by the development of CAV, and none of these patients are spared from varying degrees of this pathologic process. CAV is also referred to as transplant coronary artery disease (TCAD, TxCAD), transplant-related coronary artery disease (TRCAD), and posttransplant vasculopathy (PTV). While both atherosclerosis and CAV cause obstruction of coronary arteries and compromise coronary blood flow, these conditions have little else in common; therefore, the term *transplant atherosclerosis* is no longer an appropriate one for

the histopathology and the clinical and laboratory features of CAV.

The clinical presentation of CAV covers a wide spectrum, ranging from asymptomatic endothelial dysfunction in its mildest form to acute graft failure and death at the other extreme [1–16]. In between, there reside varying degrees of ventricular diastolic and systolic dysfunction, exercise-intolerance, dyspnea and other symptoms of heart failure, varying symptoms of myocardial ischemia (although angina pectoris is often absent), scattered small infarcts and occasional transmural myocardial infarction, cardiac dysrhythmias and near-syncope–syncope, sudden death, and death from end-stage graft failure [1–16].

CAV plays a major role in compromising the clinical course and reducing survival following cardiac transplant, and it can be viewed as occurring in three general stages [3–5, 14, 16]. First is hyperacute rejection, which results when preformed antibodies to ABO blood group antigens or to human leukocyte antigens (HLA) evoke acute, immediate rejection of the coronary vasculature of the donor heart. This is typically a catastrophic event, often starting in the operating room during the transplant procedure. Without drastic intervention, very few of these patients survive to 1 week following transplant. While aggressive interventions (e.g., high-dose immunosuppression, plasmapheresis) have been applied, there are few which are effective in reversing the intracoronary pathologic process, consisting of acute fibrin deposition and thrombus formation, marked endothelial swelling and cell death, obliterative obstruction of most of the coronary vasculature, loss of coronary blood flow and myocardial perfusion, and depending on the duration of graft survival, varying degrees of fibrinoid degeneration and destruction of coronary vessels. Urgent retransplant with a compatible donor graft, if available, remains a viable (albeit remote) option, assuming the patient (recipient) survives and remains intact to undergo retransplant. Advances in immunological testing, crossmatch testing of high-risk patients prior to transplant, and preventive therapies have reduced the incidence of this nightmare event to very rare.

The second stage occurs within the first year, typically within the first 6 months following transplant. Graft failure can occur and is mediated through the pathophysiologic cascade that follows diffuse antibody-induced injury to coronary vasculature with progressive obstruction of the coronary arteries [5, 11, 14, 16–19]. This form of CAV, now occurring in less that 7% of all heart transplants, consists of endothelial swelling and disruption, some intimal proliferation, intracoronary thrombus formation, and varying degrees of vascular and perivascular inflammation. Deposition of immune components (e.g., IgG, C3d, C4d) in small coronary arteries or arterioles can often be demonstrated with immunofluorescent staining of endomyocardial biopsy (or necropsy) specimens. Immunologic reactions directed at donor HLA or endothelial cell antigens and the graft's response to these represent the predominant mechanisms for this form of graft damage and failure [5, 11, 14, 16–24]. Patients at highest risk for this stage of CAV (± graft failure) are those allosensitized by prior transfusion of blood and blood products, pregnancy, and previous transplantation; most of these high-risk patients are identified by high reactivity to panel-reactive antigens (PRA). Left ventricular assist devices, often used to secure a favorable hemodynamic and clinical course prior to transplant, also increase pretransplant PRA titers; however, the elevated, left ventricular assist device evoked PRA in this setting does not appear to herald enhanced rejection rates or severity, acute CAV, or unfavorable clinical outcomes [25].

The third, more chronic phase of CAV develops more gradually and becomes apparent anytime after the first year following transplant [1, 4,

10, 12, 14–16], although it is not uncommon for acute coronary vasculopathy to transition directly into this more chronic form of CAV. The chronic form of CAV is mechanistically multifactorial, with immunologic factors sharing the pathologic process with nonimmunologic risks such as hyperlipidemia, insulin resistance/diabetes mellitus, systemic hypertension, renal dysfunction, atherogenic therapies, infections (e.g., cytomegalovirus), and others [3, 12, 16, 24–34]. Much of the therapy following transplant is directed at controlling as many of these CAV risks as possible, with the awareness that the impact of each risk (and its management) likely varies widely among transplanted patients. At 5 years following transplant, up to 50% of patients will have angiographically demonstrable CAV in the form of luminal lesions or narrowing of epicardial coronary arteries and/or attenuation of mid-sized to distal small vessels [1, 10, 12, 16]. Some intimal thickening of epicardial arteries is demonstrable by intracoronary ultrasound, considerably earlier in a higher percentage of patients [4, 7, 13, 14]. Intimal proliferation with an intact internal elastic lamina and paucity of calcification, both in contrast to the typical atherosclerotic lesion, are the histologic hallmarks of chronic CAV.

Cardiac allograft vasculopathy: management approach

The current standard revascularization procedures for occlusive coronary atherosclerosis (e.g., angioplasty-stent deployment, coronary artery bypass surgery) are palliative at best in the setting of CAV. This profound limitation has forced transplant cardiologists to rely heavily on preventive considerations and pharmacologic approaches to reduce the development, severity, and unfavorable clinical course of CAV.

Preventing and limiting the development of CAV

Pretransplant
From an immunological standpoint, preventive measures start prior to transplant. Needless to say, the donor heart must be ABO blood- and tissue-type compatible with the recipient. In the few instances that this consideration was violated,

hyperacute graft failure occurred with minutes of placement of the graft. To date, no therapy is available other than urgent retransplant (or perhaps replacing the rejecting heart with a total artificial heart) to rescue this unfortunate patient from the abruptly malignant immunologic reaction.

During transplant evaluation and listing, all patients undergo testing for PRA to determine the antibody reactivity level of the candidate-recipient to HLA I and II [17–20]. An elevated PRA of >10% places a patient at increased risk for acute cellular and humoral rejection. Prior transplantation, transfusion of blood and blood products, and pregnancy elevate the patient's PRA level. At most centers, an elevated PRA implicates the need to perform a prospective crossmatch between the recipient's serum and donor cells to determine the immunologic compatibility of the proposed recipient–donor interface and thus, predict the course and survival of the graft and recipient.

A number of strategies have been employed to reduce a patient's PRA level prior to transplant in an attempt to decrease short- and long-term rejection. These include avoiding transfusions, if possible, during the pretransplant waiting period, immunosuppressive therapy (e.g., cyclophosphamide, mycophenolate mofetil), intravenously administered immunoglobulin, and plasmapheresis [5, 11, 34]. There are no controlled trials comparing any of these modalities. The author has successfully decreased PRA levels of >90% to <20% with a varying combination of these measures. Whether nonimmunologic risk factors for CAV should be aggressively treated prior to transplant has not been resolved [26].

During and early after transplant

In addition, more aggressive immunosuppression at the time of transplant can eliminate or temper an acute CAV event, although the cost of such is a higher incidence of infection. Examples of this form of intervention include induction therapy with antithymocyte globulin, high-dose corticosteroid therapy, earlier and higher dosing of mycophenolate mofetil, and occasional plasmapheresis [5, 11, 34–37]. Close surveillance of endomyocardial biopsies, which in high risk patients should include immunofluorescent staining of vasculature, and of ventricular function (hemodynamics,

echocardiography) is essential in alerting clinicians to the possibility of substantial cellular or humoral (CAV) rejection prior to permanent damage to the graft and before symptoms develop; immunosuppression therapy is then adjusted to address the clinical and histologic findings.

Long-term after transplant

While the treatment of nonimmunologic contributors to CAV will not be addressed in this chapter, some of these therapies may actually have immunosuppressive properties as a component of their "pleiotropic" character. The most convincing example is the chronic administration of an HMG CoA reductase inhibitor (statin) [38–44]. Controlled trials of daily pravastatin and simvastatin administration in patients following heart transplantation demonstrated improved outcomes on several levels including survival, a lower rejection rate, and less CAV [38–43]. The improved survival has been attributed to a lower rejection rate and especially to decreased CAV. A recent follow-up publication of the pravastatin trial reported that the augmented survival and reduced CAV with continued administration of pravastatin appears to persist to 10 years after transplant [40]. The precise non-lipid-lowering mechanisms for these favorable immunologic and therapeutic effects of pravastatin and simvastatin on CAV remain to be determined, but likely involve modulation of the interface between immune reactions, inflammation, cytokines, and the endothelium [38, 43].

Employing intracoronary ultrasound, the findings of a small trial suggest that combination of calcium channel antagonism and angiotensin-converting enzyme inhibition over 1 year after transplant reduces intimal proliferation and CAV [45, 46]. At this point, it is unknown whether the reduced CAV noted for this combination is related to controlling immunologic mechanisms.

Advances in chronic immunosuppressive therapy over the past few years have had an impact on the development of CAV [47–56]. The chronic administration of mycophenolate mofetil and azathioprine was compared in a randomized trial of 650 posttransplant patients on other standard background therapy [48]. Mycophenolate mofetil effected a lower rejection rate and better survival at 1 and 5 years following transplant. A trend (but

$p > 0.05$) toward less CAV was initially reported from this study for the mycophenolate group; this finding was convincingly (statistically) established using the intracoronary ultrasound data of the trial [47, 48]. In a single center, retrospective study of 273 transplanted patients, long-term mycophenolate mofetil reduced the development and progression of angiographic CAV, compared to a previous standard antiproliferative agent, azathioprine [51]. Similar results were reported by El-Sayed *et al.* [50] in a meticulously performed angiographic study of transplant CAV. The findings of these studies, likely, explain some of the favorable clinical outcomes of mycophenolate mofetil versus azathioprine in the heart transplant population. Mycophenolate mofetil reduces the production of antibodies, inhibits the proliferation of T- and B-type lymphocytes, and impedes a number of vasculopathic mechanisms in transplanted patients [51, 52].

Small studies comparing the chronic administration of the two primary calcineurin inhibitors, cyclosporine and tacrolimus, showed conflicting results or no differences in their effects on CAV [57, 58]. Calcineurin inhibitors, in general, appear to have less impact on humoral rejection and CAV than the antiproliferative agents, mycophenolate mofetil and azathioprine, probably because the former group has less suppressive activity on B-lymphocytes and antibody production.

Sirolimus is currently the most effective agent employed on drug-eluting stents to prevent instent restenosis (reocclusion) of treated atherosclerotic lesions. In this clinical setting, sirolimus blunts intimal and smooth-muscle cell proliferation evoked by deployment of the stent. While systemic administration of sirolimus has little to no effect on instent restenosis in atherosclerosis, initial reports suggest that chronic immunosuppression with orally administered sirolimus reduces the rate of acute graft rejection and retards the development of human CAV [53–55]. Larger controlled trials are needed to document these and to establish a link between these observations and an improvement of clinical outcomes in the heart transplant population.

Eisen and colleagues [56], in a randomized, double-blind trial determined that daily administration of everolimus on background cyclosporine,

corticosteroid, and statin therapy significantly decreased CAV at 1 year following transplant compared to daily azathioprine plus the same background therapy.

Although it appears that the immunosuppressive tools are improving to prevent and limit the development of CAV, major questions remain unanswered. Long-term administration of mycophenolate mofetil, sirolimus, or everolimus is probably more effective than long-term azathioprine in preventing or slowing the development of CAV, but how do these agents compare to each other? Newer agents are still being compared to azathioprine, which should no longer be regarded as standard therapy. Are any of the newer agents more synergistic with the calcineurin antagonists in reducing rejection rate and CAV? Which agent best complements induction therapy? How will induction therapy itself impact the development of CAV? And so forth.

Treatment to reverse CAV

Reversing CAV is one of the most challenging duties of the transplant cardiologist. As noted, revascularization procedures are quite limited as long-term solutions for CAV and are, at best, palliative. Therefore, the provider is forced to consider pharmacotherapy as the principal intervention and more specifically, to employ immunosuppressive therapy as the only choice that currently may be effective in reducing CAV in the short- and long-term [50, 53, 59–61]. These patients are already on a statin for lipid control (and its other pharmacologic effects), aspirin, effective antihypertensive therapy, and so forth. The only aspect that the physician can potentially intervene upon is the immunologic component. The nonimmunologic contributors to the development of CAV should already be optimally treated; but in spite of this important consideration, these nonimmunologic interventions generally do not reverse the severity of CAV lesions.

While there are no controlled trials to guide the effort to cure or reduce CAV, there are clues in the literature to suggest that advancing immunosuppressive therapy merits strong consideration [50, 53, 59–61]. These reports also support the view that immune mechanisms play a major role in the genesis of CAV, particularly during the early posttransplant

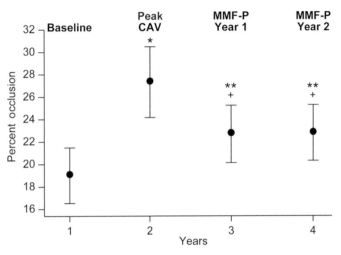

Figure 25.1 Advancing immunosuppression with combination mycophenolate mofetil—prednisone (MMF-P) significantly reduced the angiographic severity of cardiac allograft vasculopathy (CAV) 1 and 2 years after the introduction of this combination at peak CAV. Baseline represents the quantitative analysis of the same lesions 12–14 months before the detection of problematic CAV (peak). Hundred-eighteen lesions were analyzed and followed over 3–4 years in 17 posttransplant patients. $^*p < 0.01$ versus baseline; $^{**}p < 0.05$ versus baseline; $+p < 0.05$ versus peak CAV. (Adapted, with permission, from [50].)

period (<1 year following transplant). Lamich and colleagues [60] detected substantial CAV within the first year after transplantation in 24% of their patients. Augmented immunosuppression with antithymocyte globulin and 3 days of high-dose methylprednisolone on top of standard immunosuppression achieved near-complete resolution of CAV in 68% of affected patients, with an overall favorable response rate noted in 80%. Similar results were reported by Ballester et al. [59] in a smaller population. A retrospective study showed that advancing immunosuppression from daily cyclosporine and azathioprine to cyclosporine, mycophenolate mofetil, and every other day prednisone either reversed CAV or halted its progression [50] (Figure 25.1). The addition of sirolimus to standard immunosuppressive therapy effected regression of severe progressive CAV in a 33-year-old patient, 2–3 years following cardiac transplantation [53]. Pelletier et al. [61] added total lymphoid irradiation to standard immunosuppressive therapy and OKT3 to treat recurrent cellular rejection in 31 patients from 1 month to 10 years after transplant. Compared to a nonblinded, parallel control group, this intervention had a favorable effect on the short- and long-term development of CAV.

The approaches to treat and reverse CAV vary somewhat among transplant centers, with no convincing data to establish or support any one recommendation. For early CAV (within the first year), the author's usual approach has been to increase dosing of mycophenolate mofetil to ≥1500 mg twice daily and that of prednisone to 20 mg twice daily for 1 month, with stepwise decrementation over 3–6 months to 10 mg every other day. More recently, sirolimus has joined this plan at a dose of 1–2 mg daily, depending on tolerability, adverse effects, and the patient's renal function. Dosing of cyclosporine and tacrolimus is reduced with the addition of sirolimus to protect the kidneys. The author has reserved antithymocyte globulin for acute CAV-cardiac failure and for patients whose early CAV is not responsive to the approaches stated above.

For CAV that has developed over time past the first year following transplant, the author again optimizes dosing of mycophenolate mofetil, adds sirolimus at a dose range of 1 mg every other day to 2 mg daily and/or prednisone 10 mg every other day, depending on the course and severity of the CAV, adverse effects of the therapy, and concomitant renal function. Needless to say, the management of nonimmunologic cardiovascular risk factors is always optimized.

Closing comments

In spite of advances in immunosuppressive therapy over the past decade, CAV remains the major threat to overall survival of the posttransplant patient. Additional strategies to counter CAV are under study and some will merit further investigation in human cardiac transplantation [56, 62–68]. Efforts to counter this pathologic process must continue, and since allograft vasculopathy is a condition common to all transplantation, this quest is the responsibility of all who work in the area of solid organ transplantation.

References

1 O'Neill BJ, Pflugfelder PW, Singh NR, Menkis AH, McKenzie FN, Kostuk WJ. Frequency of angiographic detection and quantitative assessment of coronary arterial disease one and three years after cardiac transplantation. Am J Cardiol 1989;63:1221–6.

2 Gao SZ, Schroeder JS, Hunt SA, Billingham ME, Valentine HA, Stinson EB. Acute myocardial infarction in cardiac transplant recipients. Am J Med 1989;64:1093–7.

3 Gao SZ, Hunt SA, Schroeder JS, Alderman EL, Hill IR, Stinson EB. Early development of accelerated graft coronary artery disease: risk factors and course. J Am Coll Cardiol 1996;28:673–9.

4 Tuzcu EM, De Franco AC, Goormastic M et al. Dichotomous pattern of coronary atherosclerosis 1 to 9 years after transplantation: insights from systematic intravascular ultrasound imaging. J Am Coll Cardiol 1996;27:839–46.

5 Hornick P, Smith J, Pomerance A et al. Influence of acute rejection episodes, HLA matching, and donor/recipient phenotype on the development of 'early' transplant-associated coronary artery disease. Circulation 1997;96(suppl II):II148–53.

6 Mazur W, Bitar JN, Young JB et al. Progressive deterioration of coronary flow reserve after transplantation. Am Heart J 1998;136:504–9.

7 Yamani MH, Tuzcu EM, Starling RC et al. Computerized scoring of histopathology for predicting coronary vasculopathy, validated by intravascular ultrasound. J Heart Lung Transplant 2002;21:850–9.

8 Kushwaha SS, Narula J, Narula N et al. Pattern of changes over time in myocardial blood flow and microvascular dilator capacity in patients with normally functioning cardiac allografts. Am J Cardiol 1998;82:1377–81.

9 John R, Rajasinghe HA, Itescu S et al. Factors affecting long-term survival (>10 years) after cardiac transplantation in the cyclosporine era. J Am Coll Cardiol 2001;37:189–94.

10 Potluri SP, Mehra MR, Uber PA, Park MH, Scott RL, Ventura HO. Relationship among epicardial coronary disease, tissue myocardial perfusion, and survival in heart transplantation. J Heart Lung Transplant 2005;24:1019–25.

11 Olsen SL, Wagoner LE, Hammond EH et al. Vascular rejection in heart transplantation: clinical correlation, treatment options, and future considerations. J Heart Lung Transplant 1993;12:S135–42.

12 Costanzo MR, Naftel DC, Pritzker MR et al, and the Cardiac Transplant Research Database. Heart transplant coronary artery disease detected by coronary angiography: a multiinstitutional study of preoperative donor and recipient risk factors. J Heart Lung Transplant 1998;17:744–53.

13 Mainigi SK, Goldberg LR, Sasseen BM, See VY, Jr, Wilensky RL. Relative contributions of intimal hyperplasia and vascular remodeling in early cardiac transplant-mediated coronary artery disease. Am J Cardiol 2003;91:293–6.

14 Tsutsui H, Ziada KM, Schoenhagen P et al. Lumen loss in transplant coronary disease is a biphasic process involving early intimal thickening and late constrictive remodeling. Circulation 2001;104:653–7.

15 Muehling OM, Wilke NM, Panse P et al. Reduced myocardial perfusion reserve and transmural perfusion gradient in heart transplant arteriopathy assessed by magnetic resonance imaging. J Am Coll Cardiol 2003;42:1054–60.

16 Haddad M, Pflugfelder PW, Guiraudon C et al. Angiographic, pathologic, and clinical relationships in coronary artery disease in cardiac allografts. J Heart Lung Transplant 2005;24:1218–25.

17 Reed EF, Demetris AJ, Hammond E et al. Acute antibody-mediated rejection of cardiac transplants. J Heart Lung Transplant 2006;25:153–9.

18 Micheals PJ, Espejo ML, Kobashigawa J et al. Humoral rejection in cardiac transplantation: risk factors, hemodynamic consequences and relationship to transplant coronary artery disease. J Heart Lung Transplant 2003;22:58–69.

19 Cherry R, Nielsen H, Reed E, Reemtsma K, Suciu-Foca N, Marboe CC. Vascular (humoral) rejection in human allograft biopsies: relation to circulating anti-HLA antibodies. J Heart Lung Transplant 1992;11:24–30.

20 Rose EA, Pepino P, Barr ML et al. Relation of HLA antibodies and graft atherosclerosis in human cardiac allograft recipients. J Heart Lung Transplant 1992;11:S120–3.

21 Gullestad L, Simonsen S, Ueland T et al. Possible role of proinflammatory cytokines in heart allograft coronary artery disease. Am J Cardiol 1999;84:999–1003.

22 Hognestad A, Endresen K, Wergeland R *et al.* Plasma C-reactive protein as a marker of cardiac allograft vasculopathy in heart transplant recipients. J Am Coll Cardiol 2003;42:477–82.

23 Hosenpud JD, Everett JP, Morris TE, Mauck KA, Shipley GD, Wagner CR. Cardiac allograft vasculopathy. Association with cell-mediated but not humoral alloimmunity to donor specific vascular endothelium. Circulation 1995;92:205–11.

24 Fredrich R, Toyoda M, Czer LS *et al.* The clinical significance of antibodies to human vascular endothelial cells after cardiac transplantation. Transplantation 1999;67:385–91.

25 Joyce DL, Southard RE, Torre-Amione G, Noon GP, Land GA, Loebe M. Impact of left ventricular assist device (LVAD)-mediated humoral sensitization on post-transplant outcomes. J Heart Lung Transplant 2005;24:2054–9.

26 Cooke GE, Eaton GM, Whitby G *et al.* Plasma atherogenic factors in congestive heart failure and posttransplant (heart) patients. J Am Coll Cardiol 2000;36:509–16.

27 Kemna MS, Valantine HA, Hunt SA, Schroeder JS, Chen Y-DI, Reaven GM. Metabolic risk factors for atherosclerosis in heart transplant recipients. Am Heart J 1994;128:68–72.

28 Kapadia SR, Nissen SE, Ziada KM *et al.* Impact of lipid abnormalities in development and progression of transplant coronary disease: a serial intravascular ultrasound study. J Am Coll Cardiol 2001;38:206–13.

29 Kato T, Chan MCY, Gao S-Z *et al.* Glucose intolerance, as reflected by hemoglobin A1c level, is associated with the incidence and severity of transplant coronary disease. J Am Coll Cardiol 2004;43:1034–41.

30 Senechal M, Lemieux I, Beucler I *et al.* Features of the metabolic syndrome of "hypertriglyceridemic waist" and transplant coronary disease. J Heart Lung Transplant 2005;24:819–26.

31 Stoica SC, Cafferty F, Pauriah M *et al.* The cumulative effect of acute rejection on development of cardiac allograft vasculopathy. J Heart Lung Transplant 2006;25:420–5.

32 Benza RL, Grenett HE, Bourge RC *et al.* Gene polymorphisms for plasminogen activator inhibitor-1/tissue plasminogen activator and development of allograft coronary artery disease. Circulation 1998;98:2248–54.

33 Valentine H, Rickenbacker P, Kemna M *et al.* Metabolic abnormalities characteristic of dysmetabolic syndrome predict the development of transplant coronary artery disease. Circulation 2001;103:2144–52.

34 Lindenfeld J, Miller GG, Shakar SF *et al.* Drug therapy in the heart transplant recipient. Circulation. Part I: 2004;110:3734–40. Part II: 2004;110:3858–65.

35 Ferraro P, Carrier M, White M, Pelletier GB, Pelletier LC. Antithymocyte globulin and methotrexate therapy of severe or persistent cardiac allograft rejection. Ann Thorac Surg 1995;60:372–6.

36 Partanen J, Nieminen MS, Krogerus L, Harjula ALJ, Mattila S. Heart transplant rejection treated with plasmapheresis. J Heart Lung Transplant 1992;11:301–5.

37 Ratkovec RM, Hammond EH, O'Connell JB *et al.* Outcome of cardiac transplant recipients with a positive donor-specific crossmatch—preliminary results with plasmapheresis. Transplantation 1992;54:651–5.

38 Kobashigawa JA. Statins as immunosuppressive agents. Liver Transplant 2001;7:559–61.

39 Kobashigawa JA, Katznelson S, Laks H *et al.* Effect of pravastatin on outcomes after cardiac transplantation. N Engl J Med 1995;333:621–7.

40 Kobashigawa JA, Moriguchi JD, Laks H *et al.* Ten-year follow-up of a randomized trial of pravastatin in heart transplant patients. J Heart Lung Transplant 2005; 24:1736–40.

41 Wenke K, Meiser B, Thiery J *et al.* Simvastatin reduces graft vessel disease and mortality after heart transplantation—a four year randomized trial. Circulation 1997;96:1398–402.

42 Mehra MR, Uber PA, Vivekananthan K *et al.* Comparative beneficial effects of simvastatin and pravastatin in cardiac allograft rejection and survival. J Am Coll Cardiol 2002;40:1609–14.

43 Weis M, Pehlivanli S, Meiser BM, von Scheidt W. Simvastatin treatment is associated with improvement in coronary endothelial function and decreased cytokine activation in patients after heart transplantation. J Am Coll Cardiol 2001;38:814–8.

44 Cotts WG, Johnson MR. The challenge of rejection and cardiac allograft vasculopathy. Heart Failure Rev 2001;6:227–40.

45 Mehra MR, Ventura HO, Smart FW, Stapleton DD. Impact of converting enzyme inhibitors and calcium entry blockers in cardiac allograft vasculopathy. J Heart Lung Transplant 1995;14:S246–9.

46 Erinc K, Yamani MH, Starling RC *et al.* The effect of combined angiotensin-converting enzyme inhibition and calcium antagonism on cardiac allograft vasculopathy validated by intravascular ultrasound. J Heart Lung Transplant 2005;24:1033–8.

47 Kobashigawa JA, Meiser BM. Review of major clinical trials with mycophenolate mofetil in cardiac transplantation. Transplantation 2005;80:S235–43.

48 Kobashigawa J, Miller J, Renlund D *et al.* A randomized active-controlled trial of mycophenolate mofetil in heart transplant recipients. Transplantation 1998;66: 507–15.

49 Pethig K, Heublein B, Wahlers T, Dannenberg O, Oppelt P, Haverich A. Mycophenolate mofetil for secondary prevention of cardiac allograft vasculopathy: influence on

inflammation and progression of intimal hyperplasia. J Heart Lung Transplant 2004;23:61–6.

50 El-Sayed O, Magorien RD, Orsini A, Ferketich AK, Leier CV. Advancing immunosuppression therapy to counter the progression of cardiac allograft vasculopathy. J Cardiac Failure 2005;11:137–41.

51 Kaczmarek I, Ertl B, Schmauss D et al. Preventing cardiac allograft vasculopathy: long-term beneficial effects of mycophenolate mofetil. J Heart Lung Transplant 2006;25:550–6.

52 Rose ML, Smith J, Dureau G, Keogh A, Kobashigawa J. Mycophenolate mofetil decreases antibody production after cardiac transplantation. J Heart Lung Transplant 2002;21:282–5.

53 Ruygrok PN, Webber B, Faddy S, Muller DW, Keogh A. Angiographic regression of cardiac vasculopathy after introducing sirolimus immunosuppression. J Heart Lung Transplant 2003;22:1276–9.

54 Keogh A, Richardson M, Ruygrok P et al. Sirolimus in de novo heart transplant recipients reduces acute rejection and prevents coronary disease at 2 years: a randomized clinical trial. Circulation 2004;110:2694–700.

55 Mancini D, Pinney S, Burkhoff D et al. Use of rapamycin slows progression of cardiac transplantation vasculopathy. Circulation 2003;108:48–53.

56 Eisen HJ, Tuzcu EM, Dorent R et al. Everolimus for the prevention of allograft rejection and vasculopathy in cardiac-transplant recipients. N Engl J Med 2003;349:847–58.

57 Klaus V, Koning A, Spes C et al. Cyclosporine versus tacrolimus (FK 506) for prevention of cardiac allograft vasculopathy. Am J Cardiol 2000;85:266–9.

58 Kobashigawa JA, Patel J, Furukawa H et al. Five-year results of a randomized, single-center study of tacrolimus vs microemulsion cyclosporine in heart transplant patients. J Heart Lung Transplant 2006;25:434–9.

59 Ballester M, Obrador D, Carrio I et al. Reversal of rejection-induced coronary vasculitis detected early after heart transplantation with increased immunosuppression. J Heart Lung Transplant 1989;8:413–7.

60 Lamich R, Ballester M, Marti V et al. Efficacy of augmented immunosuppressive therapy for early vasculopathy in heart transplantation. J Am Coll Cardiol 1998;32:413–9.

61 Pelletier MP, Coady MA, Macha M, Oyer PE, Robbins RC. Coronary atherosclerosis in cardiac transplant patients treated with total lymphoid irradiation. J Heart Lung Transplant 2003;22:124–9.

62 Hershberger RE, Starling RC, Eisen HJ et al. Daclizumab to prevent rejection after cardiac transplantation. N Engl J Med 2005;352:2705–13.

63 Han WR, Zhan Y, Murray-Segal LJ, Brady JL, Lew AM, Mottram PL. Prolonged allograft survival in anti-CD4 antibody transgenic mice: lack of residual helper T cells compared with other CD4-deficient mice. Transplantation 2000;70:168–74.

64 Szeto WY, Krasinskas AM, Kreisel D, Krupnick AS, Popma SH, Rosengard BR. Depletion of recipient CD4+ but not CD8+ T lymphocytes prevents the development of cardiac allograft vasculopathy. Transplantation 2002;73:1116–22.

65 Wang CY, Mazer SP, Minamoto K et al. Suppression of murine cardiac allograft arteriopathy by long-term blockade of CD40-CD154 interactions. Circulation 2002;105:1609–14.

66 Uehara S, Chase CM, Colvin RB, Russell PS, Madsen JC. Further evidence that NK cells may contribute to the development of cardiac allograft vasculopathy. Transplant Proc 2005;37:70–1.

67 Ternstrom L, Jeppsson A, Ricksen A, Nilsson F. Tumor necrosis factor gene polymorphism and cardiac allograft vasculopathy. J Heart Lung Transplant 2005;24:433–8.

68 Koglin J, Glysing-Jensen T, Gadiraju S, Russell ME. Attenuated cardiac allograft vasculopathy in mice with targeted deletion of the transcription factor STAT4. Circulation 2000;101:1034–9.

CHAPTER 26

Role of oral pathogens in the pathogenesis of coronary heart disease

Palle Holmstrup

Background

Characteristics of periodontal disease

Because other chronic infectious diseases, including respiratory infection with *Chlamydia pneumoniae*, have been associated with the pathogenesis of coronary heart disease (CHD), much attention has recently been paid to a possible similar role of chronic oral infection in the form of periodontitis, often denoted periodontal disease (PD). However, it has to be considered that even though almost all the scientific results in this area have been established in the past decade, why much work is ahead of us before we can reach a detailed understanding and draw a firm conclusion on the relation between CHD and PD.

PD is one of the most common chronic infectious diseases caused by bacteria. The infection takes place in an anatomically unique area as being the only site in the body where nonvascularized hard tissue penetrates an outer surface covered by epithelium. The special demands for protection against microbial invasion are taken care of by a junctional epithelium attached to the tooth surface. This epithelium, in the healthy condition, seals the borderline between soft and hard tissue (Figure 26.1a). However, in the case of inflammation the epithelial structure is completely changed and as a consequence the sealing is broken. This is one of the problems behind the general health threat of the patient involved.

Since the oral cavity harbors more than 600 microbial species, there is always an infectious pressure on the area, but in case of sufficient oral hygiene, the infectious capacity is usually handled by a slight, local inflammatory infiltration and a flow of neutrophils through the junctional epithelium. If insufficient oral hygiene allows bacterial accumulation on the dental surface, the flow of neutrophils increases and a more substantial inflammatory infiltrate builds up in the area, including the presence of macrophages and lymphocytes. In this situation, clinical signs of inflammation are visible in the form of manifest gingivitis (Figure 26.1b). Without intervention, the bacteria cause breakdown of the junctional epithelial attachment, thereby creating a deepened gingival pocket. Inflammatory edema further adds to the deepening pocket. This pocket hosts numerous bacteria on the dental surface, and if not removed, the accumulating bacteria become members of an increasingly complex biofilm formation. The inflammatory response to these bacteria, which in the case of manifest PD are dominated by Gram-negative anaerobic rods, results in breakdown of connective tissue and tooth-supporting bone (Figure 26.1c). One of the clinical features associated with the disease activity is a continuing deepening of the gingival pocket, and if not treated, the tooth may become loosened and even lost, as the supporting tissue degrades while the biofilm formation in the pocket further migrates along the root surface devoid of connective tissue attachment.

It must be emphasized that the susceptibility to periodontal tissue destruction shows considerable interindividual variation, the vast majority of patients developing a chronic form of disease with

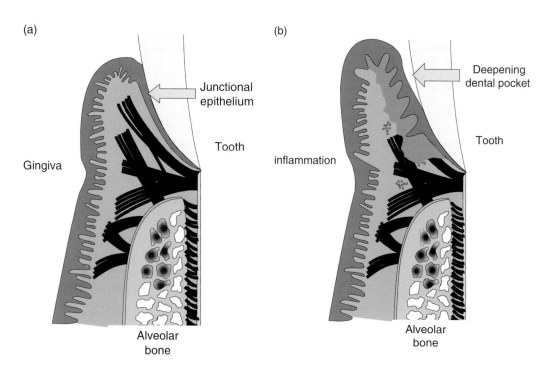

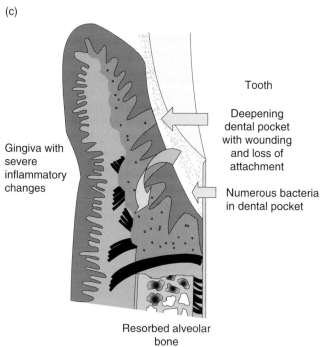

Figure 26.1 The development from healthy periodontium to periodontitis.

slight to moderate destruction while others suffer an aggressive form with rapid deterioration [1]. Presumably, this variation in disease susceptibility is due to interindividual variation of the immune response to the offending microorganisms.

An important aspect of the disease process is that persistent periodontal inflammation results in ulceration of the epithelial lining of the gingival pocket, which thereby becomes a port of entry for the bacteria present. To further understand the possible consequences of this condition, it must be considered that whereas the area of the pocket epithelium without periodontitis has been estimated to be 5 cm^2, the same area with periodontitis has been estimated to be 10–20 cm^2 due to deepening of the pockets [2].

The ongoing inflammatory process is characterized by increasing accumulation of neutrophils and macrophages. In addition, whereas the initial lesion harbors T lymphocytes, the advanced stage demonstrates a shift toward dominance of plasma cells. Not surprising, a result of their activity is increased serum levels of antibodies to the bacteria involved in the disease process. Of particular interest, for the interaction between the local periodontal inflammation and other parts of the body, is the resulting production of inflammatory mediators including important cytokines such as IL-1β, IL-6, and TNF-α. The local production of these cytokines may result in spillover to the bloodstream, thereby probably interacting with parts of the body distant from their site of origin, and this, as well as several of the above-mentioned characteristics of the periodontal inflammation, is one of the possible pathways by which PD may be significant for a number of different conditions such as CHD, diabetes, rheumatoid arthritis, and preterm birth.

Epidemiologic evidence of an association of CHD with PD

A large number of epidemiologic studies have focused on an association of CHD with PD, and cumulative evidence supports, but does not prove, a causal association [3]. Since CHD and PD are widespread conditions, an association between them is an important health issue from a preventive point of view [4]. The body of epidemiologic evidence includes longitudinal studies, case-control studies, and cross-sectional studies but due to vari-

ations in study design and measures of exposure and outcome, the results of these studies are not uniform [3, 5]. There are no published randomized clinical trials determining the effect of preventing or treating PD on cardiovascular events, rendering longitudinal studies the best form of currently existing evidence.

The majority of odds ratios (OR) in studies with significant positive results are below 2.0, which indicates low to moderate levels of association. An obvious concern with these studies is the control for confounding factors, which is particularly important when the adjusted associations are in the low to moderate range, indicated by the odds ratio below 2 [3]. However, a recent case-control study including CHD patients and controls without CHD showed an adjusted significant association of severe periodontitis with CHD among individuals younger than 60 years, the odds ratio being as much as 6.6 [4].

Pathogenic considerations

If oral bacteria are involved in the pathogenesis of CHD, a direct and/or an indirect pathway may account for the role of the microorganisms. The direct pathway is characterized by direct interaction of the microorganisms with cells or tissues in the coronary arteries involved in the CHD processes, while the indirect pathway includes interaction of the oral microorganisms with cells producing substances or mediators that may influence the CHD processes.

Direct influence of oral bacteria on CHD

Bacterial transferal to the vessels

There are reasons to assume a direct interaction of oral bacteria in the pathogenesis of CHD. It is beyond doubt that periodontal inflammation facilitates the entrance of oral bacteria into the bloodstream [6]. Due to periodontitis-associated inflammatory changes of the gingival tissue in the dental pocket, including ulcerations of the pocket epithelium, bacteremia may occur, not only as the result of invasive procedures as scaling and probing. Bacteremia may also occur after mastication and oral hygiene procedures [7, 8], and obviously multiple daily bacteremias imply a large microbial burden on the organism due to a cumulative effect [5].

The role of bacteremia, with oral bacteria, may depend on the type of bacteria transferred to the vessels. One of the important pathogens involved in PD is *Porphyromonas gingivalis*, a black-pigmented, anaerobic Gram-negative rod. DNA traces of this microorganism have been revealed in coronary and carotid atheromas [9], whereas viable organisms so far have been shown indirectly, only in one study after transferal from atheromatous tissue to endothelial cells in vitro [10, 11].

DNA traces of other bacteria, considered important in the pathogenesis of PD, have also been revealed, including *Prevotella intermedia, Actinobacillus actinomycetemcomitans, Treponema denticola, Tannerella forsythensis*, and *Prevotella nigrescens* [10, 12, 13].

It is possible that the mechanisms by which different microorganisms may interact with the atheromatous process vary. In case of bacteremia, activation of the coagulation system may account for serious consequences of CHD and stroke. Moreover, in the long-lasting atherosclerosis process, infection may have harmful, profound, and long-term effects on the arterial cell wall structure and function, lipid metabolism, and systemic inflammatory reactions [14].

Activation of the coagulation system

Interaction of oral bacteria with platelets may be an issue of significance for acute myocardial infarction, but is also important for tissues outside their site of origin, if it results in transferal of a thrombus to other organs by the blood stream. By direct interaction, *P. gingivalis* may induce thrombus formation through aggregation of platelets [15]. Platelets may also interact with supragingival plaque bacteria such as *Streptococcus sanguis*. Strains of these bacteria appear to bind selectively to platelets that result in thrombus formation [16]. Furthermore, experimental studies in rabbits treated with intravenous infusions of platelet-aggregating strains of *S. sanguis* showed larger heart valve vegetations, more signs of myocardial ischemia, and higher mortality than did injection of non-platelet-aggregating strains of *S. sanguis* [17]. Increased platelet aggregation in response to *S. sanguis* infusion was found in rabbits that were fed a high-fat diet [18].

Change of cells, wall structure, and function

A potential role for oral bacteria in several steps of atheroma formation has been demonstrated. Like *C. pneumoniae*, bacteria considered important for the pathogenesis of PD have demonstrated an ability to infect and replicate in coronary artery endothelial and smooth muscle cells in vitro. These bacteria include *Eikenella corrodens, P. gingivalis, and P. intermedia* [19]. Moreover, repeated intravenously injected *P. gingivalis* in apolipoprotein E-deficient mice have resulted in more advanced and earlier atherosclerotic macrophage-rich lesions of aorta and aortic trees than in controls [20]. Pigs fed a low- or a high-fat chow have also provided evidence that intravenously injected *P. gingivalis* are capable of inducing increased coronary and aortic atherosclerosis [21].

Several parts of the immune response have been demonstrated to be involved in the atherosclerotic process accelerated by oral bacteria. A closer simulation of the in vivo periodontitis situation by oral inoculation of *P. gingivalis* in apolipoprotein E-deficient mice resulted in exacerbation of the early stages of atherosclerosis and elevated levels of IL-6. Increased aortic expression of vascular cell adhesion molecule-1 and tissue factor antigen is indicative of a direct activation of signal transduction pathways linked to a proinflammatory response [22]. In concert with these findings, IL-1, TNF-α, and also *P. gingivalis*-induced endothelial upregulation of both vascular cell adhesion molecule-1 and intercellular adhesion molecule-1 have been demonstrated [23]. Also, innate immune recognition of invasive *P. gingivalis* has been demonstrated to accelerate atherosclerosis in apolipoprotein E-deficient mice with upregulation of toll-like receptor (TLR)-2 and TLR-4 [24]. Interestingly, the study demonstrated that immunization with *P. gingivalis* before oral challenge prevented *P. gingivalis*-accelerated atherosclerosis.

Impaired endothelial functions may be an early sign in the pathogenesis of atherosclerosis. Further knowledge of PD-associated bacterial influence on the endothelial lining comes from clinical studies of the patients with chronic PD that have revealed endothelial dysfunction based on recording of brachial artery responses to reactive hyperemia (endothelium-dependent dilatation) and sublingual nitroglycerin (endothelium-independent dilatation). An association of endothelial dysfunction with PD was further evidenced by improvement of endothelial function after periodontal treatment [25–27].

Atherosclerosis is initiated by accumulation of cholesterol in the arterial wall—a process in which macrophages play a central role, characterized by their accumulation of excess cholesterol in the form of lipid droplets, resulting in foam cell formation [28]. Thus, foam cells can affect the stability of the atheromatous plaque and lead to its rupture and following coronary thrombosis [29]. In this context it is important that *P. gingivalis*, its outer membrane vesicles as well as its lipopolysaccharide in the presence of human low-density lipoprotein (LDL), induced foam cell formation of murine macrophages in vitro. Increased doses of *P. gingivalis* resulted in higher levels of foam cell formation. Consequently, *P. gingivalis*, or its vesicles released into the circulation from sites with PD, may deliver virulence factors to the arterial wall to initiate or promote foam cell formation in macrophages, and thereby contribute to the development of atheromas [30, 31]. The significance of *P. gingivalis* for lipid accumulation in the aorta has been further explored in New Zealand white rabbits, in which lipid accumulation correlated with the severity of PD, which had been induced by it [32].

For the above processes to run as a part of early atheroma formation, recruitment of monocytes to the endothelial lining of blood vessels is important [33]. A possible role for *P. gingivalis* in this recruitment process has been suggested because it was able to induce monocyte chemoattractant protein-1 secretion of human umbilical vein endothelial cells in vitro [30].

Taken together, the experimental studies are all indicative of bacteremia with the periodontitis-associated bacteria *P. gingivalis*, resulting in activation and profound changes of the endothelial lining of the arteries to which the bacteria are distributed. Moreover, through oral and intravenous administration, the bacteria are able to accelerate the development of atherosclerosis, a process in which several parts of the immune system are taking part.

Indirect influence of oral bacteria on CHD

Lipid metabolism

A key role of serum lipid levels as a CHD risk factor is well established, and it is interesting that studies have demonstrated significant impact of PD on serum lipid metabolism. Dysregulation of serum lipid metabolism may be due to release of cytokines such as IL-1 and TNF-α from inflamed periodontal tissue. In the PD patients, total cholesterol was raised 8%, LDL 13%, and triglycerides were raised 39% [34]. In a number of additional cross-sectional studies, PD was also associated with elevated levels of total cholesterol, LDL, and triglycerides as well as decreased levels of high-density lipoprotein (HDL) [34–38].

Furthermore, a study including periodontal treatment indicated that periodontitis may diminish the antiatherogenic potency of HDL and thereby increase the risk for CHD; moreover, this influence may be reversed after periodontal treatment [39].

Systemic inflammatory reactions

There are several ways by which periodontal inflammation may interfere with the process of atheroma formation. PD is mirrored in the bloodstream by increased systemic markers of inflammation, including fibrinogen and C-reactive protein (CRP) [40–42], and, importantly, periodontal treatment reduces the level of CRP [43–45]. As elevated fibrinogen and CRP is associated with increased risk of CHD [46–48], these acute phase proteins might associate the two diseases.

Persistent elevated levels of serum IgA antibodies to the important periodontal pathogens, *P. gingivalis*, and *A. actinomycetemcomitans* are able to predict cardiovascular disease incidence [39, 49, 50], thereby supporting a link between CHD and periodontal infection with these microorganisms. The systemic inflammatory reactants mentioned may be induced by spillover of inflammatory mediators, such as IL-1β and TNF-α, from inflamed periodontal lesions to the bloodstream.

Another indirect pathogenic role of periodontal bacteria might be due to the influx of inflammatory cells into large blood vessels in response to Gram-negative bacteria or their products, for instance, lipopolysaccharides, in the blood stream. The

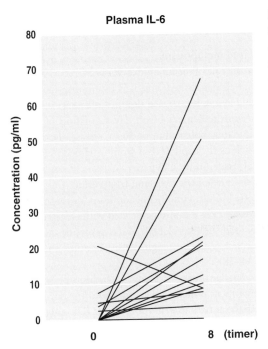

Figure 26.2 Plasma levels of IL-6 at baseline and 8 hours after bacteremia due to scaling ($n = 13$). (From [7].)

resulting synthesis of cytokines, prostaglandins, and growth factors including platelet-derived growth factor, fibroblast growth factor, and granulocyte macrophage colony stimulating factor may contribute to thickening of the arterial wall because several of these substances are atherogenic [51]. That such a mechanism may be acting was demonstrated in a recent study showing significantly elevated plasma levels of IL-6 as the result of bacteremia after scaling [7] (Figure 26.2).

Studies have demonstrated that the immune response to heat shock protein 60 (HSP60) may be involved in the pathogenesis of both atherosclerosis and PD. A recent study has suggested an autoimmune or cross-reactive CD4(+) class-II-restricted T-cell response to the human, 60 kDa, HSP60 in both PD and CHD. The study, which also investigated the expression of TLR-2 and TLR-4, further showed that TLR-4 was recognized by microbial HSP65. The authors concluded that further studies are warranted to determine if there is a common epitope within HSP60 that stimulates T-cell proliferation in both PD and CHD [52], and whether this mode of common reaction to HSP60 is an essential

link between the two diseases. Another study has shown that the antibody levels to both human and *P. gingivalis* HSP60s were the highest in atherosclerosis patients, followed by PD patients and healthy controls. Clonal analysis of the T cells revealed both human HSP60- and *P. gingivalis* HSP60-reactive T-cell populations in the circulation of patients with atherosclerosis. Also, the HSP60-reactive T cells seemed to be present in some atherosclerosis lesions, thereby suggesting that T-cell clones with the same specificity might be involved in the pathogenesis of PD and atherosclerosis [53].

The inflammatory response to a microbial challenge has been shown to possess considerable interindividual variation. Some patients respond to periodontal bacteria or their products with an inflammatory reaction, resulting in high levels of inflammatory mediators [54–56], and such a reaction may account for the rapid periodontal tissue destruction characteristic of aggressive PD. Because cytokines appear to be important for the pathogenesis of both atherosclerosis and PD, a specific phenotype characterized by high production of certain cytokines may link a risk for destructive PD and CHD, although such a background is not evidenced [5].

Conclusion

Although a possible association between PD and CHD has first been scientifically focused upon in the past decade, clinical and, in particular, several experimental studies mainly on the influence of periodontitis-associated bacteria suggest that a causal relationship between these two diseases is likely. Furthermore, as previously suggested [14] and based on the findings mentioned here, it is tempting to hypothesize that periodontal and probably other infections might explain a number of poorly understood risk factors for infarction and atherosclerosis, such as leukocytosis, hyperfibrinogenemia, hypertriglyceridemia, low HDL level, and anti-heat shock proteins, all well known sequelae of infection.

Most of the experimental studies reviewed here have dealt with the effect of the PD-associated pathogen *P. gingivalis* on the development of atherosclerosis. The crucial evidence of a causal relationship, however, needs a randomized clinical trial of long duration, involving a large number of patients, several interventions, and plenty of measured parameters—a demand which is hard to believe ever established. Until then we are referred to further unravel the processes involved in the pathogenesis of both diseases and their interactions. These studies must also include other microorganisms associated with PD.

At this point, much of the growing evidence of a causal relationship is established through experimental animal research, and although most studies do confirm the existence of PD-associated mechanisms enhancing atherosclerosis, these studies may not in detail reflect the human situation—why we are forced to be cautious in extrapolating the results to humans.

References

1 Armitage GC. Development of a classification system for periodontal diseases and conditions. Ann Periodontol 1999;4:1–6.

2 Hujoel PP, White BA, Garcia RI, Listgarten MA. The dentogingival epithelial surface area revisited. J Periodontal Res 2001;36:48–55.

3 Beck JD, Offenbacher S. Systemic effects of periodontitis: epidemiology of periodontal disease and cardiovascular disease. J Periodontol 2005;76(11 suppl):2089–2100.

4 Geismar K, Stoltze K, Sigurd B, Gyntelberg F, Holmstrup P. Periodontal disease and coronary heart disease. J Periodontol 2006;77:1547–54.

5 Holmstrup P, Poulsen AH, Andersen L, Skuldbol T, Fiehn NE. Oral infections and systemic diseases. Dent Clin North Am 2003;47:575–98.

6 Silver JG, Martin AW, McBride BC. Experimental transient bacteraemias in human subjects with varying degrees of plaque accumulation and gingival inflammation. J Clin Periodontol 1977;4:92–9.

7 Forner L, Nielsen CH, Bendtzen K, Larsen T, Holmstrup P. Increased plasma levels of IL-6 in bacteremic periodontis patients after scaling. J Clin Periodontol 2006;33:724–9.

8 Guntheroth WG. How important are dental procedures as a cause of infective endocarditis? Am J Cardiol 1984;54:797–801.

9 Chiu B. Multiple infections in carotid atherosclerotic plaques. Am Heart J 1999;138(5, pt 2):S534–6.

10 Fiehn NE, Larsen T, Christiansen N, Holmstrup P, Schroeder TV. Identification of periodontal pathogens in atherosclerotic vessels. J Periodontol 2005;76:731–6.

11 Kozarov EV, Dorn BR, Shelburne CE, Dunn WA, Jr, Progulske-Fox A. Human atherosclerotic plaque contains viable invasive *Actinobacillus actinomycetemcomitans* and *Porphyromonas gingivalis*. Arterioscler Thromb Vasc Biol 2005;25:e17–8.

12 Haraszthy VI, Zambon JJ, Trevisan M, Zeid M, Genco RJ. Identification of periodontal pathogens in atheromatous plaques. J Periodontol 2000;71:1554–60.

13 Mastragelopulos N, Haraszthy VI, Zambon JJ, Zafiropoulos GG. Detection of periodontal pathogenic microorganisms in atheromatous plaque. Preliminary results. Chirurg 2002;73:585–91.

14 Valtonen VV. Role of infections in atherosclerosis [review]. Am Heart J 1999;138(5, pt 2):S431–3.

15 Emrich LJ, Shlossman M, Genco RJ. Periodontal disease in non-insulin-dependent diabetes mellitus. J Periodontol 1991;62:123–31.

16 Herzberg MC, Brintzenhofe KL, Clawson CC. Aggregation of human platelets and adhesion of *Streptococcus sanguis*. Infect Immun 1983;39:1457–69.

17 Herzberg MC, MacFarlane GD, Gong K *et al.* The platelet interactivity phenotype of *Streptococcus sanguis* influences the course of experimental endocarditis. Infect Immun 1992;60:4809–18.

18 Herzberg MC, Meyer MW. Effects of oral flora on platelets: possible consequences in cardiovascular disease. J Periodontol 1996;67:1138–42.

19 Dorn BR, Dunn WA, Jr, Progulske-Fox A. Invasion of human coronary artery cells by periodontal pathogens. Infect Immun 1999;67:5792–8.

20 Li L, Messas E, Batista EL, Jr, Levine RA, Amar S. *Porphyromonas gingivalis* infection accelerates the progression of atherosclerosis in a heterozygous apolipoprotein E-deficient murine model. Circulation 2002;105:861–7.

21 Brodala N, Merricks EP, Bellinger DA *et al.* *Porphyromonas gingivalis* bacteremia induces coronary and aortic atherosclerosis in normocholesterolemic and hypercholesterolemic pigs. Arterioscler Thromb Vasc Biol 2005;25:1446–51.

22 Lalla E, Lamster IB, Hofmann MA *et al.* Oral infection with a periodontal pathogen accelerates early atherosclerosis in apolipoprotein E-null mice. Arterioscler Thromb Vasc Biol 2003;23:1405–11.

23 Honda T, Oda T, Yoshie H, Yamazaki K. Effects of *Porphyromonas gingivalis* antigens and proinflammatory cytokines on human coronary artery endothelial cells. Oral Microbiol Immunol 2005;20:82–8.

24 Gibson FC III, Hong C, Chou HH *et al.* Innate immune recognition of invasive bacteria accelerates atherosclerosis in apolipoprotein E-deficient mice. Circulation 2004;109:2801–6.

25 Amar S, Gokce N, Morgan S, Loukideli M, Van Dyke TE, Vita JA. Periodontal disease is associated with brachial

artery endothelial dysfunction and systemic inflammation. Arterioscler Thromb Vasc Biol 2003;23:1245–9.

26 Mercanoglu F, Erdogan D, Oflaz H et al. Impaired brachial endothelial function in patients with primary anti-phospholipid syndrome. Int J Clin Pract 2004;58: 1003–7.

27 Radnai M, Gorzo I, Urban E, Eller J, Novak T, Pal A. Possible association between mother's periodontal status and preterm delivery. J Clin Periodontol 2006;33: 791–6.

28 Brown MS, Goldstein JL. Lipoprotein metabolism in the macrophage: implications for cholesterol deposition in atherosclerosis. Annu Rev Biochem 1983;52: 223–61.

29 Libby P, Geng YJ, Aikawa M et al. Macrophages and atherosclerotic plaque stability. Curr Opin Lipidol 1996; 7:330–5.

30 Kuramitsu HK, Kang IC, Qi M. Interactions of Porphyromonas gingivalis with host cells: implications for cardiovascular diseases. J Periodontol 2003;74:85–9.

31 Qi M, Miyakawa H, Kuramitsu HK. Porphyromonas gingivalis induces murine macrophage foam cell formation. Microb Pathog 2003;35:259–67.

32 Jain A, Batista EL, Jr, Serhan C, Stahl GL, Van Dyke TE. Role for periodontitis in the progression of lipid deposition in an animal model. Infect Immun 2003;71: 6012–8.

33 Ross R. Atherosclerosis—an inflammatory disease. N Engl J Med 1999;340:115–26.

34 Losche W, Karapetow F, Pohl A, Pohl C, Kocher T. Plasma lipid and blood glucose levels in patients with destructive periodontal disease. J Clin Periodontol 2000;27: 537–41.

35 Buhlin K, Gustafsson A, Pockley AG, Frostegard J, Klinge B. Risk factors for cardiovascular disease in patients with periodontitis. Eur Heart J 2003;24:2099–107.

36 Craig RG, Yip JK, So MK, Boylan RJ, Socransky SS, Haffajee AD. Relationship of destructive periodontal disease to the acute-phase response. J Periodontol 2003;74: 1007–16.

37 Cutler CW, Shinedling EA, Nunn M et al. Association between periodontitis and hyperlipidemia: cause or effect? J Periodontol 1999;70:1429–34.

38 Katz J, Flugelman MY, Goldberg A, Heft M. Association between periodontal pockets and elevated cholesterol and low density lipoprotein cholesterol levels. J Periodontol 2002;73:494–500.

39 Pussinen PJ, Jousilahti P, Alfthan G, Palosuo T, Asikainen S, Salomaa V. Antibodies to periodontal pathogens are associated with coronary heart disease. Arterioscler Thromb Vasc Biol 2003;23:1250–4.

40 Ebersole JL, Machen RL, Steffen MJ, Willmann DE. Systemic acute-phase reactants, C-reactive protein and

haptoglobin, in adult periodontitis. Clin Exp Immunol 1997;107:347–52.

41 Pederson ED, Stanke SR, Whitener SJ, Sebastiani PT, Lamberts BL, Turner DW. Salivary levels of alpha 2-macroglobulin, alpha 1-antitrypsin, C-reactive protein, cathepsin G and elastase in humans with or without destructive periodontal disease. Arch Oral Biol 1995; 40:1151–5.

42 Shklair IL, Loving RH, Leberman OF, Rau CF. C-reactive protein and periodontal disease. J Periodontol 1968;39:93–5.

43 Glurich I, Grossi S, Albini B et al. Systemic inflammation in cardiovascular and periodontal disease: comparative study. Clin Diagn Lab Immunol 2002;9:425–32.

44 Iwamoto Y, Nishimura F, Soga Y et al. Antimicrobial periodontal treatment decreases serum C-reactive protein, tumor necrosis factor-alpha, but not adiponectin levels in patients with chronic periodontitis. J Periodontol 2003;74:1231–6.

45 Mattila KJ, Asikainen S, Wolf J, Jousimies-Somer H, Valtonen V, Nieminen M. Age, dental infections, and coronary heart disease. J Dent Res 2000;79:756–60.

46 Danesh J, Collins R, Appleby P, Peto R. Association of fibrinogen, C-reactive protein, albumin, or leukocyte count with coronary heart disease: meta-analyses of prospective studies. JAMA 1998;279:1477–82.

47 Koenig W, Sund M, Frohlich M et al. C-reactive protein, a sensitive marker of inflammation, predicts future risk of coronary heart disease in initially healthy middle-aged men: results from the MONICA (monitoring trends and determinants in cardiovascular disease) Augsburg cohort study, 1984 to 1992. Circulation 1999;99: 237–42.

48 Ridker PM, Buring JE, Shih J, Matias M, Hennekens CH. Prospective study of C-reactive protein and the risk of future cardiovascular events among apparently healthy women. Circulation 1998;98:731–3.

49 Pussinen PJ, Alfthan G, Tuomilehto J, Asikainen S, Jousilahti P. High serum antibody levels to Porphyromonas gingivalis predict myocardial infarction. Eur J Cardiovasc Prev Rehabil 2004;11:408–11.

50 Pussinen PJ, Nyyssonen K, Alfthan G, Salonen R, Laukkanen JA, Salonen JT. Serum antibody levels to Actinobacillus actinomycetemcomitans predict the risk for coronary heart disease. Arterioscler Thromb Vasc Biol 2005; 25:833–8.

51 Marcus AJ, Hajjar DP. Vascular transcellular signaling. J Lipid Res 1993;34:2017–31.

52 Hasan A, Sadoh D, Palmer R, Foo M, Marber M, Lehner T. The immune responses to human and microbial heat shock proteins in periodontal disease with and without coronary heart disease. Clin Exp Immunol 2005;142:585–94.

53 Yamazaki K, Ohsawa Y, Itoh H *et al.* T-cell clonality to *Porphyromonas gingivalis* and human heat shock protein 60s in patients with atherosclerosis and periodontitis. Oral Microbiol Immunol 2004;19:160–7.

54 Hernichel-Gorbach E, Kornman KS, Holt SC *et al.* Host responses in patients with generalized refractory periodontitis. J Periodontol 1994;65:8–16.

55 Kornman KS, Crane A, Wang HY *et al.* The interleukin-1 genotype as a severity factor in adult periodontal disease. J Clin Periodontol 1997;24:72–7.

56 Shapira L, Soskolne WA, Sela MN, Offenbacher S, Barak V. The secretion of PGE2, IL-1 beta, IL-6, and TNF alpha by adherent mononuclear cells from early onset periodontitis patients. J Periodontol 1994;65:139–46.

CHAPTER 27

Myocardial regenerative potential by stem cell transplant

Yinhong Chen, Catherine A. Priest & Joseph D. Gold

Introduction

Cell therapy, particularly that aimed at the treatment of cardiovascular disease, has progressed rapidly over the past 10 years. Multiple cell types and mixed populations of cells have been successfully transplanted in both preclinical animal models and clinical trials. Ideally, transplanted cells would form new functional myocardium to replace damaged heart tissue, although improvements in the contractility of myocardium could also be caused by other mechanisms such as increased perfusion of the damaged heart tissue.

To date, cell types used for transplantation in animal models of heart disease include autologous skeletal myoblasts (SM), blood-borne stem cells, intrinsic cardiac stem cells, fetal and embryonic cardiomyocytes, and embryonic stem (ES) cell derived cardiac cells. Many studies have shown some improvement in cardiac function, although the mechanism of improvement is not always clear. Despite these encouraging results, important challenges continue to confront investigators seeking the best therapeutic cell type. To be considered successful at repairing damaged heart tissue, the implanted cells should meet four major criteria: (1) to be able to form new cardiomyocytes; (2) to engraft into the recipient myocardium and survive for a prolonged time; (3) to form electromechanical connections with host cardiomyocytes to allow synchronous contraction; and (4) to produce stable, safe improvement in heart function. In this chapter, we will attempt to compare the myocardial regenerative potential of various cell sources, assess methods to improve cell survival in vivo, and discuss strategies to avoid host rejec-

tion. We focus on cells that are under investigation as sources of new myocardium, as opposed to cells such as bone marrow stem cells that are in clinical trials but are not thought to produce new cardiomyocytes [1].

Cell types for myocardial regeneration

Autologous skeletal myoblasts

SMs were the first cell type to be used in clinical trials attempting myocardial regeneration. Over the past 10 years, more than 40 studies have been performed that have demonstrated improvement in left ventricular (LV) function after autologous SM transplant. Menasche *et al.* [2] first demonstrated that SMs engrafted into myocardial scars enhanced both global and regional LV function. The transplanted SMs did not differentiate into cardiomyocytes but formed multinucleated, cross-striated myofibers that expressed fast skeletal myosin heavy chain (MHC) proteins, indicating a mature skeletal muscle phenotype. Grafts never expressed the intercalated disk protein N-cadherin or the gap junction protein connexin 43. Electromechanical coupling with neighboring myocardial cells did not occur [3], and there was increased risk for arrhythmogenesis. Their initial 10-patient phase I trial established the feasibility of the procedure and identified ventricular arrhythmias as potential adverse events of SM grafting. The trial also suggested that most of the myocardial scarred segments into which cells were grafted improved their contractility. This finding was deemed encouraging enough to justify the implementation of a large 300-patient

Table 27.1 Myocardial regenerative capacity of various stem cell populations.

Cell type	Sources	Markers	Engraftment and differentiation into cardiomyocytes	Express gap junctional proteins	Improve heart function
SMs [2, 3]	Muscle	Myogenic factor D (MyoD+), skeletal MHC+, α-MHC–, cardiac troponin I–, atrial natriuretic peptide–	Engraft, but do not differentiate into cardiomyocytes	No	Yes
BMDCs/ circulating stem cells [1, 5–9]	Bone marrow, cord blood, peripheral blood	CD34+, CD133+, c-kit+, Sca-1+	Short-term engraftment; little evidence for de novo cardiomyocyte formation	Unknown	Yes, short term
Intrinsic cardiac stem cells [10–12, 14]	Heart	c-Kit+, Abcg-2, Sca-1+, isl1	Engraft and differentiate into small cardiomyocytes	Yes, but electrical coupling with host myocardium unknown	Yes
Fetal or neonatal cardiomyocytes [15, 16]	Fetal or neonatal heart	MF20+, α-MHC+	Engraft as cardiomyocytes	Yes, electrically couple with host myocardium	Yes
ES-derived cardiomyocytes [32–34, 39]	In vitro cell cultures	Nkx2.5+, TnI+, β-MHC, atrial natriuretic peptide–	Long-term engraftment as cardiomyocytes	Yes, electrically couple with host myocardium	Yes

multicenter randomized efficacy trial named MAGIC (an acronym for myoblast autologous grafting ischemic cardiomyopathy) in which all the patients undergoing cardiac SM transplant received defibrillators [4]. However, this phase II study was halted after less than one-third of the patients were enrolled due to lower than predicted efficacy (http://www.bioheartinc.com/evt0406_coronay_dib), see Table 28.1.

Bone marrow-derived cells

Bone marrow derived cells (BMDCs) are a mixed population including hematopoietic, endothelial progenitor, and mesenchymal cells. There is controversy over the fate of the transplanted cells; most of the experiments have demonstrated that the frequency with which transplanted BMDCs differ-

entiate into heart muscle is negligible [1, 5]. A recent study indicated that the BMDCs were not reprogrammed and did not differentiate into cardiomyocytes but rather fused with surviving host-derived cardiomyocytes [6]. However, numerous clinical trials reported to date have described nearly identical results 4–6 months after BMDC transplantation, including a 7–9% improvement in global LV ejection fraction, significantly reduced end-systolic LV volumes, and improved perfusion in the infarcted area. In these independent clinical trials, a wide range of nonmyogenic BMDCs (28–2460 million) improved ventricular function [5], suggesting that benefit may result, in part, from mechanisms that are distinct from true myocardial regeneration. One possible mechanism of cardiac improvement in these studies may involve the secretion of paracrine factors that are cardioprotective or angiogenic [7].

Cord blood-derived cells

Umbilical cord blood contains mononuclear progenitor cells with high potential for self-renewal and differentiation. Several groups [8, 9] have shown that umbilical cord blood cells (UCBCs) could migrate into, colonize, and survive in the myocardium of infarcted animals. The administration of UCBCs substantially reduces infarct size in rats or mice without requirement for immunosuppression. The LV ejection fraction, wall thickening, and dP/dt are significantly greater in the infarcted animals that received UCBCs transplant compared to vehicle. However, the cardiac improvement appears to be due to UCBC-facilitated revascularization rather than cardiac regeneration.

Cardiac stem cells

Several different populations of intrinsic cardiac progenitor cells (CPs) exist in mouse, rat, and human hearts, including cells that are characterized by the expression of c-kit [10], Sca-1 [11], or Abcg-2 [12]. These CP populations are claimed to be distinct from one another. c-kit+ CPs are frequently found in clusters with a prevalence of approximately 1/104 mature myocytes. They are self-renewing, clonogenic, and multipotent. After injection into acutely ischemic hearts, these cells differentiate into myocytes, with characteristics of immature cardiomyocytes, and form new coronary blood vessels. In one study, ventricular function was reported to be improved significantly [10]. A second group of CPs expressing Sca-1 [11] can be induced to activate myocyte-specific gene expression in vitro. When injected intravenously into mice with myocardial infarctions, approximately half of the engrafted cells fused with host myocytes and the other half differentiated into troponin I+ and sarcomeric actinin+ myocytes. Functional effects, electrical coupling to neighboring myocytes, or capacity for cell expansion for therapeutic purposes [11] were not reported. A third class of CPs that express Abcg-2 [12] was detected as a side population in fluorescence-activated cell sorting (FACS) analysis, because of Hoechst dye efflux. These cells express the cardiogenic transcription factor MEF2. When cocultured with cardiac cells, some of the Abcg-2+ CPs began to express sarcomeric α-actinin. The cardiac regenerative potential of Abcg-2+ CPs in vivo has not been reported. Overall, an accurate and extensive comparison of these cells with regard to their characteristics and myocardiogenic potential remains to be done.

A fourth class of CPs expresses the LIM-homeodomain transcription factor islet-1 (isl1). Knock-out of isl1 leads to the absence of the atria, entire aorta and pulmonary artery, and entire right ventricle (RV) while sparing the LV [13]. Lineage-tracing experiments during heart development demonstrate that isl1+ progenitors contribute to cardiac myocyte, smooth muscle, and endothelial cell lineages. Laugwitz [14] has identified isl1+ cardiac progenitors in postnatal rat, mouse, and human hearts. Coculture studies with neonatal mouse myocytes indicate that isl1+ cells represent authentic, endogenous CPs that display high-efficiency (25%) conversion to a mature cardiac phenotype in vitro with stable expression of multiple myocytic markers, gap junctions, intact calcium cycling, and the generation of action potentials. The discovery of isl1+ undifferentiated cardiac progenitors encourages efforts to explore whether these cells can be myocardiogenic in vivo after transplantation into injured hearts. However, the acquisition of sufficient isl1+ CPs remains a challenge. More studies are required to determine whether intrinsic CPs are suitable for the large scale-up required for therapeutic purposes or if they may be sufficient only to replace the slow cardiac cell loss that occurs throughout the lifetime of the healthy organ.

Cardiac myocytes are, theoretically, the best candidate cell population to repair the damaged heart. Studies using fetal [15] and neonatal cardiomyocytes [16] in animal models of myocardial infarction or cryoinjury have shown reduced scar expansion and improved function because of the ability of the immature cells to divide and become mature functional cardiomyocytes. However, because fetal and neonatal cardiomyocytes have a limited ability to enter the cell cycle, obtaining adequate cell numbers for transplantation represents both major practical and ethical challenges.

Embryonic stem cell-derived cardiomyocytes

Optimal future therapies to repair damaged myocardium require cells that not only generate bona fide cardiomyocytes but can also be produced in sufficient quantities to treat over half a million patients a year in the United States alone (http://www.americanheart.org/presenter.jhtml?identifier=1486). ES cells derived from the inner cell mass of blastocysts have the capacity for indefinite self-renewal and the ability to undergo differentiation [17, 18] to generate numerous cell types, including cardiomyocytes [17, 19].

In 1985, Doetschman [20] first established a protocol to maintain pluripotent mouse ES (mES) cells in vitro by culturing these cells on primary fibroblast feeder layers and supplementation of the culture medium with leukemia inhibitory factor. When placed in suspension culture, these mES cells form three-dimensional aggregates (embryoid bodies) that produce multiple differentiated cell types, including spontaneously beating cardiomyocytes. In 1996, Klug *et al.* [21] generated mES cells that were stably transfected with a fusion gene consisting of the α-cardiac MHC promoter driving a cDNA encoding aminoglycoside phosphotransferase. After in vitro differentiation in the presence of geneticin, cultures that consisted of more than 99% pure cardiomyocytes were generated. These beating cardiomyocytes could be maintained for as long as 11 months. The development of more selective and efficient methods for differentiating mES cells into cardiomyocytes progressed steadily in the late 1990s, using a variety of factors. Many investigators [22–24] showed that mES-derived cardiomyocytes not only express cardiac genes but also exhibit electrophysiological and contractile phenotypes in vitro. In the mid-1990s, mES cells and mES-derived cardiomyocytes were transplanted into experimental animal models of cardiovascular disease [25]. Some groups implanted undifferentiated mES cells into rodent hearts and reported a sustained improvement of contractile function without the formation of teratomas [26, 27]; other investigators [28] found that undifferentiated mES cells form intracardiac teratomas after implantation into the hearts of syngeneic or immunotolerant rodents. Menard *et al.* [29] briefly treated mES cells with bone morphogenetic protein 2 to form "genetically selective cardiac-committed" cells and transplanted these cells (a total of 30×10^6) into infarcted sheep myocardium at 25 separate injection sites. Immunolabeling with mouse-specific β-MHC, which is considered an early cardiac cell marker, revealed that 22% of the scar area was occupied by mouse-cell-derived cardiomyocytes. These cardiomyocytes, which had apparently undergone significant in vivo differentiation after injection, exhibited well-organized sarcomeres and expressed the gap junction protein connexin 43, without evidence of cell fusion. More importantly, these cardiac-committed mouse cells improved LV function without formation of teratomas and without cellular rejection, even in nonimmunosuppressed sheep. This result provided the necessary proof of concept for implanting ES-derived cardiomyocytes to restore injured myocardium. The optimal degree of differentiation prior to transplantation and the necessary purity of the implanted cells required to avoid an unacceptable risk of teratoma formation were not explored in these studies.

In 1998, human ES (hES) cells were isolated by Thomson *et al.* [30]. Like the original mES derivations, the hES cells were initially maintained in the undifferentiated state by culture on mouse embryonic feeder layers. In early hES studies, cardiomyocytes were induced by the generation of embryoid bodies [19]. In 2001, scientists at Geron Corporation described a feeder-free system for culturing hES cells that maintained the potential of these cells to differentiate into beating cardiomyocytes [31]. The differentiated cultures could be enzymatically dissociated and enriched by Percoll density centrifugation to give a cell population that was enriched for cardiomyocytes [32]. Cells isolated from spontaneously beating areas of the culture display the structural, molecular, electrophysiological, and contractile properties of early-stage cardiomyocytes. In contrast to mES-derived cardiomyocytes, hES-derived cardiomyocytes display substantial proliferative activity, as evidenced by expression of cell cycle markers such as Ki-67, incorporation of bromo-deoxyuridine, and the frequent appearance of mitotic figures [33, 34]. However, the frequency of cardiomyocyte generation by the embryoid body method is low, and the use of animal serum (typically 20% fetal calf serum) in this process presents significant barriers to clinical use of these cells. Importantly, for future clinical use, undifferentiated hES cells are capable of maintenance and expansion in defined nonconditioned medium supplemented with growth factors [35]. After long-term culture in defined nonconditioned medium, these cells show appropriate expression of undifferentiated cell markers and maintain a normal karyotype. In addition, a method has been developed that allows the highly efficient generation of cardiomyocytes from hES cells in the absence of embryoid body formation or animal serum by the sequential application of activin A and bone morphogenetic protein 4 to monolayer cultures of undifferentiated cells [36, 37]. This method substantially increases cardiac cell differentiation and yields cardiomyocytes at an efficiency of up to 80% of total cells, without further purification. These cells express cardiac transcription factors, sarcomeric proteins and gap junctional components, manifest spontaneous contractility, demonstrate appropriate electrophysiological properties, and can be cryopreserved. These findings will permit large-scale production of hES-derived cardiomyocytes for clinical cell-based cardiac therapy.

Despite the limitations imposed by the embryoid body protocol, in vivo studies with hES-derived cardiomyocytes have been performed that show encouraging results. In 2004, Kehat et al. [38] reported that transplanted hES-derived cardiomyocytes could pace the left ventricle in swine with a complete heart block. In 2005, Laflamme et al. [33] utilized hES-derived cardiomyocytes enriched from embryoid bodies by Percoll fractionation. These cells were exposed to heat shock at 43°C for 30 minutes, 1 day prior to transplantation into the uninjured hearts of nude rats. By 4-weeks post-transplantation, grafts consisted predominantly of cardiomyocytes, expressing cardiac markers including β-MHC, myosin light chain 2v, and atrial natriuretic factor. No teratomas were observed. Heat shock improved graft size approximately threefold compared to grafts generated from cells that did not receive this treatment, suggesting that additional interventions to increase cell survival may be advantageous. Indeed, Laflamme et al. [39] have reported that additional treatments that suppress apoptosis and necrosis in the cell grafts greatly enhance survival of the transplanted cells and result in functional improvements in rat models of heart disease.

In light of improvements in the culture of undifferentiated hES cells, simplified and enhanced cardiomyocyte differentiation by these cells, and encouraging preliminary data from human ES-derived cardiomyocytes in preclinical models, these cells provide an attractive candidate for cardiovascular cell therapy.

Challenges for clinical application

Cardiac cell survival in vivo

One major hurdle that must be overcome for successful cardiac cell therapy with any cell source is to address the current low survival rate of transplanted cells. Watanabe et al. [40] found that fetal and neonatal pig cardiomyocytes and the cardiac-derived cell line HL-1 did not survive after grafting into infarcted pig myocardium. Other studies have found that engrafted cells are detected at very low frequencies in recipient animals [41–45], regardless of the cell source. Some of these studies indicated that less than 10% of transplanted cells were found in the myocardium within the first week after administration [44, 45]. Cell loss has been estimated at multiple times after transplantation. In one study [45], fewer than 25% of neonatal rat cardiomyocytes could be detected 1 day after transplantation, and at 12 weeks, fewer than 15% of the transplanted cells were identified. A similar study [44] measured the occurrence of apoptotic cells after grafting into injured or normal myocardium. In cryoinjured tissue, as many as 32% of the grafted cells were apoptotic on the first day after transplant; however, the frequency of cellular apoptosis was much lower after grafting into uninjured tissue.

Collectively, these findings suggest that the massive loss of transplanted cells, which is seen after transplant, appears to be attributable to multiple sources: cell retention in the syringe used for injection, leakage from injection sites in the initial stage, and subsequent cell apoptosis, necrotic cell death, and gradual cell loss due to the ischemic environment and host inflammatory response. Alternatively, other groups have demonstrated that cell transplantation improved short-term heart function without evidence of long-term transplanted cell survival [5]. Obviously, there is much room for improvement. Progress has been made in enhancement of cell retention, development of antiapoptotic strategies, and promotion of angiogenesis [7, 39, 46]. Hypoxia-regulated heme oxygenase-1, AKT (a serine threonine kinase), and heat shock treatment have enhanced the survival of different cell types, following administration into hearts with acute myocardial infarct [7, 39, 44, 46, 47]. Interestingly, heat shock at 43°C for 30 minutes dramatically decreased apoptosis by 54%, 1 day after transplant of neonatal cardiomyocytes [44]. The combination of angiogenic and antiapoptotic agents such as vascular endothelial growth factor and insulin-like growth factor I also increased graft cell survival [48]. Revascularization of the damaged tissue prior to cell transplant in the infarcted myocardium or incorporation of endothelial cells into the graft may be worthwhile strategies to improve the efficiency of cell-based therapy in ischemic heart disease.

Immunogenicity of stem cells

hES cells not only hold promise as an unlimited cell source for therapeutic transplantation but also display immune "privilege," suggesting that they may escape immunorejection following transplantation. hES cells express low levels of MHC-I molecules that moderately increase as the cells differentiate [49, 50]. In addition, hES cells and their differentiated progeny did not express MHC-II proteins or costimulatory molecules, and ligands for natural killer (NK) cell receptors were either absent or expressed at very low levels. When hES cells were incubated with NK cells, only limited killing by the NK cells was observed [50]. Fandrich *et al.* [51] have shown that when early isolates from rat blastocysts that resembled rat ES cells were injected intraportally into fully MHC-mismatched rats, the injected cells established partial hematopoietic chimerism and promoted long-term acceptance (> 150 days) of cardiac allografts from the same strain used to derive the rat ES-like cells without supplementary host conditioning. However, the in vivo immunogenicity of the ES cells is controversial. Some groups [28, 50, 52] have reported that MHC-I expression was significantly increased as mES and hES cells differentiated in vivo. For example, in one study, allogeneic mES

cell transplantation triggered the infiltration of T-lymphocytes and dendritic cells into the infarcted myocardium of the recipient mouse [52].

Although hES cells and their differentiated derivatives may display immunogenic profiles that are weaker than adult-derived cells, the potential for immunorejection cannot be ignored in clinical applications. Initial applications of hES-derived cardiomyocytes in the clinic will likely require conventional immunosuppressive drug regimens. Other strategies to overcome immune rejection may include establishing immunocompatible banks of hES cells that include common histocompatibility profiles, engineering a "universal cell line" that will not elicit a host response, and/or inducing immunotolerance by administering "tolerizing cells" such as immature dendritic cells derived from the same hES cell line prior to transplantation of hES-derived cardiomyocytes [53]. For individual patients, somatic cell nuclear transfer to human eggs and development of immunologically matched cell lines has been proposed as a way of generating histocompatible stem cells for the treatment of cardiac diseases [54]. The feasibility of this patient-specific approach is, however, unknown as bona fide hES lines derived from nuclear transfer have not yet been demonstrated and both the time and economics involved in generating individualized cell lines as well as differentiated cardiomyocyte preparations for individual patients may prove daunting.

Conclusion

The ultimate goal of cardiac cell-based therapy is an unlimited source of myocardiogenic cells that can regenerate and repair heart tissue. While other cell types are under evaluation, the collective data suggest that hES-derived cardiomyocytes present an attractive cell source. Large-scale production of cardiomyocytes derived from hES cells under good manufacturing practice standards appears feasible, and the engraftment of cardiomyocytes derived from hES cells after direct injection into the myocardium has been demonstrated in multiple species [33, 36, 38]. However, the extent of long-term functional improvement in various disease models must be demonstrated. One of the major challenges for cardiac cell-based therapy, regardless of the cell source, will be the development of strategies to enhance transplanted cell survival and engraftment through induction of angiogenesis and the prevention of apoptotic, necrotic, and immune-mediated cell death.

References

1 Laflamme MA, Murry CE. Regenerating the heart. Nat Biotechnol 2005;23(7):845–56.

2 Menasche P, Hagege A, Scorsin M *et al.* Autologous skeletal myoblast transplantation for cardiac insufficiency. First clinical case. Arch Mal Coeur Vaiss 2001;94(3): 180–2.

3 Reinecke H, Poppa V, Murry CE. Skeletal muscle stem cells do not transdifferentiate into cardiomyocytes after cardiac grafting. J Mol Cell Cardiol 2002;34(2):241–9.

4 Menasche P. Myoblast transfer in heart failure. Surg Clin North Am 2004;84(1):125–39.

5 Dimmeler S, Zeiher AM, Schneider MD. Unchain my heart: the scientific foundations of cardiac repair. J Clin Invest 2005;115(3):572–83.

6 Lapidos KA, Chen YE, Earley JU *et al.* Transplanted hematopoietic stem cells demonstrate impaired sarcoglycan expression after engraftment into cardiac and skeletal muscle. J Clin Invest 2004;114(11):1577–85.

7 Mangi AA, Noiseux N, Kong D *et al.* Mesenchymal stem cells modified with Akt prevent remodeling and restore performance of infarcted hearts. Nat Med 2003;9(9):1195–201.

8 Ma N, Ladilov Y, Kaminski A *et al.* Umbilical cord blood cell transplantation for myocardial regeneration. Transplant Proc 2006;38:771–3.

9 Henning RJ, Abu-Ali H, Balis JU, Morgan MB, Willing AE, Sanberg PR. Human umbilical cord blood mononuclear cells for the treatment of acute myocardial infarction. Cell Transplant 2004;13:729–39.

10 Beltrami AP, Barlucchi L, Torella D *et al.* Adult cardiac stem cells are multipotent and support myocardial regeneration. Cell 2003;114(6):763–76.

11 Oh H, Bradfute SB, Gallardo TD *et al.* Cardiac progenitor cells from adult myocardium: homing, differentiation, and fusion after infarction. Proc Natl Acad Sci U S A 2003;100(21):12313–8.

12 Martin CM, Meeson AP, Robertson SM *et al.* Persistent expression of the ATP-binding cassette transporter, Abcg2, identifies cardiac SP cells in the developing and adult heart. Dev Biol 2004;265(1):262–75.

13 Cai CL, Liang X, Shi Y *et al.* Isl1 identifies a cardiac progenitor population that proliferates prior to differentiation and contributes a majority of cells to the heart. Dev Cell 2003;5(6):877–89.

14 Laugwitz KL, Moretti A, Lam J *et al.* Postnatal isl1+ cardioblasts enter fully differentiated cardiomyocyte lineages. Nature 2005;433(7026):647–53.

15 Roell W, Lu ZJ, Bloch W *et al.* Cellular cardiomyoplasty improves survival after myocardial injury. Circulation 2002;105(20):2435–41.

16 Muller-Ehmsen J, Peterson KL, Kedes L *et al.* Rebuilding a damaged heart: long-term survival of transplanted neonatal rat cardiomyocytes after myocardial infarction and effect on cardiac function. Circulation 2002;105(14):1720–6.

17 Itskovitz-Eldor J, Schuldiner M, Karsenti D *et al.* Differentiation of human embryonic stem cells into embryoid bodies compromising the three embryonic germ layers. Mol Med 2000;6(2):88–95.

18 Amit M, Carpenter MK, Inokuma MS *et al.* Clonally derived human embryonic stem cell lines maintain pluripotency and proliferative potential for prolonged periods of culture. Dev Biol 2000;227(2):271–8.

19 Kehat I, Kenyagin-Karsenti D, Snir M *et al.* Human embryonic stem cells can differentiate into myocytes with structural and functional properties of cardiomyocytes. J Clin Invest 2001;108(3):407–14.

20 Doetschman TC, Eistetter H, Katz M, Schmidt W, Kemler R. The in vitro development of blastocyst-derived embryonic stem cell lines: formation of visceral yolk sac, blood islands and myocardium. J Embryol Exp Morphol 1985;87:27–45.

21 Klug MG, Soonpaa MH, Koh GY, Field LJ. Genetically selected cardiomyocytes from differentiating embryonic stem cells form stable intracardiac grafts. J Clin Invest 1996;98(1):216–24.

22 Muller M, Fleischmann BK, Selbert S *et al.* Selection of ventricular-like cardiomyocytes from ES cells in vitro. FASEB J 2000;14(15):2540–8.

23 Maltsev VA, Wobus AM, Rohwedel J, Bader M, Hescheler J. Cardiomyocytes differentiated in vitro from embryonic stem cells developmentally express cardiac-specific genes and ionic currents. Circ Res 1994;75(2):233–44.

24 Fijnvandraat AC, van Ginneken AC, de Boer PA *et al.* Cardiomyocytes derived from embryonic stem cells resemble cardiomyocytes of the embryonic heart tube. Cardiovasc Res 2003;58(2):399–409.

25 Dinsmore J, Ratliff J, Deacon T *et al.* Embryonic stem cells differentiated in vitro as a novel source of cells for transplantation. Cell Transplant 1996;5(2):131–43.

26 Min JY, Yang Y, Converso KL *et al.* Transplantation of embryonic stem cells improves cardiac function in postinfarcted rats. J Appl Physiol 2002;92(1):288–96.

27 Hodgson DM, Behfar A, Zingman LV *et al.* Stable benefit of embryonic stem cell therapy in myocardial infarction. Am J Physiol Heart Circ Physiol 2004;287(2): H471–9.

28 Swijnenburg RJ, Tanaka M, Vogel H *et al.* Embryonic stem cell immunogenicity increases upon differentiation after transplantation into ischemic myocardium. Circulation 2005;112(9 suppl):I166–72.

29 Menard C, Hagege AA, Agbulut O *et al.* Transplantation of cardiac-committed mouse embryonic stem cells to infarcted sheep myocardium: a preclinical study. Lancet 2005;366(9490):1005–12.

30 Thomson JA, Itskovitz-Eldor J, Shapiro SS *et al.* Embryonic stem cell lines derived from human blastocysts. Science 1998;282(5391):1145–7.

31 Xu C, Inokuma MS, Denham J *et al.* Feeder-free growth of undifferentiated human embryonic stem cells. Nat Biotechnol 2001;19(10):971–4.

32 Xu C, Police S, Rao N, Carpenter MK. Characterization and enrichment of cardiomyocytes derived from human embryonic stem cells. Circ Res 2002;91(6):501–8.

33 Laflamme MA, Gold J, Xu C *et al.* Formation of human myocardium in the rat heart from human embryonic stem cells. Am J Pathol 2005;167(3):663–71.

34 Snir M, Kehat I, Gepstein A *et al.* Assessment of the ultrastructural and proliferative properties of human embryonic stem cell-derived cardiomyocytes. Am J Physiol Heart Circ Physiol 2003;285(6):H2355–63.

35 Xu C, Rosler E, Jiang J *et al.* Basic fibroblast growth factor supports undifferentiated human embryonic stem cell growth without conditioned medium. Stem Cells 2005;23(3):315–23.

36 Gold J, Hassanipour M, Police S *et al.* Directed differentiation of cardiomyocytes from human embryonic stem cells: characterization and transplantation. In: *Abstract, 4th ISSCR Annual Meeting*, Toronto, Canada, 2006: 59.

37 Xu C, Police S, Hassanipour M *et al.* Human embryonic stem cells maintained in non-conditioned medium have capacity to differentiate into cardiomyocytes: progress towards the clinic. In: *Abstract, 4th ISSCR Annual Meeting*, Toronto, Canada, 2006:236.

38 Kehat I, Khimovich L, Caspi O *et al.* Electromechanical integration of cardiomyocytes derived from human embryonic stem cells. Nat Biotechnol 2004;22(10):1282–9.

39 Laflamme MA, Gold J, Xu C *et al.* Combinatorial anti-death cocktail improves survival of engrafted human embryonic stem cell derived cardiomyocytes within infarcted hearts. In: *Abstract, Molecular Mechanisms of Cardiac Disease and Regeneration, Keystone Symposium*, Sante Fe, NM, 2006:59.

40 Watanabe E, Smith DM, Jr, Delcarpio JB *et al.* Cardiomyocyte transplantation in a porcine myocardial infarction model. Cell Transplant 1998;7(3):239–46.

41 Scorsin M, Hagege AA, Dolizy I *et al.* Can cellular transplantation improve function in doxorubicin-induced heart failure? Circulation 1998;98(19suppl):II151–5; discussion II155–6.

42 Toma C, Pittenger MF, Cahill KS, Byrne BJ, Kessler PD. Human mesenchymal stem cells differentiate to a cardiomyocyte phenotype in the adult murine heart. Circulation 2002;105(1):93–8.

43 Taylor DA, Atkins BZ, Hungspreugs P *et al.* Regenerating functional myocardium: improved performance after skeletal myoblast transplantation. Nat Med 1998;4(8):929–33.

44 Zhang M, Methot D, Poppa V, Fujio Y, Walsh K, Murry CE. Cardiomyocyte grafting for cardiac repair: graft cell death and anti-death strategies. J Mol Cell Cardiol 2001;33(5):907–21.

45 Muller-Ehmsen J, Whittaker P, Kloner RA *et al.* Survival and development of neonatal rat cardiomyocytes transplanted into adult myocardium. J Mol Cell Cardiol 2002;34(2):107–16.

46 Reinecke H, Zhang M, Bartosek T, Murry CE. Survival, integration, and differentiation of cardiomyocyte grafts: a study in normal and injured rat hearts. Circulation 1999;100:193–202.

47 Tang YL, Tang Y, Zhang YC, Qian K, Shen L, Phillips MI. Improved graft mesenchymal stem cell survival in ischemic heart with a hypoxia-regulated heme oxygenase-1 vector. J Am Coll Cardiol 2005;46(7):1339–50.

48 Yau TM, Kim C, Li G, Zhang Y, Weisel RD, Li RK. Maximizing ventricular function with multimodal cell-based gene therapy. Circulation 2005;112(9 suppl):I123–8.

49 Draper JS, Pigott C, Thomson JA, Andrews PW. Surface antigens of human embryonic stem cells: changes upon differentiation in culture. J Anat 2002;200:249–58.

50 Drukker M, Katz G, Urbach A *et al.* Characterization of the expression of MHC proteins in human embryonic stem cells. Proc Natl Acad Sci U S A 2002;99(15):9864–9.

51 Fandrich F, Lin X, Chai GX *et al.* Preimplantation-stage stem cells induce long-term allogeneic graft acceptance without supplementary host conditioning. Nat Med 2002;8(2):171–8.

52 Kofidis T, deBruin JL, Tanaka M *et al.* They are not stealthy in the heart: embryonic stem cells trigger cell infiltration, humoral and T-lymphocyte-based host immune response. Eur J Cardiothorac Surg 2005;28(3):461–6.

53 Fairchild PJ, Cartland S, Nolan KF, Waldmann H. Embryonic stem cells and the challenge of transplantation tolerance. Trends Immunol 2004;25(9):465–70.

54 Wakayama T. On the road to therapeutic cloning. Nat Biotechnol 2004;22(4):399–400.

CHAPTER 28

Bioflavanoids and dietary anti-inflammatory actions: role in cardiovascular diseases

Simin Bolourchi-Vaghefi & Amy Galena

Introduction

Inflammation as a cause of cardiovascular disease

World Health Organization reported that about 80% of cardiovascular deaths occurred in low to middle income countries of the world in 2001, and by 2010, heart disease will be the leading cause of death in developing countries [1]. In the United States, the cost of heart disease and stroke was estimated to exceed $394.00 billion by 2005 [2]. Lifestyle factors including fat content and composition of diet (saturated and trans fats), percent of body fat, lack of exercise, obesity, hypertension, smoking, and stress are known to elevate total blood cholesterol, low-density lipoprotein (LDL), and tri-acylglycerol. These factors have been extensively researched and reported as predisposing and/or causing atherosclerosis and cardiovascular disease (CVD).

Researchers are now concentrating on inflammatory factors that initiate injuries and damage to the endothelial tissues, causing accumulation of oxidized-LDL-loaded monocytes proliferating endothelial tissues of the arteries resulting in plaques and fatty streaks. Thus, inflammation-related contributing factors are recognized as underlying cause of CVD. Atherosclerosis, a metabolic disease of nutritional origin, plays a main role in the development of CVD. Inflammation occurs during every stage of atherosclerosis, reduction of which reduces the risk of the disease. Many pathophysiological factors may increase inflammation in the arteries.

Oxidized lipoproteins, dyslipidemia, hypertension, diabetes, obesity, and infection are a few examples [3].

The inflammation markers like C-reactive protein (CRP) can predict incidences of CVD better than serum cholesterol levels or LDLs [4] can. In this chapter, the effects of above risk factors on CVD and dietary factors that may prevent damage to the circulatory system will be considered. The nutrients and non-nutrient dietary agents that protect against CVD by modifying or preventing the risk factors are also discussed.

Dietary factors as causes of inflammatory damage in cardiovascular diseases

Dietary markers of cardiovascular diseases

Atherosclerosis is an inflammatory disease caused by chronic injury to the endothelial lining of the arteries with inflammatory responses. These injuries may be due to smoking, hypertension, infectious microorganisms, physical injury, reactive oxygen species (ROS), oxidized LDL, or elevated plasma homocysteine. As a result, endothelial tissue becomes more permeable and can attract monocytes and other inflammatory and immune cells. Production of nitric oxide (NO) is reduced by the injured endothelium, causing constriction of blood vessels at the site of plaque formation. The reduced NO production may cause thrombosis. It may also promote adhesion of platelets and leukocytes, compounding the problem. Dietary habits contributing to these risk factors include high-fat diet with a high content of saturated and trans fats, specially in the fast and fried foods, low intakes of fruits, vegetables, olive oil, fish, whole grains, tree nuts, and a high meat and fat consumption.

The factors that cause endothelial dysfunction and inflammation include CRP, interleukin-6 (IL-6), E-selection, and soluble intercellular adhesion molecule-1 [5–8]. Other factors like nuclear factor-κB (NF-κB) released in the cytoplasm by the presence of ROS initiate transcription of genes by the nucleus for cytokines and growth factors, and adhesion molecules also play a role in causing inflammation.

C-reactive protein (CRP)

CRP, an indicator of inflammation, is a better predictor of CVD than LDL cholesterol. It also provides prognostic information for the risk of metabolic syndrome. High-sensitivity assays show that CRP levels of <1, 1–3, and >3 mg/L correlate to low-, moderate-, and high-risk groups, respectively, for potential CVD. A cardiovascular event is most likely to occur among individuals with a high LDL and an elevated CRP. However, a low-LDL cholesterol (below 130 mg/dL) and a CRP level >3 mg/L fall into the high-risk category, indicating a stronger effect of CRP and simpler method to predict occurrence of CVD.

In epidemiological studies, CRP has predicted incidents of myocardial infarction (MI), peripheral arterial disease, sudden cardiac death, and stroke better than those predicted by blood lipid profiles. In stable and unstable angina, patients undergoing angioplasty, and acute coronary syndromes, CRP levels have also predicted risk of both recurrent ischemia and death. CRP is a pentraxin, synthesized in the liver, comprising five 23-kDa subunits with a long half-life. It plays a main role in the inherent immune response and has demonstrated its place as a reliable indicator of atherothrombosis disease. A recent review describes at least 16 studies from the United States and Europe that support the use of CRP as a strong predictor of cardiovascular events. CRP is not affected by risk factors such as age, smoking, cholesterol levels, blood pressure, diabetes, or gender.

CRP could help screen individuals as high-risk, who might benefit from diet and lifestyle changes, and perhaps will be added to the lipid panel in the clinical setting. Even though many diet and lifestyle interventions are known to reduce cardiovascular risk and are linked to a lower CRP, it is not yet proven that reducing CRP will reduce cardiovascular events [4].

Inflammatory responses and role of dietary intervention

Inflammation plays a major role in all stages of atherosclerosis. Inflammation begins with endothelial dysfunction from atherogenic triggers and oxidized LDL, causing amplified expression of atherogenic signal molecules. These include the Vascular Cell Adhesion Molecule-1 (VCAM-1), Monocyte Chemoattractant Protein-1, (MCP-1) growth factors, macrophage colony stimulating factor, interferon γ, InterLeukin-1(λ), IL-1, IL-6, TNF-α. These molecules permit the adhesion of monocytes and T lymphocytes to the arterial endothelium and into the intima. T lymphocytes unite with macrophages in the intima and secrete inflammatory cytokines that may stimulate proliferation of vascular smooth muscle cells that enhance plaque development and thrombogenic potential [9].

Dietary intervention exerts its effect at the cellular level to reduce inflammation and atherosclerosis by inhibiting the synthesis and release of endothelial cell adhesion molecules such as proinflammatory cytokines. Omega-3 fatty acids and their metabolites slow vascular smooth muscle cell proliferation [10]. Moreover, n-3 fatty acids may enhance parasympathetic tone and acetylcholine, the main vagal neurotransmitter, which not only inhibits the release of proinflammatory cytokines, but also stimulates the production of anti-inflammatory cytokine IL-10 [11].

Hyperhomocysteinemia and cardiovascular diseases

Elevated serum levels of homocysteine have been recognized as one of the risk factors for CVD. The level of homocysteine in the blood of patients with MI was shown to be greatly elevated [12]. Although the mechanism of effect of homocysteine is still not elucidated, it is suggested that it may stimulate proliferation of smooth muscle [13], slow endothelial NO activity, interfere with production of endothelial-derived relaxing factor, and induce cardiovascular fibrosis [14, 15]. Deficiencies of three B vitamins folate, B-6, and B-12 can cause mild hyperhomocysteinemia. Severe form of this abnormality is a result of genetic defects in enzymes involved in metabolism of amino acids [16]. Folic acid in the diet or folate supplementation, alone or with B-6 and B-12, may reduce the blood level of homocysteine. Folate is abundant in green leafy vegetables. The Western dietary habits unlike Eastern and Mediterranean's do not encourage consumption of large amounts of green leafy vegetables. However, folate fortification of wheat products in the past few years and including green leafy vegetables in the daily foods can reduce the risk of hyperhomocysteinemia.

Lipids

When consumed in the context of Western dietary habits of high protein, high fat with low intakes of fruits, vegetables, and fiber as well as low levels of physical activity, diets high in saturated fat trans fat and low in mono- and polyunsaturated oils can elevate blood levels of triacylglycerol, LDL, and total cholesterol and lower high-density lipoprotein (HDL). Deficiency of antioxidants and phytochemicals due to low fruits and vegetables intake facilitates LDL oxidation and endothelial infiltration, setting the stage for atherosclerosis. The positive influence of n-3 polyunsaturated fatty acids in reducing inflammation due to the high consumption of fish and olive oil [17] is well studied.

Preventive effects of anti-inflammatory substances in foods

Fruits and vegetables

The antioxidant and anti-inflammatory effects of vitamin C (ascorbic acid) [18], tocopherols (vitamin E), and β-carotenes in fruits and vegetables are well recognized [19]. Adequate intake of vitamin K in green vegetables can be protective against CVD by its role in regulation of blood coagulation [20]. Vitamin D supplement given to patients with congestive heart failure reduced inflammatory cytokine profile. Vitamin D may serve as an

anti-inflammatory agent in this disease [21]. Folate in green leafy vegetables reduces blood homocysteine concentration. Dietary components such as phytochemicals, polyphenols, flavonoids, and alcohol also reduce blood homocysteine.

Fruits and vegetables contain numerous other nutrients and non-nutrient components—some medicinal, some nutritional in nature—that benefit health and prevent diseases. The effects and mechanisms of action of these substances are subject of intensive research at present, and some interesting results are discussed here.

Fruit and vegetable consumption, in many studies, have shown to be inversely related to most risk markers for CVD. Data from the National Heart, Lung, and Blood Institute Family Heart Study show an inverse association of consumption of fruits and vegetables to serum levels of LDL cholesterol in men and women [22]. An inverse association between consumption of fruits and vegetables and risk of CVD and all-cause mortality in the general US population has also been observed [23]. A combination of high intakes of fruits and vegetables and low intake of saturated fat was more protective against coronary heart disease and mortality than the effect of each alone in aging men [24]. Diets high in fruits, vegetables, nuts, whole grains, and fish but moderate in alcohol, with a low ratio of saturated to polyunsaturated and no trans fat, have inverse associations with plasma concentration of markers of inflammation and endothelial dysfunction [25]. Followers of this type of diets are getting more fiber, folate, vitamins, and minerals and are physically more active than population who typically consume Western type diets, high in meat, fat, and fast foods. Moderate alcohol consumption is reported to decrease risk of atherosclerosis. These observations indicate that the components of the food categories in these diets positively influence health of the individual and prevent increased blood concentrations of the risk factors for CVD.

Root and Anderson [26] show that traditional Mediterranean diet can reduce the risk factors of CVD by different nutrients exerting their specific effects, such as (a) moderate alcohol (red wine) may improve endothelial function and lower inflammation, (b) risk of cardiac arrhythmia is reduced by consumption of fish and fish n-3 fatty acids, and (c) monounsaturated fatty acids in those diets may reverse or inhibit blood clothing process. Additionally, these types of diets are very high in fiber, which may reduce the intake of excess calories in the form of fat, trans fat, and sugar. These diets are also very high in antioxidants, phytochemicals, carotenoids, flavonoids, etc., which prevent tissue oxidation and inflammation.

In a study using LDL receptor–/– apolipoprotein B transgenic mice, Adams *et al.* [27] showed that feeding freeze-dried peas, green beans, broccoli, corn, and carrots to mice for 16 weeks reduced incidence of "aortic atherosclerosis, as estimated by cholesterol ester content" 38% as compared with control mice on the regular mice diet. Elevation of other plasma factors identified to cause atherosclerosis was also reduced in vegetable-fed mice. Although the researchers were unable to explain the pathways that affected the results obtained, they believe that this study confirms the fact that the Mediterranean diet (containing 30% green and yellow vegetables) can help prevent atherosclerosis in humans as well.

A fruit- and vegetable-rich Mediterranean diet provides phytochemicals that contain strong antioxidants activities. When used as purified forms, singly or in combinations, α-tocopherol, β-carotene, and vitamin C in clinical research did not provide any protection against CVD. Some of these dietary antioxidants such a γ-tocopherol, however, have shown limited protection by reducing ROS and inactivation of NF-κB. However, lower incidence of atherosclerosis in consumers of Mediterranean diet is a proof that combination of the above nutrients in the diet has preventive effects. The essential polyunsaturated fatty acids, such as n-3 fatty acids, α-linolenic acid, eicosapentaenoic, and docosahexaenoic acid, in spite of being both oxidant and antioxidant, have suppressive response to inflammation [28].

Women either on high intakes of vegetables and fruits (10 servings/day) or on low intakes (<3.5 servings/day) showed a significantly reduced lipid peroxidation, but only high vegetable and fruit intake reduced DNA oxidation in women. The researchers emphasized that the degree of antioxidant activity of plant foods depended on the state of oxidations of serum lipids of participants in the study at the time of participation, which were not uniform in all subjects [29]. Consumption of trans fatty acids by

healthy women has been shown to have positive correlation with systemic inflammatory markers [30].

CRP levels in serum are positively related to most of the known risk factors of CVD such as obesity, physical inactivity, diabetes, smoking, and hormone replacement therapy. The mechanism of action of CRP has not yet been determined. It is evident that both dieting and exercise have strong effect in reducing CRP levels, thus lowering the risk. Inflammation proteins are produced in adipose tissue of obese individuals, cause low-grade systemic inflammation related to C3 concentrations in adolescents, and are related to total and abdominal obesity [31]. With the increased childhood and adolescent obesity, the future risk of increased CVD is certain if obesity trends are not immediately addressed.

Following results indicate the roles of a few individual fruits, showing their anti-inflammatory benefits: supplementation of the diet of men and women with 280 g/day Bing sweet cherries selectively modulated concentrations of CRP, NO, and RANTES. The researchers suggested that cherries have a role in management and prevention of inflammatory disease and by including cherries in the diet, the risk can be reduced [32]. In another study, consumption of cherries marginally decreased CRP and NO, but did not change the TNF-α. It was concluded that "compounds in cherries may inhibit inflammatory pathways" [33].

Pomegranate fruit being a rich source of polyphenolic compounds has a strong antioxidant property. Supplementation of pomegranate juice in apolipoprotein-deficient mice diet reduced their macrophage oxidative stress and cholesterol flux, and delayed the development of atherosclerosis. A tannin fraction isolated from pomegranate juice showed a significant antiatherosclerotic activity [34]. Antioxidant polyphenols of olive oil and red wine in Mediterranean diets, when taken at nutritionally relevant concentrations, have antiatherogenic effect. The phytochemicals in olive oil and red wine were incubated with human umbilical vein endothelial cells for 30 minutes; only oleuropein, hydroxytyrosol, and resveratrol—having antioxidant activity—reduced monocytoid cell adhesion to stimulated endothelium, as well as vascular cell adhesion molecule-1 mRNA and protein. This effect can partially explain atherosclerosis protection by Mediterranean diets [35].

With scientists developing and introducing new genetically engineered functional foods, which improves or increases the nutrient value of foods beneficial to human health [36], CVDs will be prevented more effectively, when these foods get approved for human consumption, since these foods will be higher in nutrients which may help reduce risk factors for elevated markers of tissue inflammation

The antiatherogenic properties of selected food groups are discussed below.

Whole grains

Research data suggest that consumption of three servings of whole grain foods per day reduces the risk of coronary heart disease (CHD) by 20–30%. Whole grain foods contain fiber, vitamins B and E, minerals (calcium, magnesium, potassium, phosphorus, selenium, zinc, and iron), antioxidants, lignans, phytic acid, phenolic acid, and other antioxidants and phytochemicals. Bran and germ of whole grains confer risk reduction benefit in relation to CHD. Jensen *et al.* [37], in following 42,850 male professionals, found an inverse association between whole grain intake and the incidence of CHD. This association became stronger in those who added bran to their whole grain diet. Ajani and coworkers reported similar result from data obtained in National Health and Nutrition Examination Survey (NHANES). Based on data from NHANES 1999–2000 with 3920 subjects, participants with higher consumption of fiber/day had lower concentration of serum CRP [38]. Other investigators have found same inverse associations between intake of fiber and Serum CRP [39].

The mechanism of action of whole grains and bran has not been elucidated, but it is speculated that high fiber in whole grains renders them low-glycemic-index foods, displacing caloric foods, preventing obesity [40] and diabetes [41], and lowers the concentration of blood cholesterol, reducing the incidence of CHD. Whole grain foods are very high in soluble fiber and upon intake increase soluble fiber in the gastrointestinal tract, enough to reduce serum cholesterol levels significantly. They also provide ample amounts of antioxidants, both water- and fat-soluble. All these factors are responsible for lowering risk of CHD [42].

Soy

Consumption of soy products, containing isoflavones is shown to be beneficial in reducing circulating CRP, but is not effective in reducing other biomarkers of inflammation. Soy protein has beneficial effects on endothelial function in postmenopausal women, which is independent of antioxidant effects [43, 44]. Soy isoflavones play a role in reducing hypertension in men and women [45]. The role of soy isoflavones in reducing blood lipoproteins is controversial. It is speculated that the ability to convert soy isoflavones to equol, which is a more potent estrogenic isoflavone, varies among individuals [46] and those who can naturally produce equol can benefit from soy products in reducing their blood lipoproteins and the risk of CVD.

Garlic

Garlic has been recognized as a therapeutic food since the inception of human history. It has been recorded in the Near and Middle Eastern, and African civilization's medical records for the treatment of variety of diseases like heart disease, cancerous tumors, and headache. In the past few decades, scientific interest in the role of garlic in prevention and cure of diseases has been a reason for explosion of research to determine the effective components, active elements, and mode of action of garlic constituents. Some of the proven effects of garlic are inhibition of enzymes involved in lipid synthesis, leading to lowered blood cholesterol, decreasing platelet aggregation, prevention of lipid peroxidation in erythrocytes and LDLs, inhibition of angeotensin-converting enzyme, and increase in antioxidant status.

Garlic contains both fat- and water-soluble sulfur-containing phytochemicals, responsible for its therapeutic and preventive effects. These compounds have antithrombotic, lipid-lowering [47], antioxidation [48], antitumoral [49] properties, and immunomodulatory effects. Garlic constituents can increase T lymphocyte blastogenesis and phagocytosis [50] and modulate cytokine production [51]. S-allylcystein from aged garlic extract (AGE) inhibits NF-κB. [52]. Extracts from dried garlic powder and diallyl disulfide modulate production of IL-1β and TNF-α in human blood by lipopolysaccharide [53]. Yeh and Yeh. [54] showed that AGE reduces the blood levels of homocysteine in rats.

Increase in aortic stiffness due to aging and pressure can be slowed by chronic garlic powder consumption, and elastic properties of aorta in elderly can be protected. It is suggested that active constituents of garlic may activate NO synthesis and thus restore impaired endothelial function [55]. In a group of patients on statin drugs, when AGE was given as an addition to statins, patients showed a significant slowing of calcification of coronary arteries [56]. It is suggested that this effect may be due to overall effect of AGE in reduction of multiple risks involved in progression of CHD. Hyperhomocysteinemia was reduced and endothelial function improved by administration of AGE to the patients [57].

From above evidences it can be concluded that the once culturally accepted benefits of garlic in maintaining health and/or preventing/curing disease have been scientifically proven. In reducing certain risk factors for CVD, garlic and its products can play a helpful role—either alone or as an adjunct to medical and pharmacological treatment of heart diseases.

Tree nuts

Tree nuts, in general, and walnuts, in particular, positively effect prevention of CVD by preventing LDL oxidation [58], in turn, lessening the formation of plaques due to infiltration of the arteries' endothelial cells by foam cells. Containing a high percentage of polyunsaturated fatty acids, mostly linolenic acid (n-3), linoleic acid (n-6), and tocopherols, as well as a high content of fiber and polyphenolic compounds, arginine (lysine/arginine ratio of 0.16), a precursor of NO, folate, and tannins, they have great cardioprotective properties. When they are a part of diet, walnuts reduce serum LDL [59, 60] and increase HDL [61]. Large prospective human studies have demonstrated that daily consumption of small amounts of walnuts results in a dose-response-related inverse association of relative risk of CVD [62]. Tree nuts, being good part of vegetarian and Mediterranean diet, contribute an important health benefit and disease prevention effect to the attributes of those diets.

Grapes and wine polyphenols and their effects in cardiovascular disease

Alcohol

Epidemiologic studies reveal that individuals with moderate wine consumption enjoy significant reductions in all-cause and cardiovascular mortality compared to nondrinkers or excessive drinkers. Moderate ethanol intake improves lipoprotein metabolism and lowers cardiovascular mortality risk [63]. Although the benefits of the polyphenols from fruits and vegetables are increasingly accepted, consensus on wine is developing more slowly. Scientific research has demonstrated that the molecules present in grapes and wine alter cellular metabolism and signaling, thus reducing arterial disease. Is it the alcohol or the phytochemicals in grapes that prevent atherosclerosis is not completely understood. This is a topic of very active research by the investigators.

Polyphenols in grapes: resveratrol

Red wine and red grapes are rich sources of antioxidant polyphenolic compounds. Dietary polyphenolics, with antioxidant activity, play a role in preventing coronary heart disease, inflammation, and mutagenesis leading to carcinogenesis [64]. Grapes, wines, and grape byproducts contain large amounts of polyphenolic compounds, mostly flavonoids, at high concentrations of 1000–1800 mg/L. Their presence and structure are affected by grape variety, sun exposure, vinification techniques, and aging [65].

The majority of grape polyphenols are present in the skins of seeds. Lipoproteins are highly specialized transporters of lipids and lipophilic compounds. Wine influences lipoprotein biology through its ethanol and polyphenol content. Ethanol consumption stimulates hepatic lipogenesis and increases plasma triacylglycerols. Polyphenols prevent platelets aggregation, facilitating the transport of lipoproteins through the bloodstream.

Resveratrol is a nonflavonoid trihydroxystilbene and is a major constituent of a variety of edible plant products, including grapes and peanuts [66]. It can also be found in grape wines as well as in other fruits and vegetables. Given that it is present in grape skins but not in grape flesh, white wine contains small amounts of resveratrol compared to red wine [67]. Wallerath *et al.* [68] incubated human umbilical vein endothelial cells with resveratrol for 24–72 hours and measured endothelial nitric oxide synthase (eNOS). This method was chosen because resveratrol was previously reported to act as an agonist at the estrogen receptor. They discovered that resveratrol can bind to and activate gene transcription by the estrogen receptor subtypes alpha and beta in estrogen-sensitive tissues and cell lines. Resveratrol can stimulate the expression of the *eNOS* gene, leading to an enhanced production of bioactive NO. These effects could contribute to the cardiovascular protection effect of resveratrol. However, Soleas *et al.* showed that tissue resveratrol concentrations after red wine consumption were inadequate to suggest that this single compound was the most important contributor to the physiological effects of red wine [69].

Resveratrol has been found to have anti-inflammatory role, protecting endothelial tissue by interfering with NF-κB signaling pathway, known to regulate the expression of genes responsible for inflammation [70]. Resveratrol also protects against proinflammatory TNF-α, a cytokine modulating endothelial function [71]. Harvard, BIOMOL researchers showed resveratrol to be the most potent molecule that triggers activity of a gene called *SIRT1*, increasing its activity by 13-folds. It was speculated that this benefit derived from activation of *SIR*-like genes. Paganga *et al.* [72] equated the antioxidant activity in 1 glass of red wine (150 ml) to that found in 12 glasses of white wine, 2 cups of tea, 5 apples, 5 100-g portions of onion, 5.5 portions of eggplant, 3.5 glasses of black currant juice, 500 ml of beer, 7 glasses of orange juice, or 20 glasses of apple juice. Red wine is thus a concentrated source of dietary phenolic acids and polyphenols.

Wine polyphenols are clearly capable of interrupting or slowing lipid oxidation in vitro and interrupting autocatalytic chain reactions of polyunsaturated lipids chemically by trapping free radicals as a stable phenoxyl radical. Many of the compounds in wine are redox active, and many are known to slow lipid oxidation in vitro [73]. Some polyphenols exhibit antioxidant and free-radical-scavenging properties. Plaque formation was reduced 30–50% in cholesterol-fed rabbits consuming red wine, red wine solids, or grape proanthocyanidin [74]. In another animal study,

(+)-catechin, the predominant flavanol in red wine, reduced plaque in an atherosclerotic, oophorectomized guinea pig model, when fed in amounts equivalent to the total polyphenols consumed by moderate wine drinkers [75]. These data support the hypothesis that lipoprotein stability is affected by the consumption of polyphenols and that this protection correlates with reduced atherosclerotic plaque in animals.

The solution to the most important question whether wine polyphenols can slow lipid oxidation in vivo was to measure the susceptibility of LDL isolated from subjects before and after the consumption of wine, but results from such studies are highly variable. The approach is currently limited by lipoprotein separation methodologies because phenolic acids and polyphenols are water-soluble and the methods used to isolate LDL invariably remove soluble plasma constituents [76]. The current cautious view among the scientists is that moderate wine consumption is protective against atherosclerosis, so is inclusion of red grapes in the diet.

Flavonoids in cocoa, green tea, black tea, and coffee

Cocoa

Purified cocoa procyanidins, when incubated with human whole blood samples inhibited platelet activation and aggregation. Cocoa flavanols may also affect blood clotting by effecting eicosanoids and synthesis of prostacyclin and leukotriene C4, D4, and E4 that cause inflammation as well as vasoconstriction in endothelial cells [77]. Therefore, it is postulated that consumption of moderate amounts of chocolate can beneficially affect the ratio of eicosanoids that can reduce inflammation and inhibit blood clotting, thus reducing risk of cardiovascular incidences.

Cocoa products containing flavon-3-ols decrease proinflammatory cysteinyl leukotrienes concentration in plasma of human subjects. Sies *et al.* [78] investigated the effects of cocoa polyphenols on inhibition of human 5-lipooxygenase, the key enzyme in synthesis of leukotriene. They proved that (−)-epicatechin and other cocoa flavon-3-ols are inhibitory at the enzyme level, thus conferring antileukotriene action in vivo. In a double-blind crossover study, human subjects received a cocoa beverage containing high and low levels of flavon-3-ols. The NO-dependent, flow-mediated dilution of brachial artery and concentrations of nitroso compounds in plasma were measured. They found that the ingestion of high flavonoids containing cocoa significantly increased plasma concentration of nitroso compounds and flow-mediated dilation of the brachial artery. They concluded that flavonoids, by enhancing the NO bioactivity, may reverse endothelial dysfunction. They believe oxidative modification of LDL to be "crucial for atherogenesis and one of the mediators is the proinflammatory proatherogenic enzyme myeloperoxidase." It was found that (–)-epicatechin or other flavonoids in micromolar concentrations suppress peroxidation of lipids in LDL by myeloperoxidase when physiologically relevant concentration of nitrite, a metabolite of NO, was present. Thus adverse effects of nitrite and peroxynitrite, metabolites of NO, were attenuated.

Tea

(–)-Epigallocatechin gallate and quercetin, flavonoids in green and black tea, are shown to inhibit apoptosis induced by H_2O_2 "through modulating the expression of apoptosis-related Bcl-2 and Bax in endothelial cells." Chio et al. [79] suggested that tea flavonoids (–)-epigallocatechin gallate and quercetin prevent the accumulation of intracellular oxidants and nuclear trans activation of p53 in the cells exposed to H_2O_2, pointing to not only antioxidant nature of these flavonoids but also more complex involvement in survival signaling of the cells. Tea flavones also neutralize NO and peroxynitrite, nitrate tyrosine forming 3-nitrotyrosine which can be found in atherosclerosis lesions. For practical purposes, a cup of tea contains 166–193 mg of a combination of catechins (24–40 mg), flavonols, and flavones (8–15 mg), thearubigins (~80 mg), and theaflavins (7–15 mg) [80].

Coffee

There are conflicting opinions on the effect of coffee on the risk of cardiovascular health. Here, we examined two reports which showed that coffee drinking does increase the risk of CVD. Effect of coffee consumption on biomarkers of inflammation in men and women was investigated by Zampelas et al. [81]. These investigators studied 3042 randomly selected men and women and found that there was linear dose–response relationship between drinking coffee and all inflammatory markers, as compared to non coffee drinkers. Men drinking 200-ml coffee/day showed 30% higher CRP, 50% higher IL-6, 12% higher SAA, and 28% higher TNF-α concentration than those who did not drink coffee. The inflammatory markers in women showed a sharper increase due to coffee drinking. Coffee-drinking men had only 3% higher white blood cell count. White blood cell count was significant when men who drank 400-ml coffee were compared with those who drank no coffee. Vlachopoulos et al. found a linear relation between coffee drinking and aortic stiffness and wave reflection. They suggest that these changes may be due to promotion of inflammation in aortic endothelial wall because of consumption of coffee. Nevertheless, the changes have detrimental effect and increase the risk of CVD [82].

Carotenoids

Lycopene and cardiovascular diseases

Intake of fruits and vegetables may help in reducing CVD by the presence of many protective factors like antioxidants, non-anti-oxidant phytochemicals, carotenoids, fiber, potassium, magnesium, vitamins, and other still to be discovered substances in fruits, specially brilliantly colored ones like berries, tomatoes, melons, citrus fruits, etc. It is generally agreed that consumption of whole foods will be more beneficial than the individual nutrients. Carotenoids are strong antioxidants, providing valuable protection against tissue oxidation at the cellular levels. Lycopene, a carotenoid, was shown to act as a hypocholestrolemic agent in the J774A.1 macrophage cell line by inhibiting HMG-CoA reductase pathway [83]. Rao and Agarwal [84] observe that lycopene is a potent antioxidant that prevents atherogenesis and carcinogenesis by protecting critical molecules such as lipids, LDLs, proteins, and DNA.

In vitro studies have shown that lycopene inactivates hydrogen peroxide, scavenges and deactivates NO, thiyl, and sulphonyl radicals. Being highly lipophilic, lycopene is found within cell membranes and other lipid components of the cell. Thus, it is expected to have maximum ROS scavenging effect in the lipid environment of the cells. It has been shown to have a very high antioxidant effect in protecting

2, 2′-azo-bis (2, 4-dimethylvaleronitrile)-induced lipid peroxidation of the liposomal membrane. Lycopene also protects lymphocytes against NO_2- induced membrane damage and cell death, twice as effectively as β-carotene.

Rissanen et al. [85] showed that when adjusted for energy, nutrients, fiber, folate, vitamins C, E, and β-carotene, lycopene "attenuated the protective effect of intake of fruits, berries, and vegetables against mortality; thus it may be the main protective nutrients in these foods." Accordingly they indicate that energy-adjusted intake of vitamins C and E, folate, and lycopene from fruits, vegetables, and berries is responsible for 28% of protection against all-cause mortality. Intake of folate and vitamins C and E explains 36% protective effect against cardiovascular mortality. They also reported that maximum oxygen uptake by the subjects during the exercise test had a strong correlation with intakes of fruits, berries, and vegetables and that men consuming higher amounts of plant products had a healthier lifestyle and included exercise in their daily life.

Preventive role of lycopene in CVD can be due to the fact that hydrocarbon carotenoids including β-carotene and lycopene are transported by LDL. Therefore, because of the position of these carotenoids in the LDL molecule, they can protect LDL from oxidation [86]. Studies have also shown that adipose tissue concentration of lycopene is associated with protection against MI.

Fuhrman et al. [87] reported the non-antioxidant function of lycopene both in vitro and in vivo in humans. By adding lycopene to macrophage cell lines in vitro, they showed a decrease of 73% in cholesterol synthesis and an increase in LDL receptors. Incubation of cells with lycopene caused 34% increase in degradation of cell LDL and about 110% increase in LDL removal. In a human study with 6 men, they showed 14% reduction in plasma LDL when feeding 60 mg/day of lycopene—equal to the amount of lycopene in 1 kg of tomato/day—without any significant change in plasma HDL concentration in the subjects. They suggested about 30–40% reduction in risk of MI as a result of consuming a high amount of lycopene regularly.

Romanchik et al. [88] enriched LDL samples isolated from serum of 5 subjects, with β-carotene, lycopene, and lutein. They found that when copper-mediated oxidation of LDL was used, before substantial amounts of lipid peroxidation products were formed, carotenoids were destroyed in the samples. This experiment further provided evidence of antioxidant functions of these carotenoids.

Rissanen et al. [89] reported that the serum lycopene was inversely related to incidences of acute coronary events and stroke. They also observed that as the serum concentration of lycopene increased by 0.01 μmol/L, the risk of acute coronary incidences and stroke was lowered by approximately 4%. In using Cox proportional hazards model adjusting for the above factors, men in the lowest quartile of serum lycopene concentration had a 3.3-fold higher risk of acute coronary events and stroke compared with the rest of the subjects.

Concentration of lycopene in the adipose tissue also has an inverse relationship to the risk of MI. Gomez-Aracena et al. [90] reported that the risk of MI for the highest quintile of the adipose lycopene concentration was 60% lower than the lowest quintile. This was after data were adjusted for age, family history of coronary heart disease, and cigarette smoking. Results of data from the total multinational, multicenter EURAMIC study confirmed this finding. The risk of MI was 48% reduced in men who had the highest concentrations of lycopene in their adipose tissue biopsies as compared with the men with the lowest levels of lycopene in their adipose tissues [91]. The results of these studies emphasize the importance of the dietary carotenoids especially lycopene in protecting against CVDs in men and women.

Conclusions

The bioflavanoids and other phytochemicals with their anti-inflammatory actions, including natural antioxidants, are present in plant foods as natural protectors of nutrients in foods and have proven protective against degenerative diseases. In order to receive adequate natural bioflavanoids, phytochemicals, and antioxidants in foods, more fruits, vegetables, whole grains, and tree nuts must be consumed along with a diet low in saturated and trans fats, and adequate in proteins. Heart diseases are number-one killer in the West. It is becoming one in other countries of the world due to aggressive marketing tactics of Western dietary products. People of the developing countries—although their cultural diet is high in natural foods containing effective deterrents of degenerative diseases—are adopting Western type diet and lifestyle. Nutrition scientists are advocating Mediterranean type foods and Eastern lifestyle for the Western consumers to prevent CVD. As the world is shrinking and the media are effective messengers, if the sound nutritional practices and lifestyle of the East along with advanced preventive and curative methods of combating disease in the West can be advocated and adopted by all, the degenerative diseases can be controlled.

It must be emphasized to the health professionals that nutrition education, especially inclusion of fruits, vegetables, whole grains, and tree nuts in meals and snacks is imperative. These foods loaded with phytochemicals and antioxidants included in daily diet can reduce/prevent degenerative diseases especially CVD.

References

1 World Health Organization (WHO). Cardiovascular disease (CVD): facts. Global strategy on diet, physical activity and health. Available from www.who.int. Accessed March 2005.

2 National Center for Chronic Disease Prevention and Health Promotion (CDC). Preventing heart disease and stroke. Available from www.cdc/gov./nccdphp/ bb_heartdisease. Accessed March 2006.

3 Paoletti R, Poli A, Cignarela A. The emerging link between nutrition, inflammation and atherosclerosis. Expert Rev Cardiovasc Ther 2006;4:385–93.

4 Ridker PM. Clinical application of C-reactive protein for cardiovascular disease detection and prevention. Circulation 2003;107:363–9.

5 Ross R. Atherosclerosis, an inflammatory disease. N Engl J Med 1999;140:665–73.

6 Hwang SJ, Ballantyne CM, Sharret AR et al. Circulating adhesion molecule VCAM-1, ICAM-1, and E-selection in carotid atherosclerosis and incident coronary heart disease cases. The Atherosclerosis Risk in Community (ARIC) Study. Circulation 1997;96:4219–25.

7 Luc G, Brad JM, Juhan-Vogue et al. C-reactive protein, interleukin 6, and fibrinogen as predictors of coronary heart disease: the PRIME Study. Arterioscler Thromb Vasc Biol 2003;23:1255–61.

8 Ridker PM, Morrow AD. C-reactive protein, inflammation, and coronary risk. Cardiol Clin 2003;21:315–25.

9 De Caterina R, Zampolli A, Del Turco S et al. Nutritional mechanisms that influence cardiovascular disease. Am J Clin Nutr 2006;83:421S–6S.

10 Engler MM, Engler MB. Omega-3 fatty acids: role in cardiovascular health and disease. J Cardiovasc Nurs 2006; 21:17–24.

11 Das UN. Beneficial effect(s) of n-3 fatty acids in cardiovascular diseases: but, why and how? Prostaglandins Leukot Essent Fatty Acids 2000;63:351–62.

12 Stampfer MJ, Malinow MR, Willett WC et al. A prospective study of plasma homocysteine and risk of myocardial infarction in US physicians. JAMA 1992;268:877–81.

13 Tsai JC, Perrella MA, Hsieh CM et al. Promotion of vascular smooth muscle cell growth by homocysteine: a link to atherosclerosis. Proc Natl Acad Sci U S A 1994;91:6369–73.

14 Tyagi SC. Homocyst(e)ine and heart disease: pathophysiology of extra-cellular matrix. Clin Exp Hypertens 1999;21:181–98.

15 Moat SJ, Lang D, McDowell IFW et al. Folate, homocysteine, endothelial function and cardiovascular disease. J Nutr Biochem 2004;15:64–79.

16 Aguillar B, Rojas JC, Collados MT. Metabolism of homocysteine and its relationship with cardiovascular disease. J Thromb Thrombolysis 2004;18:75–87.

17 Root M, Anderson JJB. Dietary effects of nontraditional risk factors for heart disease. Nutr Res 2004;24:827–38.

18 Wannamethee SG, Lowe GDO, Rumley A et al. Association of vitamin C status, fruit and vegetable intakes, and markers of inflammation and homeostasis. Am J Clin Nutr 2006;83:567–74.

19 Watzel B, Kulling SE, Moseneder J et al. A 4-week intervention with high intake of carotenoid-rich vegetables and fruit reduces plasma C-reactive protein in healthy, non-smoking men. Am J Clin Nutr 2005;82:1052–8.

20 Geleijnse JM, Vermeer C, Grobbee DE et al. Dietary intake of menaquinone is associated with a reduced risk of coronary heart disease: the Rotterdam study. J Nutr 2004;134:3100–5.

21 Schleithoff SS, Zittermann A, Tenderich G et al. Vitamin D supplementation improves cytokine profiles in patients with congestive heart failure: a double-blind, randomized placebo-controlled trial. Am J Clin Nutr 2006;83: 754–9.

22 Djousse L, Arnett DK, Coon H et al. Fruit and vegetable consumption and LDL-cholesterol: the National Heart, Lung, and Blood Institute Family Heart Study. Am J Clin Nutr 2004;79:213–7.

23 Bazzano LA, He J, Ogden LG et al. Fruit and vegetable intake and risk of cardiovascular disease in US adults: the first national health and nutrition examination survey epidemiological follow-up study. Am J Clin Nutr 2002;76:93–9.

24 Tucker KL, Hallfrisch J, Qiao N et al. The combination of high fruit and vegetable and low saturated fat intakes is more protective against mortality in aging men than

either alone: the Baltimore Longitudinal Study of Aging. J Nutr 2005;135:556–61.

25 Fung TT, McCullough ML, Newby PK *et al.* Diet-quality scores and plasma concentrations of markers of inflammation and endothelial dysfunction. Am J Clin Nutr 2005;82:163–73.

26 Root M, Anderson JJB. Nutr Res. Special Issue, Part 2: Cardiovascular Health. Nutr Res 2004;24.

27 Adams MR, Golden DL, Chen H *et al.* A diet rich in green and yellow vegetables inhibits atherosclerosis in mice. J Nutr 2006;136:1886–89.

28 Simopoulos A. Omega-3 fatty acids in inflammation and autoimmune diseases. J Am Coll Nutr 2002;21:495–505.

29 Thompson HJ, Heimendinger J, Diker A *et al.* Dietary botanical diversity affects the reduction of oxidative biomarkers in women due to high vegetable and fruit intake. J Nutr 2006;136:2207–12.

30 Mozaffarian D, Pischon T, Hankinson SE *et al.* Dietary intake of trans fatty acids and systemic inflammation in women. Am J Clin Nutr 2004;79:606–12.

31 Warnberg J, Nova E, Moreno LA *et al.* Inflammatory proteins are related to total and abdominal adiposity in a healthy adolescent population: the AVENA Study. Am J Clin Nutr 2006;84:505–12.

32 Kelly DS, Rasooly R, Jacob RA *et al.* Consumption of Bing sweet cherries lowers circulating concentrations of inflammation marker in healthy men and women. J Nutr 2006;136:981–6.

33 Jacob RA, Spinozzi GM, Simon VA *et al.* Consumption of cherries lowers plasma urate in healthy women. J Nutr 2001;133:1826–29.

34 Kaplan M, Heyek T, Raz A *et al.* Pomegranate juice supplementation to atherosclerotic mice reduces macrophage lipid peroxidation, cellular cholesterol accumulation and development of atherosclerosis. J Nutr 2001;131:2082–89.

35 Carluccio MA, Siculella L, Ancora MA. Olive oil and red wine antioxidant polyphenols inhibit endothelial activation: antiatherogenic properties of Mediterranean diet phytochemicals. Arterioscler Thromb Vasc Biol 2003;23:622-9.

36 Rein D, Schijlen E, Kooistra T *et al.* Transgenic flavonoid tomato intake reduces C-reactive protein in human C-reactive protein transgenic mice more than the wild-type tomato. J Nutr 2006;136:2331–7.

37 Jensen MK, Koh-Banerjee P, Hu FB *et al.* Intakes of whole grains, bran and germ and risk of coronary heart disease in men. Am J Clin Nutr 2004;80:1492–9.

38 Ajani UA, Ford ES, Mokdad AH. Dietary fiber and C-reactive protein: findings from National Health and Nutrition Examination Survey data. J Nutr 2004;1181–5.

39 Ma Y, Griffith JA, Chasan-Taber L *et al.* Association between dietary fiber and C-reactive protein. Am J Clin Nutr 2006;83:760–6.

40 Liu S, Willett WC, Manson JE *et al.* Relation between changes in intakes of dietary fiber and grain products and changes in weight and development of obesity among middle-aged women. Am J Clin Nutr 2003;78:920–7.

41 Montonen J, Knekt P, Jarvinen R *et al.* Wholegrain and fiber intake and the incidence of type-2 diabetes. Am J Clin Nutr 2003;77:622–9.

42 Anderson JW. Whole grain and coronary heart disease: the whole kernel of truth [editorial]. Am J Clin Nutr 2004;80:1459–60.

43 Hall WL, Vafeiadou K, Hallund J *et al.* Soy-isoflavone-enriched foods and inflammatory biomarkers of cardiovascular disease risk in postmenopausal women: interaction with genotype and equol production. Am J Clin Nutr 2005;82:1260–8.

44 Steinberg FM, Guthrie NL, Villablanca AC *et al.* Soy protein with isoflavones has favorable effects on endothelial function that are independent of lipid and antioxidant effects in healthy postmenopausal women. Am J Clin Nutr 2003;78:123–30.

45 Rivas M, Garay RP, Escanero JF *et al.* Soy milk lowers blood pressure in men and women with mild to moderate essential hypertension. J Nutr 2002;132:1900–2.

46 Setchell KDR, Brown NM, Lydeking-Olsen E. The clinical importance of the metabolite equol—a clue to the effectiveness of soy and its isoflavones. J Nutr 2002;132:3577–84.

47 Silagy C, Neil A. Garlic as a lipid lowering agent—a meta-analysis. J R Coll Physicians Lond 1994;28:39–45.

48 Wei ZH, Lau BHS. Garlic inhibits free radical generation and augments antioxidant enzyme activity in vascular endothelial cells. Nutr Res 1998;18:61–70.

49 Agarwal KC. Therapeutic actions of garlic constituents. Med Res Rev 1996;16:111–24.

50 Salmon H, Bergman M, Bessler H *et al.* Effect of a garlic derivative (alliin) on peripheral blood cell immune responses Int J Immunopharmacol 1999;21:589–97.

51 Hodge G, Hodge S, Han P. *Allium sativum* (garlic) suppresses leukocyte inflammatory cytokine production in vitro: potential therapeutic use in the treatment of inflammatory bowel disease. Cytometry 2002;48:209–14.

52 Ide N, Lau BH. Garlic compounds minimize intracellular oxidative stress and inhibit nuclear factor κ-B activation. J Nutr 2001;131:1020S–6S.

53 Keiss HP, Dirsch VM, Hartung T *et al.* Garlic (*Allium sativum* L.) modulates cytokine expression in lipopoly-saccharide-activated human blood thereby inhibiting TN-κB activity. J Nutr 2003;133:2171–75.

54 Yeh YY, Yeh SM. Homocysteine-lowering action is another potential cardiovascular protective factor of aged garlic extract. J Nutr 2006;136:745S–9S.

55 Breithaupt-Grogler K, Ling M, Boudoulas H, Belz GG. Protective effect of chronic garlic intake on elastic

properties of aorta in elderly. Circulation 1997;96:2649–55.

56 Budoff M. Aged garlic extract retards progression of coronary artery calcification. J Nutr 2006;136:741S–4S.

57 Weiss N, Ide N, Abahji T *et al*. Aged garlic extract improves homocysteinemia-induced endothelial dysfunction in macro and microcirculation. J Nutr 2006;136:750S–4S.

58 Anderson KJ, Teuber SS, Gobeille A *et al*. Walnut polyphenols inhibit in vitro human plasma LDL oxidation. J Nutr 2001;131:2837–42.

59 Abbey M, Noakes M, Belling GB, Nestel PJ. Partial replacement of saturated fatty acids with almonds or walnuts lowers total plasma cholesterol and low-density lipoprotein cholesterol. Am J Clin Nutr 1994;59:995–9.

60 Zambon D, Sabate J, Munoz S *et al*. Substituting walnuts for monounsaturated fat improves the serum lipid profile of hypercholestrolemic men and women: α randomized crossover trial. Ann Intern Med 2000;132:530–46.

61 Levedrine F, Zmirou D, Ravle A *et al*. Blood cholesterol and walnut consumption: a cross-sectional study in France. Prev Med 1999;28:333–9.

62 Feldman EB. The scientific evidence for a beneficial health relationship between walnut and coronary heart disease. J Nutr 2002;132:1062S–1101S.

63 German JB, Walzem RL. The health benefits of wine. Annu Rev Nutr 2000;20:561–93.

64 Lopez-Velez M, Martinez-Martinez F, DelValle-Ribes C. The study of phenolic compounds as natural antioxidants in wine. Crit Rev Food Sci Nutr 2003;43:233–44.

65 Krueger CG *et al*. Grape seed and grape skin extracts elicit a greater antiplatelet effect when used in combination than when used individually in dogs and humans. J Nutr 2002;132:3592.

66 Stewart JR, Artime MC, O'Brian CA. Resveratrol: a candidate nutritional substance for prostate cancer prevention. J Nutr 2003;133:2440S–3S.

67 Gao X, Xu YX, Divine G *et al*. Disparate in vitro and in vivo antileukemic effects of resveratrol, a natural polyphenolic compound found in grapes. J Nutr 2002;132:2076–81.

68 Wallerath T, Deckert G, Ternes T *et al*. Resveratrol, a polyphenolic phytoalexin present in red wine, enhances expression and activity of endothelial nitric oxide synthase. Circulation 2002;106:1652–8.

69 Soleas GJ, Diamandis EP, Goldberg DM. Resveratrol: a molecule whose time has come? And gone? Clin Biochem 1997;30:91–113.

70 Manna SK, Mukhopadhyay A, Agarwal BB. Resveratrol suppresses TNF-induced activation of protein-1 and apoptosis: potential role of reactive oxygen intermediates and lipid peroxidation. J Immunol 2000;164:6509–19.

71 Sedgwick JD, Riminton DS, Cyster JG, Korner H. Tumor necrosis factor: a master regulator of leukocyte movement. Immunol Today 2000;21:110–3.

72 Paganga G, Miller N, Rice-Evans CA *et al*. The polyphenolic content of fruit and vegetables and their antioxidant activities. What does a serving constitute? Free Radic Res 1999;30:155.

73 Agarwal DP. Cardioprotective effects of light-moderate consumption of alcohol: a review of putative mechanisms. Alcohol Alcohol 2002;37(5):409–15.

74 Cishek MB, Galloway MT, Karim M, German JB, Kappagoda CT. Effect of red wine on endothelium-dependent relaxation in rabbits. Clin Sci 1997;93:507–11.

75 Zern TL, West KL, Fernandez ML. Grape polyphenols decrease plasma triglycerides and cholesterol accumulation in the aorta of ovariectomized guinea pigs. J Nutr 2003;133:2268–72.

76 Pal S *et al*. Red wine polyphenolics increase LDL receptor expression and activity and suppress the secretion of ApoB100 from human HepG2 cells. J Nutr 2003;133:701.

77 Schramm DD, Wang JF, Holt RR *et al*. Chocolate procyanidins decrease the leukotriene-prostacyclin ratio in humans and human aortic endothelial cells. Am J Clin Nutr 2001;73:36040.

78 Sies H, Schewe T, Heiss C, Kelm M. Cocoa polyphenols and inflammatory mediators. Am J Clin Nutr 2005;81:304S-12S.

79 Chio YJ, Jeong YJ, Lee YJ *et al*. (–)-Epigallocatechin gallate and quercetin enhance survival signaling in response to oxidants-induced human endothelial apoptosis. J Nutr 2005;135:707–13.

80 Riemersma RA, Rice-Evans CA, Tyrrell RM *et al*. Tea flavonoids and cardiovascular health. Q J Med 2001;94:277–82.

81 Zampelas A, Panagiotakos DB, Ptsavos C *et al*. Association between coffee consumption and inflammatory markers in healthy persons. Am J Clin Nutr 2004;80:862–67.

82 Vlachopoulos C, Panagiotakos DB, Ioakeimidis N *et al*. Chronic coffee consumption has detrimental effect on aortic stiffness and wave reflection. Am J Clin Nutr 2005;81:1307–12.

83 Fuhramn B, Elis A, Aviram M. Hypocholesterolemic effect of lycopene and β-carotene is related to suppression of cholesterol synthesis and augmentation of LDL receptor activity in macrophage. Biochem Biophys Res Commun 1997;233:658–62.

84 Rao AV, Agarwal S. Role of antioxidant lycopene in cancer and heart disease. J Am Coll Nutr 2000;19:563–9.

85 Rissanen TH, Voutilainen S, Virtanen JK *et al*. Low intake of fruits, berries, and vegetables is associated with excess mortality in men: the Kuopio ischemic heart disease risk factors (KIHD). J Nutr 2003;133:199–204.

86 Goulinet S, Chapman MJ. Plasma LDL and HDL subspecies are heterogeneous in particle content of tocopherols and oxygenated and hydrocarbon carotenoids.

Relevance to oxidative resistance and atherogenesis. Arterioscler Thromb Vasc Biol 1997;17:786–96.

87 Fuhrman B, Elis A, Aviram M. Hypocholesterolemic effect of lycopene and β-carotene is related to suppression of cholesterol synthesis and augmentation of LDL receptor activity in macrophage. Biochem Biophys Res Commun 1997;233:658–62.

88 Romanchik JE, Harrison EH, Morel DW. Addition of lutein, lycopene or beta-carotene to LDL or serum in vitro: effect on carotenoid distribution, LDL composition and LDL oxidation. J Nutr Biochem 1997;8: 681–8.

89 Rissanen TH, Voutilainen S, Nyyssonen K *et al.* Low serum lycopene concentration is associated with an excess incidence of acute coronary events and stroke: the Kuopio ischemic heart disease risk factor study. Br J Nutr 2001;85:749–54.

90 Gomez-Aracena J, Garcia-Rodriguez A *et al.* Antioxidants in adipose tissue and myocardial infarction in a Mediterranean area. The EURAMIC study in Malaga. Nutr Metab Cardiovasc Dis 1997;7:376–82.

91 Kohlmeier L, Kark JD, Gomez-Garcia E *et al.* Lycopene and myocardial infarction risk in the EURAMIC study. Am J Epidemiol 1997;146:618–26.

Index

301